NATIONAL ASSOCIATION OF EMS PHYSICIANS

Prehospital Systems and Medical Oversight

NATIONAL ASSOCIATION OF EMS PHYSICIANS

Prehospital Systems and Medical Oversight

Edited by

ALEXANDER KUEHL, M.D., M.P.H., FACS

Director, Emergency Medical Program,
The New York Hospital
New York, New York

Associate Professor of Clinical Surgery and
Clinical Public Health,
Cornell University Medical College
New York, New York

Second Edition

formerly titled *EMS Medical Directors' Handbook*

with 85 illustrations

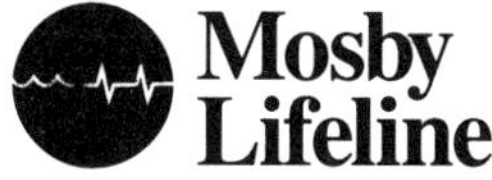

St. Louis Baltimore Berlin Boston Carlsbad Chicago London Madrid
Naples New York Philadelphia Sydney Tokyo Toronto

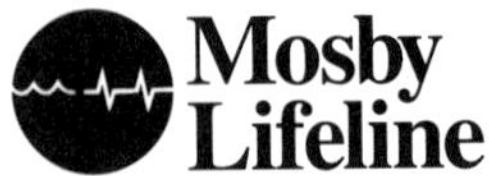

Dedicated to Publishing Excellence

Executive Editor: Claire Merrick
Assistant Editor: Ross Goldberg
Editorial Assistant: Carla Goldberg
Project Manager: Carol Sullivan Wiseman
Production Editor: Christine Carroll
Senior Designer: Betty Schulz
Manufacturing Supervisor: Kathy Grone
Cover Design: Jim Brimeyer

SECOND EDITION

Formerly titled *EMS Medical Directors' Handbook*

Previous edition copyrighted 1989

Printed in the United States of America

Composition by Carlisle Communications, Ltd.
Printing/binding by Maple-Vail Book Manufacturing Group

Mosby-Year Book, Inc.
11830 Westline Industrial Drive
St. Louis, Missouri 63146

Library of Congress Cataloging in Publication Data
Prehospital systems and medical oversight/National Association of EMS Physicians;
edited by Alexander Kuehl.—2nd ed.
p. cm.
Rev. ed. of: EMS medical directors' handbook. 1989.
Includes bibliographical references and index.
ISBN 0-8016-6580-9
1. Emergency medical services—Administration—Handbooks, manuals, etc.
I. Kuehl, Alexander. II. National Association of EMS Physicians (U.S.) III. EMS medical directors' handbook. (DNLM: 1. Emergency Medical Services—organization & administration. WX 215 P9236 1994)
RA645.5.E497 1994
362.1'8'068—dc20

94 95 96 97 98 / 9 8 7 6 5 4 3 2 1

Authors

Beth Lothrop Adams, M.A., R.N., EMT-P
Adjunct Assistant Professor of Emergency Medicine,
The George Washington University School of Medicine and Health Science,
Washington, D.C.

James G. Adams, M.D., FACP
Captain, United States Air Force;
Vice Chairman, Department of Emergency Medicine,
Wilford Hall USAF Medical Center,
Lackland AFB, Texas;
Adjunct Assistant Professor of Medicine,
Division of Emergency Medicine,
University of Pittsburgh School of Medicine,
Pittsburgh, Pennsylvania

James Atkins, M.D., FACP
Professor of Medicine,
University of Texas Southeastern;
City of Dallas EMS Medical Director,
Dallas, Texas

James J. Augustine, M.D., FACEP
Associate Director, Emergency Department,
Miami Valley Hospital;
Associate Clinical Professor of Emergency Medicine,
Wright State University,
Dayton, Ohio

Robert Bass, M.D.
Director, EMS Bureau,
Department of Fire and EMS;
Associate Professor of Emergency Medicine,
Georgetown and George Washington University,
Washington, D.C.

Leo V. Bosner, M.S.W.
Emergency Management Specialist,
Federal Emergency Management Agency,
Washington, D.C.

Odelia Braun, M.D., FACEP
Associate Clinical Professor of Medicine,
Department of Medicine,
University of California, San Francisco;
Medical Director, San Francisco Fire Department,
City and County of San Francisco,
San Francisco, California

John F. Brown, M.D., FACEP
Lt. Commander, United States Navy;
Fellow, Emergency Medical Services,
Arizona Emergency Medicine Research Center,
Tucson, Arizona

Brenda Marie Bruns, M.D., M.S.M.
Medical Director, Emergency Medical Services District,
Alameda County Health Care Services Agency,
Oakland, California;
Medical Director, Quality Assurance,
Mercy Life Care Ambulance Co.,
Burlingame, California

Richard Carmona, M.D.
Director, Trauma Services,
Tucson Medical Center;
Assistant Professor of Surgery,
University of Arizona Health Sciences Center,
Tucson, Arizona

C. Gene Cayten, M.D., M.P.H.
Director, Surgery,
Our Lady of Mercy Medical Center,
Bronx, New York;
Consultant, Surgery,
Westchester County Medical Center,
Valhalla, New York

Jeffery J. Clawson, M.D.
President, National Academy of Emergency Medical Dispatch;
Medical Director, Gold Cross Ambulance Service,
Salt Lake City, Utah

Alisdair Keith Thurburn Conn, M.D.
Chief, Emergency Services,
Massachusetts General Hospital,
Boston, Massachusetts;
Assistant Professor of Surgery,
Harvard Medical School,
Cambridge, Massachusetts

Keith Conover, M.D.
Attending Staff, Department of Emergency Medicine,
Mercy Hospital of Pittsburgh;
Clinical Assistant Professor, Division of Emergency Medicine,
University of Pittsburgh,
Pittsburgh, Pennsylvania

Lynne Susan Cooper, J.D., M.A.
Attorney, Health Care Law Department,
Bower and Gardner, Attorneys-at-Law,
New York, New York

Arthur Cooper, M.D., FACS, FAAP, FCCM
Associate Professor and Chief of Pediatric Surgical Critical Care,
College of Physicians and Surgeons of Columbia University,
Harlem Hospital Center,
New York, New York

Elizabeth Criss, R.N., B.S.N.
Senior Research Associate, Section of Emergency Medicine, Department of Surgery,
University of Arizona;
Base Hospital Coordinator, Emergency Department,
University Medical Center,
Tucson, Arizona

Steven J. Davidson, M.D., M.B.A., FACEP
Professor of Emergency Medicine and Division Chief of EMS,
Medical College of Pennsylvania;
Medical Director, Philadelphia Fire Department and Philadelphia Regional EMS
City of Philadelphia,
Philadelphia, Pennsylvania

Norm Dinerman, M.D., FACEP
Chief, Emergency Service,
Eastern Maine Medical Center,
Bangor, Maine

Joseph J. Fitch, Ph.D.
President, Fitch and Associates, Inc.,
Kansas City, Missouri

George L. Foltin, M.D., FAAP, FACEP
Director, Pediatric Emergency Service,
Bellevue Hospital Center;
Assistant Professor of Clinical Pediatrics,
New York University School of Medicine,
New York, New York

Raymond L. Fowler, M.D., FACEP
Chairman, Department of Emergency Medicine,
HCA Parkway Medical Center,
Lithia Springs, Georgia;
President, National Association of EMS Physicians,
Pittsburgh, Pennsylvania

George Garnett, M.D.
South Region EMS Medical Director,
Soldotha, Alaska

Lorraine Maria Giordano, M.D., FACEP
Medical Director, Emergency Medical Services,
New York City Emergency Medical Services,
Maspeth, New York

Michael R. Gunderson, REMT-P
Director of Research and Education,
Office of the Medical Director,
Pinellas County Emergency Medical Services,
Largo, Florida;
President, Acute Care Foundation,
Tampa, Florida

Daniel Grant Hankins, M.D., FACEP
Senior Associate Consultant, Division of Emergency Medical Services,
Mayo Clinic;
Assistant Professor, Department of Medicine,
Mayo Medical School,
Rochester, Minnesota

William E. Hathaway, M.S.
Instructor, University of Maryland Baltimore County,
Emergency Health Services Program,
Catonsville, Maryland

Mark S. Johnson, M.P.A.
Chief, Emergency Medical Services Section,
Alaska Department of Health and Social Services,
Juneau, Alaska;
Chairman, EMS Communications Committee,
National Association of State EMS Directors,
Carlsbad, California

Kristi L. Koenig, M.D.
Assistant Professor, Medicine,
University of California, San Francisco,
San Francisco, California;
EMS Co-Director, Emergency Medicine,
Highland Hospital,
Oakland, California

Jennifer Leanning, M.D.
Medical Director, Health Centers Division,
Harvard Community Health Plan,
Brookline, Massachusetts

G. Patrick Lilja, M.D., FACEP
Medical Director, Emergency Trauma Services,
North Memorial Medicine Center;
Clinical Associate Professor of Family Practice and Community Health,
University of Minnesota Medical School,
Minneapolis, Minnesota

Ronald B. Low, M.D., M.S.
Associate Chairman of Emergency Medicine,
SUNY Health Sciences Center,
Kings County Medical Center,
Brooklyn, New York

Michael Madsen, D.O.
Emergency Physician,
Department of Emergency Medicine,
Tutality Community Hospital,
Hillsboro, Oregon

Norman E. McSwain, Jr., M.D. FACS
Professor of Surgery,
Tulane Medical School,
New Orleans, Louisiana

Steven A. Meador, M.D.
Assistant Professor of Medicine,
Director of Emergency Medical Services,
The Milton S. Hershey Medical Center,
The Pennsylvania State University,
Hershey, Pennsylvania

Jeffery T. Mitchell, M.D.
Clinical Associate Professor,
University of Maryland,
Baltimore County Emergency Health Services Program,
Catonsville, Maryland

David L. Morgan, M.D.
Assistant Professor, Division of Emergency Medicine,
Department of Surgery and Internal Medicine,
University of Texas Southwestern Medical Center,
Dallas, Texas

John Lawrence Mottley, M.D., M.H.S.A., FACEP
Associate Professor, Emergency Medicine,
Boston University School of Medicine;
Executive Director, Boston Emergency Medical Services,
City of Boston Health and Hospitals,
Boston, Massachusetts

Anthony Charles Mustalish, M.D., M.P.H. FACEP, FAPRM
Assistant Professor of Surgery and Public Health,
Cornell University Medical College,
New York, New York

Michael Osur, EMT-P
EMS District,
Alameda County Health Care Services Agency,
Oakland, California

Laurie Ann Otto, M.D.
Former Associate Medical Director, Milwaukee County Paramedic Program and EMS Fellow,
Department of Emergency Medicine,
Medical College of Wisconsin,
Milwaukee, Wisconsin

Jerry Overton
Executive Director,
Richmond Ambulance Authority;
Clinical Instructor,
Medical College of Virginia,
Richmond, Virginia

James O. Page, J.D.
President, JEMS Communications,
Carlsbad, California

Gustave Pappas, B.S., EMT-P
NYS Regional Faculty Instructor;
Emergency Medical Service,
New York City—Health and Hospital Corporation,
New York, New York

Paul E. Pepe, M.D., FACEP, FCCP, FCCM, FACP
Associate Professor, Departments of Medicine, Surgery, and Pediatrics,
Baylor College of Medicine;
Director of Emergency Medical Services,
Houston, Texas;

James Pointer, M.D., FACEP
Assistant District Director,
Emergency Medical Services,
Costal Physicians Services of Broward County;
EMS Physician,
North Broward Medical Center,
Pompano Beach, Florida

Carl Joseph Post, B.A., M.A., Ph.D., EMT-D (NY)
Associate Director, Graduate EMS Program,
School of Health Sciences,
New York Medical College,
Valhalla, New York;
Assistant Professor at Large, Graduate School,
Medical School, School of Humanities,
Hahnemann University,
Philadelphia, Pennsylvania

Ernest Pretto, M.D.
Assistant Professor, Intervention Resuscitation Research Center,
Department of Anesthesiology and Critical Care Medicine,
University of Pittsburgh Medical School,
Pittsburgh, Pennsylvania

Edward M. Racht, M.D.
Associate Chief, Internal Medicine Section of Emergency Medical Services,
Medical College of Virginia;
Medical Director, City of Richmond EMS,
Richmond, Virginia

Howard David Reines, M.D.
Chief of Surgery
Medical College of Virginia,
Richmond, Virginia

Matthew M. Rice, M.D., J.D., FACEP
Chairman, Department of Emergency Medicine,
Madigan Army Medical Center,
Fort Lewis, Washington;
Assistant Clinical Professor, Department of Emergency Medicine,
Uniformed Services Health Sciences University,
Bethesda, Maryland

Steven J. Rottman, M.D., FACEP
Professor of Medicine, Division of Emergency Medicine,
UCLA Medical Center,
Center for Prehospital Care,
Los Angeles, California;
Medical Director, Burbank Fire Department,
Burbank, California

Joseph L. Ryan, M.D., FACEP
Medical Director, Pinellas County Emergency Medical Services;
President, Emergency Medical Services and Acute Care Foundation,
Largo, Florida

Sam Senturia, M.D.
Instructor in Medicine,
Cornell University Medical College;
New York, New York

Carol J. Shanaberger, Attorney-at-Law, EMT-P
EMS Liaison, Board of Medical Examiners,
State of Colorado

John E. Spoor, M.D., FACEP
Director Emergency Services, Chief Emergency Medicine,
Mary Imogene Bassett Hospital,
Cooperstown, New York;
Associate Clinical Professor, Department of Medicine,
Columbia University, School of Physicians and Surgeons,
New York, New York

Jack L. Stout, B.A.
The Fourth Party, Inc.,
West River, Maryland

Robert Swor, D.O., FACEP
Clinical Instructor, Department of Surgery,
University of Michigan,
Ann Arbor, Michigan;
EMS Coordinator, Department of Emergency Medicine, William Beaumont Hospital,
Royal Oak, Michigan

Mike Taigman, EMT-P
Corporate Director of Quality Improvement,
Med-Trans,
San Francisco, California

Peggy Trimble, B.S.N., M.A.
Director, Regional Training Site-Medical,
Army National Guard,
Annville, Pennsylvania

Terence D. Valenzuela, M.D.
Associate Professor, Surgery,
University of Arizona College of Medicine,
Tucson, Arizona

Michael P. Wainscott, M.D., FACEP
Assistant Professor and Director of Medical Education,
Surgery, Division of Emergency Medicine,
University of Texas Southwestern Medical Center at Dallas;
Faculty, Emergency Department,
Parkland Memorial Hospital,
Dallas, Texas

Bruce John Walz, Ph.D.
Assistant Professor, Department of Emergency Health Services,
University of Maryland Baltimore County,
Catonsville, Maryland

Katherine H. West, B.S.N., M.S.Ed., CIC
Assistant Professor, Department of Emergency Medicine,
George Washington University School of Medicine,
Washington, D.C.;
President, Infection Control/Emerging Concepts, Inc.,
Springfield, Virginia

Richard C. Wuerz, M.D.
Assistant Professor of Emergency Medicine,
The Pennsylvania State University College of Medicine;
Associate Director, Prehospital and Flight Services,
The Milton Hershey Medical Center,
Hershey, Pennsylvania

Donald M. Yealy, M.D., FACEP
Assistant Professor and Director of Research,
Department of Medicine, Division of Emergency Medicine,
Texas A & M University Health Sciences Center;
Senior Staff Physician, Department of Emergency Medicine,
Scott and White Memorial Hospital Clinic,
Temple, Texas

Stanley M. Zydlo, J.D., M.D., FACEP
Chairman Emergency Department;
Medical Director Northwest Community EMS System,
Northwest Community Hospital,
Arlington Heights, Illinois;
Chairman, Chicago EMS System—P.M.D. Consortium,
Chicago, Illinois

Contributors

The following individuals have been individually noted by one or more of the authors for their significant contributions toward the successful completion of this text.

Juanita N. Abston
Adrian Anast, Ph.D.
R. Jack Ayers, Jr.
Nicholas Bensten, M.D.
Russel B. Biezick, M.D.
Allan Braslow, Ph.D.
Christine Carroll
Richard T. Cook, M.D.
Michael K. Copass, M.D.
Kathy L. Cornwell
Daniel Culhane, M.D.
Donald G. Curry, M.D.
Jack Delaney, EMT-P
Gayle Dunsmore
Terry V. Fotre
Ross Goldberg
Lenard Hudson, M.D.
Kevin Kelly
Barbara Knight
Robert Knopp, M.D.
Jon R. Krohmer, M.D.
Ronald L. Krome, M.D.
Marion Lyver, M.D.
Robert R. Maisel, M.D.
Dan Mayer, M.D.
John B. McCabe, M.D. FACEP
John McMahen, M.D.
Nina Meher-Homji
James J. Menegazzi, Ph.D.
Claire Merrick
William Metcalf, EMT-P
Laura Michalowicz, B.S.N
Gregory Michels
Barbara A. Mikulski
Iris Morales
Virginia G. Mork, M.D.
Georgia O'Gilvie-Rose
Maria Ongsiako, M.D.
Jeanne Payett
Lenora Payne
Franklin Pratt, M.D.
Cecilia Reilly
David E. Rogers, M.D.
William R. Roush, M.D.
Susan Schnall, B.S.N.
G. Tom Shires, M.D.
Kathleen M. Stage
Ronald D. Stewart, M.D.
Thomas W. Turbiak, M.D.
Charles Weigel, M.D.
Kenneth A. Williams, M.D.
Roger W. Yurt, M.D.

In Memoriam

David Natt, M.D.

New York City Emergency Medical Service

Associate Medical Director (1989–1992)

EMS Fellow (1988–1989)

Foreword

Emergency Medical Services (EMS) is the practice of the evaluation and management of patients with acute traumatic and medical conditions in the out-of-hospital environment. This practice is carried out by skilled technicians, operating under the medical oversight and guidance of knowledgeable physicians. It is to these EMS physicians that this text is dedicated.

The National Association of EMS Physicians (NAEMSP) is committed to the support of the EMS medical director. The peculiarities of the practice of medicine in the EMS environment require a broad spectrum of unique medical knowledge. Further, the limitations of evaluation and management implicit in this environment demand that EMS physicians carefully study their particular system and offer only treatment regimens appropriate for the field.

The types of patient care cases that lie at the origin of EMS systems are those relating to heart disease and trauma. It became clear during the middle of this century that the rapid stabilization and transport of these patients could positively impact morbidity and mortality. Hence, EMS systems of gradually increasing complexity were created to apply emerging medical care concepts to patients in the field.

As we now celebrate the fourth decade of cardiopulmonary resuscitation and the third decade of formal federal involvement in the creation and support of EMS systems, it is appropriate to reflect on the broad list of requirements for the successful practice of EMS. A glance at the index of this text is instructive to the newcomer to EMS medical direction. Clearly, EMS systems require a sophisticated structure including appropriately constructed legislation, provision for services and training of technicians, standards for medical direction, funding programs, interplay within the medical community, infectious disease considerations, disaster management, and much more.

NAEMSP offers this text as a service to both new and experienced EMS medical directors. Under the careful guidance of Dr. Kuehl, one of the founding fathers of NAEMSP, a group of EMS experts has been assembled to proffer approaches to the many issues facing EMS. It is the hope of the organization that the information contained herein will be of service to the members of NAEMSP and the EMS community at large.

Thus we come to the practice of prehospital and disaster medicine. A branch of medicine becomes unique when an assembled body of knowledge is recognized as reflecting that specialty and none other. To this writer, it seems that EMS has become just such a unique style of practice.

The successful evaluation and management of emergency patients in the out-of-hospital environment requires the walking of a thin tightrope by all members of the EMS system. The medical director must establish appropriate protocols and provide for on-line direction where indicated. Prehiring screening must be performed to assure that new personnel are trained according to standards. Ongoing training based on real-time quality management procedures must be implemented. Adherence to treatment protocol must be dynamically applied. Application and inculcation of new medical standards must be judiciously controlled. The myriad individual entities that make up the practice of prehospital and disaster medicine must each have adequate attention lest a single lapse in some aspect cause a patient to suffer unnecessarily.

For in the final analysis, it is only for the increase of the human condition that we labor. We in EMS therefore must dedicate our efforts to resolving those factors making up our milieu that may be in conflict with this effort.

Dynamic, dedicated, and qualified medical directors are perhaps the essential vitality required to assure that we can be of the best possible service to our patients. It is to this end that this text is devoted.

Raymond L. Fowler, M.D.
President,
National Association of EMS Physicians

Preface

At its 1986 meeting, the National Association of EMS Physicians (NAEMSP) clearly and forcefully articulated the need for a textbook that would address the medical aspects of designing, implementing, and operating EMS systems. Those medical aspects of EMS systems are defined broadly by both that organization and by the editor. This textbook represents the product of a 5-year, interdisciplinary effort to collate the thoughts, recommendations, and predictions of many EMS professionals not all of whom are physicians.

Prehospital Systems and Medical Oversight expands upon the *EMS Medical Directors' Handbook*. The entire text is crafted to be read from cover to cover, although it may be used as a definitive reference on specific issues. Some issues and topics are discussed repeatedly in the text, and each additional citation adds another dimension to the concept. If after completing the text, the neophyte EMS medical director feels simultaneously stimulated, concerned, and confident, the authors have accomplished what they set out to do. Parenthetically, many readers will find the text to be a useful companion reference to the National EMS Medical Directors' Course and Practicum.

Although every attempt has been made to provide a broad and varied array of solutions to common problems that the EMS physician is likely to encounter during the various phases of EMS system development, no two EMS systems are exactly alike; solutions that are successful in one jurisdiction may not be practical, possible, or even legal in another. The reader is cautioned to use the ideas and approaches described herein simply as suggestions for guiding the evolution of a system rather than absolute templates for local system design. Of course a number of problems apparently still defy solution.

As the science of prehospital and disaster medicine has matured, so has the terminology used to describe it. Terms such as "medical control," "advanced life support (ALS)," and "disaster" originally were used to describe relatively simple concepts that quickly became increasingly complicated. In addition, regional variations in usage gradually developed. "ALS" in Montana was different than "ALS" in Maryland; "disasters" in New York City were different than "disasters" in Hope, Arkansas; and "medical control" was defined differently by every state legislature. As the authors of the individual chapters of this text described the past, analyzed the present, and predicted the future, it became painfully apparent that new terms needed to be invented and old words required more precise definitions. For example, to continue to arbitrarily differentiate between "basic and advanced life support" no longer made sense because all prehospital care requires medical oversight and in reality is a continuum from fundamental first aid through the most sophisticated intervention.

Rigorous EMS philosophers and educators have attempted to more precisely define "medical control," "medical direction and medical command" since the terms initially were coined circa 1960. In the previous edition of this text the authors recognized that "on-line" and "off-line" "medical control" had come to mean many different things and that modern prehospital medicine required standard national terms. Specifically, neither "off-line" nor "on-line" ever adequately described the hands-on patient care pro-

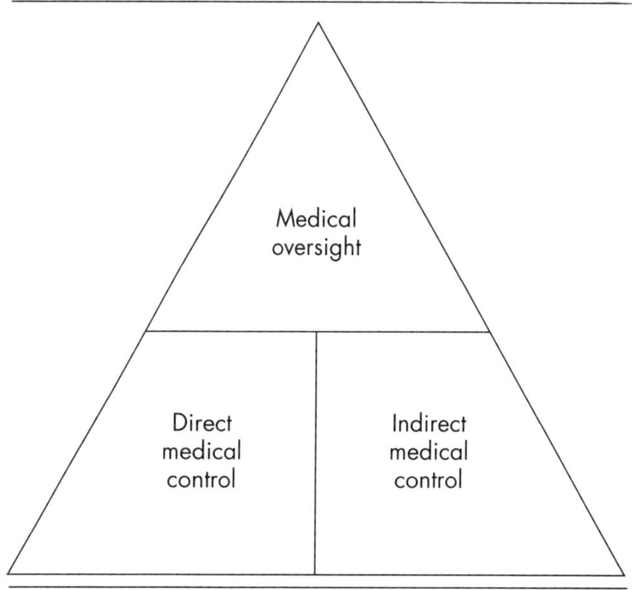

vided by the EMS medical directors of the 1980s. Therefore the term "direct medical control" was chosen to describe all activities in which the physician was contemporaneously providing *or* supervising patient care. The term "indirect medical control" was reserved for those activities that were removed by time or function from the immediate care of the patient. It is clear that both of those activities could be delegated to others by the physician ultimately and finally responsible. The term for that ultimate medical, legal, and moral responsibility in this text is "medical oversight."

In the sections of this text addressing catastrophic events and multiple casualty incidents the authors propose a more encompassing and descriptive lexicon. Undoubtedly, that terminology will evolve further with both time and experience; that is as it should be.

Before 1981, no physicians exclusively devoted their practices or their careers to EMS medical oversight. Although a slowly expanding number of jurisdictions have established full-time EMS medical director positions, most local and regional EMS systems rely on either dedicated practicing physicians or the chairpersons of regional EMS medical advisory groups as their medical directors. For the foreseeable future, most EMS physicians will continue to provide medical oversight as an adjunct to their more traditional practices of medicine; in most cases there will be only modest renumeration. Although it is the expressed intent of the editorial leadership to promote the concept of full-time EMS medical directors, we recognize that most readers have significant professional and personal responsibilities beyond prehospital and disaster medicine.

Nevertheless the number of physicians in full-time EMS medical director positions is growing, as are the variations in EMS system administrative and medical structure. At one extreme the physician director is responsible for all of the medical and operational aspects of EMS; at the other, the physician is simply an informal advisor to the EMS administration, the fire chief, the board of directors, or the regional medical advisory committee. The degree of actual authority of the physician over medical matters also varies. Occasionally the medical authority of the physician is absolute; more common, medical oversight policies and protocols are implemented only after the advice and consent of local physicians and administrators.

Undeniably the practices of prehospital and disaster medicine are becoming more complicated, more standardized, and more formalized; appropriately the medically and legally responsible physicians are exercising greater authority over the entire range of medical oversight issues. Needless to say, there are occasionally heated debates over whether issues such as response time targets, length of duty shifts, and dispatch policies are "medical issues." Unfortunately, some physicians who wish to expand the scope of medical oversight do not appreciate that with additional authority and responsibility also come increased accountability and liability. Indeed, in 1994 there are at least two instances in which an entire EMS medical oversight committee is being taken to court over untoward patient outcomes following prehospital care, naturally both are in New York City.

Over the last decade the general community of emergency physicians has grown significantly more comfortable with its responsibility to include prehospital medical oversight as an integral part of residency curricula and of the American Board of Emergency Medicine certification criteria. In addition, emergency physicians have recognized that the simple acts of receiving and caring for ambulance patients should not and do not empower them to publicly criticize the medical practice of those physicians charged with prehospital medical oversight. Recognition of prehospital and disaster medicine as a subspecialty of emergency medicine or perhaps even as a separate specialty of medicine likely will emerge before the next millennium. We trust that this text both expands and defines the knowledge base that is framing that evolving medical practice.

This textbook is divided into five discrete sections. Section One presents the reader with a broad overview of EMS, focusing particularly on the historical background, legislative underpinnings, and those basic structural issues that must be addressed relatively early in the planning and developmental process.

Section Two introduces and develops the concept of medical oversight, presenting first an historical perspective and then the varied philosophies and mechanisms for the provision of medical oversight. This section challenges the reader to widely expand the horizons of medical involvement in EMS and admittedly emphasizes a philosophy of public health rather than one of public safety or even one of emergency medicine.

Section Three weaves both factual information and unsupported opinion from a variety of disciplines into a loose credo that will be of assistance to even the most experienced medical director in creating the shared paradigm that is the hallmark of a truly successful system. More so than with the other sections of the text the chapters of Section Three are replete with apparent internal contradictions and oxymorons; however, on close reading and analysis none are entirely incorrect.

Section Four addresses the specific operational issues that virtually every EMS physician will be expected to quickly identify, intelligently evaluate, and adeptly solve. In many cases the rubric is embarrassingly thin; the limited references reflect the immaturity of our specialty rather than any shortcomings on the part of the individual authors.

The text ends with a unique and comprehensive glossary that has already been recognized as a driving force in the standardization of the diverse terminology used to describe EMS operations throughout the world. After understanding the terms, the novice medical director should be able to speak and understand our new and evolving language; however, some regional dialects are not included, and a few of the definitions are perilously close to being arbitrary. Before starting to read the text, the reader should peruse the glossary so that both student and teacher are familiar with the vocabulary.

The Epilogue of the Handbook was a serendipitous accident that we intentionally did not duplicate in this text; luckily, much of the material and the insight of that original Epilogue is found in Section Three. Dr. Dinerman has successfully reprised the soaring spirit of that philosophical creation. The Epilogue to the second edition is less spectacular but equally introspective and marginally more optimistic; it simply encourages the reader to broadly and openly view the future of EMS medical oversight from the vantage point of the present, tempered moderately by the accumulated wisdom of the past.

Finally, on a personal note, over the last 15 years, my daughter like EMS has grown from adolescence to young adulthood. Even now she is occasionally puzzled as to why a small group of physicians tilted at windmills, formed NAEMSP, created the National EMS Medical Directors' Course, and struggled with the various editions of this book. The following anonymous verse, brought to my attention by Jay Fitch, best expresses what I would tell her.

Alexander Kuehl, M.D., M.P.H., FACS

The Bridge Builder

An old man going a lone highway
Came at the evening cold and grey
To a chasm vast and wide and steep
With waters rolling cold and deep.
The old man crossed in the twilight dim
The sullen stream held no fear for him
But he turned when safe on the other side
And built a bridge to span the tide
Old man, said a fellow pilgrim near
You're wasting your strength with building here
Your journey will end with the ending day
You'll never again cross this way
You've crossed the chasm deep and wide
Why build this bridge at eventide?
The builder lifted his old grey head
Good friend on the path I have come he said
There followeth after me today
A youth whose feet must pass this way
The chasm that was naught to me
To that fairhead youth may a pitfall be
He too must cross in the twilight dim
Good friend, I am building this bridge for him.

Anonymous

Contents

Section One *System Elements*

1 History, 3
2 Response Phases, 28
3 System Models, 32
4 Urban Systems, 35
5 Rural Systems, 40
6 Wilderness, 47
7 Military Systems, 59
8 Legislation, 66
9 Funding Strategies, 76
10 System Design, 81
11 Levels of Providers, 98
12 Medical Interventions, 105
13 Communications, 118
14 Emergency Medical Dispatch, 125
15 Data Collection, 153
16 Evaluation, 158
17 Research, 168

Section Two *Medical Oversight Elements*

18 Medical Oversight, 181
19 Indirect Medical Control, 186
20 Direct Medical Control, 196
21 Quality Management, 217
22 Risk Management, 247
23 Education, 253
24 Authorization and Empowerment, 267

Section Three *Interpersonal Elements*

25 Ethical Issues, 247
26 Legal Issues, 280

27 Prehospital Providers in the Emergency Department, 294
28 Prehospital Providers, 300
29 Nurses, 307
30 Volunteers, 316
31 Discipline with Due Process, 321
32 Leadership and Team Building, 334
33 Critical Incident Stress Management, 339
34 Political Survival, 345

Section Four *Operational Elements*

35 Infectious Diseases, 353
36 Inappropriate Use, 363
37 Refusal of Prehospital Care, 375
38 Bystander Physicians, 381
39 Resuscitation Issues, 388
40 Automated External Defibrillation, 399
41 Air Medical Transport, 407
42 Interfacility Transports, 414
43 Pediatric Issues, 420
44 Hazardous Materials, 431
45 Multiple Casualty Incidents, 441
46 Catastrophic Events, 447
47 Diversion and COBRA Issues, 454
48 Regionalization and Designation of Medical Facilities, 465
Epilogue, 472
Glossary, 477

Section One

System Elements

This first section describes the historical development of EMS, the basic system models, the legislation that enabled the evolution of modern EMS systems, the structure of a generic EMS response, and the demands of specific types of EMS systems. Organizational and political strategies for the development of systems is detailed, including recommendations encompassing the choices of funding methodologies, system design, levels of providers, medical interventions, communication techniques, and dispatch algorithms.

The concluding chapters of this section, which address data collection, prehospital care report design, evaluation, and research, provide a context for those functions that are often poorly thought-out during the initial stages of system planning, as well as a stimulus to the reader to aggressively incorporate them at the inception of system implementation.

1

History

Anthony C. Mustalish, M.D., M.P.H., FACEP, FACPRM
Carl Post, B.A., M.A., Ph.D., EMT-D

Over the last 25 years, emergency medical services (EMS) in the United States has undergone major expansion, development, and change. The object of neglect before 1966, EMS has progressed and improved, since receiving emphasis by public and private agencies, resulting in the development of innovative systems, multiple levels of providers, and a new specialty in medicine. Although the events were partially due to the application of a systematic approach, the adoption of clinical breakthroughs, the integration of the hospital and prehospital phases of emergency medical care, and heightened political and public awareness, in a real sense the advances evolved naturally. There was neither supporting evidence nor a shared paradigm.

This chapter analyzes the historical development of EMS, discusses philosophical and social events that fueled change, and reviews major trends. The chapter is constructed around the watershed years of 1966, 1973, and 1982.

Before 1966

Prehospital care has existed since man learned to hunt and make war. Early hunters and warriors provided care for the injured. Although the methods used to staunch bleeding, stabilize fractures, and provide nourishment were primitive, the need for treatment was undoubtedly recognized. The basic elements of prehistoric response to injury still guide present prehospital EMS programs. Among these elements was the recognition of a need for action, which led to the development of medical and surgical emergency treatment techniques and the evolution of a system of communication, treatment, and transport to reduce morbidity and mortality.

One of the earliest known medical documents, the *Edwin Smith Papyrus,* written in 1500 BC, vividly describes triage and treatment protocol.[11] Reference to prehospital emergency care is also found in the *Babylonian Code of Hammurabi* where a detailed protocol for treatment of the injured is described.[50] In the Old Testament, Elisha breathed into the mouth of a dead child and brought the child back to life.[42] The Good Samaritan not only treated the injured traveler but also instructed others to do likewise.[48] Greeks and Romans had surgeons present during battle to treat the wounded. Chariots were available to transport them to hospitals set up nearby.

The most direct root of modern prehospital systems is found in the efforts of Jean Dominique Larrey, Napoleon's chief military physician. Larrey developed a prehospital system in which the injured were treated on the battlefield and horse-drawn wagons were used to carry them away.[34]

To quote Larrey directly: "At Limbourg, our advanced guard had a brisk engagement with the King of Prussia. The remoteness of our ambulances deprived the wounded of the requisite attention . . . we found it most impossible to bring off our wounded who fell into the power of the enemy . . . I was authorized to construct a carriage which I called the flying ambulance."[12] In 1797 Larrey built "ambulance volantes" of two or four wheels to rescue the wounded. Larrey had introduced a new concept in military surgery: early transport from the battlefield to the aid stations and then to the frontline hospital.

One can speculate that Napoleon's contemporaneous and brilliant battlefield innovation of light, highly mobile artillery sparked Larrey's creativity, much in the same way that modern physicians modified the military use of helicopters into medical evacuation roles. Larrey also initiated detailed treatment protocols such as the early amputation of shattered limbs to prevent gangrene, just as Napoleon codified his military dictums and civilian laws.

The Civil War marked the origin of the first organized prehospital system in the United States.[33] Learning from the lessons of the Napoleonic and Crimean Wars, military physicians led by Joseph Barnes and Jonathan Letterman established an extensive system of prehospital care. After several early catastrophes, the Union Army trained medical corpsmen to provide treatment in the field. In addition, a transportation system, which included railroads, was developed to bring the wounded to medical facilities.[70] As documented by Walt Whitman[73] and James Brady, the facilities were primitive; many wounded died in agony, more often from dysentery, malnutrition, and infection than an immediate result of their wounds.[63]

Throughout the first half of the nineteenth century few organized programs of prehospital care existed for civilians. The medical experiences of the Civil War stimulated the beginning of urban ambulance services in the United States and England. The first ambulance systems in cities such as Cincinnati, New York, London, and Paris during postwar years. The early prehospital care advocates, often solitary and criticized, recognized the need for a prehospital system to care for patients in workplaces, at home, and on urban streets. Injuries caused by runaway horses, fires, and other aspects of nineteenth century urban life resulted in suffering and often death for those who were either left unattended or transported in a slow and painful manner.[11]

Edward Dalton, Sanitary Superintendent of the Board of Health in New York City, established a city ambulance program in 1869. Dalton, a former surgeon in the Union Army, spearheaded the development of urban civilian ambulances to permit greater speed, enhance comfort, and increase maneuverability on city streets.[35] On the ambulance there was medical equipment such as splints, bandages, straitjackets, and a stomach pump, as well as a medicine chest of antidotes, anesthetics, brandy, and morphine. By the turn of the century, interns, themselves a new concept, accompanied the ambulance; often, care was rendered on the scene and the patient left at home. Ambulance drivers had virtually no formal medical training.

One of the best descriptions of a turn of the century urban ambulance service comes from Emily Barringer, the first woman ambulance surgeon in New York City. Her descriptions are still timely. For example, "Aside from the permanent personnel of the ambulance house, there was a most interesting collection of people who 'dropped in' there for a chat; . . . these various men exchanged confidences and formed plans. It was there in the ambulance house that the reporters would surely drop in for the 'inside dope' about any inpatient matter, be it politics, murder, or accident."[8]

Further development of urban ambulance services continued in the years before World War I. Electric, steam, and gasoline-powered carriages were used as ambulances. Calls for service were generally processed and dispatched by the individual hospital, although improved telegraph and telephone systems with signal boxes throughout New York City were developed to connect the police department and the hospitals.[35]

During World War I, the introduction of the traction splint for the stabilization of patients with leg fractures by Thomas led to a decrease in morbidity and mortality. Between the two wars, ambulances were dispatched by mobile radios. In the 1920s in Roanoke, Virginia, the first volunteer rescue squad model was begun. The Virginia Beach EMS, with more than 200 members, remains the largest volunteer EMS organization in the United States.

After the American entry into World War II, the military demand for physicians pulled the interns from ambulances, resulting in a marked alteration and deterioration of prehospital care. Physicians never returned to ambulance duty in the United States. Instead the postwar ambulances, in effect poorly equipped vehicles or hearses, usually responded to emergencies staffed by untrained personnel able to provide only minimal treatment on the scene. Half the ambulances were operated by mortuary attendants, most of whom had never taken even a first aid course.[7] The primary function was to transport the patient to the hospital in a horizontal position.

Throughout the 1950s and 1960s, two geographic patterns of ambulance service evolved. In cities, hospital-based ambulances gradually coalesced into more centrally coordinated citywide programs usually administrated and staffed by the municipal hospital or fire department. In rural areas, funeral home hearses were sporadically replaced by a variety of units operated by the local fire department or a newly formed rescue squad. In urban and rural areas a few profit-making providers continued to deliver transport services and occasionally even contracted with local government to provide emergency prehospital services and transport. In most rural venues there was minimal coordination among providers and little integration of prehospital services with medical facilities.

Before 1966, very little legislation and regulation applicable to ambulance services existed. Responding providers had relatively limited formal training, and physician involvement at all levels was minimal. Although a gradual evolution would have continued, a number of factors intersected in the mid-1960s, which stimulated a revolution in prehospital care.

Interest in prehospital care was stimulated by breakthroughs in medical treatment simply because at least something could be done. Closed chest cardiopulmonary resuscitation (CPR), reported as successful in 1960 by Kouwenhoven,[43] was quickly adopted as the medical standard for cardiac arrest in the prehospital setting. New evidence that CPR, pharmaceuticals, and defibrillation could save lives immediately created a demand for providers of those interventions in both the hospital and the prehospital environments.

Throughout the 1960s, fundamental understanding of the pathophysiology of potentially fatal dysrhythmias expanded significantly. CPR, pharmaceutical intervention, and electrical defibrillation were first carried out by physicians. In 1966, Pantridge and Geddes documented the use of a mobile coronary care unit (CCU) ambulance for prehospital resuscitation of patients in Belfast. Their treatment protocols, originally developed for the treatment of myocardial infarction in intensive care units, were quickly moved into the field.[61] Because the medical team was often with the patient at the time of cardiac arrest, the success rate was a remarkable 20%.

1966: A Turning Point

The modern era of prehospital care in the United States began in 1966. In that year the recognition of an urgent need, the crucial element necessary for aggressive development of prehospital systems, was heralded by the National Academy of Sciences-National Research Council (NAS-NRC) report. NAS-NRC is a private organization chartered by Congress to provide scientific advice to the Federal government. "Accidental Death and Disability: The Neglected Disease of Modern Society," documented the enormous failure of the US health care system to provide even minimal care for the emergency patient. Prehospital services were accurately described, in absolute terms and in comparison with care available to military personnel in World War II and the Korean conflict, as primitive and woefully inadequate. Treatment protocols, trained medical personnel, rapid transportation, and modern communications such as two-way radios and emergency call numbers were all identified as necessities simply not available to civilians.[20]

The NAS-NRC report identified key issues and problems facing the United States in providing emergency care. Twenty-four recommendations were proposed that would serve as a blueprint for EMS development. Its summary report (see box) listed factors contributing to the inadequate status of the US emergency care system.[20]

It is worth quoting this document extensively not only because it details the prehospital emergency care problem, but also because it establishes a benchmark to measure subsequent progress and change.

DEATHS: Accidents are the leading cause of death among persons between the ages of 1 and 37; and they are the fourth leading cause of death at all ages. Among accidental deaths, those due to motor vehicles constitute the leading cause for all age groups under 75. Since 1903, when the "horseless carriage" toll assumed significance, there have been more than 6,500,000 deaths from accidents in this country, over 1,690,000 involving motor vehicles. In 1965, the accident death toll was approximately 107,000 including 49,000 from motor vehicles, 28,500 at home, and 14,100 at work. Deaths from traffic injuries have increased annually; 10,000 more were killed in 1965 than in 1955, and the increase from 1964 to 1965 was 3 percent. Seventy percent of the motor vehicle deaths occurred in rural areas and in communities with populations under 2500.

Despite increasing mechanization, death rates from work accidents in manufacturing have decreased in the past 33 years, from approximately 37 accidental deaths per 100,000 workers in 1933 to a rate of 20 per 100,000 in 1965. This reduction is due largely to education, training, and surveillance of industrial workers, and elimination of hazardous machinery in industrial plants. Similar efforts should be directed to the increasing millions of drivers and to vehicles.

The tragedy of the high accidental death rate is that trauma kills thousands who otherwise could expect to live long and productive lives, whereas those afflicted with malignancy, heart disease, stroke, and many chronic diseases usually die late in life. Thus many more millions of productive man-years are lost owing to deaths from accidents than from chronic diseases among older persons. The human suffering and financial loss from preventable accidental death constitute a public health problem second only to the ravages of ancient plagues or world wars. In one year alone vehicle accidents kill more than we lost in the Korean War, and in the past 60 years more Americans have died from accidents than from combat wounds in all of our wars. In the 20–year period from 1945 through 1964, there were over 97,000 accidental deaths among military personnel, predominantly caused by motor vehicles.

DISABILITY: The total number of nondisabling injuries treated at home, in doctors' offices, in out-

Inadequacies of Prehospital Care in 1966

1. The general public is insensitive to the magnitude of the problem of accidental death and injury.
2. Millions lack instruction in basic first aid.
3. Few are adequately trained in the advanced techniques of cardiopulmonary resuscitation, childbirth, or other life-saving measures, yet every ambulance and rescue squad attendant, policeman, fire fighter, paramedical worker, and worker in high-risk industry should be trained.
4. Local political authorities have neglected their responsibility to provide optimum emergency medical services.
5. Research on trauma has not been supported or identified at the National Institutes of Health on a level consistent with its importance as the fourth leading cause of death and a primary cause of disability.
6. The potentials of the US Public Health Service Program in accident prevention and emergency medical services have not been fully exploited.
7. Data are lacking on how to determine the number of individuals whose lives are lost through injuries compounded by misguided attemps at rescue and first aid, absence of physicians at the scene of the injury, unsuitable ambulances with inadequate equipment and untrained attendants, lack of traffic control, or the lack of voice communication facilities.
8. Helicopter ambulances have not been adapted to civilian peacetime needs.
9. Emergency departments of hospitals are overcrowded, some are archaic, and there are no systematic surveys on which to base requirements for space, equipment, or staffing for present, let alone future, needs.
10. Fundamental research on shock and trauma is inadequately supported; medical and health-related organizations have failed to join forces to apply knowledge already available to advanced treatment of trauma, or educate the public and inform Congress.[20]

From *Accidental death and disability: the neglected disease of modern society*, National Academy of Sciences, Washington, DC, 1966, National Academy Press.

patient clinics or in emergency departments is unknown. In 1965, disabling injuries numbered over 10,500,000 including 400,000 that resulted in some degree of permanent impairment. It is estimated that the number of United States citizens now physically impaired by injuries is over 11 million, including nearly 200,000 persons who have lost a leg, a foot, an arm, or a hand and 500,000 with varying degrees of impaired vision.

COSTS: In 1965, accident costs totaled about $18 billion, including wage losses of $5.3 billion, medical expenses of $1.8 billion, administrative and claim settlements of $3.6 billion, property loss in fires of $1.4 billion, property damage in motor vehicle accidents of $3.1 billion, and indirect cost of work accidents of $2.8 billion. The total approaches the current national annual appropriation for conducting the war in Vietnam.

MEDICAL LOAD: The care of accident cases imposes a staggering load on physicians, paramedical personnel, and hospitals. Approximately one of every four Americans suffers an accident of some degree each year. Of the more than 52,000,000 persons injured in 1965, although many were treated at home or at work, most received medical attention in physicians' offices or in outpatient or emergency departments of hospitals. It is estimated that in 1965 more than 2,000,000 victims of accidental injury were hospitalized; they occupied 65,000 hospital beds for 22,000,000 bed-days and received the services of 88,000 hospital personnel. This exceeds the number of bed-days required to care for the 4 million babies born each year or for all the heart patients and it is more than four times greater than that required for cancer patients. Approximately 1 of 8 beds in general hospitals in the United States is occupied by an accident victim.[20]

The 1966 NAS-NRC document also cited hospital emergency departments as being woefully inadequate. Although there were more than 7000 accredited hospitals, very few were prepared to meet the increased demand that developed between 1945 and 1965. From 1958 to 1970, the number of emergency department visits increased from 18 million to more than 49 million.[20] In addition, emergency departments were staffed by the least experienced personnel, who had little education in the treatment of multiple injuries or critical medical emergencies. Efforts of the American College of Surgeons (ACS) and the American Academy of Orthopedic Surgeons (AAOS) to improve emergency care were largely unsuccessful because medical interest was essentially nonexistent.[16,17,37,38]

The 1966 NAS-NRC document was the first to recommend emergency facilities be categorized: "The current dictum that an ambulance should deliver a patient to the nearest emergency unit is no longer acceptable. In the absence of a descriptive categorization of the level of care that might reasonably be expected at a facility, neither the patient nor the ambulance driver can judge which facility is adequate to the immediate need."[20] The report further suggested emergency units might be categorized as the following: an advanced first aid facility, a limited emergency facility, a major emergency facility, or an emergency facility combined with a trauma research unit.[20]

The NAS-NRC report emphasized aggressive clinical management of trauma. It suggested that local trauma registries develop data bases concerning the natural history and epidemiology of trauma, the establishment of a national computerized central registry, and studies on the feasibility of designating select injuries to be incorporated in the epidemiologic reports of the Public Health Service. Additionally, changes were recommended to address legal problems, for autopsies of trauma victims, and for disaster response reviews. Finally, trauma research was emphasized with the ultimate goal of establishing a National Institute of Trauma.[20]

Another problem identified in the report was the broad gap between existing knowledge and operational activity. For example, the mortality rate for injured soldiers reaching medical facilities in World War I was 8%, in World War II it was 4.5%, and it was less than 2% in Vietnam.[19,39] The dramatic improvement in military survival was attributed to appropriate ambulance services, trained personnel, adequate communication systems, and strategically located treatment facilities. Yet in the mid-1960s, these components were missing from civilian services. Although communication with astronauts was possible, mobile communication with ambulances was not yet regarded as integral to EMS.

The NAS-NRC report did not appear out of thin air. The President's Commission on Highway Safety[65] had previously published a report titled "Health, Medical Care, and Transportation of Injured," which recommended a national program to reduce deaths and injuries caused by highway accidents. Its findings were complemented by and consistent with the later NAS-NRC report. The recommendations in both documents were used when the Highway Safety Act of 1966 was drafted. This law established the cabinet-level Department of Transportation (DOT) and gave it legislative and financial authority to improve EMS. Specific emphasis was placed on developing a highway safety program, including standards and activities for improving both ambulance service and provider training.[56]

The Highway Safety Act also authorized funds to develop EMS standards and implement programs that would improve ambulance services. Matching funds were provided for EMS demonstration projects and studies. All states were required to have highway safety programs in accordance with the regulatory standards promulgated by the DOT. The standard on EMS required each state to develop regional EMS systems that could handle prehospital emergency medical needs. Ambulances, equipment, personnel, and administration costs were funded by the highway safety program. Regional financing, as opposed to county or state funding, was a new concept that would be echoed in federal health legislation throughout the remainder of the decade.[56]

1966 to 1973

Encouraging matching funds from state and local governments, as well as private sources, the Highway Safety Act served as a catalyst for targeting millions of dollars toward EMS development. Between 1968 and 1979 the DOT contributed more than $142 million to regional systems under the EMS standard. Ten million dollars was spent between 1967 and 1979 on more than 50 research projects dealing with three major areas: development ($584,000), demonstrations ($4.9 million), and studies/surveys ($5.3 million). Contract obligations to the DOT included specific criteria for the EMS use of helicopters, ambulance design, EMS communication systems, and EMS system development.[27,40,58]

Other federal EMS initiatives during this period included the designation of the Health Services and Mental Health Administration (HSMHA) as the lead agency for EMS within the Department of Health, Education, and Welfare (DHEW). In 1972, $16 million was awarded by HSMHA to areas of Arkansas, California, Florida, Illinois, and Ohio to develop model regional EMS systems. The purpose of those demonstration projects was to compare various approaches to emergency medical care so other localities could develop their own systems. Typically, politically influential areas were chosen for the projects, which were federally financed operations as much as they were demonstrations.[41,68]

In 1969 the Airlie House Conference proposed a hospital categorization scheme.[18] The AMA Commission on EMS urged facility categorization and published its own, which identified staffing, equipment, services, and personnel types.[14] This became known as "horizontal categorization." Although categorization was supported by professional and hospital associations, many hospitals and physicians feared hospitals in lower categories would suffer a loss of prestige, patients, or reimbursement. The EMS demonstration projects developed a categorization scheme based on hospitalwide care of specific disease processes. Known as "vertical categorization," it was ultimately embraced by many regional programs as a major theme in the development of EMS systems.

By the late 1960s, drugs, defibrillators, and personnel were available to improve prehospital care. Fortunately, space age telemetric technology was also available, so responders with limited medical training did not have to interpret rhythm strips. As early as 1967 the first physician responder mobile programs metamorphosed into "paramedic" programs using physician-monitored telemetry. These new programs combined existing clinical knowledge, evolving technology, and available personnel to define the ultimate clinical product; obviously, there were great geographic variations in approach.[46,53] However, if automated external defibrillators had existed in 1967, the evolutionary path of prehospital providers in the United States may have been very different.

The "Heartmobile" program, begun in 1969 in Columbus, Ohio, initially consisted of a physician and three EMTs; yet, within 2 years, 22 highly trained (2000 hours) paramedics provided field care and the physician's role had become supervisory. Paramedics performed lifesaving techniques with physician supervision, resulting in a cardiac arrest survival rate similar to that obtained by physicians alone. Similarly, in Seattle, physicians supervised highly trained paramedics, increasing the survival rate from 10% to 30% for prehospital patients whose presenting rhythm was ventricular fibrillation. In Dade County, Florida, the rapid response time of mobile paramedic units was effectively combined with hospital physician direction via radio and telemetry for the first time.[53] In Brighton, England, non-physician personnel provided field care without direct medical control. Electrocardiographic data were recorded continuously to permit retrospective review by a physician.[46]

National professional organizations such as the American College of Surgeons (ACS), the American Association of Orthopaedic Surgeons (AAOS), the American Heart Association (AHA), and the American Society of Anesthesiologists (ASA) in concert with other groups provided extensive medical input into the early development of EMS. New organizations were formed to focus on EMS, including the Commission on EMS of the AMA, the Committee on Community Emergency Health Services of the American Hospital Association, the American Trauma Society, the Emergency Department Nurses Association, the Society of Critical Care Medicine, the National Registry of Emergency Medical Technicians, and the American College of Emergency Physicians (ACEP). Before 1973 such groups exerted significant but uncoordinated forces toward the reorganization, restructure, improvement, expansion, and politicization of EMS.[4,10,14,18]

The Robert Wood Johnson Foundation (RWJF) allocated $15 million for EMS-related activities in 1974, the largest single contribution for the development of health systems in the United States ever made by a nonprofit foundation. Forty-four areas received grants of up to $400,000 to develop EMS systems.[66] This money was to encourage communities to build regional EMS systems emphasizing the overall goal of improving access to general medical care. The program recognized that many patients had difficulty getting immediate and appropriate assistance in an emergency situation and that a reduction in the time between initial need and the provision of care offered tremendous lifesaving potential. RWJF estimated that more than 90,000 lives could be saved each year through prompt medical treatment of trauma victims. The money was provided over a 2-year period to establish new demonstration projects and develop regional emergency medical communications systems.[67]

In 1972 the NAS-NRC published, "Roles and Resources of Federal Agencies in Support of Comprehensive Emergency Medical Services," which asserted that the federal government had not kept pace with efforts by professional and lay health organizations to upgrade EMS. The document endorsed a vigorous federal government role in both the provision and upgrading of EMS. It recommended that President Nixon express concern about the magnitude of the accidental death and disability problem and that he propose action by the legislative and executive branches to ensure optimum universal emergency care. Furthermore, it urged interdepartmental coordination in identifying federal resources for delivery of emergency services, as well as the integration of all those responses into a single division of the DHEW, which would have primary responsibility for the entire emergency medical program. Finally, it recommended that the focal point for local emergency medical care be at the state level and that all federal efforts be coordinated through regional EMS programs.[15] This set the stage for the new EMS regional programs to directly conflict with both the counties and the states.

1973: The Emergency Medical Service System Act

By 1973 several major lessons had emerged from the demonstration projects and the various studies undertaken during the preceding 7 years. Although the federal initiative had been limited to the five 1968 DHEW regional demonstration projects, significant progress had been made toward clearly defining a potential program goal. The projects proved that a regional EMS system approach could work; however, they did not prove that a regional approach was necessarily the best.

By early 1973 many national organizations supported further federal involvement both in establishing EMS program goals and providing direct financial support. The first efforts at passing federal EMS legislation were defeated, but a later, modified EMS bill passed with support from numerous public and professional groups. President Nixon vetoed this bill in August 1973. The standard conservative philosophy was that EMS was a service that should be provided by local government and that the federal government should neither underwrite operations nor purchase equipment. Additional congressional hearings led to the reintroduction of a bill proposing an extensive federal EMS program, based on the rationale that individual communities would not be able to develop regional systems without federal encouragement, guidelines, and funding. Finally, in November 1973 the Emergency Medical Services System Act was passed and signed. It was added as Title XII to the Public Health Service Act, wherein it addressed EMS systems, research grants, and contracts. It also added a new section to the existing Title VII concerning EMS training grants.[29]

Although the law was amended to reauthorize expenditures in 1976, 1978, and again in 1979, its goal remained to encourage development of comprehensive regional EMS systems throughout the country. The available grant funds were divided among the three major portions of the EMS System Act:

Section 1202—Feasibility studies and planning
Section 1203—Initial operations
Section 1204—Expansion and improvement
Section 1205—Research

Applicants were encouraged to use existing health resources, facilities, and personnel. The EMS regions were ultimately expected to become financially self-sufficient; therefore a phase out of all federal funding was targeted for 1979, but later extended to 1982. Funding for operations, research, and training from 1973 to 1979 is presented in Table 1-1. Table 1-2 displays funding authorized under the EMS System Act through fiscal year 1982.

The program was administered in the DHEW through the Division of Emergency Medical Services (DEMS). David Boyd, the medical director of the Illinois demonstration project was named the director. The law and subsequent regulations emphasized a regional systems approach, a trauma orientation, and required that each funded system address the 15 components listed in the box on p. 10. Appendix I of this chapter describes each component as prepared by the DHEW and published as part of its revised *Program Guidelines* in 1979. Medical oversight was addressed neither in 1973 nor in 1979.

Although the EMS System Act and its subsequent regulations encouraged a degree of medical over-

Table 1-1. History of EMS Authorizations and Appropriations

Purpose	Authorized($)	Appropriated ($)
Fiscal year 1974:		
Services	30,000,000	17,000,000
Research	5,000,000	3,300,000
Training	10,000,000	6,600,000
TOTAL	45,000,000	26,900,000
Fiscal year 1975:		
Services	60,000,000	32,500,000
Research	5,000,000	4,500,000
Training	—	—
TOTAL	65,000,000	37,000,000
Fiscal year 1976:		
Services	35,000,000 5,003,000	29,700,000
Research	5,000,000	3,925,000
Training	10,000,000	—
TOTAL	55,003,000	33,625,000
Fiscal year 1977:		
Services	45,000,000	33,200,000
Research	5,000,000	3,925,000
Training	10,000,000	6,000,000
Burn program	5,000,000	3,000,000
TOTAL	65,000,000	46,125,000
Fiscal year 1978:		
Services	55,000,000	36,625,000
Research	5,000,000	3,000,000
Training	10,000,000	6,000,000
Burn program	7,500,000	3,000,000
TOTAL	77,500,000	48,625,000
Fiscal year 1979:		
Services	70,000,000	36,625,000
Research	5,000,000	3,000,000
Training	10,000,000	3,000,000
Burn program	10,000,000	3,000,000
TOTAL	95,000,000	45,625,000

From the Committee on Labor and Human Resources: United States Senate 96th Congress, 1st Session. Rep No 96-102, In: *United States Senate Hearing report,* 515-516, Feb 28, 1979, Washington, DC, 1979, US Government Printing Office.

Table 1-2. Authorizations of Appropriations for Emergency Medical Services Programs

	1980 ($)	1981 ($)	1982 ($)	Totals ($)
Services	40,000,000	40,000,000	40,000,000	120,000,000
Research	3,000,000	3,000,000	3,000,000	9,000,000
Burn trauma or poison	3,000,000	3,000,000	3,000,000	9,000,000
Training	4,000,000	4,000,000	4,000,000	12,000,000
TOTALS	50,000,000	50,000,000	50,000,000	150,000,000

From Committee on Labor and Human Resources: United States Senate 96th Congress, 1st Session Report No 96-102, In: *Hearing report,* 504, Feb 28, 1979, Washington, DC, 1979, US Government Printing Office.

sight, the focus was on the project medical director who, in retrospect at least, seems far removed from the practice of prehospital medicine.

1974 to 1981

The 15 essential EMS components may have been flawed, but the concept that an EMS chain of survival was only as strong as its weakest link was correct. In early 1974, DHEW officials began implementing the legislative mandate. Adopted from earlier experiences the basic principles were that (1) an effective and comprehensive system must have resources sufficient in quality and quantity to meet a wide variety of demands and (2) the discrete geographic regions established have sufficient populations and resources eventually enabling them to become self-sufficient.

Each state was to designate a coordinating agency for statewide EMS efforts. Ultimately, 304 EMS regions were established nationwide. Table 1-3 demonstrates the status of regional EMS activity in 1979. Of the 304 geographic areas, 22 "no activity" and 96 "section 1202 planning" areas represented 118 regions not in operation. As early as 1979, 17 regions were fully functional and independent of federal money.

In 1979 testimony was given before the congressional committee considering extension of funding. DHEW officials stated that 291 of the 304 regions had received funding under Title XII, 258 (covering 159.5 million people) had completed the planning process, and 206 (covering 150 million people) had either completed or were in the development phase.[49]

In the regulations, Boyd, strictly interpreted the congressional legislative intent of the EMS System Act to mandate that all communities adopt the 15 essential components. Regions were limited to five grants; with each year of funding, progress toward more sophisticated operational levels was expected. By the end of the third year of funding, regions were expected to have basic life support (BLS) capabilities; and advanced life support (ALS) capability was expected at the end of the fifth year. The use of BLS and ALS terminology in the regulations spread widely. However, the original definitions that responded

Table 1-3. Regional Activity: 1979

Status of EMS activity	Regions (No.)
No activity	22
Section 1202 planning	96
Section 1203 (1st year) establishment	50
Section 1203 (2nd year) establishment	68
Section 1204 (1st year) improvement	39
Section 1204 (2nd year) improvement	12
Completed eligibility	17
TOTAL	304

From Committee on Labor and Human Resources: United States Senate 96th Congress, 1st Session Report No 96-102, In: *Hearing report,* 508, Feb 28, 1979, Washington, DC, 1979, US Government Printing Office.

The Fifteen Essential EMS Components (1973)

1. Manpower
2. Training
3. Communications
4. Transportation
5. Facilities
6. Critical care units
7. Public safety agencies
8. Consumer participation
9. Access to care
10. Patient transfer
11. Coordinated patient record keeping
12. Public information and education
13. Review and evaluation
14. Disaster plan
15. Mutual aid

Table 1-4. Grant Activity Provided by the EMS System Act

Fiscal Year 1974

Eighty-five grants covering 126 regions and serving a population of 88,200,000 were awarded in the amount of $17,000,000.

Section of act	Grants (No.)	Regions (No.)	Amount ($)	Population served
1202	53	90	2,250,000	63,000,000
1203	21	27	10,400,000	18,900,000
1204	11	9	4,350,000	6,300,000
TOTAL	85	126	17,000,000	88,200,000

Fiscal Year 1975

One hundred and sixteen grants, covering 174 regions and serving a population of 121,890,000 were awarded in the amount of $32,242,800.

Section of act	Grants (No.)	Regions (No.)	Amount ($)	Population served
1202	56	82	4,617,000	57,400,000
1203	49	66	19,500,000	46,200,000
1204	11	26	8,125,000	18,290,000
TOTAL	116	174	32,242,000	121,890,000

Fiscal Year 1976

Fifty-two grants, covering 63 regions and serving a population of 44,100,000 were awarded in the amount of $29,115,300.

Section of act	Grants (No.)	Regions (No.)	Amount ($)	Population served
1202	—	—	—	—
1203	41	51	21,836,475	35,700,000
1204	11	12	7,278,825	8,400,000
TOTAL	52	63	29,115,300	44,100,000

Fiscal Year 1977

Eighty-three grants, covering 99 regions and serving a population of 69,300,000 were awarded in the amount of $32,775,000.

Section of act	Grants (No.)	Regions (No.)	Amount ($)	Population served
1202	14	21	986,563	14,700,000
1203	44	54	21,767,304	37,800,000
1204	25	24	10,021,133	16,800,000
TOTAL	83	99	32,775,000	69,300,000

Fiscal Year 1978

Ninety-four grants, covering 100 regions and serving a population of 70,000,000 were awarded in the amount of $36,027,800.

Section of act	Grants (No.)	Regions (No.)	Amount ($)	Population served
1202	12	14	930,000	9,800,000
1203	53	61	23,589,791	42,700,000
1204	29	25	11,508,009	17,500,000
TOTAL	94	100	36,027,800	70,000,000

From Committee on Labor and Human Resources: United States Senate 96th Congress, 1st Session Report No 96-102, In: Hearing report, 510-511, Washington, DC, 1979, Feb 28, 1979, US Government Printing Office.

directly to the EMT-A and paramedic levels of training quickly became elusive as variations in the EMT-A and paramedic levels emerged. An additional year of funding was authorized as the 1202b program for planning. Table 1-4 shows a summary of the grant activity provided by the EMS System Act.

Developing the geographic regions required to secure federal funding through the EMS System Act usually required new EMS legislation at the state level. The state laws developed throughout the 1970s varied markedly in regard to the issues of medical oversight, overall operational authority, and financing. In some states, physician direction was required, in others, medical oversight was not even mentioned. Often, the responsibility for coordinating activities was assigned to a regional EMS council of physicians, prehospital providers, and consumers; commonly, the physician input was somewhat removed from the medical mainstream.

Personnel

Lack of appropriately trained emergency personnel at every level of care had been identified as early as 1966 in the NAS-NRC document.[20] After 1973, extensive effort and money were directed at correcting this educational deficiency resulting in significant achievements. By 1978 the Emergency Medical Training Program, authorized under Section 789, provided more than $18 million for the training of more than 200,000 emergency care providers and 12 million citizens in CPR. This was a significant accomplishment considering that just 10 years earlier there were essentially no CPR-trained personnel.

At this time, serendipity played a role. A large number of medical corpsmen, physicians, and nurses who understood that trained non-physicians could perform lifesaving tasks were returning from Vietnam. Many also believed rapid transport and early surgery could save civilian trauma victims.

Physicians. In 1966 the NAS-NRC document stated: "No longer can responsibility be assigned to the least experienced member of the medical staff, or solely to specialists who, by the nature of their training and experience, cannot render adequate care without the support of other staff members."[20] Thus the importance of physician leadership and training in EMS was identified early. During the 25 years following World War II, increasing demands for care were placed on hospital emergency departments. This resulted from the increase in medical specialization, the decline of general practitioners, the increase in hospital-based technology, the greater expectations of the public, and the increase in health insurance support for emergency care. Not surprisingly, during the 1960s a branch of medicine evolved to deal with the critically ill. The academic discipline and scientific rigor necessary to define a separate medical specialty began to develop. In 1968 ACEP was founded by physicians interested in the organization and delivery of emergency medical care. By 1979 ACEP membership had exceeded 9500 physicians and reached 15,300 in 1991. Paradoxi-cally, by 1990, 80% of emergency department visits were for non-emergency care or for care that previously would have been given in a physician's office, 15% were emergencies requiring immediate attention, and only 5% were critical.

Even before 1966 the ACS had established standards and provided specific training for surgeons in the management of trauma. A number of physicians and centers had also attempted to improve education in trauma, but these early efforts had little impact. However, with increasing public awareness of a national crisis, groups of emergency medicine physicians began developing training programs.

In 1970 the first emergency medicine residency was established at the University of Cincinnati and the first Department of Emergency Medicine in a medical school was formed at the University of Southern California. Soon the directors of medical school hospital emergency departments founded the University Association for Emergency Medical Services. Between 1972 and 1980 more than 740 residents completed training programs in 51 emergency medicine residencies throughout the country.[6,28,47] The first major step toward certification as a specialty occurred in 1973 when the AMA authorized a provisional Section of Emergency Medicine. In 1974 a Committee on Board Establishment was appointed, and a liaison Residency Endorsement Committee was formed.[47] Further impetus toward expansion of the residency program in emergency medicine occurred with the formation of the American Board of Emergency Medicine (ABEM) in 1976.[3] Before that time there was some hesitancy to create residency programs that might not lead to board certification.

Although RWJF had supplied some money for physician education, major financial support developed when the 1976 EMS amendments provided funds for training the three major EMS personnel components: emergency physicians, emergency nurses, and emergency medical technicians. Ten million dollars was authorized for training physicians in fiscal years 1977, 1978, and 1979; 29 programs received funding for training. In 1978 alone, more than 4000 trainees were supported in medical schools, residencies, and continuing medical education. In the 1970s, mid-career education was important in the effort to produce emergency medicine specialists. The growth of residency programs between 1970 and 1993 is seen in Table 1-5.

Table 1-5. Growth in Accredited Emergency Medicine Residency Programs and Approved Positions 1970-1993

Year	Accredited Programs	Approved Positions
1970	2	3
1975	32	165
1980	51	410
1993	100	2378

From the Society of Academic Emergency Medicine and Association of American Medical Colleges.

In September 1979, emergency medicine was formally recognized as a specialty by the AMA Committee on Medical Education and the American Board of Medical Specialties. At that time the emergency medicine physician was defined as one trained to engage in (1) the immediate and initial recognition, evaluation, care, and disposition of patients in response to acute illness and injury, (2) the administration, research, and teaching of all aspects of emergency medical care, (3) the direction of the patient to sources of follow-up care as required, (4) the provision, when requested, of emergency but not continuing care to in-hospital patients, and (5) the management of the emergency medical system for the provision of prehospital emergency care.[3] ABEM gave its first certifying examination in 1980, which incidentally did not touch on any areas of prehospital care. In 1991, 901 fellows were inducted bringing the total of board certified emergency physicians to more than 6900.[1]

While emergency medicine, emergency nursing and prehospital care were all nourished by the funds distributed between 1973 and 1982, the interest of ACEP in EMS activities lagged, perhaps because individual physician interest lagged. The first full-time EMS medical director was not appointed until April 1981; previously, all had been part-time, and some had simply been functionaries. Shortly thereafter, cities like Salt Lake City and Houston followed New York's lead and appointed full-time EMS medical directors. Even then, EMS physician as a career choice was perceived by many emergency physicians as limiting and perhaps threatening.

Prehospital Providers. Before 1966 there had been little national, state, or local regulation of ambulance personnel; anyone with a driver's license could answer emergencies. In response to both the 1965 report from the Presidential Commission on Highway Safety and the 1966 NAS-NRC study, Congress passed the Highway Safety Act in 1966, which included funds to develop a training course curriculum for the new position of Emergency Medical Technician-Ambulance (EMT-A). The 70-hour curriculum originally published by the AAOS in 1969 has been updated several times, and also published in other texts.[2] The EMT-A curriculum became the mainstay of training in most states, but actual certification was required in a few.

The 200 people who took the EMT-A course in 1969 were the first ambulance personnel trained to a national standard. The new profession was further defined and officially recognized as an occupational specialty by the Department of Labor in 1972. EMT-A and the more extensive Emergency Medical Technician-Paramedic (EMT-P) were the main educational and operational levels of prehospital care during the early 1970s.

Although the EMT-A concept did not require physician input, the paramedics, who had originally grown out of the physician mobile CCU response programs, were essentially physician-extenders; this concept remained either undeveloped or unadopted by many states. The two types of prehospital providers developed more or less independently. The EMT-A quickly became a nationally recognized standard. Although initially paramedic training differed markedly from locality to locality, the DOT eventually produced a national curriculum. As early as 1973, the practice of the EMT-A was called BLS and the practice of the paramedic, usually trained first as an EMT-A, was labeled ALS.

Because of the great differences in training requirements between the two levels, many local jurisdictions and states quickly developed intermediate levels (EMT-I), which further blurred the already fuzzy distinction between BLS and ALS. By 1979, formally recognized prehospital providers existed at dozens of levels of training from 70 to 2000 hours; the degree of medical supervision required was at least as variable.[46]

By 1982 there were approximately 100,000 providers trained at the EMT-A level with a large portion providing emergency care. The EMT-A was trained to provide the most elemental emergency care at the scene and during transport to the hospital. Such first aid skills include CPR, control of bleeding, ventilation, oxygen therapy, fracture management, extrication, and transport of the patient. The educational requirements of the EMT-A grew to 81 hours of didactic lectures, skills training, and hospital observation; most of the 11-hour increase was devoted to use of the pneumatic antishock garment (PASG). After working for 6 months, graduates were allowed to take a national certifying examination administered by the National Registry of Emergency Medical Technicians (National Registry). Founded in 1970, the National Registry developed a standardized examination for EMT-A personnel as one requirement for maintaining registration. Many states recognized National Registry registration for purposes of reciprocity, but most still required additional state certification.[10]

The paramedic provided sophisticated medical intervention to patients at the site, and in some early systems either transported or accompanied the patient to the hospital.[53] Paramedic practices became somewhat more formalized with the adoption of the DOT EMT-P curriculum. In 1982, EMT-P training ranged from a few hundred to 2000 hours of educational and clinical experience. Typical clinical skills included cardiac defibrillation, endotracheal intubation, venipuncture, and the use of drugs. Their use was based on interpretation of history, clinical signs, and rhythm strips. Telemetric and voice communications with physicians were usually required. In the early days of paramedicine, extensive "on-line" medical control was usually mandatory for all calls. However, with time, the requirements for direct medical control were modified by the introduction of protocols allowing for greater use of standing orders.[31] However, a great deal of variation in the use of direct medical control remained. As early as 1980, paramedics in decentralized systems like New York's used many clinical protocols, most of which had few indications for mandatory direct medical control. On the other hand, as late as 1992, centralized systems like the Houston Fire Department's used only one protocol (cardiac arrest), which did not require instruction from direct medical control.

The concept of EMT-Intermediate (EMT-I) evolved as a provider level located somewhere between EMT-A and EMT-P. EMT-I used the EMT-A intervention's as well as some of the more advanced EMT-P techniques. A standardized national examination for the intermediate level was approved in June 1980 by the National Registry. Airway management, IV therapy, fluid replacement, rhythm recognition, and defibrillation were the most common EMT-I skills. The intermediate level was created to provide traditional paramedic skills to the patient without hundreds of hours of provider training and to build a stepwise progression from EMT-A to EMT-P. Many states developed several levels of EMT-I, often in a modular progression with formal bridge courses.

In 1979, a body was established to evaluate and accredit EMT-A and EMT-P training programs. Seven organizations, including ASA, ACEP, ACS, the American Academy of Pediatrics, the National Association of Emergency Medical Technicians (NAEMT), and the National Registry, sponsored the formation of the Joint Review Committee on Educational Programs for the EMT-Paramedic (JRCEMT-P) and agreed to review curriculum, registration, and certifying requirements. The JRCEMT-P developed criteria by which training programs were evaluated. Accreditation was offered through the AMA Council on Allied Health Education (CAHEA) made up of two representatives from each of the seven sponsoring organizations. Later, the JRCEMT-P was integrated with the CAHEA. By March 1993, 88 EMS educational centers were accredited by CAHEA and four states mandated CAHEA approval for individual EMS training programs. In October 1993 the AMA was withdrawn from the CAHEA oversight process.

Public Education

CPR training advanced as the minimum level of training needed; it was well accepted, as evidenced by participation in training programs throughout the country. As early as 1977 a Gallup Poll reported that 12 million Americans had taken a CPR course and another 80 million were familiar with the technique and wanted formal training.[33] The success of public training was documented by many studies.[24,51] Various training programs developed, and the issues of who to train when and how to improve retention continued to be explored. In the early 1980s, approaches to public CPR training included the following concepts[51]:

- Saturation concept—training enough people to guarantee training of several citizens in each neighborhood
- High-risk concept—training families of high-risk individuals
- Selected citizen concept—combining home and geographic saturation with concomitant training of high-risk groups
- Civil servant concept—training all police, fire department, and other constantly present individuals
- Public school concept—making CPR part of the curriculum in certain grades at all public schools

Communications

Before 1973 there were few communication systems available for emergency medical care. Only 1 in 20 ambulances had voice communications with a hospital, a universal telephone number was not operational, and telephones were not available on highways and rural roads, where most accidents occur. Centralized dispatch was uncommon and there were problems in communications because of community resistance, cost, and insufficient technology. With the DOT funding, major steps were taken toward overcoming the communication problems. National conferences, seminars, and public awareness programs advocated diverse methodologies for EMS communication systems. A communications manual published in 1972 provided technical systems information.[58] In 1973 the 9-1-1 universal emergency number was advocated as a national standard by the DOT and the White House Office of Telecommuni-cations. The Federal Communications Commission established rules and regulations for EMS communication and dedicated a limited number of radio frequencies for emergency systems. In 1977 the DHEW issued guidelines for a model EMS communications plan.[26]

The impact of these efforts was obvious in the evaluation statements of the 183 EMS regions studied in 1978. Sixty-two percent of the projects reported use of the 9-1-1 number covering 18.5% of the country and 34.1% of the population. Central dispatch of ambulances present in 40% of the regions involved more than 60% of all ambulances. Forty-eight percent of patients transported were managed by ambulance providers overseen by physicians. By 1979, 79% of all ambulances in the country had two-way voice communication systems.[5]

As early as 1983 the realization that transmission of biotelemetry would become superfluous had taken root. In addition, full-time EMS medical directors slowly began to comprehend the importance of more structured call receiving, patient prioritizing, and vehicle dispatching. Physicians were forced to seriously look at EMS operational issues that had previously been seen as neither critical nor medical.[45]

Transportation

Transportation of the critically ill or injured patient rapidly improved after 1973. Although national standards for ambulance equipment were developed in the early 1960s, a 1965 survey of 900 cities reported that less than 23% had an ordinance regulating ambulance services, an even smaller percentage required an attendant other than the driver, and only 72 cities reported training at the level of an American Red Cross advanced first aid course, the nearest thing to a standard ambulance attendant course before the advent of EMT-A in 1969.[36]

The hearses and station wagons used in the 1960s did not allow personnel room to provide CPR or other treatments to critically ill patients. The vehicles were designed to carry coffins and horizontal loads, not a medical team and a sick patient. In the mid-1960s, two reports focused national attention on the hazardous conditions of the nation's ambulances.[20,69] In addition to inadequate policies, staff, training, and communications, ambulance design was faulty and equipment absent or inadequate. Morticians ran 50% of the ambulance services because they owned the only vehicle capable of carrying patients horizontally. No U.S. manufacturer built a vehicle that could be termed an ambulance.

As early as 1970, the DOT and the ACS had developed optimal ambulance design and essential equipment recommendations.[30,57] In 1973 the DHEW released the comprehensive article, "Medical Requirements for Ambulance Design and Equipment," and a year later the General Services Administration issued federal specifications KKK-A 1822 for ambulances.[68] Although the KKK specifications were originally developed for government procurement contracts, local EMS agencies were often politically obligated to meet or exceed the specifications when ordering new ambulances. A 1978 study of 183 EMS regions described the status of ambulance services within 151 of the regions. Only 65% of the 13,790 ambulances in those regions met the federal KKK standards. Eighty-one regions used paramedics and 72 had some type of air ambulance capability. Response time was often longer than 10 minutes in urban areas and as much as 30 minutes in rural areas.[5]

Hospitals

When awarding grants for EMS under the EMS System Act, the DHEW required regions to develop standards and guidelines for categorization of emergency departments in the following eight critical clinical groups: (1) trauma victims, (2) burn victims, (3) spinal cord injury victims, (4) poisoning victims, (5) acute cardiac victims, (6) high-risk infants, (7) alcohol and drug, and (8) behavioral emergency victims. Patients from these categories comprised most of the 5% of ED patients with significant emergency medical problems.

Regions were required to identify the most appropriate hospital to manage each of the specific clinical problems. A planned transfer mechanism was essential to this system because often patients in the wrong hospital could be transferred to the appropriate hospital only with established written protocols.

A 1979 summary report on categorization, transfer agreements, and CCU plans stated that 91% of the EMS regions had implemented a categorization scheme for the eight critical clinical groups according to national standards. Eighty-two percent of the projects had transfer agreements providing effective triage and transportation of critically ill patients to the appropriate hospital. Critical care patient categories had been developed in 82% of regions.[5]

In reality, only a small portion of emergency facilities were functionally categorized and in many cases the system did not work as described on paper. Hospital administrators resisted losing control, physicians feared losing clinical judgment, and both feared losing patient revenues. The DHEW used EMS hospital categorization effectively to restructure acute patient distribution along the lines of clinical capability rather than market share.

1978: EMS at Midpassage

Between 1966 and 1978, EMS systems development, which progressed on many fronts, stimulated change at all levels of emergency care. Most of the deficiencies identified by the 1966 NAS-NRC report were attacked and significant progress was made in many areas. Local and state governments, private foundations, nonprofit organizations, and professional groups contributed economic resources and political support. Leadership was strong from the DOT, the DHEW, and a variety of nonprofit nongovernmental agencies including the RWJF, ACS, AAOS, ACEP, and ACT Foundation.

By 1978, as a result of broad-based interest, many original problems and questions had come into focus. There was still tremendous geographic unevenness among EMS systems regarding distribution of services, access, availability, quality, and quantity of resources. Basic questions concerning the effectiveness of the various components, system designs, goals, and relationships still existed. There was also the issue of the availability of future funding. Research had addressed a few questions, but the results were not yet available on most long-range issues because EMS systems were completing the growth phase and had not matured enough for comprehensive evaluation.

In 1978, NAS-NRC released a report called "Emergency Medical Services at Midpassage," which described, "EMS in the United States in midpassage (as) urgently in need of midcourse corrections but uncertain as to the best direction and degree." The report recommended "research and evaluation directed both to questions of immediate importance to EMS system development and to long-range questions. Without adequate investment in both types of research, EMS in the United States will be in the same position of uncertainty a generation hence as it is today."[25] Those words were prophetic; they identified in 1978 the major issue to confront EMS in 1993. The report documented coordination problems among various government agencies focusing particular concern on the multiple standards promulgated as a condition of funding. Some of the standards were conflicting; often, they had never been evaluated.[25]

The 1978 report sharply criticized how the EMS System Act was implemented by the DHEW. Financing, design, management, regulation, and evaluation of EMS systems remained in doubt.

Coordination

Between 1974 and 1982 there were various sources of federal and private funds, and each grant often came with a new set of requirements. The DOT established standards for ambulance design, provider training, and other transportation elements while the DHEW announced seven critical care areas as the basis for the systems approach and 15 components as modular elements for EMS design. A variety of private organizations also produced standards. For example, with regard to the technique of CPR both the American Red Cross and the AHA established slightly different standards, criteria, and training requirements. Fortunately, adherence to these "voluntary" standards usually was not required by law.

By 1978, some states still had not enacted EMS legislation whereas others had legislated exactly what prehospital providers could do, thereby hampering the flexibility needed for successful local development. Lack of national conformity or agreement precluded the development of universally accepted national standards in most areas of EMS.

On October 26, 1978, a memorandum of understanding was signed by the DOT and the DHEW describing each organization's responsibilities relating to development of EMS systems.[52] The agreement was an attempt to coordinate government activities and assign national level responsibility for EMS development and direction. The DOT, in coordination with the DHEW, was to "develop uniform standards and procedures for the transportation phases of emergency care and response." The DHEW was responsible, in coordination with the DOT, for developing "medical standards and procedures for initial, supportive, and definitive care phases of EMS systems." Research and technical assistance were to be performed cooperatively, and both agencies agreed to exchange information and "establish joint working arrangements from time to time."[52]

Because the roots, constituencies, and operating philosophies of the agencies were markedly different, the 1978 agreement quickly failed. Over the four subsequent years an intense civil war was fought. Critical care medicine was shunted aside, and prehospital providers were standardized by highway engineers.[64]

Financing

Toward the end of the 1970s, concern over future financing grew among those involved with development and operation of EMS. Federal, state, local, and private money had financed systems nationwide; however, the federal phaseout had been planned since the program's inception in 1973. By 1978, termination of federal funding was imminent, and the potential impact on operations and future development began to raise concerns.

The 1976 and 1979 amendments to the EMS System Act reflected concerns about future funding and had consequently demanded evidence of financial self-sufficiency as one basis for further support. Significant disagreement in describing financial self-sufficiency of the nation's EMS systems was apparent in the testimony and documents provided by the various agencies. The DOT estimates of nonfederal monies spent between 1968 and 1980 ranged up to $800 million. The DHEW estimates were similar as seen in Table 1-6, which summarizes nonfederal support.

In 1979, the DHEW officials estimated in testimony that 90% of the regions with paramedic capability had achieved financial self-sufficiency by 1978 and that 90% of those in the 1203 developmental phase would achieve self-sufficiency between 1980 and 1986.[26] The comptroller general published, "Progress in Developing Emergency Medical Services Systems," which described progress in many EMS regions but also cited considerable inconsistency in the degree and duration of support provided by community resources.[21]

In 1979 the comptroller general testified on the financial status of the national EMS regions after analyzing grant applications under the 1976 amendments. Regions were required to document commitment by local governments to continue financial support after federal funds were terminated under Title XII. Only 25 applications were properly endorsed by local government and only six had developed a specific financial plan.[21] By the 1980s, the discrepancy between the DHEW and the comptroller general's estimates of financial self-sufficiency of EMS systems suggested serious unrecognized difficulties in the continued underwriting of EMS systems.

The financial demands on an EMS system were considerable and related to four major elements; prehospital care, hospital care, communications, and management. The specific costs varied by community. The original 1966 NAS-NRC report estimated that ambulance services total about one fourth of total EMS system costs, 75% of which was for pesonnel. Communications costs varied from 7% to 35% of total cost depending on whether there was integration with existing public services and whether completely new systems needed to be established. Although management costs were high during the development phases, they were expected to account for less than 2% of the total cost during the operational phase.[25]

Table 1-6. Emergency Medical Services State and Local Government Funds

Fiscal year	Source of funds: State	Local	Total
1975	19,846,273	189,744,871	209,591,144
1976	29,902,517	200,389,021	230,291,538
1977	30,914,371	234,346,879	265,261,250
1978*	35,687,486	270,791,685	306,479,171

Modified from Division of Emergency Medical Services: testimony before the Subcommittee on Health and Scientific Research Committee on Labor and Human Resources, Feb 28, 1979, 33, *United States Senate hearing report*, Department of Health, Education, and Welfare, 1979.

*A survey for fiscal year 1978 shows that $306,479,171 were provided from state and local government funds for the support of emergency medical services, including training of personnel as appropriate.

Health insurance did not keep pace with EMS costs, which presented a real problem for EMS providers. Health care benefits were often limited to hospital care and had maximum fixed reimbursements. For example, 20% of Blue Cross patients were not covered for emergency transport and of those covered one third were only covered after an accident. By 1982, the rapid development of EMS systems throughout the country had improved emergency care without providing long-term funding. Summarizing these early financial issues in 1978, the NAS-NRC wrote, "Availability of advanced emergency care throughout the nation is a worthy objective, but the cost of such services may prohibit communities from obtaining them."[25]

System Design

In 1981 the nation was still moving toward developing a regional network of EMS systems based on the decisions made in the late 1960s; however, patients, clinical providers, and support personnel already had new and different needs. EMS had been directed to treat the critically ill and injured, yet 95% of patients were not in critical condition. Increasingly, the perceptions of the individual providers varied from the realities of the job. Moreover, the concepts forming the basis for system design, funding guidelines, program development, and implementation were unproven. EMS research was just underway and was unable to answer even the most basic questions, including critical long-term issues addressing ultimate system configuration.

Research

Between 1974 and 1979, $22 million was appropriated for EMS related research. The National Center for Health Services Research (NCHSR) in coordination with the DHEW, funded various clinical and systems research projects. During the 1979 legislative hearings, testimony from the DHEW and the leadership of academic research centers stressed the need for continued EMS research. Annual reports from the DHEW detailed the type of research underway, questions being studied, and the scope of long-term and short-term research projects funded under Section 1205 of Title XII.[54] These projects included, "methods to measure the performance of EMS personnel, evaluate the benefits and the costs of advanced life support systems, examine the impact of categorization efforts, determine the clinical significance of response time, and explore the consequences of alternative system configurations and procedures."[9] Other projects focused on, "developing systems of quality assurance, designing and testing clinical algorithms, and examining the relationships between Emergency Departments and their parent hospitals (including rural-urban differences)."[9]

Even after President Reagan took office and the Senate majority was Republican, the Center for the Study of Emergency Health Services at the University of Pennsylvania urged continued support of EMS research, "dollars spent in EMS research have a great potential to help control rising health care costs, [and can] have a significant and visible effect in preventing death and enhancing the quality of patient life following emergency events."[13] The Center suggested research identifying EMS cost control potentials because the phasing out of federal funds coupled with the effects of local tax revolts would certainly reduce financing. As the 1980s progressed, the demand for more efficient, effective systems would become universal. Managers of EMS systems, just like their counterparts elsewhere, needed to know which components of the system were crucial and which could be deleted if funding was limited. In the case of EMS, answers to those questions were anything but clear.

1981: The Omnibus Budget Reconciliation Act

Late in the summer of 1981 President Reagan signed comprehensive cost containment legislation that converted 25 Department of Health and Human Resources (DHHR) funding programs into seven consolidated block grants.[39] EMS was included in the Preventive Health Block Grant along with seven other programs such as Rodent Control and Fluoridation. In effect, individual states were left to determine how money from the block grants would be distributed. Although existing EMS programs were temporarily guaranteed minimal support, a state could later decide to withdraw all block grant money from one or more regional EMS programs. This concept, simply a fundamental premise of conservative federal government, evolved quite differently in each of the states.

The 1976 "Forward Plan for the Health Services Administration" made it clear that by 1982 all federal EMS System financial support would end, and regional EMS programs would be the responsibility of the regional health system agencies. The federal role was to be "one of technical assistance and coordination."*

1982 to 1993

The public health initiative for developing a national EMS system came to a gradual, quiet, and unceremonious demise after 1981. The remnants of the old DHEW (now the DHHS) program were left to die-off slowly under the cloud of confusion occasioned by Preventive Health Block Grants formula. In most, but not all, states EMS regional programs were lost in the shuffle of competing health programs while President Reagan and his budget director were systematically eliminating federal support for all such programs. In fact, in most jurisdictions the regional EMS momentum present throughout the 1970s simply evaporated. Paradoxically, some individuals involved in EMS saw the end of the DHEW era as cause for rejoicing because escape from the excessive, capricious, and specious regulations might allow the development and implementation of alternative innovative approaches.[60] Unfortunately, freedom to explore new methodologies was often akin to being disinherited and cast out into the world at a fragile age.

After the 1980 elections, the thrust of the federal government for most of the previous 50 years was changed beyond all recognition; the cadre of federal officials left to administrate the remaining programs had to cooperate with each of the 50 states. As federal guidance and funding diminished, a clear nationwide consensus was no longer a requirement for action; each state now had an intrinsic right to

*Department of Health Education and Welfare: *The forward plan for the health services administration,* 1976, US Government Printing Office.

govern areas such as EMS. Occasionally the new paradigm strengthened the state EMS agency; too often, however, EMS definitions gradually lost whatever precision had previously existed and became a baffling array of conflicting elements. Organizations such as the National Registry, the NAEMT, and the National Association of State EMS Directors tried to preserve some semblance of an infrastructure; while attendance lagged and membership sagged, national EMS organizations struggled to survive and keep EMS alive as a discrete cause. Some state EMS agencies managed to keep the momentum by sponsoring well-attended statewide provider conferences.

Like EMS, other industries were deregulated. Airlines, saving and loans, and the telephone company were all permitted to compete in the marketplace. Succeeding, if only in the short-term with dwindling resources became the norm. Deregulation as a path to true competition and a higher quality product found fruition in voluntary standards to reorganize EMS adopted by NHTSA in the mid-1980s.

In 1984, the Emergency Services Bureau of NHTSA was instrumental in creating the American Society for Testing and Materials (ASTM) Committee F-30. Through ASTM, NHTSA sought to legitimize the promulgation of standards in many areas of EMS. The standards branch of ASTM was based in Philadelphia, and through a complex consensus process standards were arrived at in many different industries including construction and building. As of 1993, over 7000 assorted standards had been developed through the ASTM process. Although these standards have no federal mandate, they are often enforced at the local level, for example, in building codes. Since a confusing, but enthusiastic beginning in 1984, more than 30 EMS-related standards have been developed, including those for the EMT-A curriculum, rotary and fixed-wing medical aircraft, and EMS system organization. This last document outlines the roles and responsibilities of state, regional, and local EMS agencies. During the ASTM process, competing interests often balloted against one another achieving an innocuous consensus. Established and desirable regional variations were lost in the generic rubric of documents on training, communication, evaluation, and finance. The resultant standards, although mandated by no authority, were considered by several state legislatures when state EMS laws were revised.

The F-30 Committee prospered as long as physician involvement was evident and decisive; but it was clearly NHTSA's decision what standard to expedite and when. The National Registry, NAEMT, and other interest groups joined the physicians, each to protect themselves. Although many physicians and physician groups eventually tired of the F-30 exercise, NHTSA preserved some semblance of a central authority; however, the real significance of the standards remains unclear.

State EMS agencies often patronized the DOT and the ASTM exercise because there was still the possibility of money at the end of the highway safety rainbow. Building for the future, or even sustaining the present, meant maintaining visibility of those applying for matching funds from the Governor's Highway Safety Council. Unfortunately, EMS in the 1980s was a "low priority" for the Highway Safety Council, a striking reversal from a decade earlier.

As early as 1983, NHTSA began trying to wear the mantle associated with the old DHEW program. Many of the evaluation staff were hired on a part-time basis to promote use of EMS management information systems. Management conferences were arranged for regional EMS system grantees. Saddled with growing financial problems under block grants, few could attend. In 1988, NHTSA tried to organize electronic exchange of information among surviving EMS clearinghouses. Three years of posturing came to nothing when hopes of private-public cooperation in EMS were shattered by withdrawal of the largest private clearinghouse. Because NHTSA had no mandate to promote specific programs on a nationwide basis, it was left to the states.

Training was not much different. Physician organizations backed one brand of trauma life support, but provider groups supported another. The American Red Cross, the National Safety Council, and a number of local EMS organizations prospected in the citizen CPR and first aid responder business. Most states developed their own "home-grown" provider curricula, even when provider levels were identical to those in neighboring states.

In 1986, within a decentralized federal government, NHTSA's newest and least likely role was that of standard bearer for trauma EMS system research. From 1982 to 1992, outcome measurement gradually lost relevance. Many jurisdictions and providers simply refused to underwrite the cost for "knife and gun club" specialty centers. Proofs that the system might work were supplanted by more palatable concepts. Faced with economic dislocation and cost shifting, traumatologists found themselves studying quality assurance, population-based research, and the statistical nuances of an outcome study conducted at a large number of hospitals nationwide. NHTSA evolved into the handmaiden of the CDC, awarding grants to researchers defining the structure of EMS and trauma care in the 1990s.

The federal agencies began the 1990s with the following three general areas of EMS interest:

(1) enhancing and revitalizing training standards with particular emphasis on the EMT-B level (the new term of EMT-A), (2) promoting information exchange through a computerized network of EMS information clearinghouses, and (3) encouraging trauma center designations, a negligible amount of injury control research, and some vague notions of trauma-EMS systems research. These activities actually culminated in 1990 with the passage of the Trauma Care Systems Planning and Development Act, which raised EMS, once again a subset of trauma, to a greater level of national awareness.[72]

It would be incorrect to view the period from 1982 on as simply stagnate. It might be better characterized as a time when centrifugal forces played havoc with attempts by the federal government and national organizations to define and standardize EMS. Managers, visionaries, and guardians of disciplinary parochialism were kept off balance by the fact that neither a geographic center nor a discrete EMS development philosophy emerged. Across the country, local activists battled others in pursuit of diminishing funds. Zealous idealism metamorphosed into an earnest and businesslike focus transforming EMS leaders and providers into hardened idealists with a passion for survival. By 1992, patients had clearly emerged as customers, and by the inauguration of President Clinton, EMS was just as conceptually unified, standardized, efficient, expensive, and confused as the rest of American health care.

The Clinton health care plan of 1993 barely mentioned ambulance services and did not address EMS systems at all.

EMS Physicians

Throughout the 1970s, emergency physicians and the fledgling national ACEP supported the visibility and strength federal money gave regional EMS programs. Unfortunately, by 1983, emergency physicians and the embryonic state chapters of ACEP, like most everyone else, had evolved into competitors for the same resources and recognition. Local physicians, EMS medical directors, and provider agencies were often at odds with each other. The new breed of EMS medical directors needed a forum to exchange ideas and ACEP, unfortunately, had not been receptive. In 1982 and 1983, the last unrestricted vestiges of block grant funding allowed the New York EMS agency to gather a few proponents of strong EMS medical oversight to better define the emerging field of prehospital medicine, especially in the complicated urban environment. The brotherhood of these few individuals responsible for the medical stewardship of their respective systems was immediately self-evident. After a series of organizational meetings, the National Association of EMS Physicians (NAEMSP) was created in 1985 with Stewart as its first president. Originally based in South Carolina, NAEMSP ultimately found a permanent home in Pittsburgh. As the importance of EMS to local government grew and NAEMSP focused attention, existing groups like ACEP and the Society for Academic Emergency Medicine once again emphasized and encouraged EMS activities among their members.

Training

The DOT began the 1980s urging EMS agencies to adopt EMT-I as a less expensive alternative to EMT-P. In the middle of the decade, some administrators began advocating greater use of First Responders to obviate the need for expensive EMT-A (soon to become EMT-B) refresher training. If volunteers did not have time to refresh their skills then it made sense to some to require less skill. Something was literally better than nothing. New Jersey experimentally grandfathered roughly half its 20,000 first aid providers to the EMT-A level, totally missing the point that provider tasks, teaching objectives, curriculum, and appropriate classroom hours must be determined in a logical, rational progression.[64]

An alternative approach came to force between 1988 and 1992. Although EMT-P could continue approximating the level of a junior-grade physician extender in the field, a new EMT-B curriculum could serve as an abbreviated version—in which reasoning and presumptive diagnosis took a backseat to treatment algorithms. During the first 3 years of the 1990s, NHTSA struggled to reframe the old EMT-A curriculum. Without knowing how this "new" provider level would fit into the larger system or individual states, the process was flawed; many saw it as yet another overt attempt to encumber local options with overly precise national standards. Although it was clear no one knew exactly how much EMS was enough, the National EMS Training Blueprint Project Task Force (sponsored by the National Registry and chaired by Drew Dawson) began the definition process early in 1993.[55]

The driving issues surrounding training in the early 1990s were increasingly related to medical and technologic advances and the aging of the providers themselves. After 20 years it had finally become logically, if not scientifically, clear that early defibrillation saved a proportion of people in cardiac arrest. It was not bystander CPR, paramedic ambulances, generic ALS, defibrillation in 10 minutes, nor the shocking of asystole that saved lives; it was simply defibrillation of ventricular fibrillation in less than 5 or so minutes that lead to the 30% or

40% save rates that had become the benchmarks of "good" EMS systems. Faster was better. Transporting ambulances were irrevelant. If defibrillation took more than 6 or 7 minutes, the results were depressing. Simply getting the newly developed automated external defibrillators to the right patients with the fastest provider became a goal.

The original EMS providers, who had started in 1970, were getting older. Although there were a few jobs in administration, dispatch, and education, by 1993 many of the most experienced and dedicated field providers were arriving at an intellectual, physical, and emotional dead-end. Reforming EMS practice and education was obviously much more daunting than simply writing a "new" EMT-B curriculum or defining "optimal" provider levels; what was lacking in 1993 was an operational and educational career ladder.[44,71]

Communications

Jeff Clawson, a fire surgeon from Salt Lake City, was a clear exception to the mood of uncertainty prevailing in the 1980s. He was among the first EMS medical directors to explore the communications centers, and emergency medical dispatching quickly came of age. Clawson reasoned that too much *ad hoc* medical information confused prearrival instruction and priority dispatch issues and, therefore, interfered with the appropriate provision of both.

Beginning in Utah and accelerating throughout the world, during the early 1980s, Clawson and others used logic, software, and field experience in making the initial dispatcher call tantamount to the first tier of the EMS system response. In essence, a "first" First Responder with a zero response time. *Ad hoc* human responses were replaced by algorithms. Coupled with technologic advances, such as automatic vehicle locators and computer-aided dispatch systems, many traditional causes of dispatch and response errors or delays vanished.

Transportation

Laissez-faire and voluntary standards served as hallmarks for EMS transportation from 1983 to 1990. Because ambulances were expensive and difficult to replace, more than half of EMS providers remained fire department–based. During that period, EMS began to become both professional and rational. Partly an outgrowth of priority dispatch came the need and ability to analyze how quickly and in what mode EMS vehicle response was required. Once again medical input was key. Also recognized as significant medical and risk management concerns by 1990, were issues of ambulance operations, safety, and optimal mode of response.

Hospitals turned toward more dramatic ventures whenever possible and EMS took to the air from 1983 on, dwarfing contemporaneous efforts by law enforcement. Growth of the aeromedical aspect of EMS was facilitated by an industry consolidation in the mid 1980s; there ceased to be an important distinction between public and private after that time. Several new national organizations focused on the aeromedical aspects of medicine, nursing, and operations; each developed and trumpeted its own standards.

By 1990 the solution to the golden hour, medical evacuation helicopters, were available to most trauma centers and many rural rescue units. Care delayed was no longer care denied, but it cost millions to run even a modest life-flight operation. EMS systems operating on a regional basis worked out the best possible local arrangements, but relatively few aeromedical ventures were financially successful. Often, differences in state law and insurance reimbursement were key to the success or failure of a specific program. Like land ambulances, the air ambulances occasionally crashed thus seriously diminishing their overall cost effectiveness.

Facilities

Researchers tried predicting outcomes and defining severity to justify enormous medical bills. By the 1990s, the trauma center designation criteria of the 1980s were being challenged and undermined. In most systems every reasonably sized hospital with the desire to be a trauma center was designated as such. Urban blight and crime waves tied to inexpensive drugs like crack ensured that unreimbursed urban use would not be a problem.

A related problem for EMS providers was the passage of the 1985 COBRA legislation aimed at penalizing emergency departments for refusing patients, either overtly or through diversions tied to the classic wallet biopsy.[22] In some jurisdictions the poor were legally diverted by ambulance to the public hospital.

The partial fragmentation of EMS by the development of a pediatric subgroup was predictable, but was a problem nevertheless; just as pediatric emergency medicine emerged, so did pediatric EMS. Obviously, issues went beyond clinical to political and financial. During the early 1990s, pediatric EMS was one of the only areas of EMS with enough political support and strength to garner significant funding. Other subsets of EMS may be similarly successful in the future.

Summary

During the last 20 years of the twentieth century, EMS providers experienced a sudden and at times brutal evolutionary process. Once a popular community resource, EMS was now asked to justify its very existence, usually resulting in service cutbacks, capital reductions, reconfiguration of vehicle fleets, and revisions of provider levels.

If the first few years of the 1990s were a dark age for EMS, then there were also isolated points of light portending a future renaissance. EMS physicians increasingly joined other EMS professionals in the quest to redefine and reframe EMS. This expanding physician involvement in clinical prehospital medical research as well as in the planning and operating of prehospital systems was a hopeful sign. Professional organizations established guidelines and fostered discipline in research methodologies.

These actions are already resulting in change, increased medical accountability, and better assessment of prehospital therapy. Prehospital professionals jointly evaluate protocols, procedures, and practices, perhaps to discard some and enhance others. Financial constraints, legal issues, and community expectations are also forcing reassessment and refinement of how and what EMS is doing. Federal legislation and case law are mandating accountability of all medical practices; therefore, a sound scientific and medical basis is being demanded for the clinical practice of prehospital care. Research establishing this medical basis is now emerging as a major priority.

The financial considerations of the 1990s continue to be major factors in EMS development and operations. Public policy and opinion influence decisions affecting staffing, coverage, equipment, and operations. However, spending more money does not always result in better care. Operational and basic research assist in making decisions that result in more efficient and higher quality systems. Those responsible for EMS system financing must understand the rising operational costs brought about by higher wages, increased personnel, greater demand, and expanding technology. For EMS to be accessible, new financing mechanisms, perhaps tied to a national health program or a variety of managed care programs, must be developed quickly.

After more than 25 years of rapid growth, change, and progress, medical directors' key issues of concern as EMS enters the mid-1990s are system design, management, economics, and effectiveness. System analysis and evaluation are still necessary and underfunded. EMS researchers and evaluators must continue investigating system problems to answer questions being asked by EMS managers, medical directors, and legislatures as they develop and mandate the EMS systems of the future.

Of course, the irony is that most of the newly invented tools can be used by any EMS provider; yet few providers can independently supply all the operational components required in a given system. Our society has not yet learned that the cost of EMS failure is significantly greater than the cost of EMS success. Unlike the past, the future of EMS belongs to the efficient and the innovative. Supporting evidence and a shared paradigm are required.

REFERENCES

1. *ACEP News,* 15, Dec 1991.
2. American Academy of Orthopaedic Surgeons: *Emergency care and transportation of the sick and injured,* ed 1, 1969, The Academy.
3. American Board of Emergency Medicine: *Eligibility requirements,* Adopted June 27, 1976.
4. American Heart Association, National Academy of Sciences, National Research Council: Cardiopulmonary resuscitation, *JAMA* 198:372-379, 1966.
5. Answers to questions submitted by members of Subcommittee on Health and Scientific Research of the Committee on Labor and Human Resources, In: *United States Senate hearing report,* 98-100, Feb 28, 1979.
6. Anwar AH, Hogan MH: Residency-trained physicians: where have all the flowers gone? *JACEP* 8(2):85, 1979.
7. Barkley KT: The history of the ambulance, *Proceedings, International Congress of the History of Medicine* 23:456-466, 1974.
8. Barringer ED: *Bowery to Bellevue,* New York, 1950, WW Norton & Co.
9. Boyd DR: *Emergency medical services system evaluation,* Statement submitted to the Subcommittee on Health and Scientific Research, Committee on Labor and Human Resources, In: *United States Senate hearing report,* 47-57, Feb 28, 1979.
10. Boyd DR, Edlich RF, Micik S: Systems approach to emergency care, Norwalk, CT, 1983, Appleton-Century-Crofts.
11. Breasted JH: *Bull Hist Med* 3:58-78, Chicago, 1923.
12. Brewer LA: Baron Larrey 1766-1862, *J Thorac Cardiovasc Surg* 92:1096-1098, 1986.
13. Cayten GC: Testimony to the Subcommittee on Health and Scientific Research of the Committee on Labor and Human Resources, In: *United States Senate hearing report,* 156-166, Feb 28, 1979.
14. Commission on Emergency Medical Services: Recommendations of the conference on the guidelines for the categorization of hospital emergency capabilities: 1971, American Medical Association.
15. Committee on Emergency Medical Services: *Roles and resources of federal agencies in support of comprehensive emergency medial services,* Washington, DC, 1972, National Research Council.
16. Committee on Trauma: Minimal equipment for ambulances, *Bull - Coll Surgeons* 136, July-Aug 1961.
17. Committee on Trauma: Minimal equipment for ambulances, *Bull Am Coll Surgeons* 92-96, March-April 1967.
18. Committee on Trauma: *Recommendations for an approach to an urgent national problem:* Proceedings of the Airlie Conference on Emergency Medical Services, Airlie House, Warrenton, VA, May 5-6, 1969, Chicago, 1969, American College of Surgeons, American Academy of Orthopedic Surgeons.
19. Committee on Trauma: Standards for emergency department in hospitals, *Bull Am Coll Surgeons* 112-125, May-June 1963.
20. Committee on Trauma and Committee on Shock: *Accidental death and disability: the neglected disease of modern society,* Sep

1966, Washington DC, Fifth printing by the Commission on Emergency Medical Services, Jan 1970, American Medical Association.

21. Comptroller General of the United States: *Progress in developing emergency medical services systems,* HRD 76-150, July 13, 1976.
22. *Consolidated Omnibus Budget Reconciliation Act of 1985,* Public Law 99-1, Washington, DC, 1985.
23. Duncan LC: *Civil war: the Medical Department of the US Army in the civil war,* Washington, DC, 1910, US Government Printing Office.
24. Eisenberg MS, Berger L, Hallstrom A: Epidemiology of cardiac arrest and resuscitation in a suburban community, *JACEP 1979.*
25. *Emergency medical services at midpassage,* Washington, DC, 1978, National Research Council.
26. Emergency Medical Services Division, Department of Health, Education, and Welfare: HSA 77-2036, March 1977.
27. *Emergency medical services 1966-1979: program review and fact sheet,* presented before the Subcommittee on Health and Scientific Research Committee on Labor and Human Resources, March 22, 1979, *United States Senate hearing report,* 267-299, Feb 28, 1979.
28. Emergency Medicine Residents Association: *A survey by EMRA,* May 1980.
29. *EMS System Act of 1973,* Public Law 93-154, Washington, DC, 1973.
30. Essential equipment for ambulances, *Bull Am Coll Surgeons* 55(5):7-13, 1970.
31. *Essentials and guidelines of an accredited educational program for the emergency medical technician-paramedic,* Essentials adopted 1978, guidelines approved 1979, Joint Review Committee on Educational Programs for EMT-Paramedics.
32. Federal specifications: ambulance-emergency care vehicle, Specification KKK-A-1822, Jan 2, 1974, US General Services Administration.
33. The Gallup Poll, *Field Newspaper Syndicate* June 30, 1977.
34. Garrison FH: *An introduction to the history of medicine,* Philadelphia, 1929, WB Saunders Co.
35. Haller JR, John S: *J Emer Med* 8:743-755, 1990.
36. Hampton OP: Present status of ambulance services in the United States, *Bull Am Coll Surgeons* 177-178, July-Aug 1965.
37. Hampton OP: The systematic approach to emergency medical services, *Bull Am Coll Surgeons* Sep-Oct 1968.
38. Hampton, OP: Transportation of the injured: a report, *Bull Am Coll Surgeons* 55, Jan-Feb 1960.
39. Heaton LD: Army medical services in Vietnam (guest editorial), *Mil Med* 131:646-647, 1966.
40. Highway safety program manual, *Emergency medical services* vol 11, Washington, DC, Jan 1969, US Department of Transportation.
41. Jelenko, Frey CF: *Emergency medical services: an overview,* Bowie, MD, 1976, The Brady Co.
42. 1 Kings 17: 17-24.
43. Kouwenhoven WB, Jude JR, Knickerbocker GB: Closed chest cardiac massage, *JAMA* 173:1064, 1960.
44. Kuehl AE: Form should follow function, *JEMS* 18(2):42, 1993.
45. Kuehl AE, Kerr JT: Urban EMS systems, *Am J Emerg Med* 5:217, 1984.
46. Lewis R et al: Effectiveness of advanced paramedics in a mobile coronary care system, *JAMA* 241:1902-1904, 1979.
47. Liason Residency Endorsement Committee: American College of Emergency Physicians, Information supplied, June 5, 1980.
48. Luke 10:25-37.
49. Lythcott GI: Statement before the Subcommittee on Health and Scientific Research Committee on Labor and Human Resources, In: *United States Senate Hearing report,* 24, Feb 28, 1979.
50. Major RH: *A history of medicine,* vol 1, Springfield, Ill, 1984, Charles C Thomas.
51. McElroy CR: Citizen CPR: the role of the layperson in prehospital care, *Topics in Emergency Medicine* 1(4):37, 1980.
52. Memorandum of understanding between the US Department of Transportation and the US Department of Health, Education, and Welfare: *Procedures relating to Emergency Medical Services systems,* Washington, DC, Oct 26, 1978.
53. Nagel E et al: Telemetry medical command in coronary and other mobile emergency care systems, *JAMA* 214:332-338, 1970.
54. National Center for Health Services Research: *Research management series,* Emergency Medical Services Research Projects and Research Methodology, Department of Health, Education, and Welfare.
55. National EMS Training Blueprint (working draft) Columbus OH, 1993, National Registry.
56. *National Highway Safety Act of 1966:* Public Law 89-564, Washington, DC, 1966.
57. National Highway Traffic Administration: Ambulance design criteria, Washington, DC, May, 1971, US Government Printing Office.
58. National Highway Traffic Safety Administration: *Communication: guidelines for emergency medical services,* Sep 1972, US Department of Transportation.
59. *The Omnibus Budget Reconciliation Act of 1981,* Public Law 97-35, Washington, DC, 1981.
60. Page J: *History and Legislation Panel,* EMS medical directors' course, Phoenix, March 25, 1993.
61. Pantridge JF, Geddes JS: Cardiac arrest after myocardial infarction, *Lancet* 1:807-808, 1966.
62. Pantridge JF, Geddes JS: A Mobile intensive care unit in the management of myocardial infarction, *Lancet* 2:271-273, 1967.
63. Pollack P: *The Picture history of photography,* London, 1963, Thames and Hudson Inc.
64. Post CJ: *Omaha orange: a popular history of EMS in America,* Boston, 1992, Jones and Bartlett.
65. President's Commission on Highway Safety: *Health, medical care, and transportation of injured,* US Government Printing Office, 1965.
66. The Robert Wood Johnson Foundation: *Special report,* Number 2, 1977.
67. The Robert Wood Johnson Foundation, National Competitive Program Grants for Regional Emergency Medical Communications Systems Administered in Cooperation with National Academy of Sciences: *Program guidelines,* 1973.
68. Roemer R, Kramer C, Frink JE: *Planning urban health services: jungle to system,* New York, 1975, Springer Publishing Co Inc.
69. Summary report of the task force on ambulance services, Washington, DC, April 1967, National Academy of Sciences, National Research Council.
70. Surgeon General's Office: Cir No 9, Washington, DC, 1877, US Government Printing Office.
71. Suter RE: Academic EMS, *JEMS* 18(4):15, 1993.
72. *Trauma Care Systems Planning and Development Act of 1990,* Public Law 101-590, Washington, DC, 1990.
73. Whitman W: *Complete poetry and collected prose,* 1982, The Library of America.

Appendix I

Scope and Specificity of Each Component in EMS Systems

1. *Manpower*—An adequate number of health professionals, allied health professionals, and other health personnel including ambulance personnel, with appropriate training and experience to provide EMS on a 24-hour a day basis, 7 days a week, within the service area of the system.

The major manpower elements to be considered are:

- First Responders—fire, police, and other public safety elements
- Communicators—EMS dispatcher
- Emergency Medical Technician-Ambulance (EMT-A)
- EMT-Intermediate (EMT-I)
- Emergency Medical Technician-Paramedic (EMT-P)
- Registered Nurses—Emergency Department
- Registered Nurses—Critical Care Units
- Paramedic and/or Nurse MICU Coordinators
- EMS Physician Consultants
- EMS Project Director
- EMS Systems Coordinators
- EMS Systems Consultants

2. *Training*—The provision for appropriate training (including clinical training) and continuing education programs, which (1) are coordinated with other programs in the system's service area, which provide similar training and education and (2) emphasize veterans of the Armed Forces with military training and experience in the health care field and of appropriate public safety personnel in such areas.

"Appropriate public safety personnel" includes police, firemen, lifeguards, park rangers, and other public employees charged with maintaining the public safety.

3. *Communications*—Provisions for linking the personnel, facilities, and equipment by centrally coordinated communications systems so that requests for emergency health care services will be handled by a facility which (1) utilizes emergency telephonic screening, (2) utilizes or will utilize the universal emergency telephone number 9-1-1, and (3) will have direct communication connections and interconnections with the personnel, facilities, and equipment of the system and with other appropriate emergency medical services systems.

The system should include a command and control center which would be responsible for establishing those communication channels and allocating those public resources essential to the most effective and efficient EMS management of the immediate problem. The center should have the necessary equipment and facilities to permit immediate interchange of information essential for both the system's resource and medical management and control.

The communication elements should include:

- *Access providing public interface with the emergency resource system:*
  - 9-1-1
  - Alternative single access number
  - Provisions for auditory handicapped individuals
  - Provision for multilingual access
- *Resource Management Function:*
  - Central dispatch or centrally coordinated dispatch
  - Coordination of EMS and other public services
- *Medical Control Function:*
  - Medical communications between field personnel and resource hospital for diagnosis, treatment, and triage

Modified from Emergency Medical Services Systems Program Guidelines: HSA 79-2002, August, 1979.

- *Hospital to Mobile:*
  - Basic voice
- *Hospital to Hospital (resources, associate):*
  - Basic voice
  - Advanced biomedical telemetry (optional)

The supervising medical control resource facility (communication base) must be responsible for monitoring all ALS communications and notification of other receiving hospital(s) so that they will be aware of the problem, and can assume responsibility for the care of the patient immediately upon arrival to their facility.

This supervising facility is responsible for field decisions of triage and transportation of a patient to an appropriate facility or to a special care unit in accordance with previously developed patient triage/transfer guidelines and agreements.

4. *Transportation*—This component shall include an adequate number of necessary ground, air, and water vehicles and other transportation facilities properly equipped to meet the transportation and EMS characteristics of the system area. Such vehicles and facilities must meet appropriate standards relating to location, design, performance, and equipment; and the operators and other personnel for such vehicles and facilities must meet appropriate training and experience requirements.

The elements of transportation should include:

- **Ground—Basic Life Support**
  - Radio communication providing for vehicle control, medical control, and consultation
  - Ambulance vehicles meeting GSS (KKK-A-1822) specifications and including equipment recommended by the American College of Surgeons
  - At least two EMT-As
  - Ambulance locations permitting (for 95% of all calls) a maximum of a 30-minute accurate response time in rural areas
  - Tiered response arrangement of vehicles
- **Ground—Advanced Life Support Elements**
  - All elements of a ground basic life support capability
  - At least two EMTs trained beyond the EMT-A level to address specific clinical items in the medical service plan
  - Advanced communications to provide advanced biomedical telemetry (optional)
  - Additional equipment as appropriate
- **Other**
  - Helicopters
    1. Primary response—unique use depending on geographical constraints
    2. Secondary response—30- to 150-mile transport radius
  - Fixed Wing—greater response for 150-mile transport radius
  - Water—special geographical considerations
  - Snow Mobile—special geographical considerations

5. *Facilities*—This component shall include an adequate number of designated easily accessible emergency medical service facilities which are collectively capable of providing services on a continuous basis. They must have appropriate, nonduplicative, and categorized capabilities which meet appropriate standards. All emergency receiving facilities must be categorized horizontally utilizing American Medical Association criteria and vertically utilizing national professional organizations' criteria for emergency critical care.*

The strategy and process for utilizing the criteria for designation of participating facilities for critical care within each region and the specialty facilities outside the region must be stated in the application. Plans for upgrading/downgrading emergency department personnel and equipment must be coordinated with other health care facilities and planning organizations in the region and based upon patient origin and distribution studies. There should be emplasis on upgrading critical care capabilities through consolidation and use of nonduplicating facilities resources.

Elements for facilities consideration include:

- Regional categorization with accepted state or national criteria with at least one Category II hospital providing 24-hour physician coverage in the emergency department in each EMS region
- Regional EMS Advisory Groups to plan and carry out the categorization plan. These groups should include hospital administrators, physicians, nurses, other providers, and health system planners
- Regional plans for mutual agreement of facility categorization and designation of critical care capabilities, transfer agreements, and resource sharing

6. *Critical Care Units*—This component requires providing access (including appropriate transportation) to specialized critical medical care units. These units should be the number and variety necessary to meet the demands of the service area and are to include trauma, burn, spinal cord injury, poisoning, acute cardiac, high-risk infant, and behavioral emergencies. The grantee must provide for the inventory

*American College of Surgeons (ACS), American Burn Association (ABA), American Association of Poison Control Centers (AAPCC), American Heart Association (AHA), American College of Pediatrics (ACP), and American Psychiatric Association (APA).

and categorization and designation by name of critical care capability (units, centers, program units) for specific critical patient groups. Plans must delineate the responsibility for identifying and providing transfer of specific patients.

Standard critical care capability must be identified for the seven patient categories in regions with such capabilities, and where necessary in distant regions. Facility projected needs assessments of care resources must be documented at least annually. This would include resources within the region and in other distant EMS regions. EMS projects must review the need for further centralization and expansion, and in some cases initiate decentralization as appropriate by patient impact studies.

7. *Public Safety Agencies*—The grantee will take appropriate actions to ensure the participation of public safety agencies to include police, fire departments, lifeguards, park rangers, and other appropriate public safety personnel, as First Responders and/or EMT's within the EMS system.

Provision must be made for effective utilization of appropriate personnel, facilities, and equipment of each public safety agency in the area, with sharing of resources and personnel as appropriate. "Effective utilization" means the integration of public safety agencies into standard EMS and disaster operating procedures of the regional system. It also includes the shared use of personnel and equipment, such as helicopters and rescue boats, appropriate for medical emergencies.

Public safety agency personnel are most frequently the first responders to an emergency patient. The EMS system must , therefore, work with these agencies to ensure the use of special equipment, proper training of staff, linked communications, and the development of cooperative operating procedures demonstrating appropriate coordination and mutual aid plans for day-to-day operations as well as during major disasters.

8. *Consumer Participation*—The EMS system must make provisions in its systems management and take appropriate action to ensure that persons residing in the area who have no professional training or experience participate in policymaking for the system.

Evaluation should be based upon the parameters found in Chapter IV.

9. *Access to Care*—All patients will have access to the EMS system without prior inquiry as to the ability to pay. This access must be assured for the ambulance services, initial general hospital, secondary transport to critical care units, and rehabilitation centers. The system should provide the means to monitor for restrictive measures that may eliminate any person or group of people from equal quality of services within the region. Agreements for admission should be negotiated between hospitals and ambulance services within the EMS region by the completion of the BLS system period and likewise for the ALS system period.

10. *Patient Transfer*—The EMS system shall provide for transfer of patients to facilities which offer definitive follow-up care and rehabilitation as is necessary to effect the maximum recovery of the patient.

The transfer of emergency patients from the emergency site to the emergency department of the general hospital critical care unit and rehabilitation centers is all within the scope of a total EMS system. The components of training, transportation, categorization, recordkeeping, and others all interrelates to this continuum of care.

The transfer agreement is necessary to facilitate communication and cooperation of physician providers within the system. Written arrangements between referring and receiving physicians for each of the critical groups must be documented by physician sign off for acceptance and participation. These transfer agreements from individual rural physicians to individual central critical care physicians must be established and be an integral part of an operating EMS system.

Areawide prehospital treatment and triage protocols must be established by councils of physician providers for the various specialty patient groups and are essential for completion of a Basic Life Support system.

11. *Coordinated Patient Recordkeeping*—Each EMS regional system shall take to provide for a coordinated patient recordkeeping system which shall cover the treatment of the patient from initial entry into the system through his discharge from it. This includes the prehospital, hospital, and critical care unit care within the system. Data elements shall be consistent in patient records used in follow-up care and rehabilitation of the patient; it shall be developed to ensure that emergency patients can be tracked through the system, and used to measure the system's change in efficiency in delivering emergency care.

The minimal patient records necessary for the EMS system are the dispatcher records, the ambulance records (ALS and BLS), the emergency department, and critical care records.

12. *Public Information and Education*—The EMS system shall provide programs of public education and information for all people in the area so they know about the system, how to access it, and how to use it properly.

Residents and visitors to the area need to know or be able to learn immediately how to access EMS. It should also stress the general dissemination of information on appropriate methods of self-help and first aid and the availability of first aid training programs in the area.

13. *Review and Evaluation*—The DHEW requires the grantee to provide information regarding the periodic, comprehensive, and independent reviews and evaluations to the extent and quality of the emergency care services provided in the EMS system's service area.

Therefore, the grantee will provide the DHEW with a written plan of how an objective review and evaluation is to be conducted within the EMS region. Such a plan shall include the appropriate identification of funds, staff, plans, and programmatic activities to be evaluated. The grantee will deliver a report of such review and evaluation within the period of the grant.

14. *Disaster Plan*—The EMS systems must have a plan to assure that they will be capable of providing emergency medical services in the system's service area during mass casualties, natural disasters, or national emergencies.

The EMS system is not the regional health disaster organization. It is the emergency medical organization that will work with other agencies during a disaster to provide emergency medical care. The EMS system must be linked to the local regional and state disaster plans and participate in exercises to test disaster plans.

15. *Mutual Aid*—Each EMS system must provide for the establishment of appropriate arrangements with other EMS systems or similar entities serving neighboring areas for the provision of emergency services on a reciprocal basis where access to such services would be more appropriate and effective in terms of the services available, time, and distance.

Arrangements among EMS regional systems and similar entities serving neighboring areas shall be written agreements, signed by individuals authorized to act for the respective parties with respect to such agreements, and reviewed and re-evaluated at least once a year. Such agreements should cover the exchange of service coverage, communication linkages, licensure and certification, and reimbursement.

2

Response Phases

Michael R. Gunderson, REMT-P

A complex sequence of events takes place when an EMS system responds to an emergency. This chapter describes steps that occur when state-of-the-art EMS systems are activated. The chapter also discusses corollary issues in system operations and new technologies that could have a significant impact on how systems perform in the future.

Pre-Arrival

Public Education

Public education can be considered the first phase in an EMS response. The public must have some idea what EMS is, what it is for, how to access it, and what to do before it arrives. Prevention programs are often focused toward trauma and cardiac issues. Public education in system access includes information regarding the appropriate circumstances and methods by which EMS should be requested.

System Access

It is extremely difficult for the public to recall different emergency phone numbers for different communities and different emergency needs. Such problems are exacerbated for travelers. The 9-1-1 program simplifies and expedites the process of getting help in emergent situations through the use of a universally recognized telephone number, thereby improving access to all emergency services including police, fire, and EMS. It has already been implemented with great success in a large portion of the United States.

The 9-1-1 computer systems are available in two general configurations. The basic systems provide the 9-1-1 phone number, with free access from pay telephones, linked to a public safety answering point (PSAP). The enhanced 9-1-1 systems have the benefit of being tied into computer files that automatically advise the PSAP staff of the location and name registered to the phone from which the call was made. This offers a significant clinical advantage by enabling timely responses to callers who cannot effectively communicate their needs. This may include persons with airway or breathing problems, altered levels of consciousness, and small children.

Once a 9-1-1 PSAP is contacted, the call taker determines what type of emergency services are required—police, fire, EMS, or any combination thereof. The medical director assures that the process used to make such determinations is clinically sound and consistently applied. To this end, PSAP protocols are typically employed. Most communication centers have call takers and dispatchers. Call receiving operators (CRO) primarily answer telephones and interact with callers. Dispatchers primarily talk on radios and interact with emergency personnel. This strategy accommodates a higher capacity for simultaneous emergency calls. Many systems subdivide the dispatch task even further by using separate dispatchers for police, fire, and EMS functions. In many cases the police, fire, or EMS dispatchers are not in the same facility as the CROs. Once CROs have determined which agency is needed, callers may be electronically transferred from the computer terminal of the CRO to the terminal of the agency dispatchers for more detailed questioning.

Emergency Medical Dispatcher

When the primary need is for EMS the PSAP call taker transfers the call to an emergency medical dispatcher (EMD). The EMD asks the caller specific sets of questions that allow efficient and reproducible information gathering and clinical decision making. The most basic issues for the EMD include determining number of patients, their age, if they are conscious, if they are breathing, their location, and verifying the call back number.

With confirmed patient locations, the EMD determines which EMS resources are needed and by which modes of response, emergency (hot)—with lights and sirens, immediate (cold)—without lights and sirens, or delayed—no emergency or immediate response required for transfer from hospital to home. This is referred to as the response configuration and the response mode. The options for response configurations include vehicles staffed and equipped in varied fashions. The chosen response may be a combination. Assuming the availability of First Response units and ambulances, a patient who has suddenly collapsed and is not breathing would be sent both types of units each traveling to the scene in the emergency mode. Less obvious cases would require additional questions based on the specific situation to determine the response configuration and mode. The EMD also tries to determine the nature of the call in case any special equipment may be needed and whether or not it is safe for field crews to enter. After the response configuration and mode are determined, the EMD provides the caller with prearrival instructions guiding the caller in providing basic first aid while rescuers are en route.

Emergency Vehicle Deployment

Two general models exist for emergency vehicle deployment, static and dynamic. Static deployment models use stations, not necessarily buildings, located throughout the service area. Vehicle locations remain the same between calls, excluding travel to and from the call. This is the method traditionally used by fire departments.

The most common dynamic model is system status management (SSM). It considers patterns in locations of calls for the particular time of day, day of week, and time of year. Vehicles are then placed at locations that optimize the system's ability to respond to those call patterns.

The choice between these two models has a dramatic impact on the work environment of the crews. Although it is more comfortable for crews to respond from stations, response time is measurably improved when crews remain in their vehicles and are located at key intersections. The system must decide if vehicle deployment policy decisions will be made for the comfort and convenience of the crews or for the clinical needs of patients. The physician responsible for medical oversight must have input in such decisions given the significant impact on patient care.

Multi-tiered systems use a hybrid approach. Fire apparatus provide First Responder services, and ambulances operate under SSM for transport service. A hybrid approach can also be used in a purely ambulance system; some units can be permanently stationed and others dynamically deployed. To improve resource use under SSM, ambulances are often equipped with automated vehicle locator (AVL) systems. The AVL system interfaces with the computer-aided dispatch (CAD) system, placing a symbol on an automated map display in the dispatch center that corresponds to the location of each unit in real-time. The symbol reveals the ambulance number and its status. This technology may also allow the crew to see their location and the location of the call on an electronic map on a computer monitor located next to the driver. When a call is received the CAD compares the location of available units in the system with the location of the call. Based on that comparison the CAD suggests the closest available unit and the most appropriate route. The EMD then accepts or rejects the recommendation of the CAD and selects an ambulance for the call. Meanwhile, the navigation computer in the ambulance is tracking its real-time location and is updating the CAD by radio.

On-Scene

First Responder Interventions

First Response agencies are called simultaneously with ambulances when the response configuration protocols indicate that they are needed. The First Response units are often fire trucks but may include police units in some communities. The First Responders typically provide basic service and automated external defibrillation as well. The First Responder crews may be certified at a formal First Responder level or at the EMT-A level.

Medical Interventions and Oversight

When the ambulance arrives the crew (First Responders, EMT-Bs, EMT-Is, or EMT-Ps) are given verbal and written reports on the situation from the initial response crew. The providers integrate themselves into the scene, using First Responders as needed. If the First Responders are not needed, they return to service so they may be available for other calls. The providers generally operate under two levels of protocols. The first level consists of standing orders, which they may carry out before establishing radio contact with direct medical control. The second level consists of anticipated interventions, which may be carried out only with authorization from direct medical control.

The main purpose of direct medical control via radio during patient care is to provide a real-time quality assurance mechanism. The field provider presents a verbal report, including the history, physical examination, field impression, interventions performed and planned, destination, rationale for the destination, and the estimated time of arrival at the destination. Direct medical control then decides if the plan and destination are appropriate and provide feedback and consultation. Direct medical control may be provided by receiving hospitals, designated hospitals, or designated staff equipped with portable radios. Direct medical control staff usually consists of physicians but occasionally incorporates specially trained and qualified nurses or EMS providers.

The impact of direct medical control on patient outcome has not been established. Consequently, some EMS systems allow providers to operate almost entirely on standing orders. Even in such situations they are usually provided a mechanism to consult with direct medical control at their discretion.

Transport and Transfer of Care

The timing of transport depends on the situation. In those cases in which definitive or stabilizing care may be provided in the field, transport is usually delayed until such care is initiated. Such situations may include administration of nebulized bronchodilators for mild to moderate wheezing, splinting of isolated fractures, or application of spinal immobilization. In cases in which definitive or stabilizing care is not available in the field, transport is initiated as soon as possible. These are commonly referred to as "load-and-go" situations. Examples of load-and-go candidates include patients with absolute indications for trauma center care and patients with suspected myocardial infarction for potential emergency department administration of thrombolytics. Consultation with direct medical control is often helpful when destination decisions are complicated by conflicts among patient wishes, the need for early intervention at the closest facility, and the ability of hospitals to accept patients.

Policies for notifying receiving emergency departments of incoming patients vary considerably among systems. The basic objective is to facilitate preparations, such as setting aside the appropriate type of bed, calling for additional resources, and obtaining past medical records.

Acquisition, Transfer, and Analysis of Data

When the patient is brought into the emergency department, the crew must provide adequate verbal and written reports to the staff. In most situations this will be the emergency department nurse but may include the emergency department physician.

One of the most striking impacts of EMS computerization has been the introduction of electronic or paperless forms. A number of hardware and software developments have improved the devices, which are almost the size and weight of standard EMS report clipboards. Interaction between the clinician and the paperless form is becoming as easy as writing on the computer screen with a special pen that selects items from lists and converts hand-writing into computer text characters. The many advantages in this pen-based computer technology over traditional forms include the ability to provide real-time quality assurance functions, real-time reference guide access, multiple reports, graphic tools, indexed menus, automatic hand-printing recognition, and a host of other features, making documentation more efficient, reliable, and complete.

The recording of information in real time is a significant problem in the field. Crews find it difficult and cumbersome to log their actions and observations as they occur concurrent with patient care. Consequently, data are lost or inaccurate because of delayed entry. Computer tools are being developed that will enable crews to easily log actions and observations as they occur. The computer will automatically time stamp entries so a chronologic list of events can be generated to print at the emergency department and transfer into a comprehensive clinical EMS data base.

Progress in medicine has steadily followed the ability to monitor patients. This is understandable because medicine tends not to treat what it cannot evaluate. Hence, EMS will see the introduction of more and more physiologic monitoring technology. For reasons of simplicity and practicality, most monitoring will be noninvasive. The primary purpose will be to forewarn the clinician of trends predictive of failures in natural and therapeutic compensatory mechanisms. This will permit the clinician to proactively initiate interventions before decompensation occurs. The homeostatic systems for oxygen transport will be the highest priority for EMS monitoring. Pulse oximetry and qualitative CO_2 monitoring are already common in the field. However, continued development and implementation of these technologies requires corresponding advances in real-time data management technology that will integrate with the paperless medical record systems.

Ultimately, the data transfer among the ambulance, the emergency department, and the clinical data management system will be totally electronic and real time.

EMS crews and support personnel complete multiple copies of dozens of different forms each day. Many of these forms are then keypunched with some degree of error into computer systems or are simply filed manually, making retrieval tedious and time consuming. As new technologies in hand-held computers become more prevalent, the implementation of paperless forms in applications such as inventory, personnel, billing, and purchasing will become commonplace.

The bigger picture in EMS data management will be in the analysis phase. Quality management programs will depend on the ability to precisely measure both the patient care process and clinical outcomes. The validity, accuracy, and precision of the data offered by these new technologies will facilitate a quantum leap in analysis capabilities. EMS medical directors, managers, and most importantly the providers themselves will be able to critically review compliance to standards (processes), evaluate the results (outcomes), pose solutions (hypotheses), implement changes in standards (new processes), and reevaluate the results (new outcomes) in a continuing cycle of quality improvement.

Summary

The generic description of a modern EMS response, as outlined here, must be modified and augmented to meet different challenges faced by specific systems.

3

System Models

Raymond L. Fowler, M.D., FACEP

An EMS system is a comprehensive, coordinated arrangement of resources and functions organized to respond to medical emergencies in a timely manner. An EMS system therefore is the arrangement of services provided to the consumer requiring a physician-patient contract using prehospital personnel. An EMS system in the practical world is provided because of public desire for medical care in the prehospital environment.

Police protection, fire protection, and civil defense emerged long ago in response to public demand. The various needs of an EMS system require a different structure for the provision of services than do other public services. Furthermore, a range of motivations exist behind the provision of the service, not the least of which is profit.

Under the stimulus of these variables, many methods of providing EMS operations have evolved. Almost every locale offering services has developed an EMS operation, whether public, private, volunteer, or a mixture.

Hospital-Based Systems

Hospitals commonly operate EMS systems. They purchase equipment, hire administrative personnel, train and hire EMS personnel, and contract for medical oversight. Although hospital-based systems may be privately owned, they may also be an extension of public hospital authorities, entities that direct public monies and act on the behalf of specific geographic locations. Hospital EMS systems are usually managed in a fashion typical to hospital environments, with administrators assigned to report through the hospital administration. Generally, these systems are financially tied to the hospital.

Medical oversight in a hospital model is usually an extension of emergency medical practice within the hospital. For example, medical staff guidelines for the hospital must be followed in hospital-based EMS systems as well. Because the physician-patient contract established in an EMS system does not differ from the physician-patient contract established in the hospital, peer review of all medical care must be conducted. Malpractice underwriting guidelines of the hospital should be maintained.

Medical oversight of hospital-based systems can be excellent because it encourages familiarity and close contact between medical oversight physicians and prehospital staff. Commonly, EMS personnel provide care in the emergency department when not in the field, thus further enhancing the team relationship.

Jurisdiction-Provided Systems

Another common method of EMS provision is through a jurisdiction-based system, usually at the municipality or county level; a few state and provincial models exist. The specifics of these systems vary, with economic issues playing a major role.

EMS providers housed in fire departments are one of the most common types of jurisdictional models. Approximately one half of the EMS systems in the United States are fire-based. Fire department vehicles and personnel are usually geographically well located, available 24-hours per day, and already oriented toward protecting life.

Fire departments maintain highly structured methods of training and advancement, including regular continuing education and benefits such as retirement. EMS activities are often added without such benefits, encouraging many EMS personnel to work in fire suppression to improve their benefits. Fire suppression personnel who chose EMS often return to fire suppression because of the increased opportunity for advancement and benefits.

Changing perceptions of EMS within fire services may gradually minimize such differences.

Medical oversight is usually contracted from private physicians. An important consideration for the medical director of an EMS system based in a fire department is the dominant role of the fire chief within the local public milieu. Any EMS physician who has come to loggerheads with an established fire chief quickly discovers where the power exists. Winning battles and losing wars holds very true when dealing with the hierarchy of a county or municipal fire department.

Jurisdiction-sponsored systems are typically supported by taxes. EMS may be a line item within the fire, police, or health department budget. Further sources of revenue may include billing patients. Proper management must provide for realistic billing and pricing based on the efficient provision of service. In this era of cost control and shrinking public resources, it may be difficult to shift expenses to the users. Jurisdictions providing EMS may be of any size, from small rural towns to entire territories bound into a single system such as Puerto Rico, British Columbia, or New South Wales. The matrix of management and medical oversight varies with the geographic complexities of the system.

Privately-Run Systems

One of the oldest forms of EMS is that of the private profitmaking provider. Originating in the funeral home days, these providers have evolved into highly efficient operations. Many private EMS systems become power brokers within the local legislative arenas because of their size and political influence. Private providers learned quickly to maximize efficiency, aggressively seeking service zones within the regional emergency systems that provided a steady flow of clients.

Medical oversight of private or proprietary providers must be of the same quality as that of other types of systems. High productivity is integral to the survival of private provider systems, especially in the absence of government subsidy. Excellence in patient care, consistent with the standard of care in the community, must always be the determinant of what care the patient receives, not economic motivation.

Volunteer Systems

In some rural areas the entire system of prehospital care is provided by volunteers. In fact, a few urban and many suburban jurisdictions are predominantly volunteer-based, usually with a government subsidy and a small cadre of paid personnel. Volunteer prehospital providers have existed in some parts of the world for centuries and in the United States since the 1920s.

The political power of volunteer ambulance providers is often only slightly less than that of the volunteer fire lobby, especially in the state legislatures. As a result of that political strength, volunteer organizations in some states have not been required to meet the same standards of EMS provision and medical oversight as other providers.

Complex Systems

Many complex EMS systems have evolved, some by prospective creative effort and some by the haphazard action of providers to fills gaps in care. It is not uncommon for private and public providers to coexist in the same geographic areas with various levels of providers occupying separate yet overlapping niches in any system. Often the First Responder element will be supplied by one part of the system, such as a fire department, and the paramedics will be provided by another. Land and air transport can be delivered by yet another agent.

An interesting picture of the financial and political history of a geopolitical area can be gained by examining structural elements of the EMS system. In the city of Atlanta, for example, the northern half of the city is served by a private provider and the southern half is served predominantly by a public provider. This is due, in part, to the payor mix of the populations; over the years, economic improvements in the southern area of the city have encouraged private providers to establish themselves there as well.

Public dispatch systems often evolve to take the initial call from the patient and then, as indicated by zone or other factors, dispatch private providers by secondary contact. Such call shunting may cause potentially significant delays.

Medical oversight of complex EMS systems may be exceedingly complicated, with both indirect and direct medical control being poorly coordinated. For example, providers receiving excellent direct medical control may not receive adequate or meaningful indirect medical control from their individual service medical director. Feedback among the physicians providing indirect medical control and direct medical control may not occur. One of the most important challenges for the EMS physician in a complex system is to provide ample coordination among all aspects of medical oversight.

Summary

The basic purpose of an EMS system is the provision of prehospital medical care. Therefore, excellent medical oversight remains the essential element of a well-run EMS system. In the vast technical and political milieu of providers and patients, the duty to provide accurate and compassionate medical care must always be foremost in the minds of all members of the EMS team. There is no one optimal EMS system model; most designs can provide excellent care. Regions and jurisdictions must intelligently identify the specific EMS needs of the area and organize the system responses pursuant to those particular needs building on existing resources and history.

4

Urban Systems

Lorraine Maria Giordano, M.D., FACEP
Steven J. Davidson, M.D., M.B.A., FACEP

In the rural United States, EMS generally developed as a volunteer activity; in most cities EMS began as hospital-based ambulance services staffed by full-time career personnel. Over the last 30 years the hospital-based ambulances have, for the most part, given way to municipally sponsored fire department or third-service programs. However, a few hospital-based or hybrid urban services exist.[3] The concept of full-time professionals or at least a mixture of paid and volunteer personnel is spreading to suburban areas and will eventually develop in all but the most sparsely populated areas. The problems facing urban medical directors differ from those of their rural or suburban counterparts; the most significant differences are addressed in this chapter.

Higher Call Volume

Throughout the country a relatively large number of medically underserved individuals increasingly turn to 9-1-1 and EMS systems as their entry point to health care services. In urban systems the total call volume is higher and units are generally busier. Consequently, urban units are used more efficiently because there is less downtime. Operationally the result is an effectively lower reserve capacity when call volume increases, and patients wait for ambulances more often than ambulances wait for patients; as call volume increases, response times also increase. In low-volume systems, inactivity occurs between calls, and travel time becomes a more dominant factor in response time.

Assuming no overcrowding at the receiving hospitals, efficient urban EMS ambulance units can handle approximately one call every hour. This can be translated into a staffing pattern, depending on time of day and usage patterns, requiring one ambulance for every 40,000 people. As a general rule, early evening periods (5PM to 9PM) require nearly twice as many units as early morning periods (2AM to 6AM), and other times fall between the two extremes. Depending on citizen use characteristics, some areas require more ambulances, while others require fewer.[4] Analysis of usage patterns must be combined with continual monitoring of call volume so that a fluid system of unit redeployment meeting local needs occurs.

The increased call volume of urban areas is an advantage for research and evaluation of innovations. On the negative side, however, there is also more wear and tear on the vehicles; the street life of an urban ambulance is shorter than its rural counterpart, resulting in proportionately higher capital costs for ambulance replacement. Other recent advances increasing the efficiency of the high-volume urban system, which also contribute to increased cost, are the automatic vehicle locator (AVL) system, priority dispatch, and computer-aided dispatch terminals or printouts in all ambulances.

More Paid Full-Time Employees

In urban systems the prehospital care providers are usually paid full-time fire department or third-service employees. However, there are EMS systems in a significant number of municipalities which provide services effectively through contracted commercial ambulance operators. Full-time personnel acquire more field experience, require less refresher training, and burnout more rapidly than volunteer providers in relatively low-volume environments, unless effective stress management programs are in place. Employed providers present a myriad of labor management issues in a paid system, all of which complicate the job of the medical director. Of course, there is also a higher probability that urban EMS employees will be represented by a union, which must be factored in as well. Additionally, political relationships and equal opportunity issues are more likely to affect staffing and planning.

These realities cannot be ignored. Unions demand that skill upgrades are accompanied by labor and contract negotiations and increased salary. The larger the number of employees, the higher the absolute cost to management for salary and benefit increases. There is also greater potential for labor relation cases in a paid urban system. Issues of infection control (AIDS and TB), homelessness, and drug-related and domestic violence resulting from differences in the urban and rural case mix, point to the need for a strong employee health service. These health services must work in close liaison with the infection control departments of the hospitals to which patients are transported and with the police department to ensure safety for crews. An effective urban medical director must also develop an independent employee assistance program and a large number of crisis intervention teams to meet the physical and emotional needs of personnel and their families.

Advantages of a Tiered System

A tiered response usually makes sense in an urban EMS system. Many urban programs are two-tiered, with the more advanced and the basic tiers occasionally working for different agencies. The relatively constant stream of calls in high-volume urban systems coupled with modern priority dispatch allows for more efficient use of the more expensive and relatively scarce paramedic personnel. In a priority dispatch system, the routine dispatch of both components is not necessary except for the most serious calls or when the paramedic unit lacks transport capabilities. For example, basic providers with pneumatic anti-shock garment (PASG) capability and rapid transport may be the response of choice for trauma in an urban environment. Although a minimum of one *ambulance* is generally required for every 40,000 people, a single paramedic unit with adequate transport support and state-of-the-art priority dispatch may be adequate for up to 200,000 people.[7] Despite arguments by some for all-paramedic systems, a two-tiered system allows a given number of paramedic units to serve a large population while maintaining a rapid response time.[1]

Nontransporting First Responder or emergency medical technician-defibrillator (EMT-D) programs, which have automated external defibrillation (AED) capability, are proliferating and add yet another potential tier in many urban environments. These programs can improve survival statistics but must be tightly linked with an ambulance transport service and more advanced medical backup. Difficulties can occur if AED programs are not integrated, resulting in a lack of coordinated protocols, program management, medical oversight, or contracts.

Possibility of Using Nontransport Vehicles

Responses by personnel in nontransport vehicles require that a secondary transport capability be readily available. Where that capability exists, system efficiency may be improved by using relatively inexpensive vehicles (costing a third of the price of an ambulance) as the nontransporting responder.

It is logical to use medically sophisticated personnel in nontransport vehicles and to dispatch them to cases in which such an intervention is the type most likely necessary. The use of basic personnel in nontransport vehicles makes little sense, except when ambulances are in short supply and all advanced personnel are already in nontransport vehicles. Of course, if fire or police personnel with basic first aid, First Responder, or EMT-B training are available, the urban system should seriously consider using them as the initial tier, responding in fire apparatus or police cars.

Different Response Time Factors

Ambulance cycle times of about 1 hour are usual in both rural and urban systems; however, the system variables differ. Whereas cycle times are often extended in rural systems because of scattered population and long travel times, in urban areas they may be prolonged by vertical access requirements, traffic congestion, or the lack of immediately available ambulances because of call volume surges and extended turnaround times in overcrowded emergency departments.[10]

In overtaxed systems, dispatchers must hold calls while waiting for an available ambulance more often than in relatively low-volume systems. Delayed response outliers are not only significant patient care issues, but political and media time bombs for the urban medical director.

Because of the higher usage rates, adding ambulance resources usually has a greater positive impact on response time in an urban system than in a rural area. However, in densely populated cities, traffic congestion related to rush hours, lunchtime pedestrians, construction, more frequent mass-media events plus demonstrations, plus public and political figure appearances may limit the expected benefits of adding more ambulances.

In cities with high-rise buildings, actual response times to the patient may be significantly greater than recorded response times to the address because of difficulties in vertical access from street level. For example, a response time of 6 minutes in a low-rise locality results in quicker treatment of the patient than a 6-minute response time in a high-rise area. For the urban medical director to develop medically optimal response time goals, the high-rise factor must be considered.[10,11]

Need for Standardization of Quality Management and Education

The large number of providers in urban systems requires highly structured medical oversight and quality management. A single urban medical director should be limited to control approximately 30 providers. Because urban prehospital providers use numerous receiving hospitals, there may be a tendency for medical control to be fragmented in large EMS systems. Although this is not necessarily bad, it can be confusing if the same level of providers in a single system have different protocols, educational backgrounds, or direct medical control physicians. If state or regional protocols and education requirements are not mandated, the medical directors in urban areas should voluntarily work together and with legislators to develop minimum local standards.

Because an urban medical director may be required to supervise a large number of providers, he often lacks personal contact with the individual providers. Assuming no cohesive regional quality management program is in place, an individual providing poor patient care can get lost in the numbers and float through a large urban service. If the solution is developing multiple "surrogate" medical directors at a number of medical facilities, a confusing variability of patient care can result unless there is a predetermined consensus on training, treatment, and operational protocols. Quality management programs must be proactive and ubiquitous. All sectors, government, volunteer, and commercial, must be brought into the system. Emergent and interfacility transports must be evaluated. There is an even greater need in the more densely populated urban system than in rural areas to actively interface quality management activities with receiving hospital facilities.

Need for Complex Organization and Supervision Structure

As the number of personnel increases, the supervisory and support staff requirements also expand within the agency and systemwide. Financial issues require expertise in areas such as budget, payroll, contract negotiation, and bid processing. A separate materials management section may be necessary to coordinate purchasing and inventory. Another unit may be needed to process prehospital care reports (PCR). As call volume increases, so do insurance claims and legal exposure necessitating an expanded risk management unit and perhaps even on-site legal counsel. Not surprisingly an unwieldy bureaucracy may develop both within the agency and among the various providers; in the urban EMS system care must be taken so that neither a multitude of uncoordinated small fragmented systems nor a truly unmanageable colossus evolves.

Availability of More Medical Facilities

There are usually more hospitals, both general and specialized, in an urban system. Consequently, greater consideration should be given in choosing the most appropriate institution for a prehospital patient. This not only means that field personnel must be taught to be more discriminating in facility choices but also that the local EMS system must take the lead in evaluating and designating emergency facilities of the receiving institutions.[4]

Increased institutional competition may lead to excessive political interference in site selection, direct medical control, and post locations of active units. The urban medical director must interface with all interested parties during development of the EMS system.

Less Medical Consensus

In urban environments there are often diverse and divergent medical opinions concerning appropriate medical care in the field. The greater the number of physicians involved in protocol development, the less likelihood of consensus. Although a single, responsible medical director should have ultimate authority for approving medical protocols and responsibility for supervising prehospital care, a formal, interdisciplinary, areawide medical advisory committee is critical to assist in developing prehospital medical policies and protocols. Strong negotiating skills assist in bringing the diverse opinions to a compromise. There are few situations more demoralizing to a system and its medical director than retrospective criticism and "monday morning quarterbacking" by the medical community.

Greater Physician On-Scene Medical Presence

In many urban areas there is an increased likelihood of a physician unknown to the prehospital providers being present at the scene of an emergency. These physicians may not be licensed in the jurisdiction or may not even be capable of dealing with the medical situation at hand. Therefore, it is essential to have a structured procedure for dealing with unsolicited physician interventions at the scene.

Increased Numbers of Non-English Speaking Patients

Generally, individuals who do not speak English are concentrated in urban areas; therefore the likelihood of non-English speaking patients accessing urban EMS systems is significant. Problems for the systems are accentuated by recent immigrants who not only have minimal English skills but who are also unfamiliar with the appropriate use of the emergency health care system. The urban EMS system communication center must have a large language bank of translators readily available.

Increased Nonemergent Use

Most residents of rural and suburban areas, regardless of financial status, have access to private vehicles and use them for transportation of nonurgent problems as well as emergencies; however, in the urban setting, demand for transport to hospitals is greatest in the low income communities. Because private and public transportation are often bypassed, medical directors of urban systems experience a much higher percentage of nonemergent requests for ambulances and a greater per capita usage rate than directors in suburban and rural systems.[9]

The percentage of nonemergent calls in urban systems is reported to be between 20% and 50%, depending on the local definition and circumstances. Although nonemergent use is on the decline, it is still one of the most vexing problems for urban systems and must be aggressively addressed.[8]

Limited Use for Aeromedical Capability

Medevac helicopters are usually less important and more rarely accessed on a per capita basis in urban areas. They are used to overcome difficulties of geographic access or traffic rather than long distances. Even in dense metropolitan areas, there will be an occasional need for the helicopter medevac. Thus a degree of aeromedical capability should be developed in all EMS programs with triage, dispatch, and quality improvement oversight mandated. In urban areas, competing hospitals may attempt to develop medevac programs; however, hospital-based medevac programs should be limited and must be coordinated by the regional EMS system.[9]

Testing Disaster Plans

Although disaster planning is no less important in rural settings, the more common occurrence of multiple casualty incidents (MCIs) and even disasters in urban systems allow for the evaluation of disaster response procedures on a more frequent basis. It is important that urban systems follow standard MCI procedures when dealing with all serious incidents so that the operational procedures are familiar and routine when providers face major disasters.[5,6]

A region-specific disaster plan is essential to every EMS system, but because the spectrum and consequences of possible disasters (natural and planned) are more varied in the urban environment, urban medical directors should spend time with liaisons from other agencies developing and testing many different disaster scenarios.

Summary

Although every jurisdiction requires development of a "tailored" EMS system, the issues often differ between urban and rural systems. It should be noted that around the country and around the world, urban systems are becoming remarkably similar in design and operation.

REFERENCES

1. Braun O, McCallion R, and Fazackerley J: Characteristics of mid-sized urban EMS systems, *Ann Emerg Med* 19:536-546, 1990.
2. Cadigan R, and Bugarini D: Predicting demand for emergency ambulance service, *Ann Emerg Med* 18:618-621, 1989.
3. Cady G: EMS in the United States: a survey of providers in the 200 most populous cities, *JEMS* 17(1):75-92, 1992.
4. Cayten CG, and Longmore W: Prolongation of scene time by advanced life support in an urban setting, *J Trauma* 25:679, 1985.

5. Kerr JT, and Weiman E: The planned disaster strategy for the masses, *JEMS* 7:22-23, 1982.
6. Kerr JT, and Weiman E: NYC-EMS: disaster planning pays off, *JEMS* 9:13-14, 1984.
7. Kuehl AE, and Kerr J T: Urban EMS systems, *Am J Emerg Med* 2:13, 1984.
8. Kuehl AE, and Kerr J T: Issues in urban EMS, *Urban Health* 13:24, 1987.
9. Kuehl AE et al: Report from the second international urban EMS conference, *Am J Emerg Med* 3:564-567, 1985.
10. Lombardi G, Gallagher J, and Gennis P: Outcome of out-of-hospital cardiac arrest in New York City, *JAMA* 271:678-683,1994.
11. Lumpe D: Focuses on prehospital care, *JEMS* 17(9):21-27, 1992.
12. Pepe PE, Matsumodo CM, and Bass RR: EMS call history with-in a large urban system: geographical patterns of basic and advanced life support demands and the implications for program planning [abstract], *Ann Emerg Med* 17:409-410, 1988.

5

Rural Systems

George F. Garnett, M.D.
John E. Spoor, M.D., FACEP

As pediatrics is not just caring for little adults, a rural EMS system is not simply an urban system spread over a larger area with lower run volumes. It has lengthier response times and greater distances to definitive care.[28] A rural EMS system shares with its urban counterpart the primary goals of timely assessment, appropriate stabilization, and expeditious transport of the critically ill or injured patient. The means to that end are challenging and often found only through trial and error and with the willingness of dedicated individuals to help their neighbors. The concept of neighbor helping neighbor is not unique to rural EMS systems, but it is crucial. Developing an EMS system in a rural area presents some challenges not encountered in the urban setting. Recently, many of those difficulties were outlined in a special report to the Congress of the United States by the Office of Technology Assessment.[28] These include personnel shortages, inadequate educational opportunities, limited medical supervision, limited resources of equipment and training, limited financial resources, poor communications and public access, lengthy response times, and a preponderance of volunteer providers. Rural personnel also have fewer opportunities to gain experience and reinforce skills. New innovative teaching strategies are being used to overcome this deficit. The rural population, especially farmers, tends to be more stoic and does not use EMS services as readily. Rural residents travel poorer roads at higher speeds, use seatbelts less often, and drive four-wheel drive vehicles and pickup trucks more often, increasing the likelihood of fatalities in automotive accidents.[28] Finally, the three occupations with the highest mortality and disability rates (farming, lumbering, and mining) are commonly located in rural areas.[18] Whereas urban emergency departments are frequently called the knife and gun clubs, rural emergency departments can be considered centers of blunt trauma.

What is Rural?

Multiple definitions exist as to what distinguishes an area as rural. With respect to health care and EMS, the U.S. Congress Office of Technology Assessment published a paper defining rural areas.[26] A rural area can be a few small villages with a hospital over 100 miles away or towns of several thousand people with a multi-bed hospital nearby. The definition used by the Office of Technology Assessment in their special report included all areas not designated as a metropolitan statistical area (MSA), the term used by the Office of Management and Budget. MSAs have a densely populated urban core (called an urbanized area) with at least 50,000 residents that is part of a county or counties comprised of at least 100,000 residents.[28]

In addition, wilderness areas are considered rural. Numerous training programs have been developed for providers and physicians in wilderness EMS and caring for patients when there are prolonged transport times.[3, 8, 14, 17, 20]

Evaluating Rural EMS Needs

The first step in developing or managing a rural EMS system is to study the numbers, types and distribution of medical and traumatic emergencies, and the basic demographics. Although data have been evaluated for a few states, they should not be generalized to all rural areas. The higher demand in rural areas for ambulance services for medical conditions other than injuries is believed to be due to "the older age distribution of rural residents."[28] Ambulance calls are more likely to be "urgent" or "critical" in rural areas of Texas and South Carolina.[28] This is supported by data showing that 69% of ambulance arrivals at one rural hospital required admission to the hospital.[25] Death rates are inversely related to population density, and unintentional injuries result in death twice as often in remote rural areas than in the largest cities.[28] Such data may be difficult to obtain; however, prehospital care reports, emergency department data, dispatch records, and public health department statistics may provide insight into system development.

Once needs have been assessed, specific EMS goals can be logically established for each community in the EMS system.[28] Information from the state EMS office can help determine the appropriate level of personnel and training necessary to meet specific goals in a geographic area.

In addition, every EMS system should be part of a larger statewide system. This is particularly true in rural areas where resources for planning and provision of EMS may be scarce. Planners at the state level may not be fully aware of the specific needs or capabilities of the rural areas. The medical director must become familiar with the state EMS office, the regulations, and laws covering prehospital care and EMS systems. The medical director must also become involved in the process of developing appropriate regulations that have an impact on rural EMS.

Personnel and Training

In most rural areas the EMS system is dependent on volunteer providers often at the EMT-A or lower level. The unique problems of volunteers must be recognized. Although most volunteers have a deep commitment to public service and a caring attitude, many may not be adequately prepared by the EMS system for the stresses they will encounter. They are frequently required to make decisions concerning patient care that their training and experience does not prepare them for. They often lack adequate supervision by qualified, experienced direct and indirect medical control physicians and often have to pay out of their own pockets for supplies and training. A high turnover rate can be expected among volunteer providers. The average volunteer remains active less than 5 years.[19] In some successful rural programs common characteristics were identified, including a strong community need and social fabric, integration of sound business practices into the volunteer organization, admission criteria for volunteer members, participation and commitment of community leaders, high visibility of the service, a formal organizational structure, cohesive community environment, strong physician involvement, and good interagency relationships.[29]

In many rural areas the pool of volunteers is small and may be getting smaller.[27] It is frequently hard to maintain a cadre of volunteers available during weekday working hours.[12] Retention is of primary importance when dealing with volunteers, and ongoing recruitment is essential.

It is difficult to determine the level of training necessary for rural EMS personnel. Ideally, it is based on the expected frequency of types of emergencies; however, responders in rural areas may need additional advanced level training simply because of long transport times and prolonged patient contact. The procedures taught and used should be medically sound and show over time that they have a positive impact on patient outcome. Procedures should not be instituted just because they can be taught or performed in the prehospital arena. It is hoped the establishment of the Center for Rural Emergency Medicine at the University Hospitals of West Virginia will start a nationwide process of data collection and evaluation to determine what is needed and what really works in rural EMS systems.[1] In some areas it may be more cost-effective to educate 10 EMT-As than to train a lesser number of paramedics.[30, 32] In 1972, advanced education for rural EMTs was introduced in New York state.[23] The concept was to introduce a module of education concerning an advanced procedure to be used under specific conditions. Once the technicians mastered that process they advanced to the next module. Brief courses of instruction (initial modules of 10 to 20 hours) were followed by fairly long periods of functioning at that level, allowing the technician to become successful and confident with the procedure. It also spread the educational process out over a period of time so the levels of advanced training were completed by the time the technician was required to refresh the EMT-A course. This approach was well received by the personnel. Many of the technicians in that initial module are still actively involved in the EMS system 20 years later. Unfortunately, so many different levels of education developed across the United States that the federal government finally grouped them into a single category of Emergency Medical Technician-Intermediate (EMT-I); however the modular educational process was not allowed to continue.[33] Rather than completing each procedure with successful clinical experience before progressing to the next, each level of training must usually be completed in its entirety within a set period of time.

First Responders and EMT-Ambulances (As) are usually the foundation of a rural system.[31] Strategically spaced within a rural area, First Responders can provide early, definitive prehospital care and reduce response times significantly. If there is a need for a particular medical skill in a jurisdiction, such as automated external defibrillation (AED), it is logical and possible to teach that specific skill without the expense of developing other less valuable skills. In farming areas, it is important that prehospital personnel be taught the FARMEDIC course.[10] The medical director should be involved in these courses since extrication from farm machinery and silos can be prolonged. The special problems of manure pit extrication, injuries caused by farm animals, the organic dust syndrome, and silo filler's and unloader's disease should all be included in rural areas' EMT-A training. These are unique problems associated with farming. Rural fire departments and EMS personnel that might respond with them, need to be taught the dangers of fighting silo fires and extricating persons trapped in grain bins.

It is important that the skill levels of rural providers be upgraded only when it is appropriate for the system and area within which they function. It is possible for providers to learn advanced skills though ambulances, basic skills, medical control, or communications may be inadequate. Improved capabilities of a technician or service should be the result of a system planning process involving all types of participants, ambulance agencies, technicians, hospitals, and physicians.

Once the appropriate level of education for providers has been determined, the initial educational process and a program of continuing education must be planned and established. Remote locations frequently require that services share the use of audiovisual lectures, programmed texts, and mannequins.[2] As often as possible instruction should be given close to the homes of the providers. Remote telecommunication programs (both television and telecomputer) allow several agencies to participate in a regional presentation at the same time, while the students remain at their local facilities. At times the networks are already established in cooperative public school systems. In Idaho and Alaska, mobile EMS trauma training units providing lectures as well as psychomotor skills practice have been developed that literally drive education to the rural EMS services.[1] The New York State Health Department Office of Emergency Health Services traveled throughout the state providing education and practice in rapid extrication of motor vehicle victims.[7] It is equally important to provide appropriate continuing education programs for nurses and physicians supporting the EMS and the emergency departments. As a minimum, courses such as Advanced Cardiac Life Support (ACLS), Pediatric Advanced Life Support (PALS), Advanced Trauma Life Support (ATLS), and a medical oversight course should be made available and encouraged. Educating prehospital providers to a high-level of care does little good and may prove detrimental to relationships if local physicians and nurses cannot provide the appropriate continuum of care. New video-electronic transmission of real-time video via telephone lines allows communication between the rural facilities and larger facilities. While the patient is being evaluated and cared for at the rural facility, practitioners with needed expertise and greater resources can give advice and guidance.[9]

Prehospital providers should receive feedback on a regular basis. Recognition from the community for exemplary services should be routinely provided. Whenever possible recognition should be provided in person by the medical director or designee. It is preferable to provide a means for providers to participate in evaluation of the prehospital activities.

The term *critical incident stress management* describes the psychological and emotional support and debriefing needed following a major EMS incident.[13] In rural EMS a critical incident may occur with only one patient, especially if the patient is a child, friend, or family member of the provider. The provider looks to the medical director for emotional support and debriefing as soon as possible after a critical incident. The medical director should be specifically alert for such incidents when performing run reviews. Often the field providers do not realize the personal impact that a particular incident may have on their lives.[5]

Financial Considerations

Finances are a significant problem for all areas of EMS, especially rural systems. Numerous recommendations for federal, state, and local financing have been made.[28] All avenues should be evaluated so that volunteers and paid rural personnel are provided adequate financial support to purchase supplies and keep ambulances running. The less time and money a volunteer has to invest in fund-raising the more likely the volunteer is to be retained in the system. The National Rural Health Association determined that "EMS in rural areas have not achieved the same level of advancement that it has in urban areas. Following are just a few of the reasons why. Sparse populations covering large geographic areas make the cost of providing emergency care more expensive, state and local governments in rural areas have a lower capacity to fund programs through taxes, failing rural economies often have difficulty maintaining the public service and responding to change, rural communities don't have the volume and profit potential to operate private sector EMS services when the public support system is absent."[29] All efforts to support volunteer, part-volunteer/part-paid services, or fully paid services in rural areas should be attempted including grants and third party billing. In several states avenues for financial assistance including surcharges on insurance policies (life, health, accident, and automobile), fees on telephone access lines, and portions of all fines for vehicle infractions such as driving while intoxicated, have been tried. One possible area of funding for individual ambulance services is charging third-party reimbursers for allowable fees. This route, however, is frequently frowned on by volunteers that survive on donations, fund drives, barbecue dinners, raffles, and auctions supported locally by the people the providers serve.

Medical Oversight

The local medical director may have to travel hours to meet with the providers under his control. The remote medical director should endeavor to meet with providers frequently but must meet with them at least 4 times a year. The medical director or EMS system quality improvement coordinator should try to review cases by mail monthly providing negative and positive feedback to the providers. Before instituting such a system the review should be planned with the agencies to prevent adverse interactions resulting from any negative findings.[22] The more time the medical director is able to devote to these meetings, the more enthusiasm will be built among the prehospital personnel.

Medical oversight in a rural EMS system is complicated by long response and transport times, extreme distances, and frequently inadequate communications.[29] It is important for the medical director or the hospital to maintain direct communications with the prehospital personnel throughout patient care and transport. Transport times are long and changes in the patient's condition often occur. However, in many rural areas, communications systems are lacking and extensive use of indirect medical control is required. Standing orders and protocols for this indirect medical control need to be reviewed frequently to ensure they meet the evolving needs of the community. Reviews are most important in EMS systems using intermediate levels of advanced technicians. Protocols and standing orders should include medical care, special rescue or extrication, other specialized services, hazardous material response, when to contact direct medical control, when normal direct medical control orders can be used as standing orders in the event of communication failure, interhospital transfers, and aeromedical transports.

It is important that the medical director educate others who will have contact with the EMS system so they are aware of the providers' skills and abilities. In rural areas a physician is *not* available 24 hours a day, therefore the medical director should monitor calls via radio and be aware of the system activities as much as possible. As an alternative, on-line assistance from the emergency department or nearby EMS systems may be arranged. It is also possible to use direct telephone contact between the patient's location and the medical director of an adjacent EMS system; the use of a radio-telephone switching station allows relatively long-distance communication. These methods allow voice and bioelectronic transmission of data from the prehospital provider to a direct medical control facility or physician.

The more personally a medical director knows the providers and the system, the easier it is to determine how the system should grow and what levels of care should be authorized. The medical director, whether in control of a single prehospital service or multiple services in several counties with several hospitals providing initial and definitive care, is ultimately responsible for every patient in the system. This fact may be a significant disincentive for a physician to provide medical oversight to a rural EMS system. Consequently, many states have enacted legislation that protects physicians from civil liability when they assume medical control responsibilities.[15] In addition, familiarity with the protocols, standing orders, and providers helps relieve the sense of insecurity remote supervision often stimulates.

Communications

Providing EMS communications in rural areas can be an expensive and complicated operation requiring the assistance of technical experts and electrical engineers. Frequently, detailed advice on rural EMS communications is available from experts in the particular geographic area or the state EMS office. Multiple problems have been identified with respect to communications.[15]

Access to EMS is frequently hampered by lack of 9-1-1 services. In rural areas, emergency call boxes along highways, citizen's band (CB) radios, or very high frequency (VHF) marine radios may be used for access; however, radio dead spots and congested frequencies are frequent. Many emergency agencies in rural areas are accessed by local telephone numbers. These are often party lines meaning several households may share one line and getting to use the line may be difficult. People living in the area sometimes know the number but most new people or visitors do not have that information. Some areas advertise the number on telephone stickers.[29] In other areas calling the telephone operator (dialing zero) may access a centralized operator many miles from the area who may not have the necessary information to generate a response by the required agency. Public education in rural areas should focus on accessing the system and providing first aid and CPR until EMS arrives.

Once an emergency call is received the dispatcher must send the first responders or an ambulance to the scene. It is important that the dispatchers have had emergency medical dispatch training.[16] This training should be geared to the rural environment where there are few house numbers. Landmarks and the correct names of roads may be the only way to describe a patient's location.

Medical control communication is needed once the providers arrive but may not be available or accessible for the reasons previously noted. It is important to remember that in most medical emergencies access to direct medical control is possible with a telephone.[22]

EMS communication systems are not always planned and coordinated with other services such as police, fire, or rescue. They frequently vary in quality from area to area within a rural EMS region, and an ideal system configuration is not a reality. It is important, therefore, to consider the radio frequencies of other local providers when determining mutual aid agreements or addressing disaster plans. A comprehensive radio communications plan has been successfully implemented. It consists of a VHF mountain-top repeater system supported by the sheriff's department and an ultra high frequency (UHF) repeater system supported by the state health department. The systems are placed on mountain tops so that access is provided throughout the region.[29] One county system in New York state maintains economic support for its multichannel VHF and 10 channel UHF multiple repeater system by allowing county agencies access to some frequencies for transmission of long-distance, business phone calls. The savings in long-distance calls has helped provide financial support for the EMS radio system. The tower with the strongest signal can be manually selected by the communications control center to receive the EMS signal, which can then be repeated between the towers and transmitted to the receiving facility.

Transportation

Ideally, in rural areas, response vehicles should be located and able to transport so that most areas can be reached within a reasonable time frame. The goal should be to provide an adequate number of strategically placed ground vehicles and aircraft. Where this is not possible efforts should be made to recruit and train First Responders to provide initial stabilization until a transport vehicle arrives. It is important that there be a clear agreement between independent First Response units and transporting ambulance services concerning mutual aid responsibilities and the provision of continued care at the facility. This agreement should be written, and a copy should be approved by the medical director of the system. The level of service provided by each component should be identified and agreed on before starting the program.

In farming areas, the farmer and family should be considered first responders and should receive education in preplanning acute events, initial emergency care, and accessing EMS system. This should include painting large numbers on every farm building and putting a map of the farm in the mailbox so that EMS providers can locate them if the family returns to the injured person to provide assistance. The FARMEDIC program addresses these issues, but again the medical director needs to be involved in the process.

Aeromedical Services

In rural or wilderness areas, aeromedical evacuation is often provided by commercial airlines and governmental agencies such as state police services or Air National Guard units. It is important to educate field providers about aeromedical evacuation so they may serve as escorts when needed.[11, 21] If rotorcraft are used the prehospital personnel need to know how to properly package the patient for the type of helicopter used. The patient should be well wrapped in a blanket, and then the restraining straps to the long board should be fastened over the blanket. Rear tunnel patient access helicopters may not allow use of the lower extremity traction splint because its length may prevent closure of the rear hatch door. It is also important that personnel know the protocols for controlling access to the aircraft, the dangers involved, and the process of loading the patient. It is essential that educational programs be completed before use of these aircraft to prevent injury to the patient or providers. Aeromedical transport should also be incorporated in local and regional EMS planning and medical control systems. The mechanism and process of accessing the aeromedical service should be clearly defined within the EMS medical control protocols. The EMS medical control within the area should have the most knowledge of the regional resources, can act as a consultant, and can provide direction to prehospital services and smaller hospital facilities requesting aeromedical assistance. A patient should not be held at the scene until arrival of a helicopter if the time for transport to an appropriate facility would be shorter. The helicopter can be routed to that facility if additional transfer is required. In areas where fixed-wing aircraft are used for transport (wilderness areas or islands), it is usually necessary to initially transport the patient to a predesignated landing site.

Patient Recordkeeping

It is not unusual in rural areas for two or more services to be involved in treating and transporting a patient. In these cases, extra attention should be given to coordinating patient recordkeeping. Patient records should be easy for all prehospital responders to use. It is often best to use a series of check boxes rather than lengthy narrative reports so that copies of the primary responders' reports can be given to the secondary services without significantly delaying patient transfer. This information should be related to the receiving hospital by the primary responders so that the condition of the patient can be followed continuously throughout the course of prehospital care. Copies should be retained by the service initiating the care and the service providing transport for review by the medical director. Interfacing services should collaborate on the design and use of the form, unless there is already a systemwide or state approved form. A good recordkeeping system provides access to statistics that aid in prehospital research and rural EMS system development. The data will become crucial as quality improvement activities and research in prehospital care begin to sort the beneficial actions from those that are of no help or even harmful.

Major Incidents

All rural EMS systems should actively participate in developing and testing disaster and major incident protocols. Sooner or later every EMS system will respond to a major incident involving more patients that the system routinely handles. Planning and preparation will reduce the stress of the incident and help the providers deliver better care. In addition to having a detailed plan the entire system including hospitals and other involved facilities should participate in periodic drills (using moulaged victims) to assure that the plan and communications work. A critique of the drill including the prehospital personnel, the moulaged victims, and the hospital staff should be conducted as soon as possible. This is necessary to identify problems and obtain suggestions on how the plan can be improved. Including all persons involved provides insight not otherwise obtained and builds camaraderie and mutual respect.

Mutual Aid

Rural EMS systems should have mutual agreements not only with other ambulances, but also with other public safety agencies, extrication teams, and search and rescue groups. Often agreements need to be made with agencies such as the military, depending on their availability and the remoteness of the area. It is better to start a mutual aid response early in an incident and cancel if not needed than to start late and lose time and lives.[24]

As part of the EMS system, any rural hospital that does not have the range of services required to care for the gamut of emergencies expected in a rural setting should develop close relationships with a facility that does. This may be a neighboring rural hospital, a rural referral center, or a suburban or urban center. The time to find resources for a particular problem is not when that problem requires a rapid solution. If there are designated specialty facilities near the rural facility that provide the service, under federal legislation a patient that needs to be transferred must be accepted.[4,6] The rural facility will evaluate and stabilize the patient, receive the patient's consent, contact the facility and physician at the receiving hospital, and transfer all the necessary records. The plan for assistance from the larger facility should also include educational programs such as triage and transfer processes and protocols, the provision of ACLS, ATLS, and PALS, and other services that the smaller facility may not be able to do on their own.

Summary

All EMS systems share common goals. Rural systems tend to be less structured, coordinated, and educated in advanced emergency care techniques than urban systems. Each is characterized by its own unique set of problems, usually centered around geography and demographics. The thorough knowledge of these parameters coupled with thoughtful needs assessment will lead to a smoothly functioning rural EMS system.

REFERENCES

1. American College of Emergency Physicians: *ACEP News* 11 (4), April 1992.
2. Anderson P et al: Trauma in the country: a statewide approach to trauma skills training for rual EMTs, *JEMS* 11:61-64, 1986.
3. Applachian Search and Rescue Conference: Wilderness EMT.
4. Consolidated Omnibus Budget Reconciliation Act, 1986 and Omnibus Budget Reconciliation Act, 1989.
5. Dernocoeur K: *Street sense communication, safety and control,* Bowie, MD, Brady Communications.
6. Frew S: *Patient transfers: how to comply with the law,* 1991, The American College of Emergency Physicians.
7. Gilbertson M: Rapid extrication, Office of Emergency Medical Services, Albany, NY, New York State Department of Health.
8. Goth P, and Garnett G: *Wilderness EMT guidelines, prehospital and disaster medicine,* In press.
9. Hartman J: MEDNET. Paper presented at the symposium Rural Health care: strategies to increase access, sponsored by the American Medical Association, Chicago, Sep, 1991.
10. Hill D: FarMedic responding to rural america, *Rural Emergency Medicine,* In: *Newsletter from the American College of Emergency Physicians* 1 (3), Feb 1993.
11. Johnson M: Alaskan aire: aeromedicine in a wilderness state, *Aeromedical Journal* 2(#):11-13, 1987.
12. McHenry S: Communication at the OTA Rural EMS Workshop, Washington, DC, May 4-5, 1989.
13. Mitchell J, and Resnik H: *Emergency response to crisis,* Bowie, MD, 1981, Robert J and Brady Co.
14. National Association for Search and Rescue: *Wilderness EMT.*
15. The National EMS Clearinghouse: *Protection from liability for EMS personnel,* Lexington, KY, 1987, The National Association of State Emergency Medical Services Directors and the Council of State Governments.
16. National Rural Health Association: National rural EMS needs workshop, *JEMS* March, 1989.
17. National Society Wilderness Medicine: *Policies and procedures.*
18. Pratt DS: Occupational health and the rural worker: agriculture, mining, and logging, *Journal of Rural Health* 6 (4), Oct 1990.
19. Scalice B: More than a numbers game, *JEMS* 46-47, June, 1988.
20. Solo: *Wilderness EMT.*
21. Southern Region EMS Council: *Aeromedical evacuations in alaska: an escort training manual,* Anchorage, AK, 1985, The Council.
22. Spoor J: *Personal experience,* Unpublished data, Cooperstown, NY, M I Bassett Hospital.
23. Spoor J: Advanced training for rural EMTs (part 1 of 3), *Emergency Medical Services* 6 (5):77-78, Sep/Oct 1977.
24. Spoor J: Trauma response, beyond the ABCs, *JEMS* 12 (2), 33-36, Feb 1980.
25. Spoor J: A rural emergency medicine profile, *Rural emergency medicine.* In: *Newsletter from the American College of Emergency Physicians* 1 (3), Feb 1993.
26. US Congress, Office of Technology Assessment: *Rural areas: impacts on health care policy and research,* Washington, DC, July 1989, US Government Printing Office.
27. US Congress, Office of Technology Assessment: Rural emergency medical services workshop, Washington, DC, May 4-5, 1989.
28. US Congress, Office of Technology Assessment: *Rural emergency medical services, special report,* Stock No 052-033-011735, Washington, DC, 1989, US Government Printing Office.
29. US Department of Health and Human Services, Office of Rural Health Policy: *A study of rural emergency medical services: success and failure,* May 1990, National Rural Health Association.
30. US Department of Transportation: *Emergency medical care: a manual for the paramedic in the field,* Washington, DC, 1979, US Government Printing Office.
31. US Department of Transportation: *Emergency medical services: first responder training course,* Washington, DC, 1979, US Government Printing Office.
32. US Department of Transportation: *Emergency medical technician ambulance,* ed 3, Washington, DC, 1984, US Government Printing Office.
33. US Department of Transportation, National Highway Traffic Safety Administration: *EMT-Intermediate course guide,* 1985. The Department.

6

Wilderness

Keith Conover, M.D.

An idealized picture of wilderness EMS appears in the 1986 *Prospectus of the Appalachian Search and Rescue Conference*[17]:

> The final part of the Project will be to establish, in cooperation with local emergency medical services (EMS) and search and rescue (SAR) agencies, a regional Wilderness Emergency Medical Services System, with regionwide training, certification, communications systems, and support services. This EMS system will complement existing EMS and SAR systems providing a coordinated, statewide (or multistate) plan for dealing with wilderness medical problems in a coordinated and professional manner. It will use the most modern emergency medical knowledge and technology available, while recognizing the constraints of the wilderness environment on personnel and equipment.

Many EMS systems, even ostensibly urban ones, may need to provide care in a wilderness or similar context. Wilderness incidents may be rare, but they strain system resources and attract publicity. The prudent EMS medical director plans for such events; thus ensuring high quality patient care and favorable, publicity. Planning for wilderness EMS requires the following:

- *Wilderness-related medical training for prehospital providers:* Wilderness medical training modules are becoming standardized nationwide and can be used "as is" or adapted slightly to meet local needs. These are continuing education modules for prehospital providers of all levels and depend on previous prehospital training.
- *Search and Rescue (SAR) training for prehospital providers:* Basic SAR training is readily available from many sources such as nationwide courses or local SAR teams.
- *Physician training for medical oversight of wilderness providers:* In some cases, medical oversight of wilderness operations might be delegated to a particular physician or group of physicians. In other cases, providers may be members of a SAR team with its own wilderness-specific medical oversight and control. In either case, physicians working with wilderness providers need special training such as the Wilderness Command Physician course described later in this chapter.
- *Broad wilderness-specific standing orders:* Wilderness providers do not have reliable communications with direct medical control physcians. Therefore wilderness providers need broad, detailed wilderness standing orders. The standardized wilderness medical training modules are guidelines for creating such standing orders.

Aspects

Mountain Rescue

Mountain rescue involves more than spectacular alpine-cliff rescues. It also includes the less spectacular yet difficult rescues in the rolling mountains and foothills of the Appalachians and similar areas. The eastern United States does not have the thousand-foot vertical cliffs nor the altitude of the west, but the weather and the brush can be worse than in the Sierra Nevada. For example, one difficult, vertical rescue in Shenandoah National Park lasted 11 hours at night in fog and freezing rain.

Vertical night rescues in freezing rain are not necessary for SAR to be mountain rescue. Mountain rescue operations are graded as technical or semitechnical evacuations, depending on steepness of terrain. Technical evacuations require that rescuers be tied into the litter or otherwise protected from falling. Cliff rescue is the most common technical evacuation. Semitechnical evacuation is over terrain that requires a rope attached to the litter for belay or hauling but not so steep that rescuers must be tied into the litter. Rescuers may need to use mountain rescue techniques, specifically semitechnical evacuation, on any long, steep slope far from a road. This could be in a deep ravine, on a coastal bluff, or in the mountains. Long semitechnical evacuations have even occurred within city limits of several major cities.

Cave Rescue

Exploring caves is a popular and somewhat hazardous outdoor recreation in parts of the United States. Cave rescue has unique access problems; victims may be accessible only to rescue personnel small enough to fit through a tight crawlway, in excellent physical shape, and experienced at traveling wild caves. Vertical pits with waterfalls may need to be rigged by those experienced in choosing and rigging cave anchor points.

In cave-bearing areas of the United States, recreational caving frequently results in SAR. Although cave rescues are underreported, some 100 to 200 cave rescue operations are recorded yearly in the United States as extrapolated from 20 years of reports in the National Speleological Society's "American Caving Accidents" series. Cave rescues are long in duration, technically difficult, and offer unique medical considerations. The *Manual of U.S. Cave Rescue Techniques* is available to those who must integrate cave rescue into their EMS system.

The National Cave Rescue Commission (NCRC) assists EMS agencies in planning for cave SAR operations. The NCRC can identify cave rescue teams near cave-bearing areas for EMS medical directors. The NCRC offers classes at several levels in cave rescue. A medical director whose responsibilities include cave rescue would find the weekend NCRC "Orientation to Cave Rescue" class enlightening.

Diving Medicine

Most recreational diving accidents come to a quick resolution; either the victim survives and promptly comes to a shore facility or boat or the victim dies. In either case, those at the scene use first aid and diving training to help the victim. Because of the inability of humans to breathe underwater and the rapidity with which a sport diver may reach the surface, dive rescue teams rarely care for a live victim. In reality, most are body recovery teams. On rare occasions, a dive rescue team finds someone alive in an air pocket and effects a rescue. In such situations, rapid rescue predominates over treatment at the scene.

The National Association of Diver Medical Technicians (NADMT) sponsors a Diver Medical Technician course. Designed for providers on drilling rigs where underwater work is a daily activity, the course also applies to sport diving. Most companies with underwater construction or utility work have medical systems for their divers. The company medical and rescue resources can also be helpful outside the company; joint planning with the local EMS agency is essential to smooth operation during incidents.

Mine Rescue

Deep mine rescue like cave rescue takes place underground, but there are important differences. The environments are different; for example, cave-ins are exceedingly rare in natural caves but an ever-present danger in mines. Most mine rescue personnel are employees of a mining agency or corporation, whereas almost all cave rescue personnel are recreational cavers on volunteer cave rescue teams. Resources from mine rescue are occasionally used in cave rescue; for example the Special Medical Rescue Team, which consists of volunteer paramedics and doctors trained in mine rescue, may help with cave rescues. Sometimes, an NCRC coordinator will ask for federal mine rescue help to tunnel down to a victim trapped in a cave.

Many EMS agencies have active or abandoned mines in their areas or mutual aid areas. The EMS plan in such areas should include mine rescue coordinated with local mining companies, mine safety agencies, and possibly the Special Medical Rescue Team.

River Rescue

River rescue can be dangerous and proper training is essential to prevent unnecessary danger. Textbooks on river rescue are available and are a good starting point for the medical director. However, books are no substitute for proper field training. Several commercial organizations now offer high quality river rescue instruction.

Scope of Practice

Wilderness EMS links the fields of prehospital and wilderness medicine; neither are currently medical specialties. However, wilderness medicine has a national medical organization, the Wilderness Medical Society, and a journal, the *Journal of Wilderness Medicine.* There is a widely accepted compendium text that defines the field; electives in wilderness medicine and wilderness EMS are now being developed for medical students and residents. Wilderness medicine includes a wide spectrum of medical, paramedical, and nonmedical topics such as preventive measures for foreign travelers, definitive care of minor injuries in the wilderness, environmental exposures, improvised evacuation of patients, and the physiologic study of altitude effects.

Wilderness EMS only deals with a subset of wilderness medicine defined by the needs of medical and paramedical personnel in wilderness SAR. This includes management of patients over extended periods, treatment of exposure, trauma, shock, and infections, and the use of drugs, IVs, and other invasive procedures.

Wilderness EMS is an extension of regular EMS. The components are the same as those in an urban EMS system, but at the earlier stages of rescue providers require special wilderness training. After reaching a road or helicopter landing zone the wilderness branch of the EMS system merges with the urban or rural branch (Figure 6-1).

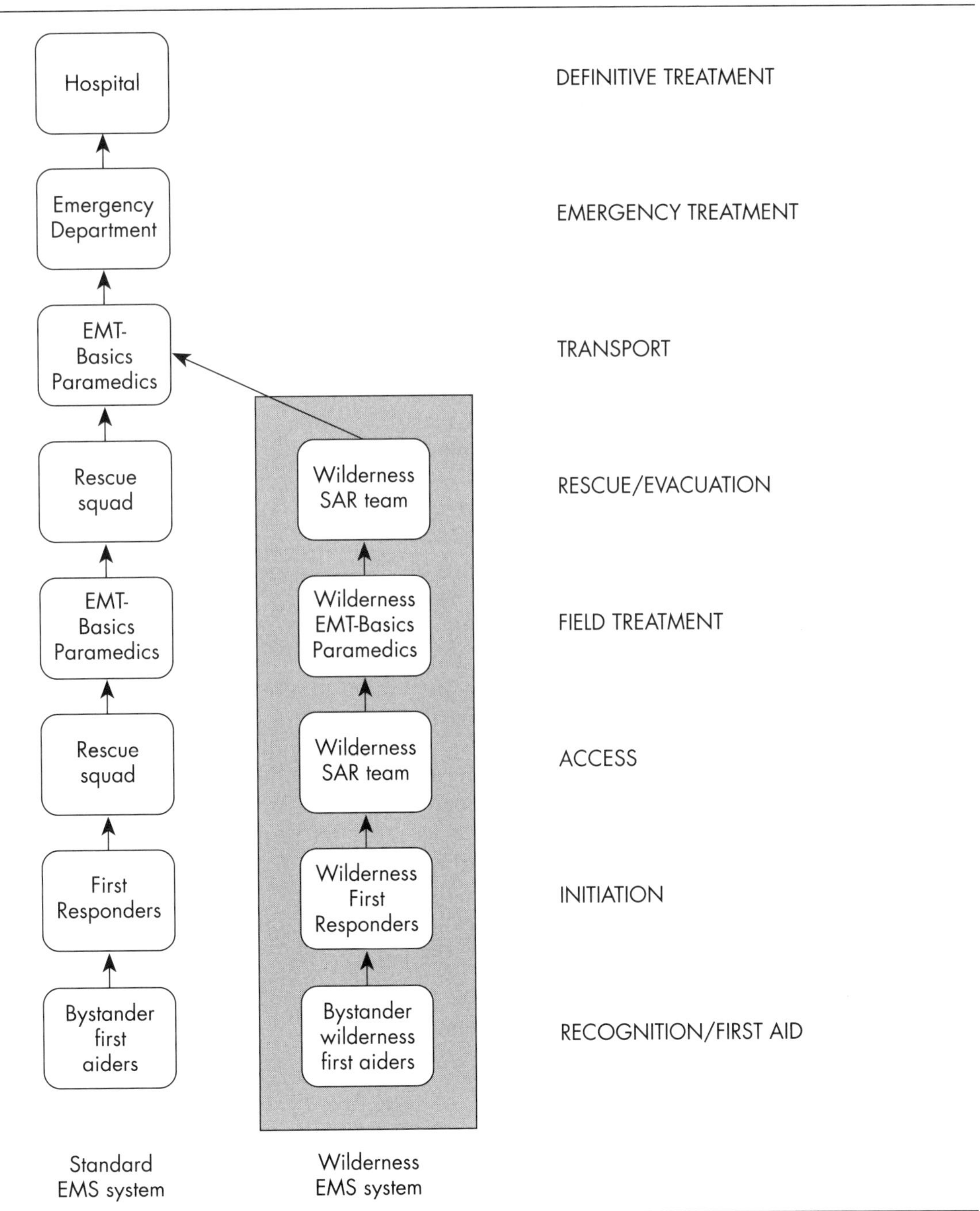

Figure 6-1. Phases of the wilderness EMS system. (Modified from Wilderness EMS Institute.)

Wilderness First Aid

An early Wilderness Medical Society document defined wilderness first aid as follows[46]:

> Backcountry First Aid can be defined as first aid rendered under conditions where immediate, definitive medical care is unavailable because of distance, adverse travel conditions, or difficulties in communications. The term "backcountry first aid," therefore, can be applied to first aid rendered at high and low altitudes, from arctic ice and subarctic tundra to forests, deserts, seashores, the tropics, and even under the seas. Small boat sailors, inhabitants of isolated villages, and victims of disasters where medical facilities and communications have been destroyed may all require "backcountry first aid." Backcountry first aid differs from the usual type of first aid and EMT training in three major ways:
>
> a. The need to learn new procedures in order to handle injuries and illnesses in which a delay of more than a few hours or days will likely cause adverse effects which outweigh the dangers of teaching such new procedures to laypersons. Standard urban protocols for these illnesses and injuries are not adequate for the backcountry setting.
>
> b. The need to deal with entirely new illnesses and injuries not seen in the urban setting.
>
> c. The need to learn basic care of an injured or ill person so that ordinary day-to-day requirements of the body will be met until definitive care is secured. These requirements include temperature control (warmth or coolness), shelter, water, food, cleanliness, psychological support, and the management of excretory functions.

There are very different ideas about the ideal wilderness first aid course. Consider the widely different contexts for wilderness first aid from afternoon hikes to expeditions in the Hindu Kush, from blisters on the heel to open femur fractures, and from Sunday afternoon hikers to medics with Mountain Rescue Association teams.

First, consider occasional hikers, climbers, cavers, hunters, or white water paddlers. Their needs exceed the content of the American Red Cross Standard First Aid class, particularly regarding environmental dangers such as hypothermia and heat exhaustion, improvised splinting and evacuation, and accessing the wilderness SAR system and EMS systems. Almost 20 years ago, the Seattle Mountaineers and the Seattle Red Cross developed a mountaineering-oriented standard first aid course. This course uses the classic booklet *Mountaineering First Aid*.

Weekend wilderness backpackers need more training than hikers in dealing with major trauma, severe illness, and common medical problems until a doctor or hospital can be reached. Most backpackers carry over-the-counter and some prescription drugs including injectable epinephrine for anaphylaxis, antidiarrheal drugs such as loperamide, and analgesics such as acetaminophen with codeine or hydrocodone. Their wilderness first aid training must deal with the appropriate use of these drugs. Teaching backpackers to use prescription or nonprescription medications has legal implications that cause some doctors and first aid instructors to cringe. However, training laybackpackers to use prescription and over-the-counter drugs appropriately makes sense. The advice to "see your doctor if the problem persists" is less than helpful when you are a day's hike from the road, especially if a common medication may be helpful. For the serious outdoors devotee, an ideal program would be (1) a wilderness-oriented American Red Cross Emergency Response course or a wilderness-oriented National Safety Council First Aid and CPR course and (2) additional instruction on using simple medications for minor problems. Several books address the need for such a program.

Wilderness Prehospital Provider

Diverse problems exist in the wilderness and standards of care are different for wilderness rescues. Prehospital providers working in the wilderness need specialized training to supplement standard EMS training.

First, wilderness providers need special training for the environment and SAR. Providers must carry out medical tasks despite severe environmental stresses such as freezing rain, blizzards, or heat. To keep the operation moving smoothly providers must interface easily into wilderness SAR operations even if not actually assisting with SAR tasks.

Second, wilderness providers need special medical training. Some problems are more common in the wilderness than on the street particularly environmental problems such as hypothermia, heat exhaustion, and heatstroke. Certain problems common to the wilderness are not discussed in traditional EMS courses including plant contact dermatitis and friction blisters. Though they may seem minor, such problems can be temporarily disabling in the wilderness. Wilderness patients may also need long-term care. For example, during extended evacuations it may be appropriate to monitor the patient's urine output with an indwelling catheter or condon drain. Infections, acetectasis, and deep venous thrombosis may become problems during an extended wilderness evacuation. Wilderness emergency medical equipment is generally limited to what the team members can carry on their backs or improvise at the scene. Providers must be trained to improvise.

Thus the wilderness provider must have EMS training, SAR training, and special training in applying EMS training in the backcountry, commonly termed a wilderness medical module (Figure 6-2).

Wilderness medical modules may be considered a certification level for providers, suggested by the current popularity of the term Wilderness EMT. However, wilderness modules are better defined as continuing education training that allows providers to function in a specialized context. EMS medical directors should ensure that providers asked to function in a specialized environment have training for that environment. For the wilderness, this includes SAR training and a wilderness medical module.

Wilderness medical modules are oriented to the outdoor environment, which is vastly different from Alaska to Texas. One might think that it is impossible to design a wilderness medical module applicable to the entire United States. However, heat exhaustion occurs in Alaska's summertime heat and hypothermia can occur during rescues at the southern tip of Texas. Developers of wilderness medical modules have found that roughly 95% of the material applies throughout the country. The few topics applicable to restricted environments such as snakebite, scorpion sting, and altitude illness require little additional time to teach.

Wilderness primary care. Wilderness providers often provide incidental medical care for team members. In wilderness rescue, sending a team member back to a search base for medical care might be disastrous; a team member or two must accompany the injured rescuer, and the depletion of the team may delay an evacuation for hours. Because mountain rescue often stresses team members to the limit, injuries and illnesses that are minor at home loom larger in the wilderness, which is another argument for wilderness providers to provide primary care for the team. Although wilderness providers need not be physicians assistants capable of providing all routine primary care services, they should be able to care for minor injuries and medical problems common in the wilderness. Physicians serving as medical advisers to wilderness EMS agencies should take this need into account when selecting training and when providing protocols and standing orders.

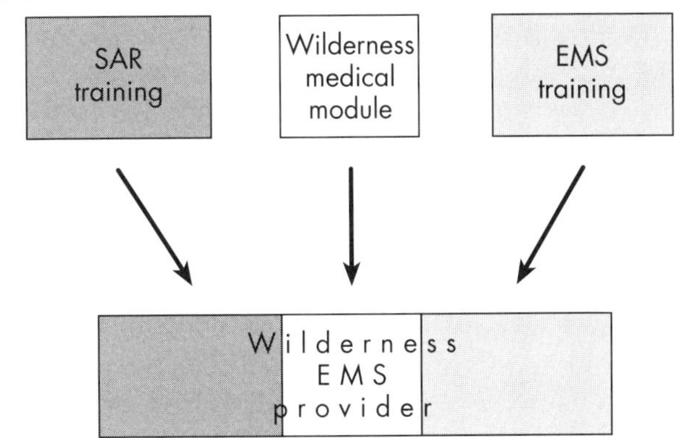

Figure 6-2. Components of wilderness EMS training. (Modified from Wilderness EMS Institute.)

Training prehospital providers to administer over-the-counter or prescription oral medications counters existing EMS training. Yet, prohibiting providers from administering simple medications when far from medical facilities makes little sense. The major question is which level of provider the medical director should permit to administer medications. Summative test results in wilderness EMT classes showed an excellent understanding of pharmacology principles and oral drug use by EMT-Bs. The choice will usually be made by the medical director and depends on the specific background training of the different levels of prehospital providers.

Jurisdiction and protocols. Since wilderness medical emergencies occur only rarely in many states, EMS agencies rarely have the special training, experience, or equipment necessary to deliver state of the art wilderness emergency care. Some wilderness SAR teams provide service to many counties or even several states. For example, the Appalachian SAR Conference (ASRC) offers SAR services in Maryland, North Carolina, Pennsylvania, Virginia, West Virginia, and the District of Columbia. For SAR team wilderness providers, it makes sense to use their special training and standing orders when caring for a wilderness patient regardless of the county, state, or EMS district. A good model is Virginia; the state EMS issues a letter granting ASRC wilderness providers permission to use their wilderness-oriented protocols and standing orders throughout the state. The providers are responsible to their own medical director.

Wilderness Provider Levels

EMS providers are currently grouped into First Responders, EMT-Bs, various types of EMT-Intermediates (EMT-Is) and Paramedics (EMT-Ps). Existing wilderness EMS modules are designed to supplement these training levels. There are two wilderness medical module levels, one for first responders and another suitable for EMTs of all levels.

Wilderness First Responder. Assume that a hiker in a state park breaks a leg and a companion hikes out for help. A park ranger calls the local SAR team then hikes to the patient who is now hypothermic. The wilderness SAR team eventually responds to evacuate the patient. The local ambulance service then transports the patient to the hospital.

Rangers are wilderness First Responders. Because they see major injuries more often than the occasional hiker, rangers should have training in the care of major problems as well as standard first aid training. They do not need training in the use of over-the-counter and prescription medications unless they patrol the backcountry for extended periods.

The standard US Department of Transportation (DOT) *Emergency Care First Responder* curriculum does not address many needs of the wilderness first responder such as improvised equipment, care of patients for extended periods and environmental illnesses, injuries, and hazards. Several commercial providers offer wilderness-oriented first responder courses that include the standard DOT curriculum. There is no accepted standard national curriculum for wilderness first responder training, but the ASTM F-30 Committee on EMS is developing a standard training guide.

Wilderness EMT. The wilderness SAR team needs training at least at the park ranger's level and preferably more. Training should be at the EMT level or higher including specialized SAR and wilderness medical training.

Though many SAR teams have certified EMTs, few operate as EMS agencies. In some areas, only members of legitimate EMS agencies may become certified, thus, members of SAR teams are excluded from full participation in the EMS system. When planning wilderness operations, medical directors should carefully integrate local SAR teams into the EMS plan. This might include helping SAR team members obtain EMS training.

The term Wilderness EMT is now common. It refers to EMTs certified at any level who function in the wilderness context and have had additional wilderness-specific training.

Prehospital Providers

Do prehospital providers need special authorization to perform emergency care in the wilderness? Before answering this question consider that proper emergency care in the wilderness may differ from proper prehospital care on the street. The following examples illustrate the differences between street and wilderness emergency care.

Open Fractures—The standard treatment with short transport times is to brush off loose dirt, cover with a sterile dressing, and transport the patient. When transportation will be delayed, proper prehospital care includes wound irrigation and oral or parenteral antibiotics.

CPR—Standard guidelines for street CPR call for resuscitation to continue until more advanced providers arrive, the patient recovers, or rescuers are exhausted and unable to continue. In the wilderness, additional help may be hours or days away. Victims of lightning strikes, hypothermia, or near-drowning may recover if CPR is administered, but most victims of wilderness cardiac arrest are unlikely to recover with CPR. In the wilderness, especially during winter or in the high mountains, continuing "until the rescuers are exhausted and unable to continue" puts rescuers at risk of death from hypothermia. Therefore, wilderness rescuers are advised to continue CPR for 30 minutes then give up if there is no response.

Shoulder Dislocations—The current procedure for street prehospital providers is "never attempt to reduce a dislocated shoulder." However, the standard treatment of a knee dislocation without a pulse is to attempt reduction.

Even with a good distal pulse, reducing an anterior shoulder dislocation in the wilderness makes good sense; at the least, it will reduce pain and suffering and it may prevent the need for reduction under general anesthesia at the hospital. When spasm has been intensifying for many hours, reduction may be impossible without general anesthesia. The Wilderness Medical Society position statement says, "The common anterior shoulder dislocation can usually be reduced without too much difficulty and the sooner this is attempted, the easier it will be."

Now, consider the question again. Do prehospital providers need special authorization to perform emergency care in the wilderness? In particular, consider the reduction of shoulder dislocations in the field.

Because prehospital providers are trained to use axial traction to straighten angulated limbs, those trained to reduce anterior shoulder dislocations should be able to do so *within the scope of their practice.*

This argument may be applied to essentially all care administered by wilderness prehospital providers. The actual care may be different in the wilderness and wilderness providers may need special training, but the scope of practice is the same. According to this argument, there is no need for special licensure of wilderness prehospital providers; their provider certification should suffice.

An objection could be made. Prehospital providers might mistake a humerus fracture and try to reduce it as they would a shoulder dislocation. This is purely a training issue; if wilderness providers are trained to properly palpate the shoulder for the characteristic deformity of an anterior shoulder dislocation and to check for the inability to touch the hand of the affected extremity to the opposite shoulder, the chances of inappropriate reduction attempts will be minimal.

However, state EMS laws and regulations differ widely. For example, in Pennsylvania EMT-Ps are only allowed to administer drugs on a list published by the state EMS office. Therefore, if following EMS regulations a paramedic could not administer oral or parenteral antibiotics to a wilderness patient with an open fracture, even if it is the accepted standard of care for a physician.

Many states have not addressed wilderness EMS in their regulations. Maine has adopted specific protocols for wilderness EMTs that differ from street EMT protocols. Virginia is considering adding wilderness EMT certification to the EMS training program and, by letter of authorization, has allowed wilderness rescue teams to use special statewide wilderness protocols that differ from standard protocols. Pennsylvania considers wilderness EMS outside regular EMS, and medical directors may establish wilderness protocols for their own EMS agencies.

Medical Oversight

The ideal physicians for wilderness EMS programs are certified by the Mountain Rescue Association, members of a wilderness SAR team, and have completed a wilderness command physician class. Because such physicians are exceedingly rare, one should compromise. An understanding of the field problems of wilderness EMS is necessary, but serving in the field is not. Therefore a wilderness EMS medical director or a physician providing direct medical control should either have an outdoor background or go through a realistic wilderness rescue orientation such as a wilderness command physician course. If cave or white water rescue are part of the wilderness EMS system, the direct medical control physicians should observe or participate in rescue simulations during their training. The wilderness EMS physician must have both a broad base of knowledge about prehospital medicine and experience with medical oversight, but need not be a full-time emergency medicine physician.

A wilderness EMS agency could opt either to operate entirely on standing orders or require direct medical control. A common approach is to specify a single hospital as the source of direct medical control. However, it is unlikely that all direct medical control physicians at a medical facility will be qualified to provide direct medical control to wilderness-trained providers. One way to ensure availability of qualified physicians is to maintain a roster of wilderness direct medical control physicians. The roster could include physicians at different hospitals or in different cities or towns.

Wilderness rescue operations take many hours, sometimes days. Thus, direct medical control of wilderness providers is much different than most direct medical control. Wilderness rescue entails an extended patient relationship. For continuity of care a single physician should provide direction for the entire rescue, although this may be impossible in practice. Because the condition of the patient will be known well before arrival, the physician can discuss the case with the emergency department physicians who will care for the patient once admitted. The wilderness direct medical control physician can consult specialists during the prehospital management of the patient. Therefore the wilderness EMS physician should be well educated regarding inhospital and prehospital management of unique problems.

Communications

In many wilderness rescues the providers must function without direct medical control. In some mountainous areas, existing medical radios are useless due to the terrain. In cave and mine rescue, VHF and UHF radios will not function. Although underground field telephones can be used sometimes, connecting them to the EMS radio may present an insurmountable technical problem. Finally, some wilderness SAR teams simply cannot afford the technology for direct medical control communications. EMS medical directors can help by proactively investigating wilderness SAR communications resources and making recommendations to wilderness SAR teams. Improving technology extends the reach of the direct medical control physician. However, EMS medical directors should establish broad standing orders for wilderness providers of all levels to use when direct medical control and advice are unavailable for extended periods.

In some jurisdictions, a physician must be in direct voice contact with the provider to legally provide orders for invasive procedures or drugs; the provider may not accept the order from a third person relaying the message. Portable repeaters are both scarce and difficult to carry up a mountain. Therefore, attended radio relays are often used in wilderness SAR operations: A member with a radio stands on top of a mountain and relays messages back and forth. This would seem to preclude direct medical control in areas requiring direct voice contact; however, there is a reasonable alternative. In the hospital, doctors often give orders by writing on the chart, but verbal orders must be taken directly by a nurse. The critical point is that the nurse or prehospital provider must receive the physician's order by a method that limits errors. A method of radio communication as reliable and well documented as written orders should allow legitimate relay of the orders. The direct medical control physician enters the order on a standard medical order form. In the physician's presence, the radio operator transmits the written order to the wilderness providers through a relay if necessary and the wilderness providers read the order back for confirmation. The wilderness providers record the orders in their log and sign off on both their log and the net control communications log at completion of the mission.

Equipment

Much standard ambulance equipment is inappropriate for the wilderness. For example, an ambulance cot is a poor choice for cliff or cave rescue. However, the underlying reasons for ambulance equipment requirements may hold clues to equipment for wilderness EMS.

Consider a wilderness "ambulance." The litter team members' booted feet are its "tires." Blistered feet or slippery shoes on a rescue team may be just as hazardous as bald tires on an ambulance. Training in foot care and proper personal equipment are essential parts of the wilderness ambulance. One might argue that the rescue team's equipment can be all team equipment with no need for personal equipment, but a quick thought about boots belies this claim. A 5-mile climb in not-broken-in "team" boots would make any rescuer a casualty. The rescuers' headlamps are the wilderness ambulance's headlights. Nighttime rescuers carrying a patient and using hand-held flashlights are probably worse off than providers in an ambulance without headlights and interior lighting.

Of course, these analogies can be carried to extremes, but they are a useful starting place for examining the equipment needs of a wilderness rescue team.

Epidemiology

Most of the hard data on wilderness trauma comes from mountaineering and caving journals. Unfortun-ately, little data are available on injuries along the trail. The statistical data available, though far from comprehensive, show that trauma is the most common emergency in the wilderness. Not surprisingly, most wilderness trauma results from a fall. Because of time factors inherent in wilderness incidents, patients frequently develop secondary complications such as hypothermia, infection, and dehydration. The periodical *Accidents in North American Mountaineering* offers the most compelling information regarding wilderness. Critiques of mountaineering accidents between 1960 and 1981 show the primary cause is human error. This includes climbing without a helmet, misuse of equipment, inexperience, and surpassing one's abilities.[41-44, 50-58] The type of injuries reported in *Accidents in North American Mountaineering* have been tabulated from 1984 to 1990 (Figure 6-3).[50]

Schussman cites climber error in 39% of accidents in the Grand Tetons from 1981 to 1986.[45] Where review board information was available, 50% had no experience or climbing experience of less than 1 year. Weather and other environmental factors influence the frequency and severity of wilderness injuries. However, available data clearly cite human error as the primary etiology of wilderness trauma; environmental factors are usually secondary. This observation applies to wilderness rescuers as well. In the wilderness, EMS personnel are their own worst enemies. Therefore, safety is the first commandment of wilderness travel and rescue. The type of injuries in Schussman's study are summarized in Figure 6-4.

One study implicated acute mountain sickness and hypothermia in about half of all climbing injuries in the Sierra Nevada mountains. The presumption is that these conditions contributed to

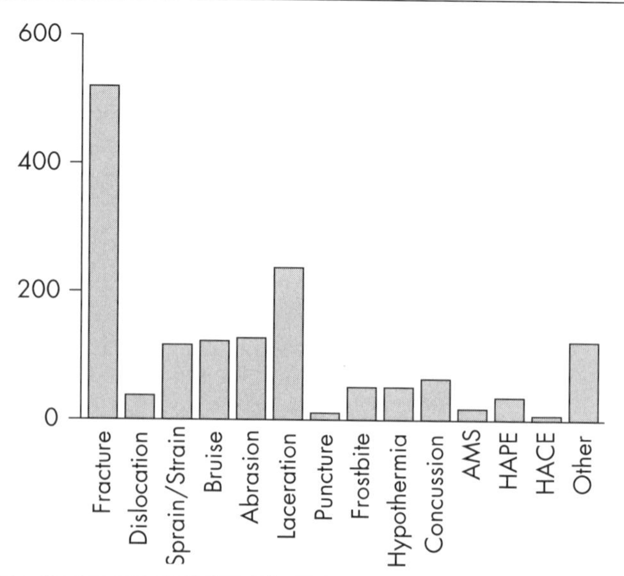

Figure 6-3. American mountaineering accidents 1984 to 1990. (Modified from Wilderness EMS Institute.)

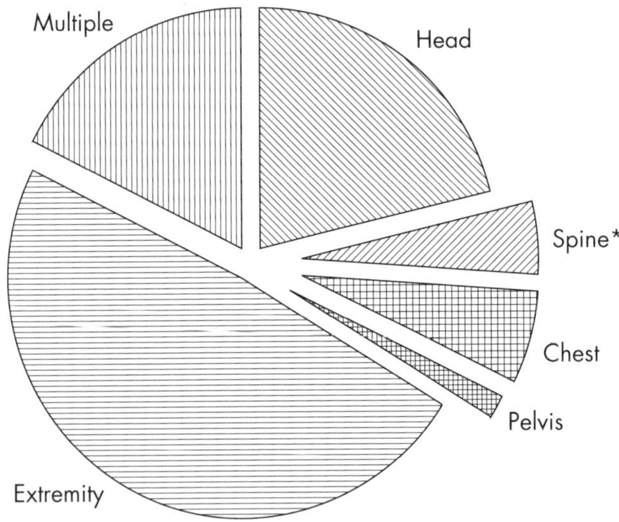

Figure 6-4. Accidents in the Grand Tetons 1981 to 1986. (Modified from Wilderness EMS Institute.)

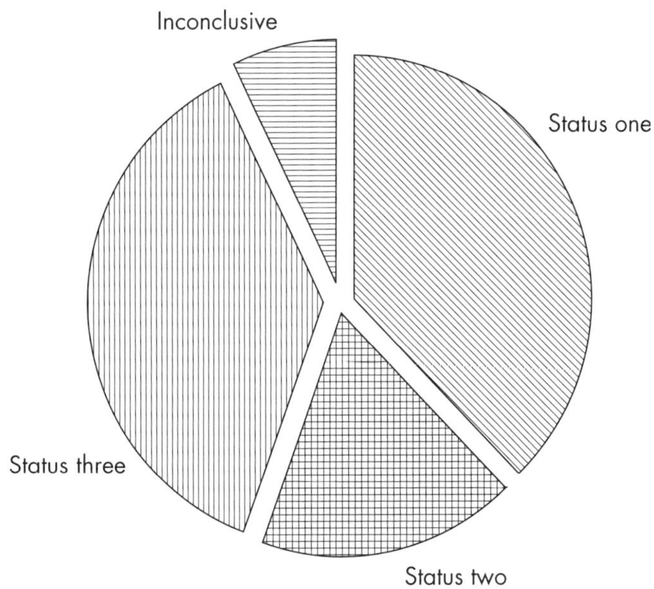

Figure 6-5. Appalachian SAR Conference 1975 to 1987 search subject status. (Modified from Wilderness EMS Institute.)

errors in judgment resulting in accidents.[35] Acute mountain sickness, hypothermia, exhaustion, and fatigue may all cloud judgment.

A study from the U.S. Outward Bound program shows injury patterns roughly similar to those cited above. The author compares the safety of outdoor recreation with that of other sports and finds injury rates similar.[39] Caving accidents also show a similar pattern.[8-12, 24-33]

Informal discussions with SAR teams in the White Mountain National Forest of New Hampshire reveal some differences. Because many older people hike and stay in the high mountain huts there, cardiac problems are more common than reflected in other wilderness SAR data. Compared with climbing injury statistics the information gathered by the ASRC regarding their SAR subjects represents a more general wilderness SAR population. Dehydration and hypothermia assume larger dimensions because many subjects were not involved in major trauma. Diabetic hypoglycemia, psychiatric problems, and epilepsy are also disproportionately represented. Injuries and burns from light aircraft crashes and gunshot wounds from hunting accidents are the major sources of trauma in their data (Figures 6-5 and 6-6).

Most EMS systems divide trauma patients into two classes, immediately life-threatening or not immediately life-threatening. Patients with life-threatening trauma decompensate very rapidly; thus the concept of "the golden hour."[14] For every half hour a patient is in shock mortality roughly doubles. The focus of urban trauma care is to save patients in danger of dying in a matter of minutes. "Scoop and run" is the appropriate treatment for urban trauma patients. All measures are geared to rapid treatment and rapid

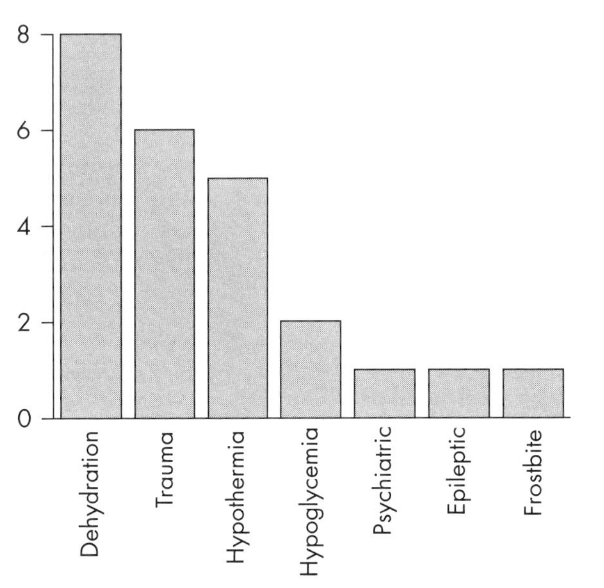

Figure 6-6. Appalachian SAR Conference 1975 to 1987 status two injury or illness. (Modified from Wilderness EMS Institute.)

transport to the operating room. For example, IVs are started en route, if at all. In the wilderness, those with severe injuries are already dead; this is simply a function of time. It takes too long for someone to walk for help and then for a team to respond. Patients, if alive when found, usually survive the evacuation.

Wilderness patients differ from urban trauma patients in other ways as well. Wilderness trauma patients always have multiple problems. Cold exposure and dehydration are common.[53] These conditions may combine with mild blood loss and rhabdomyolysis and myoglobinuria, for example, to cause acute renal failure. Hydration as well as warming and monitoring the urine color and volume are appropriate interventions that may be instituted in the field.

Wilderness trauma patients require long evacuations. Patients develop trauma complications urban providers never see such as compartment syndrome, deep venous thrombosis, decubitus ulcers, and adult respiratory distress syndrome. All trauma patients are in danger of such problems, but street providers' responsibilities end before these problems become evident.

All wilderness trauma patients have metabolic needs. For extended evacuations, especially with patients who have been lost or stranded for long periods, wilderness providers must ensure nutrition and hydration and expect elimination.

Catastrophic Events

A catastrophic event is much the same as a wilderness SAR operation. There is no shelter and exposure to heat, cold, snow, or rain are problems for victims and rescuers alike. There may be no potable water or food. Providers need overland evacuation skills because roads and streets may be impassable; and they must be ready to care for patients for a prolonged time. Local hospitals may be destroyed or overwhelmed, and doctors and nurses may be dead or injured themselves. Transportation of the sick or injured may be delayed for days, and it may take several days for a disaster medical team to set up in the area. Although victims may be trapped in ways that require special urban rescue skills, many may simply need evacuation by mountain or cave rescue techniques. As in the wilderness, providers must be self-sufficient in terms of food, water, and shelter. During the first hours to days, local medical resources will be aimed at the critically ill so prehospital providers may care for minor injuries. For all these reasons, wilderness providers are a major asset in any catastrophic event and should be included in any plan.

Wilderness Resources

Wilderness EMS is a complex topic, but there are many resources for help. Contact the resources listed below to integrate wilderness into your EMS system.

- Appalachian Search and Rescue Conference, P.O. Box 440, Newcomb Station, Charlottesville, VA 22904, (804) 674-2400 (emergency only). A large multi-team SAR organization that operates as a wilderness EMS agency in several states, and may serve as a source of advice for EMS medical directors.
- ASTM, 1916 Race Street, Philadelphia, PA 19103, (215) 299-5400. Committees F-30 on EMS and F-32 on SAR set national and international standards and actively develop standards for wilderness EMS.
- Center for Emergency Medicine of Western Pennsylvania, 230 McKee Place, Suite 500, Pittsburgh, PA 15213-4904, (412) 578-3200. The Center offers wilderness EMT and wilderness command physician training.
- Emergency Response Institute, 4537 Foxhall Drive NE, Olympia, WA 98506, (206) 491-7785. This Institute offers SAR and related training.
- Mountain Rescue Association, 2144 South 1100 East, Suite 150-375, Salt Lake City, UT 84106, (303) 567-9584. The MRA is a national wilderness rescue organization.
- National Association for SAR, P.O. Box 3709, Fairfax, VA 22038, (703) 352-1349. This Association serves as a national information resource for SAR.
- National Cave Rescue Commission, c/o National Speleological Society, Cave Avenue, Huntsville, AL 35810. (205) 852-1300 (Emergency: contact the National Rescue Coordination 1-800-=851-3051).
- Ohio Department of Natural Resources, Division of Watercraft, 1952 Belcher Drive, Building C-2, Fountain Square, Columbus, OH 43224, (614) 265-6480. The Ohio Department of Natural Resources offers a wide range of water rescue training and serves as an information resource on water rescue.
- Pennsylvania SAR Council, P.O. Box 504, Somerset, PA 15501, (814) 926-2554 (Emergency: (412) 647-7828). The Pennsylvania SAR Council is a state SAR organization.
- Rescue 3, P.O. Box 519, Elk Grove, CA 95759, 1-800-457-7283. White water rescue trainingis available from Rescue 3.

- SOLO (Stonehearth Open Learning Opportunities), RFD #1 Box 163, Tasker Hill Road, Conway, NH 03818, (603) 447-6711. SOLO is a provider of wilderness medical training.
- Special Medical Rescue Team, c/o Richard Kunkle, MD, Latrobe Area Hospital, Latrobe, PA 15650, (412) 537-1187. This SAR team specializes in mine rescue.
- Virginia SAR Council, c/o SAR Coordinator, Virginia Department of Emergency Services, 310 Turner Road, Richmond, VA 23225-6491, (804) 674-2421 (Emergency: (804) 674-2400). Information is available from the state SAR organization and SAR office.
- Wilderness Medical Associates, RFD 2 Box 890, Bryant Pond, ME 04219, (207) 665-2701 or (800) 742-2931. Wilderness medical training is provided by the WMA.
- Wilderness Medical Society, P.O. Box 2463, Indianapolis, IN 46206, (317) 631-1745. The WMS serves as a national wilderness medical organization.
- Wilderness Medicine Institute, P.O. Box 9, Pitkin, CO 81254, (303) 641-3572. The Institute is a provider of wilderness medical training.

REFERENCES AND BIBLIOGRAPHY

1. American Academy of Orthopaedic Surgeons: *Emergency care and transportation of the sick and injured,* ed 3, Chicago, 1981, The Academy.
2. Auerbach PS: *Medicine for the outdoors: a guide to emergency medical procedures and first aid,* Boston, 1986, Little, Brown & Co.
3. Auerbach PS and Geehr EC, editions: *Management of wilderness and environmental emergencies,* St Louis, 1989, The CV Mosby Co.
4. Bechdel L and Ray S: *River rescue,* Boston, 1985, Appalachian Mountain Club.
5. Bezruchka S: *The pocket doctor,* Seattle, 1988, The Mountaineers.
6. Bowman WD: CPR and wilderness rescue: when and when not to use it, *Response!* Sep:42-3, 1987.
7. Bowman WD: *The national ski patrol's outdoor emergency care: comprehensive first aid for nonurban settings,* 1988, National Ski Patrol.
8. Breisch RL, edition: *American caving accidents: 1967-70,* Albuquerque, 1974, Speleobooks.
9. Breisch RL, edition: *American caving accidents: 1972,* Albuquerque, 1975, Speleobooks.
10. Breisch RL, edition: *American caving accidents: 1973,* Albuquerque, 1975, Speleobooks.
11. Breisch RL, edition: *American caving accidents: 1974,* Albuquerque, 1976, Speleobooks.
12. Breisch RL, edition: *American caving accidents: 1975,* Albuquerque, 1977, Speleobooks.
13. Bush S: *Proposed outline: wilderness medical technician course,* Littleton, Colo, 1981, National Association for Search and Rescue.
14. Campbell JE: *Basic trauma life support: advanced prehospital care,* ed 2, Bowie, Md, 1988, Brady Communications.
15. Christensen A, edition: *Wilderness first aid: a resource manual for outdoor leaders in British Columbia,* Vancouver, BC, 1986, Wilderness First Aid and Safety Association of British Columbia.
16. Conover K: Partial draft proposal for a national wilderness medical technician program. Emergency Medicine Committee, 1980, National Association for Search and Rescue.
17. Conover K, edition: Wilderness emergency medicine curriculum development project: prospectus. Presented at the Appalachian Search and Rescue Conference, Center for Emergency Medicine of Western Pennsylvania, 1987.
18. Darvill FT: *Mountaineering medicine: a wilderness medical guide,* ed 12, Berkeley, Calif, 1989, Wilderness.
19. Farrington JD: Death in a ditch, *Bull Am Coll Surgeons* 52(3):121-30, 1967.
20. Fears JW: *Complete book of outdoor survival,* New York, 1986, Outdoor Life Books.
21. Forgey WW: *Wilderness medicine,* ed 3, Merrilville, Ind, 1987, Indiana Camp Supply Books.
22. Hudson S, edition: *Manual of US cave rescue techniques, ed 2,* Huntsville, Ala, 1988, National Speleological Society.
23. Iserson KV, edition: *Orthopedic injuries in the wilderness III: guidelines for individuals with advanced skills,* Position papers 1989, Point Reyes Station, Calif. 1989, Wilderness Medical Society.
24. Knutson S, edition: American caving accidents: 1976-79, *NSS News* 39(5 [part 2]):A1-82, 1981.
25. Knutson S, edition: American caving accidents: 1980-81, *NSS News* 41(3):99-118, 1983.
26. Knutson S, edition: American caving accidents: 1982, *NSS News* 41(10):255-65, 1983.
27. Knutson S, edition: American caving accidents: 1983, *NSS News* 42(11 [part 2]):347-58, 1984.
28. Knutson S, edition: American caving accidents: 1984, *NSS News* 43(11 [part 2]):355-67, 1985.
29. Knutson S, edition: American caving accidents: 1985, *NSS News* 44(11 [part 2]):399-410, 1986.
30. Knutson S, edition: American caving accidents: 1986, *NSS News* 45(11 [part 2]):386-98, 1987.
31. Knutson S, edition: American caving accidents: 1987, *NSS News* 46(12 [part 2]):475-90, 1988.
32. Knutson S, edition: American caving accidents: 1988, *NSS News* 47(12 [part 2]):314-34, 1989.
33. Knutson S, edition: American caving accidents: 1989, *NSS News* 48(12 [part 2]):331-49, 1990.
34. Lentz JM, Macdonald SC and Carline JD: *Mountaineering first aid: a guide to accident response and first aid care,* ed 3, Seattle, 1985, The Mountaineers.
35. McLennan JG and Ungersma J: Mountaineering accidents in the Sierra Nevada, *Am J Sports Med* 11(3):160-3, 1983.
36. National Association of Diver Medical Technicians: *Field guide for the diver medical technician,* Bay City, Tex, 1983, The Association.
37. National Highway Traffic Safety Administration: *Emergency medical services: first responder training course,* Washington DC, US Government Printing Office.
38. National Safety Council: *First aid and CPR,* Boston, 1991, Jones & Bartlett Publishers Inc.
39. Paton BC: Health, safety and risk in outward bound, *J Wildl Med* 3(2):128-44, 1992.
40. Rural Affairs Committee NAEMSP: Clinical guidelines for delayed/prolonged transport: I. cardiorespiratory arrest, *Prehospital and Disaster Medicine* 6(3):335-40, 1991.
41. Safety Committee AAC: *Accidents in north american mountaineering 1960,* New York, 1960, American Alpine Club.
42. Safety Committee AAC: *Accidents in north american mountaineering 1969,* New York, 1969, American Alpine Club.
43. Safety Committee AAC: *Accidents in north american mountaineering 1973,* New York, 1973, American Alpine Club.
44. Safety Committee AAC: *Accidents in north american mountaineering 1974,* New York, 1974, American Alpine Club.
45. Schussman LC et al: The epidemiology of mountaineering and rock climbing accidents, *J Wildl Med* 1(4):235-48, 1990.

46. Wilderness Medical Society: *Backcountry first aid workshop.* Position paper presented at Yosemite Park, November 1984, Point Reyes Station, Calif, 1984, The Society.
47. Wilderness Medical Society Prehospital Committee: Wilderness prehospital emergency care (WPHEC) curriculum, *J Wildl Med* 2(2):80-7, 1991.
48. Wilkerson JA: *Medicine for mountaineering,* ed 3, Seattle, 1985, The Mountaineers.
49. Williamson JE, edition: *Accidents in north american mountaineering 1976,* New York, 1976, American Alpine Club.
50. Williamson JE and Miskiw O, editions: *Accidents in north american mountaineering 1991,* New York, 1991, American Alpine Club.
51. Williamson JE and Reader R, editions: *Accidents in north american mountaineering 1981,* New York, 1981, American Alpine Club.
52. Williamson JE and Reader R, editions: *Accidents in north american mountaineering 1982,* New York, 1982, American Alpine Club.
53. Williamson JE and Reader R, editions: *Accidents in north american mountaineering 1983,* New York, 1983, American Alpine Club.
54. Williamson JE and Whalley E, editions: *Accidents in north american mountaineering 1977,* New York, 1977, American Alpine Club.
55. Williamson JE and Whalley E, editions: *Accidents in north american mountaineering 1978,* New York, 1978, American Alpine Club.
56. Williamson JE and Whitteker J, editions: *Accidents in north american mountaineering 1988,* New York, 1988, American Alpine Club.
57. Williamson JE and Whitteker J, editions: *Accidents in north american mountaineering 1989,* New York, 1989, American Alpine Club.
58. Williamson JE and Whitteker J, editions: *Accidents in north american mountaineering 1990,* New York, 1990, American Alpine Club.

7

Military Systems

Matthew M. Rice, M.D., J.D., FACEP
John F. Brown, M.D., FACEP

Necessity as the mother of invention is an apt maxim for the early development of military EMS. Some of the earliest EMS experience came from information and expertise gathered through medical support of military operations. A structured and organized system of early medical care and evacuation has developed to deal with the high numbers of casualties in armed conflicts. Today, we take much for granted in civilian and military emergency care systems, but organized EMS systems are a relatively recent development.

Background

Throughout much of history, the care of wounded soldiers was neglected or poorly administered. Military commanders were more concerned with tactics, troop movements, and supply. Casualties were a nuisance and given little thought. Before the eighteenth century, surgeons accompanying armies served only the nobility. The troops had to depend on comrades in arms or family. Queen Isabella of Spain was the first monarch to organize help for wounded soldiers. In 1487 at the siege of Malaga, her armies carried wounded soldiers in bedded wagons to large tent hospitals in safe areas. These ambulances were cumbersome often requiring up to 40 horses to pull them. They were stationed miles from the battlefield and frequently bogged down in muddy roads. The surgeons had to wait hours to reach the injured and then provide what little care was possible. Progressive military leaders recognized that poor medical care wasted military manpower and was demoralizing to the soldier.[4]

Systematic collection of the wounded from the battlefield began during the Napoleonic Wars. Recognizing that battlefield casualty care neared complete chaos, Napoleon appointed Jean Larrey to develop what became known as the "ambulance volantes" or flying field hospitals. These lightweight carriages and hospital facilities moved quickly to collect, transport, and care for the injured even as the fighting continued.[13] The word *ambulance* developed its true meaning. Unfortunately, few of these innovations were exported to America. The wartime lessons learned in Europe were ignored or quickly forgotten.

The first major test of US military emergency medical care was the Civil War. Between 1861 and 1865, more than 300,000 soldiers died on the Union side alone. Although battle injuries accounted for 100,000 deaths, the remainder were caused by disease. The first major battle of the war was Bull Run in 1861. It was a true disaster by most military and medical standards. Overconfident and ill-prepared the Union Army entered the battle with few ambulances or medical personnel. Litter bearers were untrained bandsmen who laid down their instruments and picked up litters. The civilian ambulance drivers drank the alcohol in their medicine chest and stayed near the battlefield only long enough to rob the wounded of their valuables. Ambulances that did not break down or had not been commandeered by officers for their personal use were often used by nonwounded panicking Union soldiers. In the Union Army's retreat, not a single wounded person was transported to the safety of Washington, DC. Fearing for their lives, many wounded men performed remarkable feats. Many walked and crawled the 27 miles to Washington including one man who had his arm amputated, one man with a large hole through both thighs and scrotum, one man with a large hole in both calves, and one man with a hole through both cheeks and his tongue. These were the lucky victims. Three days after the battle, 3000 wounded men still lay on the battlefield without food, water, or protection from the summer sun and rain. Some were without care for 6 to 7 days. Many died from lack of food, water, and basic medical care.[2]

Wars teach costly lessons. After the disaster at Bull Run the Union military realized that medical care was inadequately organized. Improvements were necessary to maintain soldier effectiveness and morale. Military commanders realized that it is easier to convince soldiers to fight when they know evacuation and medical care will be provied for the wounded. It soon became inherent in military thinking that once an army had taken the field casualty care was of high importance. Shortly after the Bull Run fiasco, the military began restructuring its haphazard wartime emergency care services into an organized system. William Hammond, the Surgeon General of the Union Army, and Jonathan Letterman, the medical director of the Army of the Potomac, were the primary agents of change.

Since the nineteenth century, military training, funding, manpower, and organization have come together in a system that has been stressed, tested, and refined. The military approach to EMS began long before civilian systems were formed in the 1960s and 1970s.

The military EMS system relies on the training of individual soldiers in preventive medicine and first aid, properly positioned care providers ranging from medics to surgeons, adequate numbers and availability of appropriate ambulances, and availability of graduated care. Rapid transport and early surgery in hospitals with sophisticated technologic capabilities made a tremendous impact on military preparedness by preventing disease, boosting morale, and conserving manpower. Through evolving technology and individual creativity, the military medical system has continually improved wartime military casualty survival rates (Table 7-1). Some estimate that more than 22,000 lives were saved in Vietnam as a result of advances beyond the medical care methods and standards of the Korean War.

The lessons learned and innovations prompted by wartime circumstances were brought to the United States by returning military medical care providers. Elements of the systems approach to emergency medical care were eventually integrated into the civilian community. This transition was slow unfortunately. Although tremendous strides were made in medical specialization, as veterans returned to their peacetime communities their experiences in Korea and Vietnam brought acceptance of organized systems for emergency care. Contributing to civilian growth were military influences and resources including medical centers and assistance to civilians such as the Military Assistance to Safety and Traffic (MAST) program. Civilian EMS services enjoyed tremendous growth during the 1960s and 1970s. Thus the military has played a large role in the establishment of the current EMS system in the United States.[4]

Table 7-1. Mortality of Battle Casualties Reaching Treatment Facilities

War	Mortality (%)
World War I	8.0
World War II	4.5
Korea	2.5
Vietnam	2.0

Current Military EMS

To understand the modern military EMS system it is important to understand military wartime and peacetime needs including military-civilian interaction. The goal of each is to accomplish a mission. The military medical system's specific mission is to "conserve the fighting strength."[1] During peacetime the mission is accomplished much as it is in the civilian EMS community, but it is drastically modified in form, procedure, and administration during conflict. The military wartime medical structure can best be understood by describing its personnel, organization, transportation, equipment, communications, and control.

Personnel

The Army provides medical assistance through a spectrum of trained personnel. From frontline medics with basic skills to sophisticated nursing, physician, administrative, and logistical support, individuals are assigned a specific job with their skills represented by an associated Military Occupational Skills (MOS) number. These descriptive numbers with associated training and skills are divided into medic level identifiers as follows.

The 91A medical specialist receives 10 weeks of training including skills equivalent to basic emergency medical technician (EMT-B) training. Additional training is provided in intravenous insertion and the care of patients with military-related problems such as nuclear, biological, and chemical warfare injuries.

The 91B-30 medical noncommissioned officer receives 12 weeks of training in addition to the basic

91A training. The training is at least equivalent to an EMT Intermediate (EMT-I). Skills include intubation, intravenous access, and advanced cardiac life support (ACLS).

The 91C practical nurse receives 36 weeks of training following 91A training. This number is equivalent to civilian Licensed Practical Nurse training.

The Air Force's version of the Army identification system is the Air Force Specialty Code (AFSC). The 90230 medical technician receives 16 weeks of training including an EMT-A curriculum and additional training similar to that given to Army counterparts. Medical technicians progress to the 90250 level by completing self-study Career Development Courses (CDC) while enrolled in on-the-job training. The 90270 level is achieved by completing 1 year in upgrade training time and additional CDCs.

In the Navy the hospital corps provides the bulk of the manpower for prehospital emergency care. Most corpsmen are classified as general duty or 8404, which is similar to the Army's 91A medical specialist. After 10 weeks of training, they usually have 1 year of inpatient care experience before working in EMS. Corpsmen, classified as 8425, act as dispatchers, First Response providers, and trainers of other personnel. All corpsmen must be EMT-A certified and must complete an emergency vehicle operator course before serving as ambulance crew members. Corpsmen can continue in specialty schools; the most relevant to EMS is independent duty training, which is 1 year in duration. These corpsmen are assigned to isolated duty stations such as small ships where they may practice medicine independent of direct physician control for long periods of time (Table 7-2).

In all branches of the uniformed services, medical direction is provided by the branch medical corps. Military physicians are required to be state licensed, and the majority are specialty board certified. Special military needs require physicians be trained and proficient in medical problems specific to their patient populations.

Military dentists actively participate in the system during wartime. In addition to their usual peacetime dental care activities, during conflict they serve as triage officers and assist with anesthesia and wound management.

The nursing corps provides EMS support in several ways. Nurses meet special criteria in critical care wartime medical missions and staff hospital ships, field hospitals, and fixed facility hospitals. Nursing personnel are also the primary trainers of hospital

Table 7-2. Navy Corpsmen Specialties Involved in Emergency Medical Services

Designator	Title	EMS component served	Length of training beyond initial 10 wks (wks)	Refresher required
8402	Submarine Force Independent Duty Corpsman	Submarines	52	Yes
8404	Medical Field Service Technician	Marine units, casualty clearing stations, ambulance services	5	No
8406	Aerospace Medical Technician	Medevac squadrons	10	No
8425	Advanced Hospital Corpsman	Ships, casualty clearing stations, field hospitals	48	Yes
8432	Preventive Medicine Technician	Field hospitals	26	No
8483	Operating Room Technician	Casualty clearing stations, field hospitals	26	No
8485	Psychiatry Technician	SPRINT (Rapid Deployment Crisis Intervention) team, field hospitals	11	No
8493	Medical Deep Sea Diving Technician	Submarines, commando diving units	11	No
8707	Field Dental Service Technician	Casualty clearing stations, field hospitals	5	No

corpsmen and medics. Physician assistants provide primary medical care with special training in trauma for wartime needs.

All levels of providers receive training in emergency care specific to military needs including treatment of chemical and radiation casualties and handling mass casualty incidents. Military hospitals and EMS systems are mandated to exercise their mass casualty capabilities several times a year; deployable assets such as ships and special support facilities have these exercises on an even more frequent and mission-specific basis.

Organization

Using basic care providers, an integrated medical care system offers each patient the most sophisticated modern medicine. Most aspects of nursing care and essentially every medical specialty are incorporated into the military medical system. In addition, unique skills are necessary to meet special requirements including aeromedical, hyperbaric, radiation, chemical, and biological warfare specialists. Though the structure and mechanism differ somewhat between conflict and peacetime needs, providing the best of care for each ill and injured patient remains the goal of military medicine.

The military recognizes the benefits of bystander first aid, first responders, triage, and early evacuation. Experience has demonstrated that morbidity and mortality can be significantly decreased through intelligent use of an organized prehospital care system, an appropriately accessed hospital system, aggressive use of technology, and a rapid evacuation system that moves patients to higher levels of care.[3] The basic concepts in military medical care are preventive medicine and self first aid. Every soldier, sailor, marine, and member of the air force is trained to prevent injury; however, if injured each is trained to administer self first aid. Individuals are also trained to assist injured members of their unit. "Buddy aid" includes airway management, hemorrhage control, splinting, and basic shock. The ability to provide medical treatment to an injured colleague is an integral part of the system. The first line of additional assistance is from combat medics or corpsmen.

In the Army, medics are assigned to each combat unit. They provide medical care and arrange transportation of the injured and ill to higher level of care aid stations. An aid station is a very mobile facility near the frontlines staffed by a physician assistant or a general medical officer and several medics. Triage, basic lifesaving procedures, and minor care are provided before the soldier is sent back to duty or evacuated to the next echelon of care, the clearing station. Limited laboratory and radiologic support is present at the clearing station as is the capability for some basic lifesaving surgery. Once again the casualty is triaged and referred to higher levels of care including mobile field and combat support hospitals or more definitive fixed facilities (Figure 7-1).[8]

As casualties move to higher echelons of care, medical support becomes more sophisticated with greater numbers of providers and more technologically advanced nursing, laboratory, radiographic, and physician support. When conditions and logistics permit, critical casualties may be transported

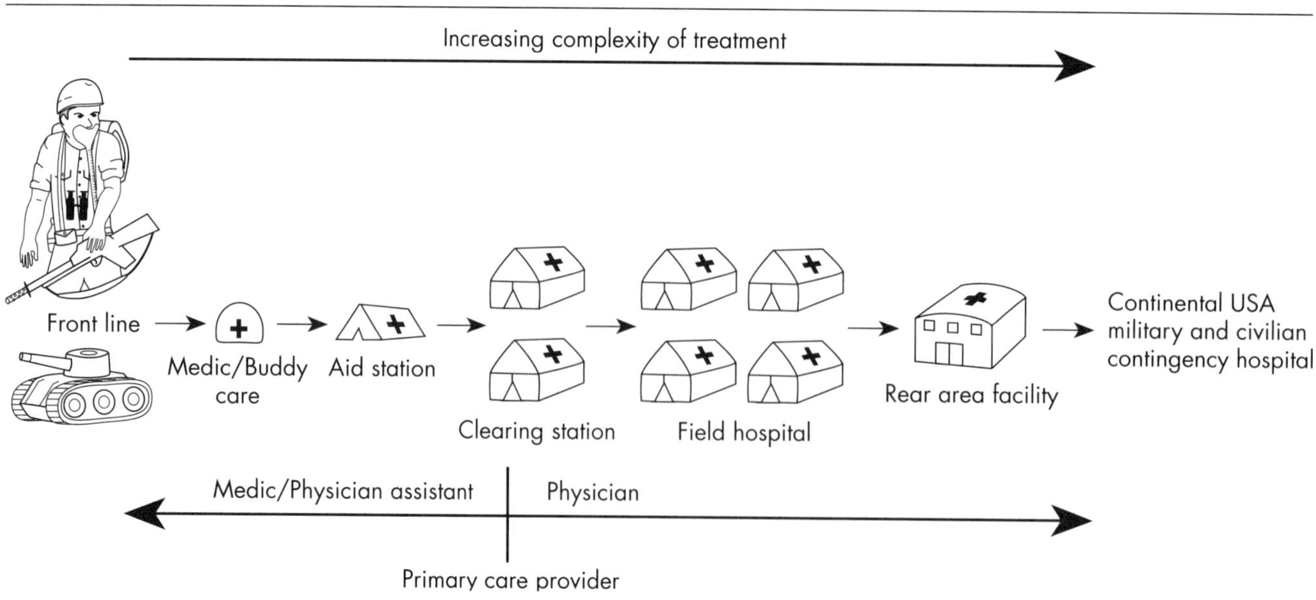

Figure 7-1. Echelons of emergency care.

directly from the site of injury to fixed hospitals, bypassing the lower levels of care. With great numbers of casualties, this is not feasible or desirable.

Transportation

Simple methods including manual carries, handheld litters, and specialized wheeled and tracked field ambulances are used for transportation from the battlefield. Other forms of transportation including trucks, specially equipped buses, ships, and even trains are also available. In addition, fixed and rotary-wing aeromedical evacuation are used extensively for wartime and peacetime needs. During peacetime, modern, state of the art ground and air equipment are used for transportation.

Equipment

Medical equipment is often limited by weight and space restrictions in initial medical care. Initial care equipment includes airway, breathing, circulatory, hemorrhage control, and splinting devices. Intravenous circulatory support and basic invasive procedures including needle and tube thoracostomies may be performed at the aid station. Simple lifesaving surgery may be performed at the clearing station, but definitive procedures are reserved for the hospitals further in the evacuation chain. Rear-area evacuation hospitals are capable of modern, sophisticated services.

Communications

Key principles in wartime care are locating patients rapidly, moving them to safety, completing triage at each level, continually performing basic life support (BLS) procedures, and moving viable patients to an appropriate higher level of care as rapidly as possible. The direct radio supervision of field providers that is common in peacetime cannot occur in battle. Radio communications in the tactical setting must be minimized for security reasons.[15] Decisions must often be made by independently functioning providers.

The organization of Navy EMS in wartime is similar to that of the Army, as illustrated in Figure 7-1. Clearing stations and field hospitals servicing the marine expeditionary forces are often collocated with combat support units to facilitate supply and evacuation logistics. There are no dedicated aeromedical assets in the marine field environment; thus, patient transportation must be coordinated with troop and supply transport units. Frequent use of helicopters may bring the patient directly to a hospital ship or primary casualty receiving ship such as an amphibious assault ship with the treatment capability of a rear-area facility. All amphibious assault ships' secondary mission is casualty care; many are capable of accommodating several hundred patients and providing advanced diagnostic and surgical services.

In the case of casualties generated by a shipboard incident, response by the ship's medical department is usually rapid and effective. The ship environment poses constraints of difficult extraction and hazardous operating conditions. Such problems are overcome by training, drills, a pervasive emphasis on safety, and ingenious ideas such as specialized stretchers, backpack transport of medical supplies to incident locations, and location of multiple satellite treatment facilities (battle dressing stations) throughout the ship. Patients with injuries or illnesses beyond the capabilities of the ship's sick bay are evacuated to a rear-area facility or major hospital ship.

Military Peacetime EMS Mission

In peacetime the EMS systems at military facilities generally follow the civilian model. Ambulances are based at hospitals or branch clinics and are staffed by corpsmen or medics with a minimum of EMT-A training. Medical control is provided by the base hospital emergency department through a combination of direct radio communication with the emergency department physician and indirect protocols. Response areas are usually limited to the bases themselves but may extend well into the surrounding community.

Interaction with the Civilian Community

Military units are supported by facilities at fixed-posts or fixed-bases. Each military base or post is a federally owned and operated enclave governed as an independent federal jurisdiction often surrounded by civilian communities. The base or post usually has its own community services such as water, waste disposal, health care, and fire and police protection. Some of these services may be purchased from or shared with the civilian community. The military is often dependent on the goodwill of neighbors; the civilian communities are often dependent on the jobs and revenues generated by the military presence. Both communities may depend on each other for a variety of services. One of these services is medical care.

Each post or base is generally responsible for its own medical care under the direction and support of a centralized military medical command. The post may depend on military BLS or ALS personnel to respond to emergencies and transport patients to a military or local civilian facility. Some military institutions have the only resources for ambulance or emergent medical care in a community and share them with the civilian population. The medical services of each post are linked to the overall military medical care system. From isolated posts, patients are referred to military hospitals at larger posts for secondary care. These posts are linked to a series of more sophisticated tertiary care medical centers each with special capabilities, consultants, and equipment. However, referral is not restricted to military systems. A patient may be referred to the closest appropriate hospital, whether military or civilian. Conversely, civilian patients may be referred to a military facility when appropriate resources are not otherwise available.

A unique feature of military EMS is the large number of overseas hospitals. Some are located in communities where EMS is poor or nonexistent. In these situations the response area may be very large and response may involve helicopter or fixed-wing assets. Transferring patients to host country facilities for further care is often difficult and necessitates attention to protocol development and maintenance of contacts with local EMS personnel.

Military hospitals often provide resources not available to the civilian community. Many serve as specialty care centers for large geographic areas. Madigan Army Medical Center in Tacoma, Washington, Brooke Army Medical Center in San Antonio, Texas, William Beaumont Army Medical Center in El Paso, Texas, and Wilford Hall Air Force Hospital in San Antonio, Texas all serve as trauma centers in their communities. Madigan is an important provider of paramedic ambulance services for an otherwise unprotected portion of Washington; it also serves as an EMS direct medical control facility. Darnall Army Hospital in Killeen, Texas is the only hospital providing sophisticated emergency services in a large area of central Texas. Brooke Army Medical Center is an important international resource for burn victims. The Armed Forces Institute of Pathology serves as an important international referral and review center for medical services. These resources and many more enhance rather than compete with civilian services.

The use of military resources for community services is exemplified by the MAST program.[11] Since 1969 the MAST program has provided military aeromedical evacuation capabilities to civilian communities. They have flown thousands of missions and transported tens of thousands of patients. This has been accomplished safely and without expense to the patients; the military has benefited by maintaining aeromedical evacuation skills.[10] Such services were the forerunners to the now prevalent civilian air-medical programs. In developing civilian programs, much was learned from military air-medical evacuation experience.[7] Since the development of civilian helicopter systems throughout the United States, the number of MAST missions has declined. This is primarily because the military may not compete with civilian free enterprise systems. Where civilian aeromedical systems exist, they must be accessed first and decline a mission before MAST may participate.

This noncompetition concept can be a major hindrance to the development of joint military-civilian EMS systems. Regulating agencies often view cooperation as competition even when it best meets the needs of the military and civilian communities.

EMS ground ambulance services are another potential area for shared resources between the military and civilian communities. In areas where the military has few medical resources the government often contracts the civilian community to provide ambulance coverage. However, many military facilities have ambulance services available for routine and emergency responses both on the post and in the surrounding community. Military ambulances must meet federal equipment standards. Likewise, prehospital providers must meet federal and state training standards. Medical control remains mostly in the hands of the military installation medical personnel. As in civilian systems the depth of medical control, institutional support of EMS, and quality and interest of the participants is relative to their commitment to quality medical care. Ironically, some excellent military EMS services stop at the boundary of the federal installation. In other areas, federal ambulances share responsibility with civilian ambulance services providing optimal use of resources. In addition, such emergency care provides excellent training and skill maintenance for military medics and physicians caring for acutely ill patients.

Some civilian communities are reluctant to approach the military for assistance or cooperative medical planning. This often leads to a loss of resources for the community and a loss of training for the military. In fact, there are numerous precedents for such joint efforts. In those areas where military resources fill a need, the civilian community should approach the military facility commander with requests for assistance. The facility commander has some authority to assist the civilian community. Authority for further assistance can be requested by facility commanders from higher headquarters. Because a large portion of the civilian community is often comprised of retired and active military personnel and their families, extending services to the civilian community benefits them and is often in the best interest of the military. However, caution must be taken not to overburden the existing military system in its military mission. Likewise, caution must be taken to avoid the perception of competition or interference in the civilian sector. Several instances have been documented in which private EMS services voiced concern over the loss of patients and revenues to government health care providers. Such complaints resulted in a pullback of military resources that previously complemented the civilian community.

The Military and the National Disease Medical System

The Department of Defense is a prime initiator, planner, and current participant in the National Disease Medical System (NDMS). Military resources are the transportation backbone for many NDMS missions. Military personnel and facilities assist in the coordination of participating hospital networks. Department of Defense leadership, medical personnel, and logistic groups may assist in relief efforts.[6,9,12]

Although not yet well-tested, the NDMS concept holds great potential for combining military and civilian medical missions. With the decreasing likelihood of large military confrontations, it seems logical to divert some of the well-organized and trained medical assets to peacetime disaster needs of the NDMS. Excellent equipment with transportation assets and organized, trained medical personnel are logical choices for future NDMS needs. This will also provide practical exercises for military contingencies.

Summary

The military pioneered systematic emergency care. Both the military and civilian sectors have come a long way in adapting wartime lessons to peacetime EMS.[9] The sharing of resources and responsibilities by civilian and military communities can improve these services even more. Because much can be learned from each other, open professional exchanges and planning to meet the needs of the ill and injured must take priority over issues of jurisdiction, sources of payment, and patient eligibility. Working from these premises, the mission and goals of both sectors may be accomplished.

REFERENCES

1. Academy of Health Sciences, US Army: *Health services support in a theater of operation,* Ft. Sam Houston, Tex, 1983, The Academy.
2. Adams GW: *Doctors in blue,* New York, 1961, Collier Books.
3. Bellamy R: The causes of death in conventional land warfare: implications for combat casualty care research, *Military Medicine* 1495:55-62, 1984.
4. Boyd D, Edlilch R, and Micik S, editors: *Systems approach to emergency medical care,* Norwalk, Conn, 1983, Appleton-Century-Crofts.
5. Department of the Army: *Soldiers manual and trainer's guide,* Washington, DC, 1985, The Department.
6. Dolicker GJ: Preparing for the worst: The challenge facing NDMS, *JEMS* 16(8):94-100, Aug 1991.
7. Dorland P: *Dust off: army aeromedical evacuation in Vietnam,* Washington, DC, 1982, Center of Military History, United States Army.
8. Duggan B: *Organization of military medical units.* In: Burkle F, editor: *Disaster medicine,* New York, 1984, Medical Examination Co.
9. Heaton LD: Army medical service activities in Vietnam, *Military Medicine* 131:646, 1966.
10. Interagency Executive Group: *Program manual for MAST programs,* Jan 1978.
11. Military Assistance to Safety and Traffic (MAST): *Emergency employment of army and other resources,* Army Regulation No 500-4, Washington, DC, Jan 1982, Department of the Army.
12. National Disaster Medical Systems: *Concept of operations,* Rockville, Md, 1991, National Disaster Medical System.
13. Richardson GR: *Larrey: surgeon to Napoleon's imperial guard,* London, 1974, John Murray.
14. Stewart MJ: *Moving the wounded: litters, cacolets and ambulance wagons, U S Army 1776-1876,* Fort Collins, Colo, 1979, The Old Army Press.
15. US Department of Defense: *Emergency war surgery: NATO handbook,* 1st revision, Washington DC, 1975, US Government Printing Office.

8

Legislation

Raymond L. Fowler, M.D., FACEP

Excellence in prehospital emergency medical management requires careful attention to EMS system structure and design at state and local levels. EMS is the provision of physician evaluation and management of prehospital emergency medicine through the employment of prehospital providers. In some systems, on-scene physician attention is a dynamic portion of patient care. However, for the most part, field personnel provide patient assessment and management in the absence of physicians. Modern parlance, especially as expressed in the mission statement of the National Association of EMS Physicians, suggests that providers' skills are generally considered extensions of the medical oversight physician's license.

EMS providers are rarely independent practitioners. They are trained in specific skills and have quite rigid descriptions of clinical conditions for which they may render patient care. EMS providers are permitted to complete their various medical duties and responsibilities as "dependent practitioners." Though they possess skills and are allowed by law to perform procedures, they can apply certain skills only through authorization by physicians either by prearranged protocol (indirect medical control) or real-time physician order (direct medical control).

All EMS providers have a specific "scope of practice." This means that they may perform only those skills delineated either in statute (written in the law) or in regulation (outlined by the department responsible under the statute for regulating these matters). Therefore, independence to "practice medicine and surgery" is not a privilege of prehospital providers who are limited to the skills mentioned.

This chapter describes how EMS providers become authorized to perform skills in the prehospital and interhospital environment. Mention is also made as to how legislation provides a legal framework for the development of EMS systems. Sample legislation that may be examined as a model for the design and implementation of EMS systems is also offered.

General Concepts

The fundamental element of an EMS system is medicine; the basic purpose is to offer relief for public cries of distress caused by acute medical conditions. The functional parameters required to operate a system such as hiring trained personnel, providing equipment, managing finances, maintaining supervision, solving problems, and being mired down in paperwork can easily relegate the "medicine" of EMS as secondary to "operations." System design and structure must revolve around the quality management of medicine.

EMS systems, like all medical provider systems, provide most hands-on medical care through technical support. EMS medical care is generally practiced in the physical absence of the physician. However, enabling legislation provides for physician assessment and treatment skills to be performed by EMS personnel. This concept has been popular in medical oversight circles for at least a decade; but as EMS providers acquire greater responsibility, it is arguably true that many physician skills are becoming field provider skills.

Some EMS legislation places other individuals between the physician and the patient. For example, in California the mobile intensive care nurse (MICN) provides prehospital care and instructs EMS personnel. The MICN is a registered nurse who is functioning pursuant to Section 2725 of the Business and Professions Code and who has been authorized by the medical director of the local EMS agency as qualified to provide prehospital advanced life support or to issue instructions to prehospital emergency medical care personnel within an EMS system according to standardized procedures developed by the local EMS agency consistent with statewide guidelines established by the authority.

In the emergency department a physician can maintain a one-on-one relationship with a patient; there is no distance between them. If the physician gives an order to the nurse some distance develops between the physician and the patient as the nurse performs the duty. It is the physician's responsibility to guard the relationship with the patient. In the field the EMS personnel work as a direct extension of the physician and in accordance with the contract established between the physician and the patient. When the physician's role in the patient care scenario falls to zero the physician's relationship with the patient is breached.

History and Development

Independent physician practice acts have been predominant in the United States for generations. Encounters including the diagnosis, disposition, treatment, and release of patients are limited to physician authority, except in states where independent practitioners such as nursing practitioners and physician assistants are authorized. In many of these excepted situations the non-physicians practice under some form of blanket authority extended to them by a licensed physician. It should be emphasized that this discussion is essentially limited to the United States and "westernized" nations in general. Many countries, especially Russia and China, utilize physicians as part of routine care in the field. Some countries require field "rotation" as a part of a physician's routine duties under a national or local medicine provision program. Such practice extension generally describes the subordinate practitioner as a dependent practitioner.

EMS is somewhat new in the long history of medical practice. The lack of physicians to respond to the scene of accidents and illnesses, the growing sophistication of extrication and transport techniques, the general lack of familiarity by physicians of field conditions, and the growing need for secondary transport to alternative levels of care are some of the reasons that lead to the increased demand for and subsequent provision of prehospital providers who were not independent practitioners.

Provision of initial patient care by technicians, especially when advanced skills such as endotracheal intubation and intravenous medications are used, generally requires the enactment of a state law enabling non-physicians to assume certain medical skills with physician oversight. Laws enacted for this purpose are deemed "enabling legislation." Other aspects of such laws enable the state, region, or locality to develop regulations to fulfill legislative goals and intent.

Enabling legislation allows non-physicians to provide specific diagnostic and treatment skills. Although all states provide some sort of EMS enabling legislation, many do not view their statutes as providing specific extension of physician licenses to the prehospital arena. This is due in part to the development of extensive EMS medical oversight long after most initial EMS statutes were set in place. Only later did EMS physicians realize that field providers were practicing skills requiring physician authorization, skill, time, and judgment and the subsequent medicolegal risk extended to the physician's themselves. In the 1980s, revised EMS statutes began to reflect that the medical oversight physician was extending his medical license and authority to the non-physician technician.

One reason for the recent formal licensure extension was the need to assure the quality of medical care through physician review and direction. Whether by clear and concise mandate or inferential statutory construction, the role of the physician is generally acknowledged as the central element of medical oversight.

Another reason for licensure extension is the merger of traditional terms advanced life support (ALS) and basic life support (BLS); differences in ALS and BLS skills have essentially disappeared. Initially, any invasive procedure requiring medical oversight was considered ALS. However, determining whether a skill is BLS or ALS depending on the risk to the patient blurs the distinction. Suctioning an airway, traditionally a BLS skill, incurs great risk to the patient if inappropriately performed. Direct and indirect medical control physicians bear the responsibility for all prehospital skills. Therefore the medical oversight is responsible for all assessment and management skills practiced by all levels of prehospital providers.

Rule-making

Newcomers to the legislative process may not be familiar with the concepts of legislative mandate and departmental rule-making. The state legislature is the collective voice of the citizens. Federal issue generally supersedes state legislative issue. The legislative voice of the state, through discussions and votes, provides laws or statutes. After the generation or modification of the statute, further definition and explanation are often required. State executive departments promulgate regulations in fulfillment of their operational roles and provide further definition and explanation. The formation of rules and regulations is an important method by which a state shapes policy to address the general instructions given under a statute.

Not uncommonly the statute may contain only a few sentences, but the rules and regulations addressing the statute may run to reams. For example, the Georgia EMS statute states that "to enhance the provision of emergency medical care, each ambulance service shall be required to have a medical adviser [and] the duties of the medical adviser shall be to provide medical direction and training for the ambulance service personnel in conformance with acceptable emergency medical practices and procedures." The Georgia Department of Human Resources rules and regulations list many headings by which the medical adviser is to perform these duties including formulation of policy and procedures affecting patient care; formulation, development, and evaluation of training objectives; establishment of quality control; and performance of liaison roles with the greater medical community.*

It is critical that the EMS physician be informed concerning state regulations relative to EMS. Meaningful input of the appropriate departments when rules and regulations are being created or changed is essential. Approaches to EMS statutes differ from state to state. What is actually written law and what is left to rules and regulations also varies significantly. For all practical purposes the statute and subsequent regulation carry the same authority. Although penalties exist for violations of either, it is far easier to modify a regulation than to amend a statute.

Sample Components of EMS Law

EMS statutes contain many elements. This section discusses in some detail concepts of selected elements that may be found in a state EMS statute.

Title

Each EMS statute has a title indicative of the content that will follow. Typical titles include Emergency Medical Services and Emergency Medical Care Personnel.

EMS is a service provided to the public similar to fire and police protection. The titles of EMS statutes make it clear that medicine is the service. There may be a medical act separate from the legislative act establishing the state medical board. The public can demand that a service be provided and the state will provide that service irrespective of existing physician medical acts. EMS legislation often emphasizes the incompleteness of existing physician practice acts. The entirety of the EMS statute could be covered under the rules established by the state medical board; however, the complexity of EMS, including personnel, management, certification, and ambulance licensure, necessitates detail that cannot be included solely in the state medical board purview. Thus the EMS statute often provides direction to a department that can manage such administrative details.

The provision of EMS is rooted in many different resources such as fire departments, other public safety agencies, and hospitals. There are private providers in the business of providing EMS. In addition, public providers were established by many counties, fire districts, rescue agencies, and municipalities. Ideally, EMS statutes create the framework for prehospital medicine to be provided by well-trained personnel, staffing carefully maintained vehicles, dispatching through controlled communications systems, ultimately providing an equitable distribution of patient calls.

Rationale

In the rationale section of an EMS statute a statement is made as to why the state legislature approved the statute. Typically it states that the legislature finds it in the public interest to assure that emergency medical services are readily available and coordinated. Occasionally the need for quality in the provision of these services is included. The complex nature of EMS makes coordination essential; it is not a given that such services are in fact highly coordinated. In general, if something that cannot take care of itself is important to the public the government will step in and ascertain the need for a law that provides regulation. This is an important justification for EMS laws. It is equally important, of course, to allow extension of physician practice to non-physician providers in the prehospital environment. However, the fact that EMS is important to the public is most commonly the actual driving force behind legislation.

The state is responsible for protecting the public interest and has broad power through the legisla-

*Georgia EMS Code Chapter 11 and Department of Human Resources Rules and Regulations Chapter 290-05-30.

tive process to carry out this duty. In general, a state may regulate anything considered in the public interest or presenting a risk to citizens. EMS is viewed by many legislatures as just such an entity that should be broadly regulated. Matters relative to EMS that may be regulated include the distribution of calls, the number of providers established in the interest of economy and efficiency, the regulation of the flow of patients to trauma centers, the provision of immunity from civil liability, and the description of who is allowed to carry out EMS duties.*

State and Local Administration

Typically, EMS statutes address the various official positions required for administration of the system.

State EMS director. Statewide professional direction of the EMS system is under the guidance of a state EMS director. There is a national organization of these directors.[†] The state EMS director is usually not a physician, though this varies from state to state.[‡] The state EMS director functions both as the manager of the office that generates state EMS policy and as the enforcer of that policy. Other duties include directing licensure, certification, recertification, and disciplinary processes. Typically the appointment is made by the governor or the director of the state health or public safety agency. Responsibilities include management of the system and medical matters. In the absence of medical training the state EMS director should not give medical opinions. It is not the purpose of the state EMS director to make quality assurance judgments regarding medical care. The need for a person with a medical background to make such judgments cannot be overemphasized; medical oversight is extremely important to EMS.

State EMS committee, council, or commission. Many state EMS statutes provide for the appointment of a state EMS governing or advising committee, council, or commission. The responsibilities, compositions, and appointments of these groups vary significantly. Progressive statutes provide for appointment of a representative group from the EMS community including physicians, fire chiefs, administrators, county commissioners, and laypersons. In California the law provides for appointment of the EMS Commission, which has direct authority to establish rules regulating the state EMS system.[§] Although the EMS Board of Tennessee is similarly structured, this centralization of power is uncommon.[‖] Alabama has a state EMS medical control board consisting of physician representatives from the state's six EMS regions. Advisory in nature, this board makes recommendations directly to the Alabama Board of Health. In New York recommendations of the state medical board are made to the state EMS council for final approval.

The direct authority of the California EMS Commission should be contrasted with states such as Georgia, where only a passing reference to an "Emergency Medical Services Advisory Council" is made in the law.[¶] The Georgia Council is appointed by the state EMS director and has no direct authority. As in many other states, recommendations are made to the regulatory agency (in this case the Georgia Department of Human Resources), which

*Georgia EMS Code Chapter 11 and Department of Human Resources Rules and Regulations Chapter 290-05-30.

†National Association of State EMS Directors.

‡The State of California mandates, "The Emergency Medical Services Authority shall be headed by the Director of the Emergency Medical Services Authority who shall be appointed by the Governor upon nomination by the Secretary of the Health and Welfare Agency. The director shall be a physician and surgeon licensed in California pursuant to the Provisions of Chapter 5 of Division 2 of the Business and Professions Code, and who has substantial experience in the practice of emergency medicine." (1979.101) The Texas statute states that the bureau shall be under the direction of a bureau chief with proven ability as an administrator and organizer and with direct experience in emergency medical services. In filling the position of bureau chief, a preference shall be given to any applicant for the position who is a physician.

§The California statue provides for a Commission on Emergency Medical Services consisting of 16 members: one physician and surgeon whose primary practice is emergency medicine, one trauma surgeon, one physician representative from the California Medical Association, a county health officer, a registered nurse, a full-time paramedic, a private provider, a representative of fire protection, an emergency physician who is knowledgeable in state emergency medical services programs and issues, a hospital administrator of a base hospital, a peace officer, two public members who have experience in local EMS policy issues, a local agency, and an active member of one of the firefighting associations. This commission has direct authority to review and approve regulations, standards, and guidelines to be developed by the EMS Authority, to advise the authority on the development of an emergency medical data collection system, to advise state health facilities, and make recommendations for further developments. The Commission may use technical advisory panels. (1799.2)

‖The Tennessee statute provides for a Board of 13 members of similar appointments to 10 above though with fewer mandated physician members. This Board approves EMS schools and curricula, promulgates regulations for the issuance of licenses and certificates of personnel, services, and vehicles, provides for hearings, and establishes standards for the amounts and types of insurance coverage required for ambulance services. It also regulates the development and operation of EMS telecommunication systems and regulates fees. The Board's rulings are advisory to the Tennessee Board of Health.

¶State of Georgia EMS Statute, Code Chapter 11.

can act either positively or negatively on those recommendations. In practice the opinions of this body are accepted as authoritative, although they require review and final approval by the Department of Human Resources, the Composite Board of Medical Examiners, or both.

Formation of rules and regulations. Many statutes provide for an element of state government to make rules and regulations that "carry out the purposes and intent of this part and to enable the authority to exercise the powers and perform the duties conferred upon it by this part not inconsistent with any of the provisions of any statute of this state."* It is not practical or logical for the statute to contain all necessary policy and procedure for the provision of EMS.

One area of great variability among EMS statutes is the amount of detail. In the California statute the specific duties of EMS personnel are enumerated, but the certification and recertification standards are left to the regulatory agency approved by the EMS Commission. However, in the Georgia law the requirements for EMT-B recertification are delineated.

Rules and regulations become the living organ of the provision and administration of EMS; and the law is the guiding force for formation of the rules. Therefore if the law states that the regulatory agency should determine certification requirements, then the rules should provide for these requirements, generally after consultation with experts and the public.

Less astute statutes provide significant operational detail in the language of the law; modifications in the scope of practice then require changes in the law through the legislative process. In Georgia, for example, all duties of EMS personnel are spelled out in the statute. Therefore the provision of defibrillation by EMT-Bs required a change in the law. The wording and detail in the writing of EMS law is critical to the progress and growth of EMS systems. Changes in regulation are much easier than changes in statute. A well-thought-out statute will need very little modification.

Regional EMS councils or coordinating entities. The impact of the 1973 EMS System Act may be traced across the country by the development of regional EMS councils.† These councils considerably influenced the training of personnel, purchasing of equipment, and the initial design and direction of EMS systems.

Fiery politics raged when state legislators addressed the issue of regional EMS councils. Many private and public providers had a stake in the channeling of patients within the EMS systems. Regional councils in many states were authorized to make such determinations of need and award response zones to various providers.

The Georgia EMS law delineates a bureaucratic process for patient routing through a "local coordinating entity." This entity operates at the regional level in the stead of the controlling board of the state regulatory agency or its designee, the Director of Public Health.‡ Therefore the regional level has guidance and policy mandates from the state. The membership of these local coordinating entities is not spelled out in Georgia law.

On the other hand, the Pennsylvania EMS law details the membership, terms, quorums, and duties. Carrying out "the emergency medical services plans" of the state and region is included in the duties. The Texas statute provides for regional EMS councils, but also allows local providers to make their cases with the county commission or local municipalities; an appeal to the state is also available. A distinct flavor of the initial organization of a state's EMS structure can be gained from analyzing the establishment of regional EMS councils.

Local EMS planning. Many EMS statutes address the need for comprehensive planning by local EMS systems. The complex and sophisticated nature of EMS is exemplified in the delineations of how local-level issues should be handled. Such issues include awarding calls and response zones to various providers, handling complaints, managing the communications system, coordinating with state emergency preparedness agencies, approving new EMS providers, initiating contracts, providing for hearings, appointing EMS medical directors, developing mechanisms for quality improvement, and assigning responsibilities to a local EMS office.

This section of EMS law is vitally important in areas where EMS personnel cannot carry out med-

*California EMS Code 1797.107: Rules and regulations. Note that the EMS Commission in California must approve all regulations promulgated by the EMS Authority.

†Public Law 93-154, Emergency Medical Services Systems Act of 1973, Title XII of the Public Health Service Act.

‡"The Board of Human Resources shall have the authority on behalf of the state to designate and contract with a public or nonprofit local entity to coordinate and administer the EMSC Program for each health district designated by the Department of Human Resources. The local coordinating entity thus designated shall be responsible for recommending to the board or its designee the manner in which the EMSC Program is to be conducted." Georgia EMS Code 31-11-3.

ical acts unless employed. Since local-level certification is provided in such areas, EMS personnel are allowed to perform their duties only when employed by an approved EMS service in the geographical area. Lack of employment means inability to carry out prehospital skills professionally. Local-level medical oversight and system design therefore become prominent parts of the provision of EMS.

Ambulance Services

EMS statutes often focus on developing methods to approve vehicles and services. The extent to which methods are covered varies. Some statutes go as far as establishing local certificate of need (CON) procedures similar to those required for hospitals and other health facilities. Others, like the California EMS statute, leave the determination of approval to the state agency or local EMS systems.

The Georgia statute includes specifics on the application for licensure, the description and location of ambulances, the duties of the license officer, the requirements for insurance coverage, the ambulance standards specifications, and the procedures for renewal, suspension, and revocation.* The Tennessee law strikes a middle ground; it requires a state EMS board to form standards for ambulance vehicles and equipment, but the licensure, permit, and certification criteria are in another section of the law.[†]

In general, EMS statutes provide for the licensure of ground, air, and water vehicles and the systems that operate them. Performance standards are often defined either in law or rules. Inspections must be conducted by a state or local government entity. A logical inclusion is a provision for the revocation of system or vehicle licenses including allowable reasons for revocation and the method for appeal. Whether ambulance regulation is directly in the law or indirectly assigned to some portion of the system varies.

Medical Oversight

Authorization of EMS personnel to carry out medical activities also varies in EMS law. Typically the need for EMS and its coordinated provision is stated in the opening rationale statement. However, statutory descriptions of EMS as the provision of medical care through others are unusual. EMS laws often do not address this concept; consequently, EMS physicians in many states lack statutory authority for medical oversight.

The Georgia statute is a good example of the medical oversight problem. Although EMS systems are required to have a medical director to "enhance the provision of emergency medical care," this physician must simply be licensed to practice medicine in the state. If a medical director cannot be obtained, the district health director should fill the role. The enumerated duties of the medical director include providing medical oversight and training for the ambulance service personnel "in comformance with acceptable emergency medical practices and procedures." Notably and commendably, the rules and regulations use that statement to layout "acceptable emergency medical practices and procedures" of the medical director.[‡]

Since EMS law often does not instruct the responsible agency to draw up medical oversight regulations, it has been argued that the agency does not have the authority to address and expand the medical oversight portion of the statute by issuing rules and regulations. However, broad interpretation of the state EMS agency's responsibilities allows for such authority. In Georgia rules and regulations have been established for trauma systems despite the absence of specific authorization.[§] Statutory modification over the years has provided for greater specificity in medical oversight.

A striking contrast is the California law, which provides for medical oversight of EMS systems through prospective creation of policy and procedure, concurrent review, direct management, and retrospective audit.[||] It further states that these are minimum standards for any system implemented in the state.

An EMS law should provide direct physician authority for medicine practiced in the field. Any

*Georgia EMS code 31-11-30 through 31-11-36.

[†]"Standards for the design, construction, equipment, sanitation, operation, and maintenance of ambulances, invalid vehicles, and for the operations and minimum emergency care equipment for emergency response vehicles shall be promulgated by the EMS board. The EMS Board may authorize standards for the licensure of air ambulance services to provide for such special personnel equipment operation and activities as may be necessary. Permits shall not be required for individual aircraft." Tennessee EMS Statutes 68-140-506.

[‡]Georgia EMS Code Chapter 11 and Department of Human Resources Rules and Regulations Chapter 290-05-30.

[§]Senate Bill 320, 1989, now Code Chapter 31-11-60.1 provided for a name change from EMS medical "adviser" to "director" and provided for the first time sufficient authority for the medical director to perform quality assurance duties. Interestingly, this bill, though passed into law, did not go into effect for 2 years until 1991.

[||]"The medical direction and management of an emergency medical services system shall be under the medical control of the medical director of the local EMS agency." California EMS Act, 1798.(a). In 1990, the California EMS statute was changed to require that each local EMS agency have a medical director. This medical director must be a physician who has substantial experience in the practice of emergency medicine. (1797.202) medical system that may hold a physician liable for the practice of medicine should provide authority for design, implementation, maintenance, and quality improvement with the statute as the final arbiter. EMS physicians must determine how prehospital medicine will be practiced. Otherwise, the medicine practiced may not be under the final control of physicians. Difficulty establishing medical oversight at the state level is caused in part by the absence of national standards on EMS medical director education and responsibility.

Prehospital Care Reports

The requirement for recordkeeping is highly variable in EMS statutes. The Georgia law states, "Records of each ambulance trip shall be made by the ambulance service in a manner and on such forms as may be prescribed by the Department through regulations. Such records shall be available for inspection by the Department at any time, and a summary of ambulance service activities shall be prepared on specific cases and furnished to the Department upon request." The rules and regulations of Georgia detail what should be included on the prehospital care reports and the summary that must be submitted to the Department on request. The need for medical record confidentiality is mentioned in many statutes.*

Communications

The federal effort to bolster EMS through the EMS System Act concentrated on providing communication equipment. Consequently the authors of state statutes usually included methods of system design and regulation for such equipment, including the regulation of frequencies and occasionally the licensing of users. The term "communications" usually includes handling public calls, such as through 9-1-1 systems, and operating radio and telephone response equipment. Advancing communications technology has caused a gradual metamorphosis of EMS statutes. Cellular equipment and satellite communication are logical targets for EMS legislation and regulation.

An important part of communications addressed in state statutes is the provision of care in the absence of radio communication with direct medical control. The California statute addresses this point extensively.[†] Some states require completion of a special report, similar to a hospital incident report, if direct medical control contact cannot be made. Georgia, in its new allowance for standing orders, requires such a report.

Providers

Another fundamental area of EMS law is the provision for EMS personnel. Some state laws mention provider levels but assign state or local authorities to define these levels.[‡] On the other hand the Georgia statute meticulously defines all levels of EMS personnel. Such statutory delineation is trying in modern EMS. Changing duties of EMS personnel may be difficult if specifics are written into statute. Defibrillation could not be added as an EMT-B skill in Georgia until the law was changed. In New York, emergency medical technician-defibrillation (EMT-D) was implemented across the state, but only under the guise of an experimental trial.

The Texas Code of 1983 progressively provides minimum skill levels for EMS technicians, but allows the state agency to determine precisely what skills EMS personnel can perform. Other states allow localities to define the care provided at a given level.

Standards found in EMS statutes include certification, recertification, continuing education, active practice requirements, services by providers working in hospitals, methods for obtaining medications, disciplinary procedures, and standards for use of standing orders.

*The subject of medical records is not mentioned in either the Tennessee statute or the rules and regulations. Medical records are not mentioned in the California statute or in the Texas statute. In Tennessee, there exists a general requirement for record-keeping in a policy statement issued under authority of regulation. In California, there is regulation providing for record-keeping under statutory authority given to the rules-making process from 1791.107.

[†]"When an EMT-P who, at the scene of an emergency, reasonably determines that voice contact or a telemetered electrocardiogram for monitoring by a physician or authorized registered nurse cannot be established or maintained and that delaying treatment may jeopardize the life of a patient, and when authorized by policies and procedures approved by the local EMS authority, the EMT-P may initiate any paramedic procedure specified in this section in which such EMT-P has received training until such direct communication may be established and maintained or until the patient is brought to a general acute care hospital ..." California Code of Regulations Title 22, Social Security, Division 9, Pre-Hospital Emergency Medical Services, Chapter 4, EMT-Paramedic, Section 100144, Scope of Practice.

[‡]The State of California allows for modification of the basic state scope of practice for paramedics by EMS medical directors at the local level. Under 1797.172, the authority and commission adopt minimum state standards for training and scope of practice. Local level medical directors may petition a committee of local EMS medical directors named by the Emergency Medical Directors Association of California for additions to a "local optional scope of practice for EMT-P's ... prior to the implementation of the addition in the local system."

The inclusion of certain items in law may make later educational change cumbersome. In Georgia, for example, state-level recertification materials are minutely delineated, including the requirement that five "different and discrete" modules be covered over five years. It is difficult to cover skills such as patient assessment and endotracheal intubation that must be reviewed annually without conflicting with the statute.*

The Indiana EMS law is extremely progressive and should be read by anyone contemplating a change in law. A state agency is responsible for drawing up recertification requirements; the result is an excellent model for EMS providers.[†]

In 1992, 17 states "licensed" paramedics. The meaning of this licensure varies from state to state. The usual interpretation is that the licensed paramedic may carry out certain skills and procedures without the approval of direct medical control. This "dependent licensure" requires various system components such as physician medical oversight to allow the use of standing orders. However, many states that allow paramedics to use standing orders simply call the process "certification." No state licenses prehospital providers as independent practitioners.

Specifics to Individual States

The flavor of various statutes is reflected in the details included. For example, "invalid cars," vehicles used for convalescent calls, are often mentioned. In the New York and Georgia laws, these vehicles are specifically not regulated by the EMS statutes.[‡]

Small counties are often excluded from law and regulation for financial reasons. The Georgia law excuses counties with populations less than 12,000.[§] The Tennessee statute excludes counties with populations less than 50,000.[||]

Good Samaritan laws and other liability limitations are included in many EMS statutes; however, in states such as Colorado the limitations are elsewhere in law.[¶] Liability for simple negligence is usually excused; however, Good Samaritan laws generally do not provide immunity from liability for gross negligence or willful and wanton misconduct.

An immunity statute in no way protects the provider from litigation, rather, it excuses the provider from liability if the individual was not guilty of gross negligence or willful and wanton misconduct. Therefore liability is generally absent if the provider acts competently within the standard of care. Occasionally, similar provisions are made for EMS medical directors or council members who serve for no remuneration.[#] The standard of care for medical oversight is far more complex than it was a few years ago. To avoid being guilty of willful and wanton negligence, EMS physicians must demonstrate the provision of reasonable medical oversight, including direct and indirect medical control, depending on the level of participation.

Regional trauma systems and other programs that divert patients to appropriate facilities are allowed in many statutes. The Georgia law was amended recently to allow EMS agencies to route prehospital patients to trauma centers. The California law includes a section entitled Regional Trauma Systems. Statutory expansion of the "regionalization" of patients with specific medical conditions is likely in the future.

Indemnification is a new concept in some statutes; providers of public services may be offered a death or disability settlement for injuries or death resulting from their jobs. It is debatable whether private providers and EMS medical directors should be included in such indemnification.

*"The continuing education requirements shall be met by annually completing one-fifth of the following five-year requirements for hours of continuing education: 50 hours for emergency medical technicians; 75 hours for cardiac technicians; and 100 hours for advanced emergency medical technicians. These five-year continuing education requirements shall be divided into five different and discrete segments or modules of equal length." Georgia EMS Code 31-11-58 (d). In 1992, an attempt was made to allow for flexibility in establishing recertification requirements for EMTs. This required a law change that would give the authority to the Department of Human Resources. The bill giving this flexibility was defeated in committee, and hence even with the recommendation of the state EMS Advisory Council, minimal annual requirements cannot be established due to the wording of the law.

[†]State of Indiana Official Rules and Regulations for the Operation and Administration of Advanced Life Support, revised September 1984, 836 IAC 2-6-4 Continuing Education Reporting Requirements.

Advanced Life Support Continuing Education Manual from the Indiana EMS Commission: "The purpose of this manual is to outline the specific continuing education requirements for the Paramedic and the Advanced EMT, and to provide the mechanism for reporting continuing education to the commission."

[‡]"This chapter shall not apply to an invalid car or the operator thereof." Georgia EMS Code 31-11-11(4).

[§]"This Code section shall not apply to any county having a population under 12,000." Georgia EMS Code 31-11-50(c).

[||]"The provisions of this part shall not apply to counties having a population of not less than 49,400 nor more than 50,000 according to the 1980 Federal Census or any subsequent Federal Census." Tennessee EMS Statutes 68-140-516(c).

[¶]Personal communication from CJ Shanaberger, JD, July 1988. "

[#]A physician shall not be civilly liable for damages resulting from that physician's acting as medical adviser to an ambulance service if those damages are not a result of that physician's willful and wanton negligence." Georgia EMS Code 31-11-8(b).

Local Ordinances

One of the most vital areas of legal control and direction of EMS is the development of local ordinances. Municipalities and counties can establish local ordinances. These decrees set rationales and structures for the performance and regulation of various matters.

If a city declares that it is in the interest of the populace to forbid the sale of alcoholic beverages within certain distances of churches, then this issue is a "local law," with various penalties for infractions thereof. Likewise, if a county determines that standards must be met by road contractors building thoroughfares within the county boundaries, then such roadways can only be built according to such specifications. Local ordinance cannot conflict with state statute. Furthermore, local ordinance often requires a complex hearing process before adoption.

Similarly, local jurisdictions may issue ordinances concerning EMS. Such standards are powerful tools for EMS medical directors and should be carefully studied and pursued. Topics that can be addressed locally include the following:

1. Direct medical control training standards
2. Indirect medical control requirements and contractual arrangements
3. Specifications for vehicles
4. Minimum response times for EMS services
5. Minimum equipment standards for vehicles
6. Minimum training standards for providers
7. Quality management requirements

The EMS medical director must carefully review the existing local ordinances in the community. Perhaps the most significant impact of the medical director is the creation of a lasting, quality local EMS ordinance that provides for physician medical control of EMS activities.

A Model EMS State Legislation Outline

- I. Title of the EMS Act and rationale for EMS provision
- II. State administration
  - A. State professional director of EMS
    - 1. Qualifications
    - 2. Powers
    - 3. Duties
  - B. State medical director of EMS (if state director is a non-physician)
    - 1. Qualifications
    - 2. Powers
    - 3. Duties
  - C. State EMS commission
    - 1. Appointments
    - 2. Responsibilities
    - 3. Authority
  - D. EMS department
    - 1. Allowance for formation of rules and regulations
    - 2. EMS department duties
- III. Regional administration
  - A. Regional EMS councils
  - B. Regional EMS medical director
  - C. Regional EMS coordinator
  - D. Provision for regional patient flow guidance
- IV. Local administration
  - A. Local EMS councils
  - B. Local EMS system directors
  - C. Local EMS medical directors
- V. Ambulance services (specifics may be relegated to the Commission)
  - A. Licensure of ground, air, and water vehicles
  - B. Standards
  - C. Inspections
  - D. Revocation of licenses
  - E. Penalties
- VI. Medical control
  - A. Authorization for physician authority and medical direction
  - B. Provision for EMS technicians to provide practitioner assessment and management responsibilities
  - C. General EMS physician qualifications and responsibilities to EMS systems
- VII. Indemnification
- VIII. Limitations on liability
- IX. Medical records
- X. Communications
  - A. Rationale: The responsibility to respond to the public cry for distress
  - B. Confidentiality
- XI. EMS technician (specifics may be relegated to the Department or commission)
  - A. Certification
  - B. Recertification
  - C. Services
  - D. Continuing education
  - E. Active practice requirements
  - F. Hospital services
  - G. Obtaining drugs for EMS services
  - H. Revocation of certificates
  - I. Penalties
  - J. Standing orders
- XII. Specifics to states
  - A. "Invalid cars"
  - B. Special provisions for small counties or large cities

Summary

The proper formation of EMS statutes, regulations, and ordinances is critical to the continued EMS system growth. However, many aspects of EMS practice are found outside the EMS enabling legislation, making the search for medical oversight authority confusing. In some states the specifics of medical oversight are not found in the statute but in the activities of a state medical board.

EMS laws should limit inclusion of matters such as personnel criteria, continuing education requirements, and specific skills and medications. Authoritative bodies of EMS physicians and other qualified personnel can then determine the responsibilities and skills of the various levels of EMS personnel.

An EMS commission including physicians practicing within the state EMS system is essential. The commission must have statutory authority relative to the EMS system. When regional systems were established the medical oversight necessary for the proper monitoring and functioning of EMS was absent. Medical oversight is necessary for all EMS providers as is statutory authority for direct and indirect medical control physicians to carry out their delegated duties.

All EMS physicians should take a dynamic role in the review of their EMS statutes to facilitate excellence in EMS practice and future growth. They must assume that liability limitation laws do not protect them unless they can demonstrate and document aggressive participation in their EMS systems.

9

Funding Strategies

Robert Swor, D.O., FACEP

Most politicians and physicians agree that prehospital emergency care is, like police and fire protection, a basic right of the people. Few, however, agree on how this service should be provided and funded. This section both reviews the methods used to fund EMS systems in the past and catalogs some of the current funding methods. Development of adequate ongoing funding for EMS systems will be a crucial issue to all EMS systems in the future.

Historical Background

Initial EMS Funding

Before the development of organized EMS systems, delivery of prehospital care was fragmented. Perhaps the largest provider of emergency care were funeral home operators, because they owned vehicles that could transport a patient on a gurney. After the publication of "Accidental Death and Disability: The Neglected Disease of Modern Society," federal funding for emergency care on the streets became a priority. Initial funds were provided through the US Department of Transportation (DOT) by the Highway Safety Act of 1966, which provided for matching grants. Funding was available for EMS components such as ambulances, communications, and personnel (Section 402), and for special demonstration projects (Section 403). This program was a catalyst for initiating EMS systems and developing public support. It usually did not stimulate development of organized EMS systems.

As interest in prehospital care increased, it became apparent that medical, pediatric, and other subspecialty patients would also benefit from a regionalized approach to emergency care. In 1972, Congress approved funds for EMS demonstration projects in five regions. The object was to show that comprehensive EMS could be supplied throughout a region.[3] The Robert Wood Johnson Foundation began funding EMS demonstration projects on EMS response systems with a well-publicized emergency medical telephone number. Grant monies were distributed to 33 regions from 1972 to 1977. A myriad of other federal projects supplied monies for training, disaster preparedness, and communications.

Emergency Medical Service Systems Act of 1973

The Emergency Medical Service Systems Act of 1973 was the first comprehensive federal support of regional EMS system development. This act enumerated 15 mandatory components of an EMS system and served as a template for program planners. The act was designed to promote development of systems "to meet the individual characteristics of each community."[3] Funding totaled $185 million over 3 years and was granted to regional "lead agencies" that disbursed funds. Each region had an average population of 700,000. Initially 303 regions were created, although not all received funding each year. Funding was disbursed in 2-year increments as follows:

Section 1202—Feasibility studies and planning
Section 1203—Initial operations
Section 1204—Expansion and improvement
Section 1205—Research

The expected level of funding for each lead agency to develop a successful and viable program was $1.5 to 1.75 million. Funding was apportioned so that 25% of all monies went to rural areas. On a per capita basis, regions received $1 for urban areas, $3.50 for rural areas, and $10 for wilderness areas. Between the program's inception in 1974 and termination in 1981, the act was amended in 1976 and 1979. Securing other sources of funding was emphasized so services could continue when federal funding ceased.

However, the chief failure of the EMS System Act was its inability to stimulate local initiatives to fund EMS. When the "feds" eventually went out of the EMS business in 1981, so did a number of programs.

Preventive Health Block Grants

Federal funding for EMS systems was cut dramatically by the federal block grant programs in the Omnibus Budget Reconciliation Act of 1981.[3] This legislation divided Health and Human Services funds into seven blocks, with EMS funding under preventive health block grants. Programs included with EMS funding were hypertension control, rodent control, rape prevention and crisis services, fluoridation, home health service, and health education. Disbursement of funds was left to the state authorities. Funds were not to be used for operation costs or equipment purchases.[3]

The purpose of the Omnibus Budget Reconciliation Act was to shift responsibility for funding EMS services to the states while still funding lead agencies to direct EMS services. The result of this policy was a significant decrease in total EMS funding from 1981 to 1983. In a General Accounting Office (GAO) survey of six states (California, Florida, Iowa, Massachusetts, Pennsylvania, and Texas), funding decreased 34% between 1981 and 1983. However, funds were increased 28% between 1983 and 1985; the concept of shifting funding to local government was a success.[18] EMS had to compete with the other constituencies included in the preventive health block for funding. In areas where EMS was not a priority or the EMS community was not aggressively garnering support, funding diminished significantly.

Cost-Effectiveness of EMS

Because of the withdrawal of federal funds for local EMS systems, developing an EMS system and funding it requires careful planning and accurate need assessment. Frequently, this assessment requires philosophical and financial decision-making. Cost-benefit ratios have been calculated using the number of lives saved after cardiac arrest as a model.[1, 7, 11] These estimates of cost-per-life-saved vary extremely ranging from $4300 after establishing a basic ambulance to $42,358 after establishing a paramedic system.[1, 7] Valenzuela reviewed cardiac arrest survival rates in Tucson, comparing cost-effectiveness of EMS programs to that of other sophisticated medical modalities.[24] Treatment of prehospital cardiac arrest compared favorably with heart, liver, or bone marrow transplants and chemotherapy for acute leukemia in cost-per-year-of-life-saved. Although the methodology for calculating these numbers is variable and complex, EMS system costs appear to be similar to other advanced medical technology costs.

System Costs

The calculation of a system's cost includes personnel, administration, maintenance, training, equipment, and facilities. Certainly the most expensive part of any paid EMS system is personnel, which totals between 60% and 90% of a typical system's cost.[8] Because of the high cost of personnel, many municipalities use fire departments, a preexisting traditionally underused resource, as primary EMS providers. From a cost standpoint this appears effective; between 65% and 70% of these agencies' requests are EMS calls.

Equipment costs are also significant. The estimated cost of a basic ambulance is between $35,000 and $40,000 and a paramedic ambulance approaches $80,000.[7] The number of units required for a given area depends on population density, response time requirements, geographic area covered, and other EMS service demands. These factors make calculating system needs difficult. For 25 mid-sized cities, Braun found an average of one ambulance per 51,223 people.[4] The average number of persons served by paramedic units ranged from 58,000 to 120,000 depending on whether a one-tier (all paramedic response) or a two-tiered (mixed response) system was used.[4] The cost of adding paramedic service to preexisting basic units (that is, pay differential for paramedics, equipment, medications, and training costs) is usually small enough that paramedics can be used exclusively to render care.[21] For municipal services, Pons argues that using a third-service rather than a fire-based service allows increased scheduling and staffing flexibility. He compared data from cities with both types of service and calculated a cost of $81 per response for third-service municipal systems and $162 per response for fire-based services.[16] Cost is only one variable in this complex equation.

The industry standard for calculating EMS service costs is the total cost of deploying a fully staffed vehicle per hour of actual service. This calculation includes operations, dispatch, and maintenance. A more complete discussion of unit costs is included in Chapter 10.

System Needs

Estimates of need are also critical in devising a system. Generally, estimates indicate that only 5% of calls are true emergencies, another 15% require urgent evaluation, and the remainder are non-emergencies. Approximately 100 medical emergencies and two or three cardiac arrests are generated per million people each day.[17] However, these numbers are obtained retrospectively and emergency responses must be provided to a much larger number of cases to ensure appropriate response times for real emergencies. Methods identifying emergency needs such as priority dispatch systems have not yet been scientifically validated; however, effective priority dispatch should reduce the number of calls dispatched as emergencies.

Estimated numbers of emergency calls are only one factor in determining need for prehospital services. Population density, proximity to local hospitals, and the age of surrounding population must be included in the equation. Because the fixed-costs of EMS systems are so high, rural and wilderness systems that operate with low volumes are extremely expensive on a per capita basis.[3] As a population ages, its need for EMS services increases. Some argue that an urban system in close proximity to hospitals might be staffed most efficiently by EMT-D personnel using automated external defibrillators. In the absence of clear data on the benefit of most advanced interventions, need becomes a philosophical question reflecting a community's demands and funds in addition to how well the medical community articulates the apparent, yet undocumented, benefits.

Current Funding

Federal

Although federal funding of EMS systems has declined since 1981, most states still receive significant federal aid. A 1992 survey showed that 35 states receive block grant funds to use for different aspects of EMS services. Another 25 receive DOT highway safety funds. Most commonly, these are provided by Section 402 of the Highway Safety Act and are used for training personnel.[19] In keeping with the intent of the block grant initiative, funds are disbursed to state agencies that may either use them for statewide administration of EMS or distribute them to local agencies.

State

State financial support is crucial to the continued viability of EMS systems. States surveyed by the GAO in 1985 showed a 50% increase in EMS expenditures since 1981.[18] Methods of funding vary substantially from state to state. The box below shows a 1991 survey of state EMS directors. Different funding mechanisms are identified including *ad valorem* tax districts; fees for vehicle registrations, driver's licenses, and traffic violations; excise taxes; and tobacco taxes. The most common of these, ad valorem tax districts, allow local communities to tax themselves for organizing and funding EMS. Fees typically range from $1 to $3 million.[12] These funds are used at the state-level or distributed to local regulatory or provider agencies. The purposes vary; funding is disbursed for training, equipment, communications, operations, and administration. Virginia returns 25% of funds collected to the county a vehicle is registered in. Some states also allocate funds for unique EMS needs; California grants $754,000 to high-tourist areas. Levels of funding are extremely variable; states spend as much as $1.20 (Alaska) or as little as three cents (California) per capita.[19]

Maryland is unique in its support of EMS and has created a statewide EMS system. Initiated in 1973 by an executive order of the governor, this system provides for training of EMS personnel, develop-

State Methods of EMS Funding

Revenue from vehicle or driver license

Colorado, Florida, Idaho, New Mexico, Virginia

Revenue from motor vehicle violations

Arizona—$2.3 million from driving while intoxicated fines and other moving violations
Florida—$5 per violation, $25 for driving while intoxicated
Indiana—drunk drivers pay uncollectible EMS fees for motor vehicle accidents they are involved in
Minnesota—$10 for failure to wear a seat belt
Mississippi—$5 per violation, $5 for bail forfeiture
Rhode Island—$1 surcharge per violation
Utah—$3 for fines or bail forfeiture

EMS service vehicle license fees

Florida, Maine, Massachusetts, New Mexico, Oklahoma

Tax Districts

Alaska, Florida, Iowa, Kentucky, Mississippi, Missouri, New York, North Carolina, North Dakota, Oklahoma, South Dakota, Texas, Utah, Wyoming

Modified from Kleinholz SB and Doeksen GA: Southern Rural Development Task Force, March 1991.

ment of a statewide helicopter emergency transport system, development of tertiary care centers for specialized medical conditions (most notably trauma care), and expansion of research facilities. A statewide 9-1-1 system has been developed as part of the program. The system is supported by the state general fund; in fiscal year 1986, funds were raised to replace helicopters with a surcharge on vehicle license fees.[14]

Local

System design depends on whether the system is public or private, urban or rural, and whether the population is affluent or impoverished. Sources of revenue include tax subsidies, patient revenues, service charges, and subscriptions. Municipal systems are supported by tax-generated revenue with funds sometimes augmented by billing for service. Some regions have special assessment for EMS services. For example, King County, Washington, passed a special county tax to fund the local EMS system.

Many systems use so-called subscription services; the populace is offered the option of subscribing for EMS care by paying an annual fee ($12 to $14 in Orange County, California).[8] Those who subscribe receive EMS services free of charge that year; others are charged on a fee-for-service basis. Other systems are supported by operating revenues of hospitals, by corporate foundations, or by surcharges. The costs of medical administration are typically borne by governmental agencies in metropolitan areas (more than 500,000 population) and by hospitals in less populated regions.[22]

Third-Party Reimbursement

The role of third-party reimbursement as a source of revenue also varies. As expected, urban areas have low levels of privately insured patients and consequently payment levels are low. In 1987, Detroit was estimated to generate only 20% of its EMS operating budget from third-party payments.[13] Orange County, on the other hand, generates 70% to 80% of reimbursements through direct billing.[8] Stout and others argue that government subsidy of EMS systems artificially lowers the cost of EMS, thereby subsidizing not only the self-payors, but also the third-party payors (see Chapter 10).

Public Utility Model

In an effort to develop cost-effective EMS services that are accountable to the public a number of systems (Pinellas County, Florida; Tulsa, Oklahoma; Oklahoma City, Oklahoma; and Fort Wayne, Indiana) have evolved under the public utility model. This model is a quasi-government system that uses a government oversight body and a private contractor to supply EMS. A government ambulance authority is established to procure equipment, manage administrative expenses, handle billings, and contract for provision of services with an ambulance provider. The ambulance provider manages the delivery of EMS services in accordance with standards established by an independent medical control board. Common features of this model include provision of all-paramedic care and single-provider provision of all emergency and non-emergency transportation, which defray the cost. Another common provision of this model is a franchise fee (typically $2 to $5 per transport) charged to fund oversight by a medical control board.

Summary

Maintaining current levels of funding for well-financed EMS systems and developing new funding sources for less supported systems will continue to be a challenge. Through legislation, many jurisdictions have instituted permanent funding mechanisms for EMS. Such legislative support is difficult to obtain because the beneficiaries of well-supported EMS care, emergency patients, are indifferent until ill or injured. Currently, third-party insurance carriers are an important source of EMS revenue and physicians involved with prehospital care should look to them for emergency care funds. As with all medical reimbursement, this source will undergo intense scrutiny as costs escalate and appropriate uses of EMS services are questioned. The continued financial support of EMS requires a visible, politically active EMS community.

REFERENCES AND SUGGESTED READINGS

1. Acton J: Evaluating public programs to save lives: the case of heart disease, *Rand Corporation Rep* R930 RC, 1973, Santa Monica Rand Corporation.
2. Best J: GAO reviews 1200 series grants, *EMS Management Advisor* 1(6):1-4, 1985.
3. Boyd DR: *The history of emergency medical services systems in the United States of America.* In: *Systems Approach to Emergency Medical Care,* Norwalk, CT, 1983, Appleton-Century-Croft.
4. Braun OE, McCallion R, and Fazackerly J: Characteristics of mid-sized urban EMS systems, *Ann Emerg Med* 19(5):536, 1990.
5. Committee on Trauma and Committee on Shock: *Accidental death and disability: the neglected disease of modern society,* Sep 1966, Washington, DC, Fifth printing by the Commission on Emergency Medical Services, Jan 1970, American Medical Association.
6. Crampton RS et al: Reduction of prehospital, ambulance, and community death rates by the communitywide emergency cardiac care system, *Am J Med* 58:155-165, 1975.

7. Cretin S: Cost-benefit analysis of treatment and prevention of myocardial infarction, *Health Serv Res* 12(3):174-189, 1977.
8. Drake L and Thompson M: *Systems design and human resources.* In: *Prehospital care, administrative and clinical management,* Rockville, MD, 1987, Aspen Publishers Inc.
9. Fry GE: *The prehospital transportation component in an EMS system.* In: *Systems approach to emergency medical care,* Norwalk, CT, 1983, Appleton-Century-Croft.
10. Grace WJ and Chadbourne JA: The mobile coronary care unit, *Dis Chest* 55:452, 1969.
11. Hallstrom A, Eisenberg MS, and Bergner L: Modeling the effectiveness and cost-effectiveness of an emergency service system, *Soc Sci Med* 15C:13-17, 1981.
12. Kleinholz SB and Doeksen GA: *State legislation for funding of rural emergency medical services,* March 1991, Southern Rural Development Health Task Force.
13. Loose C and Angell DEM: Condition Critical For EMS, *The Detroit News* April 12-15, 1987.
14. Maryland Institute for Emergency Medical Services Systems: *Annual Report,* 1986-87, The Institute.
15. O'Rourke B: *Emergency medical services system legislation.* In: *Prehospital care, administrative, and clinical management,* Rockville, MD, 1987, Aspen Publishers Inc.
16. Pons PT: Mixing fire and EMS. Presented at the National Association of EMS Physicians annual meeting, Orlando, FL, 1991.
17. Proceeding of The National Association of Emergency Medical Service Physicians annual meeting, 1985.
18. Report assesses leadership of states in providing EMS using federal grants, *EMS Communicator* 13(6):1-4, 1986.
19. State survey, *Emergency Medical Services* 21(10):167-189, 1992.
20. Stout JL: Public utility model revisited, *JEMS* 71-74, March 1985.
21. Stout JL: *Systems financing.* In Rousch WR: *Principles of EMS systems: a comprehensive text for physicians* Dallas, 1989, ACEP.
22. Swor RA and Krome RL: Administrative support for EMS medical directors: a profile, *Prehosp Disaster Med* 5(1):25-30, 1990.
23. Urban N, Bergner L, and Eisenberg MS: The costs of a suburban paramedic program in reducing deaths due to cardiac arrests, *Medical Care* 19(4):379-392, 1981.
24. Valenzuela TD et al: Cost effectiveness of paramedic emergency medical services in the treatment of prehospital cardiopulmonary arrest, *Ann Emerg Med* 19(12):1407-1411, 1990.

10

System Design

Jack Stout, B.A.

The most powerful force influencing an EMS system's ability to convert available dollars into clinical performance and response time reliability is system design. The prime directive of EMS is to provide every critical patient the best possible chance of survival without disability, given state-of-the-art prehospital care and available financial resources.

Price of Entry

EMS advocates unwilling or unable to grapple with the realities of economic efficiency, worker productivity, and the need to generate more high quality service with limited financial resources cannot be taken seriously by public officials.

Before the United States was forced to tighten its economic belt, EMS advocates could ask, "What's a life worth?" Not anymore. Public needs of equal or perhaps even greater importance (for example, prenatal care, infant nutrition, drug abuse prevention, the battle against AIDS, law enforcement, and deficit control) now compete vigorously for the limited dollars available. The country is facing a far more challenging question, "Is this the best we can do with the money we've got?"

To answer this question, EMS leaders must compare systems. For the comparison to be more than a whitewash, they must risk comparing their system's current clinical and economic performance—not with systems known to be inferior—but with the handful of renegade systems operating at the outer limits of economic efficiency.

Secret Ingredient

High-performance EMS systems enjoy the advantages of superior system design discussed in this chapter; but design alone cannot explain the startling 300% differences throughout the industry in output per dollar. Something more is involved. The secret ingredient of high-performance EMS systems was discovered by a member of the Michigan Ambulance Association. During an overview of advanced system status management (SSM) practices he exclaimed, "Why hell, there's no magic in this; it's just a bunch of hard work." Indeed.

We Are Doing It For . . . Whose Benefit?

EMS system designers and managers cannot avoid the conflict between decisions made for the patient's benefit and those made for the system's convenience. Following are four examples:

- Faced with highly predictable 400% fluctuations in time-of-day and day-of-week demand for prehospital care (usually coincident with the worst possible traffic), ambulance services staffed at or near a constant level around-the-clock cannot claim, "We are doing it for the patient."
- Faced with massive and surprisingly cyclical shifts in geographic demand concentration by time-of-day and day-of-week (that is, buildings are fixed but people move around) and the predictable AM/PM rush hour reversal of traffic flow in most urban areas, ambulance services employing fixed-post deployment methods cannot claim, "We are doing it for the patient."
- Fire departments that, in spite of declining demand for fire suppression services, refuse to provide trained first response using existing personnel or overload a limited number of costly rescue crews while millions of dollars in engine company resources stand idle cannot claim, "We are doing it for the patient."
- Volunteer services failing to guarantee fully staffed paramedic response, while pointing

with pride to 100% volunteer staffing and token user fees or no fees at all (that is, angels of mercy don't charge a fee) cannot claim, "We are doing it for the patient."

The hard truth is that the conventional wisdom of EMS system design (for example, tiered response, the specialized production strategy, 24 hour shifts in urban settings, use of fixed-post locations, the every-man-for-himself dispatch method still used by many volunteer organizations) made convenience to the system and respect for its traditions a higher priority than meeting the needs of patients. For the convenience of the system, patients have been inconvenienced—in some cases to death.

Some EMS systems designed and managed for their own convenience have attempted to offset their inefficiencies through ever-increasing local tax support. Developing a tolerance for large even massive dollar dosage, low-performance systems have become addicted to local tax support with a bizarre result. Today an imperfect but unmistakable inverse correlation exists between the level of local tax support (that is, per capita per year subsidy) and the quality of patient care. The most startling example, as of 1992 America's most heavily subsidized urban ambulance service is also its least effective—that is, the District of Columbia (DC) ambulance service.

Whether or not the latest newly appointed medical director of the DC system will overcome the system's long-standing affinity for flawed design and inefficient production methods, the fact will remain that throughout their tenure, the DC system's traditional design and production methods consumed cash at the fastest rate in the industry, while producing an internationally embarrassing level of service.

Facing the political liability of a poorly performing EMS system design, elected officials too often fail to diagnose the *system itself* as the cause and treat the symptoms. Although it is doubful that too much money causes quality of prehospital care to deteriorate, chronic symptoms of faulty system design are often misdiagnosed as financial malnutrition and treated with monetary nutrients. Over time, the EMS system designs most resistant to dollar therapy have become the most dependent. Figure 10-1 (based on 1991 data) illustrates the point.

The question is not whether an EMS system design is *capable* of consuming large sums of money, any design can. The question is whether, at any given level of financial support, one design generates more service of higher quality than other designs. This chapter presents the major elements of EMS system design that contribute to or detract from the system's ability to convert available dollars into quality prehospital care.

Fundamentals of EMS System Design

System design refers to the EMS system's underlying framework of legal, organizational, business and medical oversight structures, and financing strategy.

Limitations

System design is critically important but not all-powerful. The following are its limitations:

1. Talented and motivated people can produce good results in a bad system design, but not for extended periods of time.
2. Incompetence can produce poor results in even the best system design.
3. Talented people tend to be attracted to system designs more likely to nurture and showcase their individual talents.
4. Talented people have options because they are talented. In general, our industry's most talented managers choose to avoid employment in EMS systems that tend to nullify rather than demonstrate their abilities.
5. Good system design makes excellence possible and superior performance probable, but guarantees neither.
6. Bad system design makes excellence impossible and inferior service probable.
7. Sound system design cannot guarantee clinically appropriate and economically efficient performance; but poor system design can make consistent lifesaving performance extremely unlikely even impossible.

What System Design Determines

The term system design is uncomfortably vague. The first step in defining the concept is identifying the *direct effects* of an EMS system's design. Any EMS system's design establishes 8 major structural attributes and 28 secondary features. The 8 most important are as follows:

1. **Geographic scope.** The geographic scope of the system's *primary service area* (monojurisdictional or multijurisdictional) affects economies of scale and can determine whether less economically desirable areas can be served at all. (Note: The allocation of market rights in other utility industries deliberately grafted difficult-to-serve areas onto more economically desirable markets so a nationwide network of otherwise impossible telephone and electric power systems could develop. Although the

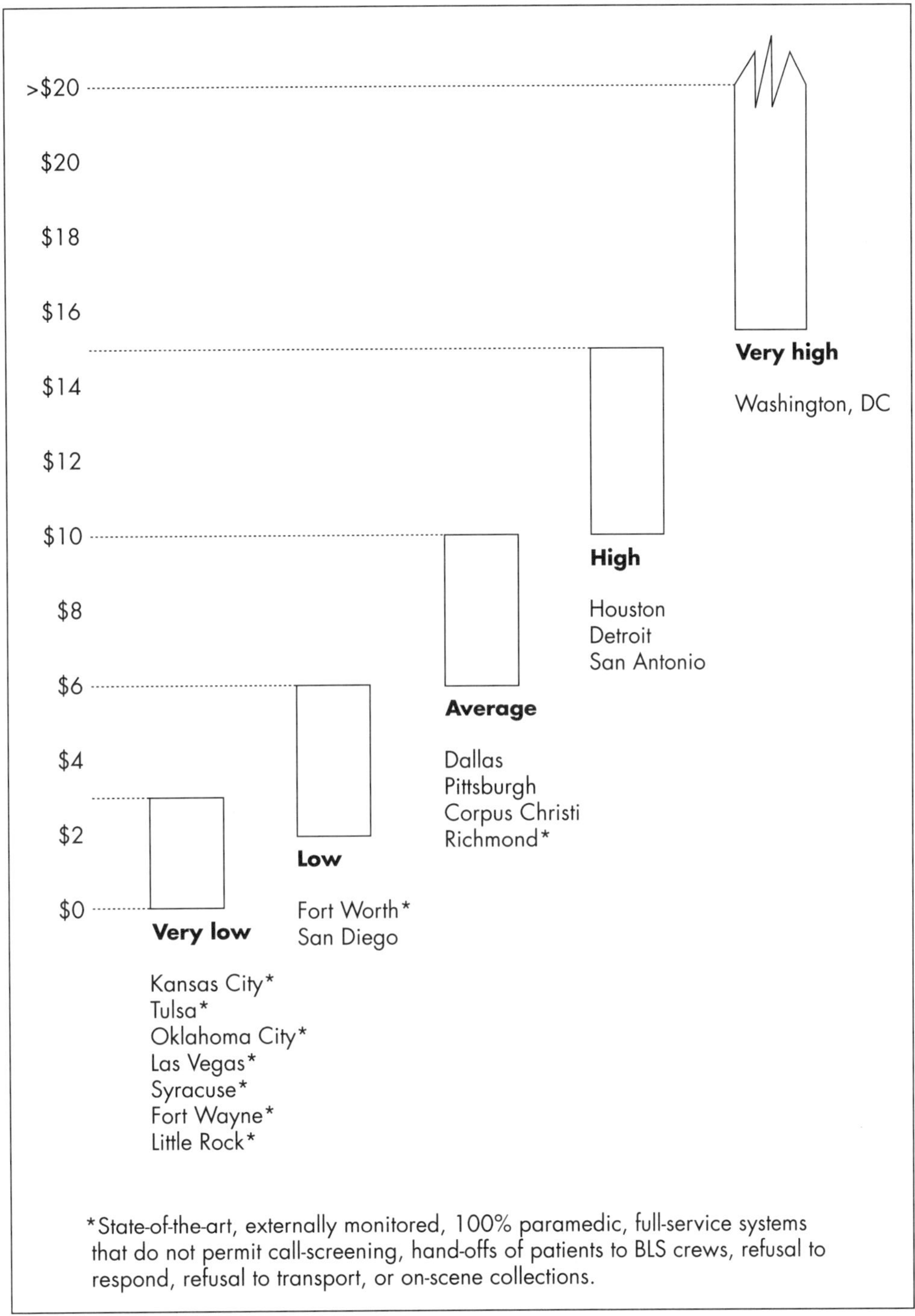

Figure 10-1. Local tax EMS sibsidy per capita per year.

ambulance service industry exhibits every characteristic of a utility industry, EMS regulators have thus far failed to learn from the success of other utility industries.)

2. **Standards setting and enforcement.** The process whereby performance standards are established (if established), monitored, and enforced is in the long run the most important aspect of an EMS system's design. In general, if this element is well-designed, it will eventually expose and correct defective aspects of the system's design.
3. **Division of functions.** Division of functional responsibilities among participating organizations (for example, EMT-D level firefighter; first response with paramedic-level private ambulance service) impacts funding requirements and revenue options, affects distribution of lia-

bility, and can enhance or dilute organizational accountability for performance results.

4. **Production strategies.** Production strategies employed (for example, the specialized production strategy vs. the flexible production strategy, engine company first response vs. rescue squad first response) establish the system's limit of worker productivity and thus more directly impact production costs and funding requirements than any other single factor including wages.
5. **Market allocation.** Selection of organizations to participate within the system (for example, bid competition, accident of history, political influence, default) sets the stage for all that follows. Oddly, only a few EMS systems deliberately award EMS market rights and responsibilities to the best-qualified organizations willing to do the job.
6. **Consequences of chronic failure to perform.** As 75 years of Soviet experience has revealed, organizations whose role in society is perceived to perpetual rather than contingent on performance, just do not try hard enough. If and how a poorly performing organization can be replaced by one more qualified is a key element of EMS system design. Not surprisingly, this feature is least likely to be applied where it is most clearly defined and readily available.
7. **Business structure.** The sources, amounts, routes, and contingencies of dollar flow into and within the system determine which organizational behaviors will be financially supported or rewarded and which will not. In many lower performance systems, these contingencies of financial reinforcement are either irrelevant to the system's reason for being or downright contrary (for example, budget increases justified by deficient performance). Market test comparisons with other systems serving similar markets and known for their efficiency can be a powerful stimulant where complacency prevails. In short the system's business structure provides or fails to provide the critical link between the public interest and organizational motivation.
8. **Caliber of management required.** Not all EMS system designs require the same caliber of management to extract the system's maximum potential. In general, policymakers must choose between low-performance designs capable of approaching their full but modest potential even if lead by managers of mediocre ability versus high-performance designs capable of achieving superior results, but requiring leadership talents well above the norm.

The last of the preceding items is in some ways the most interesting. Just as a high-performance automobile or aircraft operated at or near its limits demands a highly skilled driver or pilot, an EMS system with high-performance potential demands a higher caliber of management. Furthermore, in the same way a high-performance machine may be dangerous in the hands of a modestly skilled operator, a high-performance EMS system design can be deadly and expensive if managed by persons of modest ability and motivation.

Thus the chief advantage of low-performance EMS system designs is that their maximum performance, modest though it may be, can often be achieved by managers of limited ability. For example, what could be easier to manage than a system using level coverage staffed with 24-hour shifts and fixed-post locations? However, even where substantial subsidies are available the maximum performance of inferior designs falls far below that achieved by systems of superior design.

Origin of Current Design

Most prehospital system designs are *not* the product of policy decisions deliberately selecting certain features and rejecting others with full understanding of each option's demonstrated advantages and pitfalls. Rather, most system designs have simply evolved through a process of short-term, issue-driven policy accretion or were loosely patterned after a television series.

Fortunately a growing number of today's working EMS systems are products of informed selection of structural features that deliver the best possible chance of survival without disability using limited financial resources—the "Prime Directive." The track records of these high performance EMS systems are defining the future of EMS.

Economic Efficiency

Just as nothing impacts a system's ability to turn dollars into service more powerfully than design, nothing impacts patient care more powerfully than the system's ability to convert dollars into service. Economic efficiency and clinical effectiveness are more than related; they are absolutely interdependent.

Measuring Economic Efficiency

By shortening one or two legs of the triangle in Figure 10-2, even a poorly structured, badly managed system

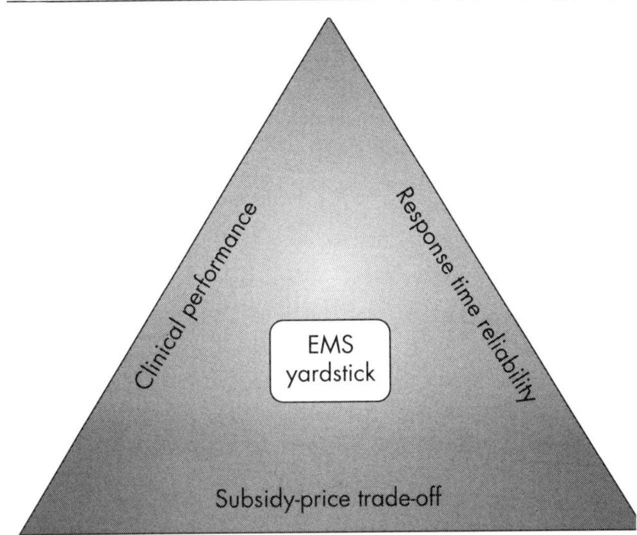

Figure 10-2: Measuring economic efficiency.

can perform reasonably well on one or two measures, creating an appearance of competence when viewed from a favorable angle. The consequences of such distortion harm the patient, the taxpayer, or frequently both. For example, an unskilled manager can limit spending by allowing clinical quality and response time reliability to deteriorate. Similarly, given enough money, even the most pathetic management team can generate something of value.

The challenge is to simultaneously generate clinical excellence, response time reliability, and economic efficiency. Meeting that challenge qualifies any system and its personnel as high-performance.

Economic efficiency among EMS systems today varies by more than 300%. That is, when compared in terms of total system cost per patient transport, total system cost per capita for service area population, or combined subsidy-cost per capita and user-fee level, some system designs consistently require more than 3 times the financial resources than others. With few exceptions, differences in system design account for differences in economic efficiency; the combination of poor system design and severe budget limitations is deadly.

Learning to Distinguish the Best from the Rest

As in most facets of human endeavor, we stand to learn the most from those in the lead. Some EMS systems ingesting huge sums of money produce service of limited quality, quantity, and reliability. Other EMS systems feed on scarce financial resources yet consistently produce high-quality service and impressive response time reliability. In nearly every case, system design accounts for the difference.

After nearly two decades testing our industry's 27 basic prehospital system designs (and hundreds of variations), design features can be isolated that are more common and sometimes universal among better performing systems and less common or nonexistent among systems performing at low levels of efficiency.

Levels of Efficiency

For purposes of examination, EMS systems can be divided into the following four categories:

- High quality with above average cost (San Antonio),
- Low quality with below average cost (most common),
- Low quality with above average cost (Washington, DC), and
- High-performance EMS systems—above average service with below average cost (Las Vegas; Syracuse; New York; Tulsa/Oklahoma City; Reno, Nevada; Fort Wayne, Indiana; Little Rock, Arkansas; Fresno, California; Fort Worth, Texas; Kansas City, Missouri; the ambulance service component of Pinellas County EMS, Florida; Clark County, Washington; the Acadia System serving rural Louisiana; the East EMS System serving rural eastern Texas; and a handful of others).

The systems in the high-performance category share key features of system design rarely associated with less cost-effective systems. Before valuable lessons can be learned from high-performance systems, it is necessary to distinguish them from the rest. Just as the acid test of a quality product lies not in its initial performance but in its long-term reliability, most EMS designs perform reasonably well while new and shiny. The question is, how will the system perform when the new wears off?

Economic efficiency and clinical performance are directly interdependent and certain system design characteristics influence and define efficiency potential. It is also necessary to understand that three broad objectives, when combined, furnish a basis for predicting and explaining the operational consequences of policy decisions affecting system design. Those three objectives are as follows:

- To establish a framework for comparing the structure and performance of any EMS system with those of any other EMS system regardless of system design.

- To develop a basic working knowledge of three measures essential to judging and comparing economic efficiency.
- To identify EMS system design elements that contribute to or detract from the system's ability to convert dollars into service.

First a method of defining, examining, and classifying EMS systems must be established that can be fairly and productively applied to any EMS system regardless of its design.

The Great Conceptual False Start of 1973

Propelled by the force of more than $300 million in federal grants, the federal government's 15 components of EMS system design sent the nation on a conceptual wild-goose chase from which we are still recovering (see p. 10).

People began to believe that systematic thinking was logical thinking. In fact, it is quite possible to think illogically in a very orderly and systematic way.

Lacking fundamental elements such as medical direction, financial structure, legal structure, a method of allocating market rights and responsibilities, or even a framework for describing performance expectations the 15 components fell short of furnishing a conceptual basis for rational EMS system development. After brief national recognition primarily for their ability to secure and spend federal grant funds the shining EMS stars of the 1970s faded. Almost without exception the high-performance systems of today were not recipients of federal EMS grants.

The 15 components failed in four ways to furnish a conceptual foundation on which a nationwide network of quality prehospital care systems could be built. First the 15 components were not developed from the patient's (that is, the customer's) point of view. Second, as a systems approach (the rage of the 1970s), the 15 component framework violated key principles of systems engineering. Third the 15 components failed to identify and organize essential elements of an effective EMS system into a useful framework. Fourth the 15 components assumed a hopelessly oversimplified view of a complex industry.

With the advantage of hindsight a far more effective conceptual framework has developed. A framework evolved from the patient's point of view encompassing essential elements of input, structure, output (process), and outcome.

EMS System Defined from the Patient's Point of View

An EMS system consists of those organizations, individuals, facilities, and equipment whose participation is required to ensure timely and medically appropriate response to each request for prehospital care and medical transportation.

Every EMS system regardless of design has two types of input; patients and money and several types of output: services such as patient assessment, extrication, defibrillation, and medical transportation. Linking input and output the system converts dollars into service. Depending on efficiency, some EMS systems generate small volumes of low quality service from a large dollar flow and others generate large volumes of high quality service from a small dollar flow.

Impact on patient outcome, the most important result of all this activity, is a function of two related but very separate factors. First, efficacy of system protocols (that is, priority dispatch protocols, medical protocols, and system status management protocols) and system compliance with those protocols. These two factors must be dealt with separately, because a defect in one factor cannot be corrected by acting on the other.

Relationship of the System to Its Environment

Past definitions of EMS systems developed from the viewpoint of the system itself. For example, systems based on the specialized production strategy define routine transport service and the financial and other resources involved as outside the system, thus avoiding comparison with systems based on the flexible production strategy. The specialized production strategy employs two, three, or even four types of ambulances each specializing in specific types of calls. The flexible production strategy employs a single ambulance staffed and equipped to respond to any type of call. Either strategy may incorporate the use of one or more types of first responder units (Figure 10-3).

Some EMS system definitions assume that callers reliably triage themselves into emergency and routine categories, dialing 9-1-1 in emergencies and a 7-digit telephone number for routine transport. The underlying assumption is that callers who do not dial 9-1-1 are not a responsibility of the EMS system because they failed to follow the access rules. Again the system escapes accountability for a huge segment of the patient population including related costs and outcomes.

The term "EMS" reflects the original assumption that emergency patients can be distinguished from non-emergency patients and that specialized production dedicated to each type of work will provide better service at a lower cost. This once conventional wisdom failed to account for patterns of demand for prehospital care and has since proved false.

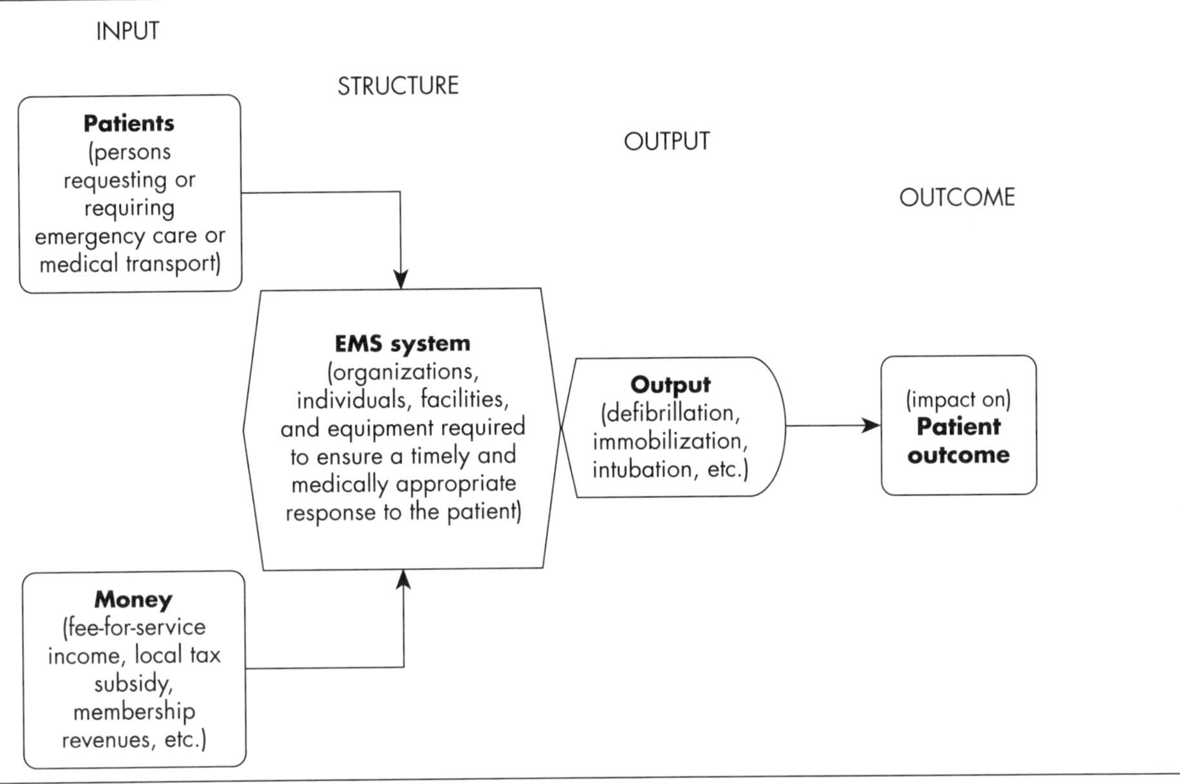

Figure 10-3. Relationship of the "system" to its environment.

Any conceptual framework subordinating the patient to the system fails to furnish a basis for fair comparison of different system types. Because the needs of the patient are not securely anchored to the system's purpose, such conceptual frameworks are not stable platforms for comparing advantages and disadvantages of system designs.

Alternatively, defining the EMS system from the patient's point of view avoids bias and apples-to-apples comparisons become possible. Before a patient-centered conceptual framework can replace the 15 components of 1973 the patients must be identified.

If an EMS system serves patients, then there must be a clear understanding of who these patients are. The following are the facts regarding consumer requests for medical assistance and transportation where a universal 9-1-1 exists for an extended period of time:

1. Slightly more than 50% of all medical requests enter the system through 9-1-1 access.
2. Slightly less than 50% of all medical requests enter the system through 7-digit telephone numbers.
3. When paramedic crews respond, 20% to 30% of 9-1-1 medical requests are found to require paramedic skills.
4. When paramedic crews respond, about 12% of 7-digit number ambulance requests require paramedic skills.
5. About 70% to 80% of 9-1-1 medical requests do not require paramedic service.
6. About 88% of non-9-1-1 medical requests do not require paramedic service.
7. Many bona fide emergency calls do not require ALS, whereas some bona fide non-emergency calls require ALS en route (for example, scheduled interfacility transport of a patient requiring advanced en route support—an increasingly common type of call) (Figure 10-4).

Thus in creating a conceptual framework for comparing EMS systems of diverse design (that is, a framework biased in favor of the patient but blind to system design), the system's response to every patient must be tracked including those failing to follow the system's telephone access rules and those the system excludes from its field of vision. If the decision to organizationally and operationally separate emergency service production from routine transport production is clinically and financially sound, only a comparison of total system performance—clinical and financial, emergency and routine—can test the proposition conclusively.

Thus in defining the system from the patient's point of view, all patients are included regardless of how they access the system, whether system managers accept or reject responsibility for their care, and whether such patients ultimately require heroic

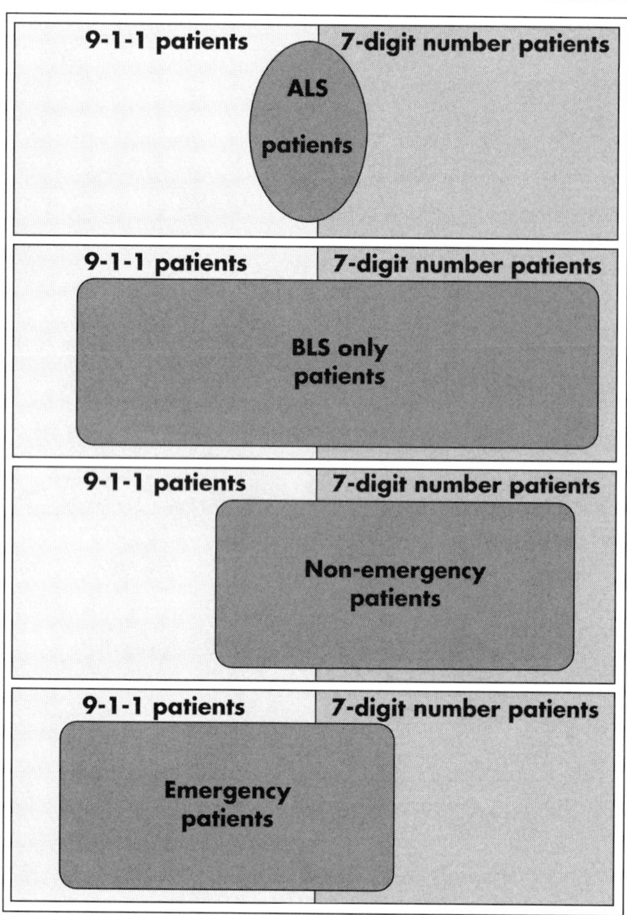

Figure 10-4. Predicting patient needs. All we know for certain is that some requests are via 9-1-1, and some are via 7-digit numbers. Figure based on data from full-service prehospital care systems serving a combined patient population of more than 300,000 patients annually. (Courtesy Wendy Jones, M.D., FACEP.)

intervention or just simple kindness and safe medical transport.

The system's most important input is the patient. The other input every system must have is money. Each of the organizations required to generate a timely and medically appropriate response to each patient's request requires funds to fuel its operation. Again the EMS system is a machine for converting dollars into service.

EMS systems regardless of design deal with two universal inputs, patients and money. Similarly, every EMS system regardless of design is a structure comprised of organizations, individuals, equipment, some type of communications networks and facilities to house functions such as fleet maintenance, training activity, control center operations, crew quarters, billing and collection activity, and other support services. Along the same line, every system has some type of information system, mechanisms of financing its operations, and a formal or informal legal structure defining organizational roles and responsibilities. Finally, almost every system has or purports to have some type of medical oversight structure, external or internal.

EMS System Matrix

The EMS System Matrix that follows provides a two-dimensional framework for documenting and comparing any system's structure and performance with that of any other regardless of design. The most important task of every EMS system is to generate a planned, coordinated, and medically appropriate response to every patient in need of its services. Thus the matrix is deliberately driven from its left vertical axis (that is, a comprehensive, sequential list of system response phases from prevention through indirect medical evaluation of the response and ongoing quality improvement).

Documenting an EMS system using the matrix is a formidable task regardless of the system's design; and therein lies its value. Using the matrix, any EMS system can be documented in detail and compared fairly with any other regardless of differences in design (Figure 10-5).

A few comments should be made regarding use of the matrix. Medical oversight items are the only elements appearing on the vertical and horizontal axes. As outputs, direct and indirect medical control require the full-range of structural components (such as a responsible organization, a legal basis, and funding) for which provision is made horizontally.

The three most important duties of medical oversight are formulating system performance specifications (that is, standards and protocols governing output performance), monitoring compliance with specifications, and action ensuring compliance as needed. Although most high-performance systems employ unified medical oversight (that is, a single medical authority in charge of all output categories), some systems still do not. Thus provision is made vertically for listing a separate medical oversight entity or specifying "none" for each output category.

Comparing Clinical Capability

To document and compare clinical capability, it is necessary to examine written protocols, personnel certification requirements, equipment standards, monitoring and quality improvement practices, patient outcome measures, and other aspects of the following system outputs on the left axis of the EMS matrix:

OUTPUTS (services)	STRUCTURE									SYSTEM STANDARDS AND PROTOCOLS
	A. Responsible organization	B. Personnel	C. Equip-ment	D. Commu-nications	E. Facili-ties	F. Info-systems	G. Finance (sources, amounts)	H. Legal basis	I. Medical over-sight	
1. Prevention and early recognition										
2. Bystander action and system access										
3. Complaint-taking function										
4. Telephone inquiry and pre-arrival care										
5. First Response dispatch										
6. Ambulance dispatch										
7. First Responder services (rescue)										
8. Ambulance services										
9. Direct medical control										
10. Receiving facility interface										
11. Indirect medical control										

Figure 10-5. EMS system matrix.

1. Prevention and early recognition (for example, seat belt awareness, feetfirst first time water safety, early recognition of cardiac symptoms)
2. Bystander action and system access
   A. CPR instruction
   B. Telephone
      1. Emergency (9-1-1)
      2. Routine (7-digit number)
3. Complaint-taking function (in 9-1-1 systems)
4. Telephone interrogation and prearrival instructions
5. First response dispatch
6. Ambulance dispatch
7. First responder services
   A. Rescue and extrication
   B. Initial medical support and assistance during transport
8. Ambulance services
   A. Life-threatening emergency calls (presumptively classified)
   B. Non life-threatening emergency calls (presumptively classified)
   C. Routine transport calls (presumptively classified)
   D. Interfacility transfers
   E. Helicopter transport (scene flights)
9. Direct medical control
   A. Electronic instructions
   B. Hands-on care by scene physicians
10. Receiving facility interface
    A. Patient exchange procedures
    B. Participation in quality assurance
    C. Equipment exchange arrangement
    D. Information exchange arrangement
    E. Selection of hospital destination

11. Indirect medical control
    A. Internal or external
    B. Advisory or authoritative
    C. Integrated or fragmented
    D. Qualifications of physicians
    E. Level of funding and staff support

Response Time Reliability

Just as a system generates reliable or unreliable clinical performance, it also generates reliable or unreliable response time performance. Figure 10-6 shows ambulance response time distributions for two systems claiming "8-minute response time reliability." Given what has been learned recently about the pathophysiology of cardiac arrest, it is clear that Oklahoma City's 8-minute *average response time* delivered life-threatening service to most patients when these data were collected. (That operator has since been replaced.)

In contrast, Tulsa's 8-minute *fractile response time* (at the 90% level of reliability) delivered a bona fide chance of survival more than 90% of the time. Because cardiac arrest is the most time critical of all calls, response time standards for first response and ambulance service are both geared to meeting the needs of patients experiencing cardiac arrest.

Average response time is not only a dangerously misleading indicator of response time reliability, it is also a clinically inappropriate goal. Deployment practices producing the most impressive-sounding average statistics are quite different from those generating 8-minute—90% fractile reliability or a less stringent rural equivalent. It is impossible to pursue the lowest possible average response time *and* the highest percentage fractile reliability; a choice must be made.

The type of report shown in Table 10-1 typifies performance by the ambulance component of the Fort Wayne, Indiana, EMS system, and is widely used by high-performance systems to track response time reliability.

Response Time From the Patient's Point of View

Response time is discussed as though what it is and how it is measured are understood. The following questions and answers summarize what paramedic response time is and is not.

Q: When does the paramedic clock start?

A: When the first request for help is received. It does *not* start when an extended telephone interrogation has been completed, when the responding

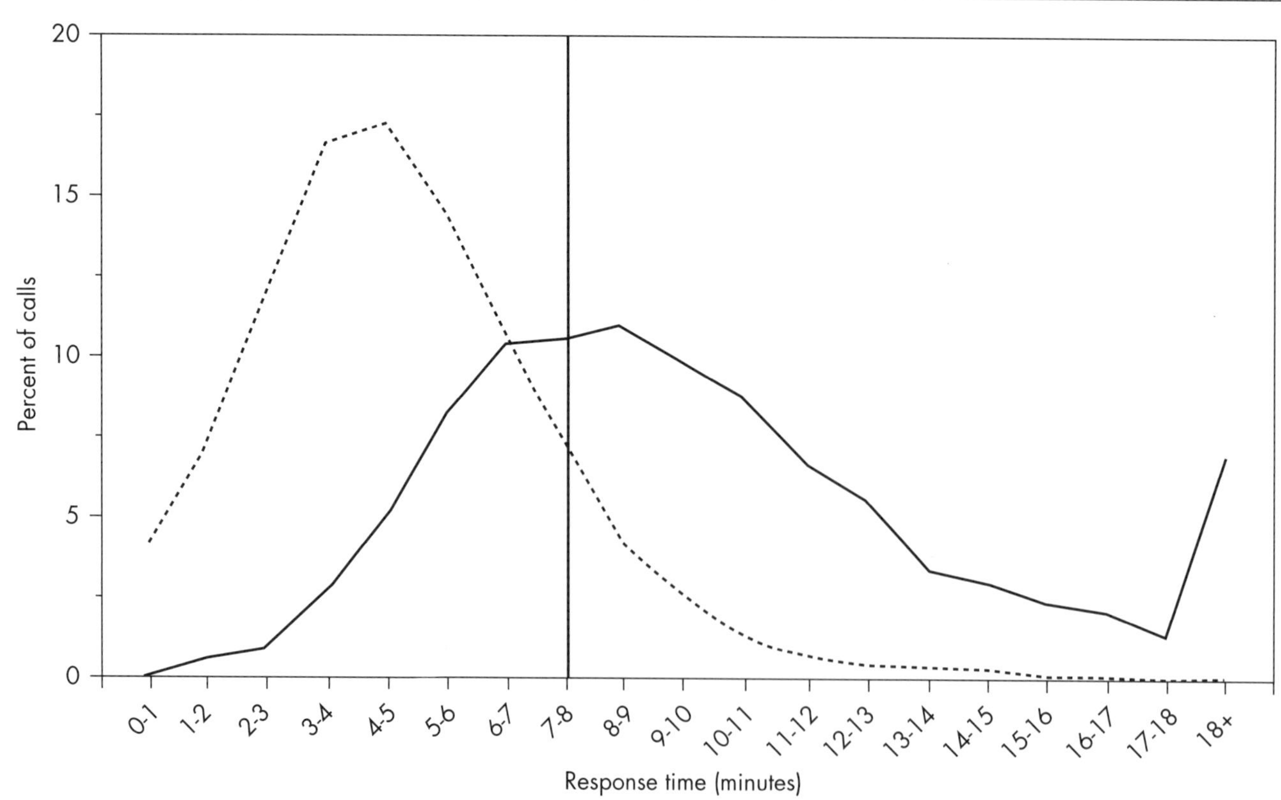

Figure 10-6. Ambulance response time distributions for two systems (Tulsa and Oklahoma City) claiming "8-minute response time reliability."

unit is alerted, when the crew acknowledges the dispatch, or when the unit starts en route.

Q: When does the paramedic clock stop?

A: When a fully staffed and equipped paramedic unit arrives on the scene. Some systems stop the clock not on arrival at the scene, but on arrival at the patient. To time-stamp this moment in large-volume systems a "patient contact" button may be programmed on a portable radio with automatic number identification capability and interfaced to the (CAD). Where automated vehicle tracking (AVT) is available the CAD also time-stamps electronic convergence of AVT and scene. It does *not* stop when a volunteer crew responds to the station, when the responding crew acknowledges the dispatch, when the unit starts en route, when the unit is within sight of the scene, when a First Responder crew arrives on the scene, when a supervisor arrives in a "flycar", or when an EMT-A mutual aid provider arrives on the scene.

Equal Opportunity

Although a fractile response time standard equalizes response time reliability among various zones, districts, or neighborhoods of the service area, it still leaves room for medically and politically dangerous geographic pockets of chronic poor performance. If the areawide standard is already stringent, requiring that standard within each zone or district will raise the systemwide standard to an unattainable level. The solution is institution and enforcement of the following standard: there shall be no chronic pattern of response time discrimination against any neighborhood, district, or zone as defined by local ordinance.

Table 10-1. Fractile Response Time Distribution

Response Time (Min.)	Runs (No.)	Total (%)	Cumulative (%)
<1	4	2.0	2.0
1-<2	8	4.0	6.0
2-<3	18	9.0	15.0
3-<4	28	14.0	29.0
4-<5	36	18.0	47.0
5-<6	40	20.0	67.0
6-<7	34	17.0	84.0
7-<8	18	9.0	93.0
8-<9	6	3.0	96.0
9-<10	2	1.0	97.0
10-<11	1	0.5	97.5
11-<12	0	0.0	97.5
12-<13	0	0.0	97.5
13-<14	2	1.0	98.5
14-<15	1	0.5	99.0
15-<15	2	1.0	100.0

How costly is response time equality among neighborhoods? The city with the longest-standing and highest expectations of response time equality among neighborhoods is Kansas City, Missouri. There 87% citywide paramedic reliability at the 8-minute level is cause for alarm, practically a crisis, and grounds for declaration of major default. The elected official from each of Kansas City's six districts expects monthly reports demonstrating that the constituents are getting their fair share of response time reliability. Adding the neighborhood standard to Kansas City's already stringent 8-minute—90% fractile standard increased annual production costs of an unusually efficient provider between $500,000 and $700,000.

But My Town is Harder

In rural Arizona, *low* population density is the excuse for extended response times, and in New York City *high* population density serves the very same purpose. Wherever response time reliability is deficient the managers have developed persuasive arguments accounting for the deficient performance. As one manager put it, "If God ran this system on the budget I've got, His response times wouldn't be any better."

It is true that call-density-per-square-mile, road systems, shape of the service area, caliber of mutual aid, traffic congestion, placement of hospitals, weather conditions, population fluctuations, and other factors define the limits of response time reliability achievable from any given operating budget. In other words, these factors determine the maximum productivity level or unit-hour utilization ratio (U/UH) at any given level of response time reliability. One of several indicators monitored by managers of high-performance systems, the U/UH ratio is calculated by dividing the number of patients transported during a given period by the number of ambulance unit-hours produced during that same period. In metropolitan areas, U/UH ratios from 0.33 to more than 0.5 are routinely generated by high-performance systems meeting the 8-minute—90% standard of reliability. However, experience has shown that the most important factor in determining maximum, realistic response time reliability at any given funding level is system status management (SSM).

Comparing System Costs

Having established a basis for comparing internal structures, clinical performance, and response time performance of different EMS system designs, attention must be given to comparisons of economic efficiency (that is, the system's ability to turn dollars into service).

Diagnosing and correcting causes of poor economic efficiency requires a working knowledge of marginal cost analysis (especially when dealing with first responder costs), amortized capital costs, the U/UH ratio, paid versus effective unit-hour production, average versus marginal unit-hour costs, economies of scale, and several other management accounting tools. Nearly as complex, revenue considerations could easily fill a book of their own.

Fortunately, a relatively simple method exists to compare system costs even if the details remain a mystery; it is the Subsidy-Price Trade-off Chart. To use this tool productively, avoid the following four mistakes made considering EMS costs:

1. **Price = Cost.** Wrong. In EMS, price (or user-fee) rarely equals cost. Because subsidies distort price structures, some of the most efficient EMS systems charge the highest user-fees, and the token charges of less efficient systems create the illusion of a bargain. Comparison of bottom-line efficiency must account for the combined effect of subsidies and user-fees in different proportions among different EMS systems. The Subsidy-Price Trade-off Chart does just that.
2. **Component Cost = System Cost.** Wrong. The cost of operating a system component (for example, 9-1-1 ambulance service or paramedic First Response) is not the cost of operating the entire system even if the managers of that component have declared it to be the entire EMS system. For example, where a subsidized government-run third-service handles 9-1-1 requests and private firms provide routine and interfacility transport the total cost of the ambulance service component includes *all* user-fees paid to private firms and user-fees and subsidy payments supporting the government-run third-service. That total does not include the costs of public education, first response, or external medical oversight if such oversight exists. Thus the total system cost to a community includes the following:

	User-fee charges (all providers, emergency and routine)
less	Bad debt and contractual allowances
plus	Local tax subsidy (ambulance service subsidy plus marginal costs of first responder services)
plus	Other subsidy (regulatory costs of medical oversight if not included in user-fees)
plus	Dollar value of allocated government overhead, facilities, and shared services ("free" legal services by a city attorney, payroll services, taxpayers' opportunity cost of uninvested working capital, allocated cost of insurance or risk pool reserves)
equals	**Total EMS system cost**

3. **More Subsidy = Better Ambulance Service.** Wrong. Subsidizing the ambulance service component of an EMS system reduces price (or user-fees) below cost. For example, assume a provider's total annual subsidy divided by its total annual patient transports is $400 (a figure typical among low-efficiency systems). Further, stipulate that this provider also charges an average user-fee (that is, base rate plus mileage and other add-on charges) of $250 per patient transport and currently experiences a 50% unadjusted collection rate (that is, unadjusted for contractual allowances). Simple arithmetic reveals that, if the subsidy stopped, this provider could theoretically survive by increasing its average user-fee to $1050. Although such an inefficent system could survive economically, it could not survive politically; someone would notice. The "zero-subsidy" user-fee level of many systems burdened with antique designs exceeds $1500 per patient transport. Thus the only effect of the ambulance subsidy is to reduce price below cost merely delaying the inevitable demise of a poorly designed system.
4. **Ambulance Subsidies Support Higher Wages.** Wrong. Although heavily subsidized government-run services pay slightly better wages than unsubsidized private services, many unsubsidized private services offer wages and benefits competitive with those paid by heavily subsidized systems. Only a fraction of subsidy payments can be accounted for by higher wages, lower user-fees, or a combination thereof. To understand these discrepancies, consider the following fairly typical example:

> If the ambulance service component of the EMS system serving Fort Wayne, Indiana, (currently at zero-subsidy) received the same per capita per year subsidy as that paid by Corpus Christi, Texas, residents (about $11 per capita per year) and these revenues were applied entirely to increase wages of field and control center personnel, every medic working in the Fort Wayne

system would earn more than $100,000 per year. Conversely, without the pay raise but given Corpus Christi's subsidy, the Fort Wayne System could operate without user-fees. The Corpus Christi system has not been singled out to overdramatize a point. In fact, subsidies ranging from $10 to $17 per capita per year are common in metropolitan areas.

The Subsidy-Price Trade-off Chart

Figure 10-7 shows the amount of money from subsidies, user-fees, or a combination of both required to sustain the ambulance service of four EMS systems. For example, in 1990 the Tulsa, Oklahoma, system was comfortably and profitably operating without local tax subsidy by charging an average total bill of $324.30. Alternatively, without charging any user-fees the city could have operated equally well with an annual subsidy of $13.61. Any combination of subsidy and user-fee charges between those extremes (as defined by the line labeled "Tulsa") would also have been sufficient.

To plot the subsidy-price trade-off line for the ambulance component of a system, obtain or estimate total payments for all emergency and routine ambulance services (including all providers the market—public and private, emergency and routine) from all sources (local tax support, private-pay patients, private third-party payors, bundled hospital payment transports, HMO contracts, Medicare, Medicaid, donated funds, subscription membership fees). Divide that total by the population of the primary service area and plot the result (that is, the total system cost per capita regardless of how financed) along the horizontal axis at the bottom of the chart. This point defines the amount of annual subsidy per capita that would sustain the system without revenue from any other source, one of two points along the system's subsidy-price trade-off line.

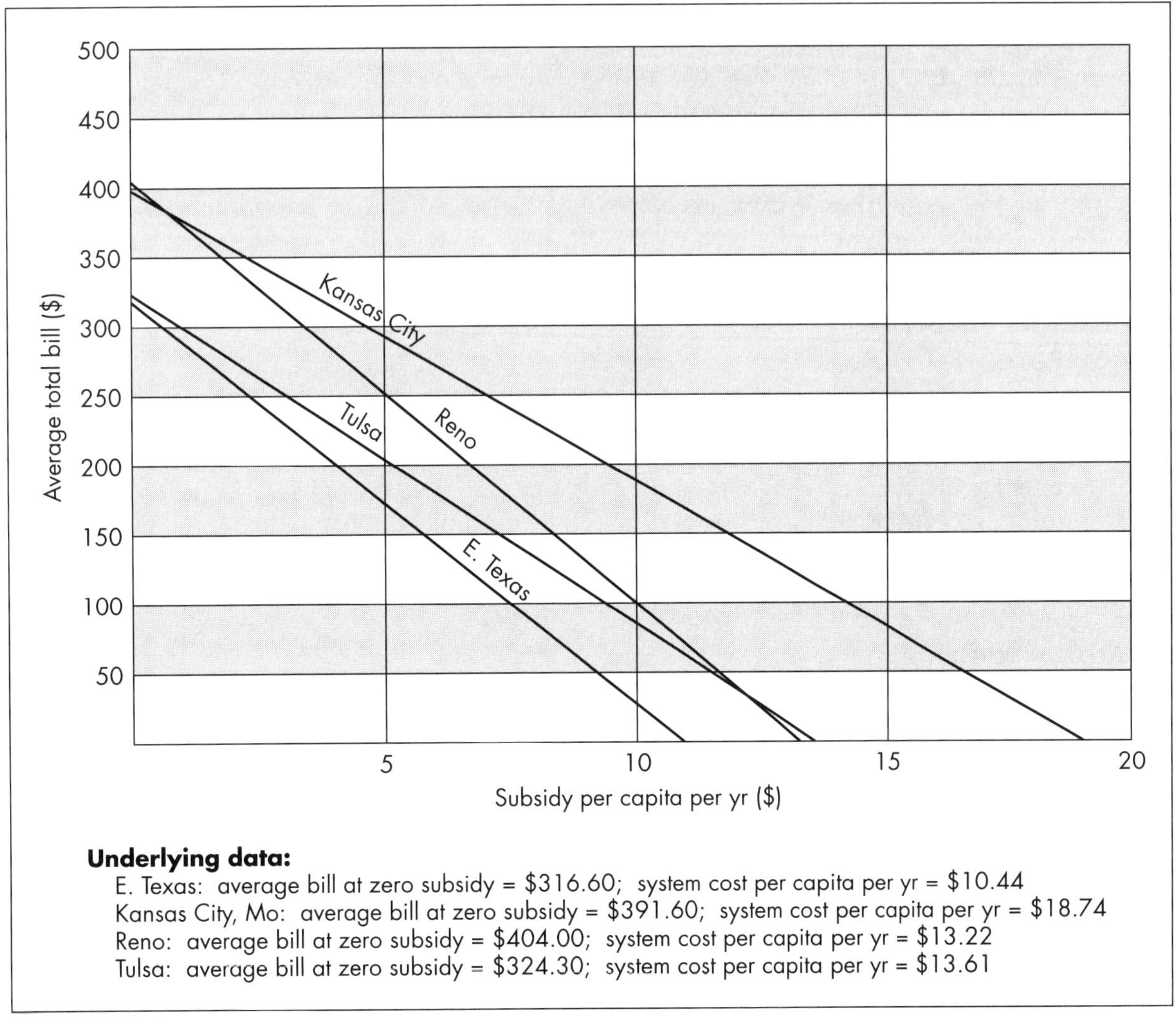

Figure 10-7. Subsidy-price trade-offs—1990 data.

Next estimate the current total average bill (base rate mileage and all add-on charges) for ambulance service in the service area. Note that number, but do not plot it on the chart yet. Estimate the current per capita per year local tax subsidy of the system's ambulance service component. Using these two numbers (the current total average bill and the current per capita per year subsidy), locate where the current total average bill intersects the current per capita subsidy and mark the spot. This point defines the system's current actual position on its subsidy-price line, the second of the two points required to draw the system's current subsidy-price trade-off line.

Now for the moment of truth. Connect the two marks, extending the left end beyond the plotted point to intersect the vertical axis. The result is the subsidy-price trade-off line. At this point many feel they have somehow misunderstood the instructions. Probably not. If the system is an urban system generating paramedic ambulance service with 8-minute—90% reliability and you plot both ends of the subsidy-price trade-off line on Figure 10-7 without extending either axis, your system is more efficient than 90% of all urban ambulance services. For example, to plot the current subsidy-price trade-off line for Washington, DC's ambulance service, it is necessary to more than triple the sample chart's vertical axis and double its horizontal axis; for New York City the vertical axis would be doubled.

Design Factors Affecting Efficiency Potential

Although a high-performance EMS system is the product of "a thousand little things done right," design characteristics of four key elements impact the system's ability to convert dollars into service. Those key elements and the most significant design characteristics of each follow.

Service Area Definition

In the same way and for many of the same reasons that it has become impossible to operate a clinically superb and financially stable stand-alone 20-bed hospital, it is increasingly difficult to operate a small ambulance service of high clinical quality. The minimum for bona fide high-performance operation is a service area population of approximately 150,000 people exclusively served (emergency and routine) by a single ambulance service provider. The average cost curve continues to decline as the population increases to about 1.2 million, still served by a single firm (Figure 10-8).

Where local populations are insufficient to generate optimum economies of scale, multijurisdictional systems (ideally, but not necessarily, contiguous) are often the answer. For example, Tulsa's Emergency Medical Services Authority, the first public utility model, handles about 68% of all patient transports in the state of Oklahoma including much rural area without local tax support.

On the other hand, a large urban service area can be made to function as poorly economically as if it were a sparsely populated rural area. By allowing multiple firms to share the same geographic market, each firm's service area remains equally large, but call-density per square mile resembles that of a rural area.

Medical Oversight

High-performance EMS systems are driven by externally imposed and enforced clinical and response time standards. In this regard, the characteristics of effective medical oversight are as follows:

External versus internal. The medical director is neither hired nor compensated by any organization whose work is the subject of medical oversight. The medical director's authority is independent of and superior to the organizations participating in the EMS system. Otherwise, it would be difficult or impossible for the medical director to fill the role of "referee" in disputes among participating organizations.

Advisory versus authoritative. On matters affecting the quality of patient care, the medical director does direct, not advise. (That is, the system design assumes that the delivery of prehospital care is the medical director's practice of prehospital emergency medicine.)

Scope of authority. A single medical director oversees all organizations and individuals participating in the EMS system. The scope of authority is systemwide and extends to all output components of the EMS matrix, all organizations in the system, and in multijurisdictional systems this authority is legally recognized by all jurisdictions served.

Funding. Effective medical direction requires a sustained commitment and continuing level of effort. The minimum funding required appears to be from \$3 to \$5 per patient transport (emergency and routine) systemwide. It is higher in smaller systems than larger systems with better economies of scale.

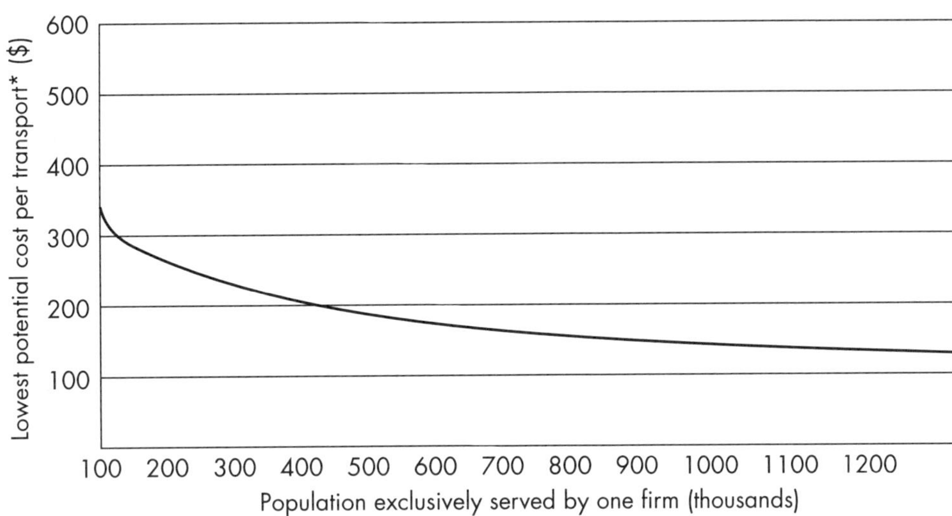

*Assumptions:

- 8-minute/90% paramedic response time reliability
- High clinical quality
- Medium productivity (0.25 to 0.40 U/UH ratio)
- Efficient unit-hour production ($50 to $80 per unit hour)
- Midwest United States cost of living
- Average difficulty of coverage

Figure 10-8. Impact of economies of scale: average cost curve.

First Responder Program

Delivered by existing fire department personnel with fire apparatus, firefighter first response is without question local government's best public service bargain (less than $27 marginal cost per response at the EMT-D level including training, fuel, medical supplies, accelerated vehicle maintenance and depreciation, and amortized costs of medical equipment). The characteristics of first response in high-performance systems include the following:

Production method. Engine company responds at the EMT-D level, no separate rescue units requiring additional personnel and vehicles. Many experts suggest that a rapid First Responder-D or EMT-D response with 10-minute—90% paramedic ambulance service will save more lives than an EMT-A response with 8-minute—90% paramedic ambulance service.[1] This is an easy trade economically and medically, that is, the amortized costs of automated external defibrillators and marginal training costs for first responders is less than the savings realized by replacing the 8-minute—90% standard with a 10-minute—90% standard. Note that the 8-minute—90% ambulance response time standard was developed before the value of early defibrillation was fully understood.

Utilization. Priority dispatch (for example, Clawson protocols) on all presumptively classified life-threatening calls, usually from 40% to 45% of 9-1-1 medical requests or about 25% of all ambulance calls (emergency and routine).

Service area. Unlike ambulance services that must respond and transport across geopolitical boundaries in conformance with medical-trade patterns, the most cost-effective form of first response is monojurisdictional. Thus in multijurisdictional EMS systems (for example, Pinellas County, Florida) each participating fire department is responsible for serving its sponsoring jurisdiction, and the ambulance service component operates regionally for best economies of scale.

Unit selection. In advanced multijurisdictional EMS systems, first response near geopolitical borders is dispatched on a "nearest-unit" basis, not on the basis of political affiliation. The Pinellas County, Florida, EMS system, with 17 participating fire departments and a single regional ambulance service provider, is highly advanced in this respect.

First—before what? No discussion of first response would be complete without raising the two following questions:

- How often are your First Responders first?
- Early defibrillation: earlier than what?

Even though fire department resources outnumber ambulance service resources, it has often proved difficult for first responders to routinely arrive before ambulance crews achieving an externally monitored 8-minute–90% standard of reliability. The Fort Worth Fire Department may deliver America's most reliable first response. As part of a system whose ambulances achieve the 8-minute standard with 90% reliability, the Fort Worth Fire Department first responders are first on the scene in approximately 80% of presumptively classified life-threatening calls.

Ambulance Service

Of all EMS system elements, ambulance service is the most costly (except where separate rescue units are used for first response), the most complex, and the most politically volatile. To make matters worse the proven principles of high-performance ambulance operation fly squarely in the face of the conventional wisdom of the 1970s.

Every ambulance service documenting externally monitored paramedic response time performance at the 8-minute—90% level of reliability while consuming a subsidy of less than $3 per capita per year exhibits the following characteristics:

Single-provider. Exclusive market rights to furnish emergency and routine ambulance service are granted to a single (often competitively selected) organization. "Cream skimming" competition is banned by local ordinance or state law. To put it more directly, elected officials designing an EMS system face a difficult but inevitable choice. They may enjoy the benefits of two of the following three features, but they cannot have all three:

- High quality ambulance service with clinically sound response time reliability.
- Retail competition and consumer choice within the market.
- Little or no local tax subsidy.

Flexible production strategy. Rather than operating specialized ambulance fleets (for example, paramedic units for really sick patients, EMT-B units for not-so-sick patients, and still other fleets providing "invalid coach" transport), high-performance systems employ a single fleet of paramedic units capable of handling any type of service request. Single-provider systems using advanced system status management practices (flexible production strategy) allow safe use of productivity levels or U/UH ratios as much as 300% higher than those found in systems relying on the specialized production strategy.

Peak-load staffing. Patient demand and traffic congestion tend to cycle predictably and coincidentally on a weekly basis. Thus rather than relying heavily on 24-hour shifts and constant staffing practices, high-performance systems carefully match supply with predictable demand and traffic pattern fluctuations for each of the 168 hours of the week, demand fluctuations are tracked at one or two standard deviations from the mean to achieve the 90% standard of reliability. Patterns of demand for EMS more closely resemble those for law enforcement than fire suppression. For the same reason urban police departments do not use 24-hour shifts, high-performance ambulance services in urban areas use few if any 24-hour shifts.

System status management. Because buildings are fixed and fires are rare, fixed-post locations make sense in deploying for fire suppression. In contrast, geographic patterns of demand for EMS cycle widely on an hourly basis with the movements of people and their changing patterns of activity. Just as high-performance EMS systems carefully study and learn the cyclical patterns of *volume* demand, they study and learn the cyclical patterns of *geographic* demand distribution and changes in traffic congestion patterns, designing and refining deployment strategies precision matched to patients' need for service. A medium-sized urban high-performance system may use more than 2000 system status plans (SSPs), one for each potential remaining level of production capacity for each of the 168 hours of the week.

Summary

Although most high-performance EMS systems employ a private contractor for delivery of paramedic ambulance services, every high-performance EMS system employs one or more fire departments in the critical role of first response. America's best and most cost-effective EMS systems blend the best capabilities of the public and private sectors. Even so, is it necessarily true that private is better when it comes to provision of paramedic ambulance service? The irrelevance of this question cannot be better illustrated than by the simultaneous truth of *all* four of the following statements:

1. Some of the best ambulance service is provided by government agencies.
2. Some of the worst ambulance service is provided by government agencies.

3. Some of the best ambulance service is provided by private firms.
4. Some of the worst ambulance service is provided by private firms.

In choosing an ambulance service provider, each jurisdiction selects from one or two local government agencies and several hundred private firms throughout the United States, several with national reputations and excellent track records serving multiple communities in several states. The rational choice is the best qualified organization willing to take on the task. If that organization's credentials and track record clearly demonstrate an ability to generate the required clinical and response time performance *from the financial resources available,* then whether that organization is a government agency or a private firm is only as important as the color of its stationery. Experience has revealed that much of what was assumed and believed during the 1970s simply was not true. Unfortunately the lessons were learned slowly.

REFERENCES

1. Lombardi G et al: Outcome of out-of-hospital arrest in New York City, *JAMA* 271:678-683, 1994.

11

Levels of Providers

James E. Pointer, M.D., FACEP

North America encompasses a wide spectrum of EMS systems, including a diversity of prehospital providers. The following four levels of prehospital providers are common in North America: First Responder, emergency medical technician-Ambulance (EMT-A), emergency medical technician-intermediate (EMT-I), and emergency medical technician-paramedic (EMT-P). Although there probably are no two states that define and train these levels similarly, national standards exist. The U.S. Department of Transportation (DOT) established curricula for the four levels with ranges of required training hours. The DOT only sets standards; it does not train or test. The National Registry of Emergency Medical Technicians (NREMT) is an independent, nongovernmental agency established in 1970. The NREMT tests and certifies EMT-Basics (equivalent to the DOT's EMT-A), EMT-Is, and EMT-Ps. NREMT requires successful completion of an approved DOT training program. Some states require NREMT certification; others perform testing and certification through a state or local agency. Table 11-1 lists training hours for the four prehospital provider levels based on DOT standards.

Despite a paucity of scientific evidence, many urban areas have established complex and sophisticated paramedic systems.[31] The term *advanced life support* (ALS) is hopelessly vague; in some localities, it refers only to the paramedic level and in others it traditionally referred to any intervention requiring a physician order. The paramedic level of care varies tremendously. Paramedics administer a variety of medications, use advanced procedures, and manage the cardiac arrest patient aggressively. Nearly all paramedic systems employ direct and indirect medical control.[22] On the other hand, basic life support (BLS) classically meant the provision of first aid, cardiopulmonary resuscitation (CPR), splinting techniques, and oxygen administration. EMT-As were often said to provide BLS care; past systems were characterized by little if any medical oversight, a superficial approach to patient assessment and treatment, and even less validating research than ALS systems. Although many rural areas do not even use EMT-As, systems that employ ambulances with two or three paramedics have become the "gold standard." To confuse the issue further, some states have an intermediate level between EMT-A and paramedic. These EMT-Is are essentially upgraded EMT-As or downgraded paramedics. The final prehospital provider level is the First Responder. These municipal or volunteer personnel deliver basic first aid and CPR until more highly trained EMTs or paramedics arrived. Until recently, First Responders were rarely subject to medical oversight, often practiced without policies or procedures, and consequently were frequently overlooked as members of the prehospital "team." Although in some cities paramedics are the initial responders, usually First Responder or EMT-A firefighters are first on the scene, followed by private, fire, or third-service ambulance providers. The box on the following page gives sample scopes of practice for the four provider levels based on DOT and NREMT standards.

A number of factors have recently changed the classification of prehospital provider levels. First the

Table 11-1. Training Hours for Prehospital Providers

Level	Didactic	Clinical	Internship	TOTAL
First Responder	40	Optional	Optional	40
EMT-A	99-104	10	Optional	109-114
EMT-I	36-75	48	48	132-171
EMT-P	212-350	232-250	256-500	700-1100

Scopes of Practice for Prehospital Providers

First Responder

CPR
First aid
Basic airway management
Patient assessment
Deliveries
Spinal immobilization
Oxygen administration
Assisted ventilation

EMT-A

Scope of First Responders and:
On-scene triage
Fracture splinting
Extrication and transport
Pneumatic Antishock Garment Application

EMT-I

Scope of EMT-A and some or all of the following:
Medical communications
Esophageal obturator airway or orotracheal intubation
Peripheral vein cannulation
Basic determination of death
Defibrillation

EMT-P

Scope of EMT-I and some or all of the following:*
Oro/nasotracheal intubation
Needle/surgical cricothyrotomy
Defibrillation
Pleural decompression
Intraosseous infusion
Drug administration including:
- Thiamine
- Dextrose/glucose
- Naloxone
- Cardiac arrest drugs
- Beta 2 agents
- Morphine/meperidine
- Diazepam/lorazepam
- Dopamine
- Verapamil/adenosine
- Glucagon
- Furosemide
- Charcoal/ipecac
- Paralyzing agents
- Diphenhydramine

*The following medications and procedures are occasionally used in EMT-P programs: thrombolytics, isoproterenol, aminophylline, nalbuphine, promethazine, nifedipine, phenytoin, procainamide, dobutamine, mannitol, isoethrane, propranolol, glucocorticosteroids, oxytocin, local anesthetics, and central vein cannulation.

urban paramedic scope of practice has greatly expanded. Even in conservative states such as California standing orders within the treatment protocols are now prevalent, and in some states local jurisdictions can enact almost any addition to the paramedic armamentarium. Second the EMT-A scope of practice has also grown; in some states it approaches that of the paramedic. The distinction between advanced EMTs and intermediate providers has blurred. Third the First Responder has arguably become the most important member of the urban prehospital team because of early defibrillation. Last and perhaps most important, fiscal times are different. Government can no longer afford prehospital systems that do not save lives *and* dollars. Research and quality control, previously alien concepts to EMS, are beginning to test the hypotheses of prehospital efficacy.

This chapter describes the levels of prehospital providers in the context of changing needs and diminishing resources. By design and necessity, EMS systems will change drastically over the next decade.

First Responders

First Responders are literally the first persons (citizens, public safety personnel, or prehospital professionals) to arrive at the scene of an emergency. In modern EMS systems the term *First Responder* refers to nonmedical public safety personnel usually firefighters or police. A number of regulatory agencies including the DOT have developed standardized Certified First Responder (CFR) training curricula. These materials provide approximately 40 hours of training in educationally straightforward formats. In the 1970s, fire departments began responding to medical calls because the decreasing incidence of fires made large budgets difficult to justify. Now, many cities have firefighters trained to either the CFR or EMT-A level. Fire department CFRs arrive before more highly trained personnel because there are usually more fire vehicles than ambulances. In most systems, more advanced personnel transport the patient to the hospital. First responders are no longer disinterested firefighters acting as gofers for paramedics. Advances in CPR education and the advent of automated external defibrillation (AED) have elevated the least-trained member of the prehospital team to, potentially, its most essential component (CFR-D).

Well-trained CFRs deliver crucial care; they perform basic patient assessment, including measurement of vital signs. This information is not only important for initial treatment but also provides a baseline for future therapy. Patients with a number of life-threatening conditions including airway obstruction, external hemorrhage, and fractures and dislocations can benefit from the skills of the CFR. These personnel can assist ventilation and give supplemental oxygen, administer CPR, and apply AED. CPR and AED are the two most important components of the scope of practice of the CFR-Ds. These are arguably the most critical procedures in prehospital care; in fact, they are the only treatment modalities that clearly improve patient survival.[26]

Numerous authors have demonstrated the benefit of CPR.[10,34] Much of this literature concerns Seattle where First Responders administer CPR, as well as a high number of private citizens. Seattle has so significantly refined its emergency response that no other area has duplicated its cardiac arrest survival rate.[35] Papers have also shown the benefit of AED in improving survival from ventricular fibrillation.[11,16] Although AED is not included in either the DOT First Responder or EMT-A curriculum, many jurisdictions have added the module for these levels. It is not uncommon for communities to double ventricular fibrillation survival rates after instituting First Responder defibrillation.[16] The AED devices are smart; the only skills required of the operator are CPR and recognition of the lack of a pulse. These skills can be learned in 4 hours. Some communities have even instituted AED programs for laypersons.[9] It is now the standard of care that automated defibrillation be integrated into EMS systems.[20]

Despite the importance of their skills, the First Responders are traditionally omitted from medical oversight or quality improvement plans. Although most EMS jurisdictions require training and retesting in automatic defibrillation, many firefighters practice other medical skills without formal standards or direct or indirect medical supervision; there are several reasons for this. First, in many communities, prehospital care other than that provided by First Responders is provided by another agency. It may be logistically, politically, or fiscally difficult for the EMS agency to regulate the fire department. Second, EMS has traditionally expended an excess of resources regulating paramedics to the detriment of EMT-A personnel and First Responders. System managers must incorporate First Responders into quality improvement plans and should consider formal medical oversight.

Basic EMTs

What applies to CFRs is even more relevant to EMT-As. EMT-As perform all the first responder skills and much more in many areas. In fact, it is becoming increasingly difficult to distinguish an advanced EMT from a paramedic. Most basic EMT-A courses require about 90 to 120 hours; however, many states and communities add training modules that can expand the curriculum to over 300 hours.[19] The personnel trained in these programs have a number of confusing letters or numbers after their EMT designation including *T* for trauma, *A* for advanced, *I* for intubation, *D* for difibrillation, and now a new *B* for basic. To make it even more difficult, some state regulations include an intermediate-level provider with a distinct set of quality improvement and medical oversight requirements. For example, California regulations allow the following three types of providers: EMT-Is, EMT-IIs, and EMT-Ps.[8] The scope of practice of the California EMT-II is between the EMT-I and the EMT-P.

In the most basic form the EMT-A scope of practice includes little more than that of the CFR. Paradoxically, many First Responders are trained at the EMT-A level. However, in some two-tiered systems, EMT-As make scene triage decisions and decide whether the patient can be safely transported to the hospital by an EMT-A unit or requires paramedic intervention and transport.[6] Other two-tiered systems respond with EMT-As and paramedics, and the paramedics make triage decisions. Although a discussion of system configuration is beyond the scope of this chapter, it is sufficient to say that in some systems the EMT-A determination of patient severity and hospital destination is essential.

System planners must exercise extreme care in developing or selecting the modules to add to the EMT-A curriculum. Medical literature supports AED as a lifesaving skill, but there is no evidence that prehospital intravenous (IV) lines alone have any effect on survival.[16] AED can be learned in 4 hours; venous cannulation requires more teaching and practice.[29] Several experts condemn the esophageal obturator airway; providers should not use it as the first choice for airway management.[2,30] Endotracheal intubation is the preferred advanced airway method, but this does not mean that every basic EMT must learn to intubate; new airway devices are coming on the market regularly. Such a decision depends on local regulation and the needs of each community.

The EMT-A curriculum is being revised. The DOT has funded a study considering a significant upgrade in the EMT-A scope of practice without a significant increase in teaching hours. Additions to the scope of practice include pharyngotracheal lumen airways, pleural decompression, subcutaneous injection of epinephrine, oral glucose administration, sublingual nitroglycerine administration, and AED. Other issues under discussion include training time, quality improvement, medical oversight, legislation, and costs. The upgrade of the EMT-A curriculum to EMT-Basic (EMT-B) is controversial. The new EMT-B curriculum was field tested and first taught in early 1994. It will quickly replace the EMT-A curriculum because the number of contact hours are essentially the same.

The inclusion of EMT-B personnel in medical oversight programs is required. Direct medical control may be crucial for EMT-A as certain advanced procedures are added. EMS administrators must develop operational and medical standards and procedures. EMT-As who triage patients, particularly in systems with categorized specialty-care hospitals, should have access to direct medical control and be subject to concurrent review and retrospective analysis. Finally, program cost is a major consideration. EMS administrators must consider resources and scientific evidence in planning prehospital programs. For example, does it make economic and medical sense for an urban community to upgrade all EMT-As to EMT-Bs if the fire department's paramedics arrive 3 minutes later? Does a town of 1000 persons with a small but adequate hospital need any prehospital care other than EMT-A trained volunteer firefighters with AED capability?[20] In the early days of EMS, curricula and scopes of practice were established by anecdote and majority vote. Today, patients and budgets require a rigorous, scientific approach.

Intermediate EMTs

The EMT-I's scope of practice lies between that of EMT-Bs and paramedics. Many of the principles applicable to this group were discussed in the section on EMT-Bs. In most states, one becomes an EMT-I either by upgrading EMT-A or EMT-B skills through training and testing in appropriate add-on modules or by training and testing at an established intermediate level. For example, California has an EMT-II designation with a scope of practice containing about half of the paramedic elements but greatly augmented over that of an EMT-A. North Carolina uses the following four levels of EMS training: EMT-B, EMT-I, EMT-Advanced Intermediate, and EMT-P.[14] Virginia has no intermediate category, but accomplishes the same goal through EMT modular upgrades. For local EMS planners, it will be better to create the EMT-I through the addition of modules than through established state regulation. DOT curricula, state regulations, and state statutes have created scopes of practice often too limited to fit local needs. The modular approach permits local medical directors to choose the skills needed for their jurisdictions. Whatever the mechanisms the usual justification for EMT-I is to provide some advanced skills in geographic areas that do not need or cannot afford paramedics. It is crucial that the reaffirmed national levels of CFR, EMT-B, EMT-I, and EMT-P be viewed locally as minimum levels rather than as ceilings. Too often in the years since 1973, state ceilings prevented innovative medical directors from adopting clinically proven advances such as AED.

The scope of practice of the EMT-I ranges from that of an EMT-A with one additional skill to near the level of a paramedic. This intermediate level varies the most from state to state in scope of practice. Although DOT adds additional patient assessment skills, administration of IV fluids, esophageal obturator airway, and medical communications to the EMT-A curriculum, many jurisdictions have augmented the EMT-I scope with one of these approaches. In many areas an intermediate can defibrillate and administer several medications. Every level of prehospital provider should perform AED. EMS administrators must provide EMT-Is with medical oversight and inclusion in the quality improvement plan. Considering the lack of scientific evidence demonstrating the efficacy of the additional skills and drug administration used by paramedics the most cost-effective prehospital system might be one that starts with the CFR and adds interventions in a modular form as needed.

Paramedics

Paramedics provide the most sophisticated prehospital care. Depending on law and local need, these providers administer an array of medications and initiate a large number of procedures. In some states, paramedics enjoy an exceptionally broad scope of practice if they are adequately trained and tested under appropriate medical oversight.[12] Paramedics have been the subject of extensive regulation and scrutiny during their short existence. The group has been required to test more frequently, complete more continuing education, and accept more direct supervision than any other health care professionals. Paramedics have often been subject to regulatory review without due process. Initially, physicians and nurses overregulated paramedics to protect their own professions, expressing concern that paramedics might replace them in certain positions. In the early days EMS planners believed that strict control and supervision would compensate for the lack of scientific validation of the paramedic scope of practice. Over the years the situation changed. Paramedics established a niche in the health care systems and are considered true professionals. Many paramedics are not just technicians; their ability and responsibility to provide complete patient assessment and technical skills often may separate them from other prehospital providers. Their scope of practice may logically expand to that of physician extender in the near future, thereby providing a crucial additional step on the career ladder.

Although the overall efficacy of advanced interventions has not been established, scientific scrutiny of many components of the paramedic armamentarium has begun. Most systems have abandoned the esophageal obturator airway as an advanced airway adjunct; researchers have shown the safety and efficacy of endotracheal intubation.[30] Careful research has shown a detrimental effect from the use of the pneumatic antishock garment (PASG) in penetrating trauma of the chest. Use of the device in *any* circumstance other than as a splint in femoral and pelvic fractures is questioned.[4,24] Researchers have demonstrated the prehospital safety and utility of a number of drugs and procedures including intraosseous infusion, rectal diazepam, morphine sulfate, naloxone, verapamil, nifedipine, and pulse oximetry.* In spite of the extensive body of literature on prehospital medications, not one has been shown to be beneficial in the prehospital arena.[28] EMS medical directors and others have begun carefully evaluating important quality improvement issues, not just structural and process standards but also outcome.[18,32] These developments and the ongoing experience of EMS systems have produced inevitable and exciting areas of controversy such as the expanding scope of practice, medical oversight, system configuration, and cost-effectiveness. The evolution of these EMS system concerns will define future prehospital care. Tomorrow's systems will only vaguely resemble those of today.

Controversies

Scope of Practice

In most systems the scope of practice has been *expanding*. Not only has the number of paramedic drugs and procedures increased, but the circumstances and conditions under which a paramedic practices have also increased. This broadened scope of practice is due to the expanding technology and the increasing numbers of available therapeutic modalities. More important, the health care community is increasingly comfortable with the use of prehospital providers and is actively searching for improvements in system cost-effectiveness. As quality improvement methods evolve, EMS planners may ask prehospital providers to perform more complex assessments and to administer a more extensive array of medications and skills. Because of shrinking health care resources, paramedics will function in wide variety of clinical arenas. Particularly in the inner city, prehospital services supplant previously existing, underfunded community health programs. Although not the original intent, paramedics often work as technicians in emergency departments and hospital wards, partly because they are well-suited to the task and the environment, but mostly because they are paid less than nurses and other medical professionals. Legislators and EMS planners will soon consider use of paramedics as physician extenders in spite of political pressure from other health professionals. Several states have established a new provider level, the emergency department technician (EDT) or emergency department paramedic (EDP). To become an EDT or an EDP a paramedic usually must have several years of field experience under the direction of an emergency physician or a registered nurse. The paramedic performs much of the field scope of practice but works directly for the hospital.[13] We may soon see the day when paramedics act as inner-city "barefoot doctors." These practitioners would still perform their prehospital duties, but they would also treat a variety of outpatient entities under protocols, perhaps obviating a trip to the hospital. A model is the Alaska Native Health Practitioner Program.

Medical Oversight

Medical oversight is also changing rapidly. Initially, almost every prehospital call required direct medical control by a physician or nurse and the telemetric transmission of electrocardiographic data. Many systems are reducing the amount of direct medical control and increasing the use of standing orders. Of course the quality improvement plan must include mechanisms for monitoring and tracking the effects of such changes. Even quality improvement has experienced a period of growth. The trend is moving away from verifying completion of forms and repetitive tape audits toward outcome audits and comparing the prehospital assessment with the emergency department diagnosis.[25,33] Although some of these changes are the result of research and improved administrative methods, many are due to cost considerations. It is simply a waste of time for a paramedic and a physician to discuss any but the essential elements of a patient's assessment and treatment. Direct medical control should be restricted to deviations from established protocol, quality improvement purposes, and information essential for system management and patient care.

*References 1, 3, 7, 15, 17, 27, 36.

The changes in medical oversight raise an important consideration. In the past, paramedics practiced under the license of the indirect medical control physician or a surrogate. Now, because of enhanced quality improvement and more standing orders the paramedic may not directly communicate with any physician. System planners must clearly delineate the license under which providers assess and treat. Virtually all states require physician medical oversight. The indirect medical control responsibility assumed by the physician must be medically and legally unequivocal; provision of direct medical control must be supervised by the system medical director.

Scene Management

Scene management issues continue to be controversial. Numerous papers on cardiac arrest affirm the importance of prehospital management of ventricular fibrillation. Because of the nature of this condition the first person to arrive on-scene with a defibrillator must use it if the patient is to have any chance of survival. It is inappropriate to transport patients in ventricular fibrillation to the hospital without first attempting electrical conversion if available. However the situation for trauma patients is not so clear-cut. Few would argue that paramedics should intubate patients who are apneic or near-apneic as a result of trauma. The efficacy of PASG and IV lines by paramedics in trauma patients has not been determined. Comprehensive studies show that PASG has a detrimental effect in penetrating chest and abdominal injuries, but there are no good data on use of this device in blunt trauma.[4,24] Infusion of IV fluids also elevates blood pressure in the injured patient. A number of papers debate the time spent by paramedics initiating an IV line on-scene, but again the data are inconclusive.[29,33] Recently, several authors came to the conclusion, based on animal lab evidence, that an elevation in the trauma patient's blood pressure before the control of hemorrhage may be detrimental.[5,21] Predictably the issue requires much more research. In the meantime, advanced airway management, hemorrhage control if needed, and rapid transport to a facility specializing in trauma care is the optimal prehospital treatment for the patient, particularly in urban areas.

Multiple Responders

The use of tiered systems is another area of controversy. A single-tiered system uses the same level of provider for all prehospital responses and transports. Thus a single-tiered system could be all EMT-A or all paramedic. A two-tiered system may use EMT-A personnel to respond and to transport lower priority patients, and paramedics to respond and to transport the more seriously ill and injured. Nontransporting fire department or police First Responders, EMT-As, or even paramedics may be dispatched first; other providers, often commercial in nature, follow to transport if necessary. Dispatch personnel must determine the appropriate provider for each patient. There are many combinations and types of one-, two-, and even three-tiered systems. Single-tiered paramedic systems offer simplicity and safety because every patient receives the benefit of paramedic attendance; however, this configuration is costly and uses highly trained personnel unnecessarily. Multitiered systems use resources more efficiently, but occasionally EMT-As respond in situations requiring more sophisticated care.[6] The use of EMT-Is as the lower tier in a two-tiered system can alleviate the problems of undertriage.

Cost

Cost-effectiveness must be mentioned because it is common to each of the controversial areas listed previously. Shrinking budgets and rising costs have stimulated cost-saving methods and the consideration of a total reconfiguration of EMS systems. For example, a two-tiered system using defibrillator-capable and advanced airway-trained First Responders and EMT-Is may be more cost-effective and efficient than a one-tiered paramedic system.[23] Prehospital providers may soon be educated to perform clinical tasks formerly reserved for physicians or physician's assistants. Urban EMS systems may not be able to respond to every call; in spite of the legal ramifications, some patients may be advised by telephone to seek medical help on an elective basis. Health care systems of the future will have to combine resources. It is not cost-effective to send two paramedics in an ambulance to assess a patient with a sprained ankle; however, one paramedic responding in a van with limited equipment and appropriate social service and medical referral back-up may accomplish more for less money. It is pointless and expensive for paramedics to consult direct medical control for every component of the scope of their practice or to rigidly perform a detailed patient history and physical exam without medical need. Better care is provided when direct medical control is required only in problem cases and standing orders are used for the majority of conditions, and when the quality improvement program is focused on outcomes and deviations from medical protocol. Because of major advances in technology and quality improvement techniques, lowering program costs can be a "win-win" situation for both the prehospital patient and the provider.

Summary

The technologic advances of the 1990s have clarified the role of prehospital care. However, much work remains in clearly proving that EMS benefits patients. On the basis of experience and the desire to provide more services efficiently, the distinction among the various levels of providers and the differences between ALS and BLS are progressively blurring. To continue advancing EMS, planners must be even more creative and flexible in system design and developing the curricula of the providers who drive those systems. In the optimal system, there may be no defined levels but rather a gradual continuum from First Responder to the ultimate prehospital provider accomplished through modules. Prehospital provid-ers armed with physician extender education and standing orders might decompress and integrate our health care systems by assessing and treating a range of conditions in both the prehospital and the hospital environments.

REFERENCES

1. Albano A, Reisdorff EJ, and Wiegenstein JG: Rectal diazepam in pediatric status epilepticus, *Am J Emerg Med* 7:168-172, 1989.
2. Auerbach PS and Geehr EC: Inadequate oxygenation and ventilation using the esohageal gastric tube airway in the prehospital setting, *JAMA* 250:3067-3071, 1983.
3. Aughey K et al: An evaluation of pulse oximetry in prehospital care, *Ann Emerg Med* 20:887-891, 1991.
4. Bickell WH et al: Randomized trial of pneumatic antishock garments in the prehospital management of penetrating abdominal injuries, *Ann Emerg Med* 16:653-658, 1987.
5. Bickell WH et al: Use of hypertonic saline/dextran versus lactated ringer's solution as a resuscitation fluid following uncontrolled aortic hemorrhage in anesthetized swine, *Ann Emerg Med* 19:463, 1990.
6. Braun O, McCallion R, and Fazackerley J: Characteristics of mid-sized urban EMS systems, *Ann Emerg Med* 19:536-546, 1990.
7. Bruns BM et al: Safety of prehospital therapy with morphine sulfate, *Am J Emerg Med* 10:53-57, 1992.
8. *California Code of Regulations* Title 22, Social Security Division 9, Prehospital Emergency Medical Services, 1991.
9. Cummins RO et al: Training laypersons to use automatic external defibrillators: success of initial training and 1-year retention of skills, *Am J Emerg Med* 7:143-149, 1989.
10. Eisenberg M, Bergner L, and Hallstrom A: Paramedic programs and out-of-hospital cardiac arrest: I. factors associated with successful resuscitation, *Am J Public Health* 69:30-38, 1979.
11. Eisenberg MS et al: Treatment of out-of-hospital cardiac arrests with rapid defibrillation by emergency medical technicians, *N Engl J Med* 302:1379-1383, 1980.
12. Garrison HG et al: Paramedic skills and medications: practice options utilized by local advanced life support medical directors, *Prehospital and Disaster Medicine* 6:29-33, 1991.
13. Garza MA, New Alabama certification: EDP, *EMS Insider* 19:4, 1992.
14. Hartley JM, Landis SS, and Allison EJ: Physicians' forum: medical direction and accountability for EMS advanced life support care in rural North Carolina, *NC Med J* 46:271-273, 1985.
15. Haynes BE, Neimann JT, and Haynes KS: Supraventricular tachyarrhythmias and rate-related hypotension: cardiovascular effects and efficacy of intravenous verapamil, *Ann Emerg Med* 19:861-864, 1990.
16. Haynes BE et al: A statewide early defibrillation initiative including laypersons and outcome reporting, *JAMA* 266:545-547, 1991.
17. Heller MB et al: Prehospital use of nifedipine for severe hypertension, *Am J Emerg Med* 8:282-284, 1990.
18. Hoffman JR et al: Does paramedic-base hospital contact result in beneficial deviations from standard prehospital protocols? *West J Med* 153:283-287, 1990.
19. Holroyd BR, Knopp R, and Kallsen G: Medical control: quality assurance in prehospital care, *JAMA* 256:1027-1031, 1986.
20. Johnson JC: Prehospital care: the future of emergency medical services, *Ann Emerg Med* 20:426-430, 1991.
21. Kowalenko T et al: Improved outcome with hypotensive resuscitation of uncontrolled hemorrhagic shock in a swine model, *J Trauma* 31:1032, 1991.
22. McSwain NJ: Medical control of prehospital care, *J Trauma* 24:172, 1984.
23. Ornato JP et al: Cost-effectiveness of defibrillation by emergency medical technicians, *Am J Emerg Med* 6:108-112, 1988.
24. Pepe PE et al: Use of MAST in penetrating cardiac injuries, *Chest* 89:452S, 1986.
25. Pointer JE et al: The impact of standing orders on medication and skill selection, paramedic assessment, and hospital outcome: a follow-up report, *Prehospital and Disaster Medicine* 6:303-308, 1991.
26. Roth R et al: Out-of-hospital cardiac arrest: factors associated with survival, *Ann Emerg Med* 13:237-243, 1984.
27. Seigler RS, Tecklenburg FW, and Shealy R: Prehospital intraosseous infusion by emergency medical services personnel: a prospective study, *Pediatrics* 84:173-177, 1989.
28. Shuster M and Chong J: Pharmacologic intervention in prehospital care: a critical appraisal, *Ann Emerg Med* 18:192-196, 1989.
29. Slovis CM et al: Success rates for initiation of intravenous therapy en route by prehospital care providers, *Am J Emerg Med* 8:305-307, 1990.
30. Smith JP et al: A field evaluation of the esophageal obturator airway, *J Trauma* 23:317-321, 1983.
31. Smith JP and Bodai BI: The urban paramedic's scope of practice, *JAMA* 253:544-548, 1985.
32. Wasserberger J, Ordog GJ, and Donoghue G: Base station prehospital care: judgment errors and deviations from protocol, *Ann Emerg Med* 16:867-870, 1987.
33. Wears, RL and Winton CN: Load-and-go versus stay-and-play: analysis of prehospital IV fluid therapy by computer simulation, *Ann Emerg Med* 19:163-168, 1990.
34. Weaver WD et al: Considerations for improving survival from out-of-hospital cardiac arrest, *Ann Emerg Med* 15:1181-1186, 1986.
35. Weaver WD et al: Factors influencing survival after out-of-hospital cardiac arrest, *J Am Coll Cardiol* 7:752-757, 1986.
36. Yealy DM et al: The safety of prehospital naloxone administration by paramedics, *Ann Emerg Med* 19:902-905, 1990.

12

Medical Interventions

Kristi L. Koenig, M.D.

The concepts of Emergency Medical Technician-Ambulance (EMT-A) and paramedic levels were independently developed in the 1960s. Initially, physicians were only marginally involved with education and medical oversight of EMT-A providers. Paramedics, on the other hand, were generally viewed as physician extenders and specific protocols were developed to govern their actions.

The development of automated external defibrillators (AED) heightened interest in providing medical control and protocols for all prehospital activities. In fact a new basic emergency medical technician (EMT-B) curriculum is being devised as a replacement for EMT-A and direct medical control is being considered for some interventions.[70] This new EMT-B curriculum may include interventions previously considered advanced. With many systems developing structured protocols for basic providers the distinction between levels is disappearing. A continuum of care is emerging; it is no longer meaningful or useful to distinguish between the two. In the future, all responders will require medical oversight. The need for direct medical control varies among levels of providers and types of systems. Although future EMT-Bs will be trained and equipped to perform advanced procedures, if a purely assessment-based format is used, that person will not necessarily understand pathophysiology as well as current advanced providers.

Protocols

Protocols are the rules that run the system. They include aspects of both direct and indirect medical control and guidelines for both administrative and clinical operations. Ideally, protocols should govern every situation a provider might encounter including clinical care given by direct medical control. Some systems are permissive concerning which provider interventions can be ordered by direct medical control; others carefully define what the physician may authorize.

In defining protocols, medical directors establishing a new system or building on an existing system must first decide *what* to treat and then *how* to treat. The specific community environment should be considered, and the protocols should be customized accordingly. For example, the average length and range of transport times will influence how aggressive on-scene treatment should be. Furthermore, protocols must be tailored to the level of the system's responders and to whether there is a tiered response. The level of responder responsible for transporting patients also influences protocol structure. The medical director must be careful not to write protocols that are impossible to follow; this error could lead to malpractice litigation.

The introduction of protocols for advanced providers closely paralleled the development of prehospital care. At first, medical care was provided by physicians, but they quickly replaced themselves with paraprofessionals. Initially, physicians only felt comfortable with significant direct medical control. Gradually, experienced providers were increasingly allowed to act under standing orders.

Standing orders are those protocols that may be carried out by prehospital providers independent of direct medical control. They are a subset of indirect medical control. Some systems operate entirely under standing orders with no requirement for direct medical control. Despite evidence suggesting that standing orders may improve efficiency of prehospital care without compromising quality, some systems do not use them at all.[46] In the majority of systems, voice communication is established with the direct medical control after the initiation of standing orders. If a system uses standing orders, they should be included in the protocols.

Establishing a Treatment Philosophy

There are a number of basic philosophical issues the medical director must resolve before choosing treatment modalities and designing specific protocols. Deciding what drug to administer encompasses only a fraction of the scope of designing protocols; emphasis is increasingly focused on overall improvement of EMS systems. For example, simply adding defibrillation capabilities is ineffective if not coupled with adequate response times. Conversely, adding First Responder defibrillation in fast response, urban systems served by paramedics may have little impact.[55] The medical director must therefore consider the overall system when developing protocols.

Diagnostic versus Symptom

The first thing the medical director must decide is whether treatment will be assessment-based or diagnostic-based. Because it is more difficult to teach providers a diagnostic-based format, the medical director may opt for an assessment-based format. The advantage of a symptom-based format is that protocols may be initiated without establishing a diagnosis, which is often difficult in the field. The classic dilemma is differentiating between congestive heart failure (CHF) and chronic obstructive pulmonary disease (COPD); the chief complaint of both may be "shortness of breath." Although it is easier to identify symptoms, a diagnostic-based format may allow more specific interventions.

Education

Another basic consideration is the level of pro-vider education the local system can support. If the medical director implements additional or more complex clinical protocols, will any additional education and cost be required? Further-more, are there resources available to implement and continue new training? For example, if after studying the clinical needs and medical evidence the EMS physician adds pediatric intubation, questions must be asked. These are listed in the box above, right.

When initiating change the medical director must also consider provider motivations such as whether the proposed changes will be readily accepted and performed. Furthermore the director must know the

Questions to Address Before Adding a New Skill

1. Are there available training institutions or other options to teach the providers this skill?
2. What is the mechanism for implementing protocol changes?
3. How will these changes be used?
4. How will these changes affect the system?
5. Will there be sufficient field experience for the providers to maintain their skills?
6. Is there a quality improvement system in place, and can it be effectively monitored?

allowable scope of practice for the given provider level. Providers cannot perform interventions prohibited by local ordinance or state law.

Safety

The safety of prehospital personnel must remain paramount when designing protocols. It may not be feasible for providers to perform certain procedures in unsafe areas or under difficult conditions. Field conditions often differ radically from hospital conditions. In New York City, for example, paramedics carry narcotics on their persons, because it is unsafe to leave them in the drug box. When patients are victims of violent crimes, providers in many urban settings wait for police to secure the scene before initiating treatment. Such factors may increase response and scene times and limit the performance of certain clinical procedures.

Specialty Receiving Centers

The medical director determines what type of specialty receiving centers (SRCs) exist in the community. Specific SRCs may be designated for clinical areas such as trauma, burn, hyperbaric medicine, replantation, toxic envenomation, spinal cord injury, neonatal, eye, behavioral, pediatric burn, pediatric trauma, chest pain, and poison. Protocols for transport to SRCs must be clear so patients can be triaged to the appropriate facilities. The goal may not be transportion of all appropriate patients to SRCs, because many patients would be brought to these centers unnecessarily. Rather the medical director must determine what degree of triage to SRCs is appropriate. For example, if one trauma patient out of 100 needing immediate surgery is missed, is this reasonable? Field triage criteria are usually modified to fit the degree of acceptable undertriage. The percent of patients overtriaged will then be accepted. Research may lead to improved methodologies for field decision-making.[78]

If SRCs are used in a system, excessive overtriage and triage of patients for economic reasons must be avoided. Furthermore, unstable patients may not be candidates for transport to SRCs. For example, a hypotensive patient with severe chest pain might benefit more from transport to the closest ED, rather than a "chest pain" SRC. With the advent of national health care reform and increased implementation of managed care plans, destination decisions must not be adversely affected by the fear of lack of treatment authorization at non-plan facilities.

Treatment and Transport

Other considerations include the questions of which patients can refuse transport and which patients the providers can refuse to transport.[38] These are difficult medical, legal, and ethical issues. Therefore the protocols should state at what point direct medical control must be involved in difficult transport and clinical decisions. The protocols should also indicate when patients must be transported against their will. The medical director must be familiar with local laws regarding patients' rights.

There are several other philosophical questions regarding patient rights. For example, suppose a patient wishes to be transported to the hospital where his or her private physician practices, bypassing other appropriate facilities. Because the hospital of choice is not the closest, how will the resources of the entire system be affected? Will the ambulance be unnecessarily out of service for a long time? What if the patient is having chest pain or becomes unstable en route? To limit liability and provide the best care for the most patients, methods to answer these questions must be delineated in protocols.

Consider a case in which the provider arrives on-scene and feels that the patient does not have an emergency. In some systems, police or other First Responders may cancel the prehospital response because either the patient's condition is not an emergency or the patient is dead. There is an inherent danger in allowing personnel with limited medical training to make such determinations. Although many systems have sufficient resources to transport all patients who request it, in some systems the limited resources would be quickly overwhelmed. It must be decided whether any provider can refuse to transport a patient and if so under what circumstances. A procedure must be developed to prevent individual variance, increased liability, or suboptimal patient outcomes. The role of paramedics is being expanded in some systems to include nontraditional care rather than transportation of all pat-ients.[32] Such services could include immunizations, primary care, identification of at-risk elderly or domestic violence patients, and referrals to clinics or social services for patients lacking true emergencies.

Withholding Treatment

The discussion of when it is appropriate to withhold or discontinue treatment of prehospital patients is increasingly relevant. Because of limited resources and growing attention to cost-effectiveness, some systems have implemented treatment protocols that provide for the discontinuance of care in those cases considered futile.[10,14,21,29,52] For example, in San Francisco, patients in asystole are pronounced in the field.[88] Recent studies suggest that continued resuscitation efforts for victims of cardiopulmonary arrest for whom prehospital resuscitation has failed are not worthwhile, except in patients with primary cardiac arrest and persistent ventricular fibrillation or patients with severe hypothermia.[12,35,53] Potential problems such as body removal delays and access to grief support counseling must be anticipated. As with any protocol the medical director should seek medical, political, and legal advice.

To simplify transport decisions concerning patients in arrest, it may help to categorize patients as "medical," "blunt-trauma," or "penetrating trauma." Medical arrest patients can be divided further according to their initial cardiac rhythms. For example, a patient with a long downtime and a presenting rhythm of asystole may be a candidate for pronouncement in the field. In the case of penetrating trauma, it may be beneficial to transport those in asystole to the nearest trauma center, especially if pericardial tamponade is suspected. The blunt-trauma victim in arrest might best be pronounced in the field. In some systems, patients with unstable airways are transported to the closest receiving center regardless of any other classification. These issues must be decided systemwide in conjunction with local physicians representing a broad range of specialties. Both the providers and direct medical control must have written guidance and understanding concerning the medical director's philosophy on the transport of "dead" patients.

All circumstances under which resuscitation may be abandoned or withheld must be clearly defined.

Thus medical directors must also address the issue of do-not-resuscitate (DNR).[57] DNR plans are currently designed for terminally ill patients who do not wish to be aggressively treated. A DNR directive is necessary when a friend or relative summons an ambulance for a terminally ill patient near death or in cardiac arrest. Often, state law requires prehospital providers to initiate resuscitative measures even against the known wishes of the patient. Since 1991, patients participating in the DNR system in Orange County, California, have been given green, plastic arm bands that are readily identifiable by prehospital providers.[72] The bands are distributed by private physicians and strictly controlled by the Orange County EMS Agency. When an ambulance is summoned for a patient enrolled in the DNR plan, providers may not initiate resuscitative measures. Procedures such as airway suctioning are performed to provide patient comfort. In some states, DNR patients are given Medic Alert bracelets and standardized documentation.

There are prehospital situations in which further medical care is futile, but social circumstances prohibit declaring death in the field. For example, if a large crowd is observing the providers, it may be necessary to remove the patient from the scene before declaring death and terminating resuscitative efforts. If the medical director recognizes the value of such an approach, it should be spelled out in protocols.

Level of Provider

A system-specific decision must be made concerning the level of provider sent to each call. Some systems work with only paramedics, some use EMT-As, and others send Certified First Responders (CFRs) to the scene. Some systems mix the levels of response, either within units or separated tiers.[14,52] Although it is simplest to send paramedics on all calls, it may be financially prohibitive. Even if this were possible, it is unlikely that ambulances could be positioned to provide optimal response time to all victims of cardiac arrest. Conversely, if there were unlimited resources and a paramedic could be placed on every corner, there would not be enough critical patients for the providers to maintain their psychomotor and assessment skills.

In the future, EMT-B personnel may be equipped with most of the medical interventions shown to improve patient outcomes but currently used only by paramedics. Even today, EMT-As with defibrillation capabilities (EMT-Ds) decrease the need for paramedics. If Eugene Nagle, a father of paramedicine, had an AED in 1968, would he have labored to teach firemen how to read an ECG monitor?

Vehicles

In a tiered system, matching provider level with vehicle type can be complicated. Should paramedics use nontransport vehicles so they can leave quickly when their interventions are not required? If so, suppose a paramedic is first on the scene and finds a critical patient in need of immediate transport? The protocol must indicate when paramedics can transport in the "fly car." What actions would the medical director take if a stable patient is being transported and a call from a critical patient located en route to the hospital comes in? Should ambulance personnel be forbidden, permitted, or required to stop and assess the critical patient?

Hot versus Cold

Another operational issue to address when writing a protocol is whether response vehicles should be sent to the scene with lights and siren (hot) on every call.[21] This is unnecessary and is a potential danger to prehospital providers and the public. The same question applies to transport from the scene to the hospital. Certainly if a patient is medically unstable, rapid response and transport may be appropriate, but what about transporting a patient who is stable? For example, suppose a patient experiencing chest pain has reasonable vital signs but appears to have a cardiac origin of his pain. Is rushing the patient to the hospital in a speeding ambulance with lights and siren likely to exacerbate the patient's condition? Should the patient be slowly and quietly (cold) transported? The answers to these questions depend in part on transport distances and medical probabilities. The best way to decrease prehospital time may be careful organization of the response itself rather than driving fast. The medical director must specify in each protocol whether the providers should respond and transport patients hot or cold.

Use of National Standards

One approach in designing protocols is to conform with national standards such as Advanced Cardiac Life Support (ACLS) guidelines. However, as long as the medical director has garnered local medical agreement, adherence to nationally endorsed guidelines is not imperative. For example, the decision to use high-dose epinephrine, which has not been incorporated into ACLS protocols, is an option some systems use. Obviously the medical evidence must support such decisions. Another example is the continued use of the pneumatic antishock garments (PASG) for penetrating chest trauma after the publication of evidence to the contrary.

Telemetry

The medical director must decide if electrocardiographic (ECG) transmission is required.[20,28] In systems that use only standing orders, telemetry of ECG leads is not mandated. The decision to require radio contact and transmission of ECG rhythm strips depends on the level of prehospital provider training, sophistication of clinical protocols, length of transport times, and the type of patients encountered. Systems that use telemetry usually transmit single ECG leads. However, as interest in the use of prehospital thrombolytic agents has grown, some physicians have added the capability to transmit a complete 12-lead ECG.[6,23,37,51] The medical director must evaluate the impact of and the need for data transmission in the specific system. Ideally the decision should be based on a cost-benefit analysis. Telemetry is still required by law in some states.

Scene Time

Another issue to consider when designing protocols is scene time.[24,34,98] The medical director must decide when providers should "load-and-go" and when further scene treatment may be appropriate. Certainly, in the case of major trauma some medical directors feel that scene time should be kept to a minimum, although transport may be unavoidably delayed for patients that require extrication. The optimal solution may not be to "scoop-and-run," but rather to "scoop-and-treat," that is, to begin treatment en route.

In the case of a medical arrest the issue of optimal scene time is more complicated. There may be little more treatment possible in the hospital than in the field. Early transport of the patient may simply delay appropriate ACLS interventions. Obviously, certain procedures such as defibrillation should be performed immediately in the field. However, the goal of the prehospital provider should be to stabilize patients as quickly as possible then transport them to the hospital for definitive care. To determine how quickly providers should leave the scene, the medical director must decide if they have what the patient needs, then modify the corresponding protocol accordingly.

The prehospital providers may not be able to "scoop-and-run" in all appropriate situations. When providers are forced to remain on the scene because they do not have a destination or accepting facility, lack a transport vehicle, or have a prolonged extrication, the medical director must decide whether *ad hoc* deviations in the protocols are allowed. A case in point is the rare necessity for a field amputation, which is a procedure outside of the paramedic scope of practice in most systems.[56] Although some argue that a degree of vagueness can be useful, experience indicates that it is best to incorporate all reasonable possibilities in the protocols so that there is consistency and accountability in each situation.

Direct Medical Control

The medical oversight must be certain that all direct medical control physicians in the system know and understand the basis of the protocols. Protocols must address whether prehospital providers are allowed to administer the patient's own medications such as nifedipine or insulin; this determination must be codified.

For clinical protocols the medical directors must determine if and when direct medical control is required. They must also decide under what circumstances direct medical control can override existing protocols.[44,86,97] The permissiveness of the protocols is based on the sophistication of the direct medical control and the philosophy of the local EMS system medical director. There are certainly cases in which deviation from protocols might provide better patient outcomes. However, allowing direct medical control to routinely deviate from the protocols is clearly undesirable and patently risky. No drug should be ordered by direct medical control without an approved protocol and the appropriate education of providers.

Rather than allowing direct medical control to independently deviate from existing protocols, many medical directors include optional sections in the clinical protocols. In this way, uniformity can be maintained in educating providers, while still allowing for individual physician judgment. The system medical director is ultimately responsible for all aspects of indirect and direct medical control. Some directors interpret protocols as rough guidelines; others feel protocols should be strictly adhered to at all times. Certainly the specific interpretation must be clear to the direct medical control physicians. Furthermore, when there is deviation from a protocol a mechanism for retrospective review of the direct medical control deviation should exist.

Summary of Treatment Philosophy

Finally, protocols must be customized and endorsed according to the community standard or consensus. National or statewide protocols usually cannot be applied to a system without review, modification, and local approval. Once all philosophical and operational issues have been considered the system medical director develops the specific language for that system. Of course, protocols need constant revision and each change takes time to implement.

Establishing Specific Treatments

This section will not cover every clinical protocol, but it will discuss some of the areas of specific clinical controversy that the medical director encounters when designing and seeking approval for treatment protocols.

Airway and Breathing Management

A controversial area of prehospital medicine is how airways should be managed. Options for the medical director include exclusive use of one type of airway or use of several types. There are many airway adjunct devices available, including oral endotracheal tubes (ET), nasal ET, esophageal gastric tube airways (EGTA), esophageal obturator airways (EOA), percutaneous transtracheal ventilation devices (PTV), surgical tracheal devices, and combitubes. Because patients often can be ventilated without an airway adjunct, protocols should state when adjuncts are indicated or required. The protocols will differ for adult and pediatric populations. The medical director may choose to use nasogastric tubes as an adjunct in children. Although the literature is controversial on which method of airway management is best, ET intubation is usually the method of choice in the hospital and there is little reason to believe any other method would be medically superior in the field.[1,59,79,84,85] Yet a national survey of airway practices with data from 1989 indicates that 81% of the responders used EOA or EGTA.[58] Presumably the reason ET intubation is not universally used is difficulty in training and maintaining intubation skills. The combitube is an option that may come into greater use.[5]

An advantage of ET intubation is that several medications can be given through the ET tube. These medications include naloxone, atropine, diazepam, epinephrine, and lidocaine. Because intravenous (IV) access can often be difficult in the prehospital arena, ET administration of drugs is frequent. Further studies are needed to determine the optimal dosing and dilution of medications. It is not yet clear that standard drug doses will be effective when used with devices that block the esophagus. The ACLS guidelines recommend tripling the ET tube dose.[27]

If ET intubation is used, the medical director should also consider whether the providers should be allowed to use anesthetic or paralytic drugs to facilitate intubation.[82] For example, succinylcholine is used in the Portland system. Protocols must specify when such agents can and must be used; they are dangerous if given inappropriately.

Management of reactive airway disease is constantly changing in the hospital; these changes should be reflected in the prehospital setting. The measurement of peak flow as a determinant of treatment is currently out of favor. Because of the low therapeutic-to-toxic ratio and decreased benefits, use of aminophylline has declined as well, especially in patients with COPD.[83]

The beta-agonists most commonly used in the field to treat reactive airway disease are metaproterenol and albuterol. Albuterol is probably the best choice because of its decreased cardiac side effects. Thus it is being considered for the new EMT-B curriculum. Dosing inhaled beta-agonists for children can be difficult. If a normal adult dosage is available, the nebulizer is held up to the child and 15 to 20 breaths are taken. This method gives an adequate dose as a result of the child's smaller tidal volume. Larger doses also appear safe. The current *EMS for Children Guidelines* recommend using continuous albuterol until a positive effect is seen.

Another medication the medical director may choose to include is isoproterenol. Although this medication has fallen out of favor in the treatment of cardiac patients, it can be lifesaving in a pediatric asthmatic patient. However, it would probably be unnecessary in an EMS system with very short transport times.

Although they do not replace more traditional assessments of adequate oxygenation, two airway adjuncts are increasingly common and deserve special mention. First, pulse oximetry has multiple uses and is already common on ambulances in New York City. Second, end-tidal CO_2 devices are now inexpensive and can be lifesaving.[33,74]

An airway procedure that may be included is cricothyrotomy.[74] Modalities used less frequently are the Heimlich valve and the McSwain dart.[64] Skills maintenance may be problematic because relatively few patients require these specialized procedures.

Management of Cardiac and Circulatory Emergencies

Asystole is the worst possible initial rhythm.[80] In systems such as Orange County, California, prehospital providers are instructed to routinely defibrillate patients presenting in asystole. The patient may actually be in fine ventricular fibrillation, and defibrillation almost certainly will not harm a "dead" patient. In other systems, it is routine for the providers to check lead placement and then confirm asystole in two separate ECG leads before defibrillation.[22] This helps prevent potentially dangerous use of electricity on a patient who may simply have misplaced leads.

Some ACLS medications have fallen out of favor. However, before removing these drugs the medical director should consider whether prehospital providers should be educated in their other uses. For example, sodium bicarbonate is no longer commonly used in cardiac resuscitations unless it can be shown that the patient has a profound acidosis.[3,16] However, in the case of severe cardiac toxicity from a tricyclic antidepressant overdose if the patient is deteriorating in spite of other supportive measures the medical director may include a direct medical control option allowing the use of intravenous sodium bicarbonate as a first-line therapy.[45]

Another medication gradually removed from the ACLS protocols is calcium. Yet in the case of a known calcium channel blocker overdose or a renal failure patient in or near cardiac arrest, this medication may improve outcome. It should therefore be considered for inclusion in the armamentarium of the prehospital provider, perhaps not to be used through a standing order but rather as a physician option.

The dose of a medication commonly used for cardiac arrest patients has recently come into question. The so-called high-dose epinephrine ranges from 5 to 15 mg.[16,17] Although this increased dose of epinephrine is being studied, it has not been proven to be beneficial in the prehospital setting and may be detrimental.[17,73,76] Preliminary results indicate that even though more "hearts" are resuscitated the patients are brain-dead. High-dose epinephrine is not routinely recommended in the most recent ACLS guidelines.[27]

There is at least one system in which medical oversight is convinced that this higher-dose regimen improves patient outcome, therefore the providers have been directed to give the higher dose of epinephrine.[68] Because providers may be unfamiliar with this dose and do not carry high-dose vials of epinephrine this order may create confusion. It is imperative that the system medical director is aware and approves of all actions taken by the direct medical control physicians.

Another modality relatively new to the prehospital arena is thrombolysis for patients with acute myocardial infarction (MI).[7,19,36,37,51] Certainly in a patient without contraindications, thrombolytic agents should be administered as early as possible. There is evidence that identification of thrombolytic candidates in the prehospital setting reduces the time to treatment, thereby improving outcome. It is not yet clear whether the risks and difficulties of implementing thrombolytic therapy in the field will outweigh its benefits. Such a protocol may prove most beneficial in a system with relatively long transport times.

Aspirin is another agent currently recommended in the setting of acute MI, and it is used in some systems. Aspirin and thrombolytic agents should not be ordered without a protocol; and before new protocols and procedures are implemented there must be a general consensus among the physicians in the community. Obviously, education of the providers is necessary before implementing any protocol change.

The use of antidysrhythmics in the treatment of cardiac emergencies is controversial. The indirect medical control physician may choose to strictly follow the ACLS guidelines in designing the protocols or modify them based on community needs. The use of lidocaine prophylactically deserves special mention. Some medical directors have written protocols that support lidocaine administration to any patient suffering from an acute MI. However, several studies demonstrate that prophylactic lidocaine in the prehospital setting does not favorably effect patient outcome.[39,42] Antidysrhythmic agents such as bretylium tosylate or procainamide are used in addition to lidocaine in some systems. The use of external cardiac pacemakers is also being explored in some systems.[8,26,41,96] "Thump pacing" may be considered as well.

Many studies show that the cardiac patient with an initial rhythm of ventricular fibrillation and a short "downtime" has the best outcome.[25,40,99,100] To this end there has been much interest in upgrading the capabilities of EMT-As so that they are also capable of defibrillating, thus creating the so-called EMT-D. EMT-Ds are equipped with AED. The use of EMT-Ds has already improved patient outcome.[16,25,40,93,101] Ideally, First Responders who arrive on-scene before more highly trained personnel should also be trained and equipped with AED such as is the case with police officers in some systems. New methods (such as interposed abdominal compressions) and devices (such as "toilet plunger CPR devices") are constantly being studied. The medical director must keep abreast of the current literature and decide what is appropriate for the system.

A cardiac protocol that deserves consideration addresses the treatment of congestive heart failure (CHF) or acute pulmonary edema (APE). There has been a trend away from morphine (MS) as a first line treatment of CHF toward a more liberal use of nitrates. The prehospital study that examined the treatment of patients with presumed APE compared the following four regimens: nitroglycerin (NTG) plus furosemide, MS plus furosemide, NTG plus MS, and a combination of all three. The authors found that NTG is beneficial in the prehospital management of APE. MS and furosemide may not add anything and may be potentially deleterious.[43]

Some physicians are hesitant to allow providers to use NTG before contacting direct medical control, because it is difficult to distinguish between CHF and COPD. In the case of a very ill prehospital patient the protocol may allow for both NTG and bronchodilators. When CHF is suspected, furosemide may also be used; however the optimal dose is not well-established. When determining the prehospital dose, it is beneficial to have prehospital personnel obtain a history of prior use and dosage. Pressor agents such as dopamine or dobutamine may also be used in low cardiac output states; however, it may be difficult in the prehospital setting to determine whether the patient is volume depleted or in cardiogenic shock.

The prehospital management of supraventricular tachycardias (SVT) encompasses several options. If the patient is unstable, cardioversion is recommended. However, in the field this is a frightening procedure that must be carried out under less than ideal conditions. Some studies have examined the use of verapamil to treat SVT in the prehospital setting.[75] This medication appears to be efficacious; however, side effects such as hypotension may occur. There is some evidence that pretreatment with calcium blunts this decrease in blood pressure without affecting the antidysrhythmic effects.[38,69,87,103] Other possible prehospital treatments for paroxysmal SVT include vagal maneuvers, PASG, overdrive pacing, and other drugs. In older patients, who are at higher risk for cerebral embolism from carotid sinus massage, alternate types of vagal maneuvers may be preferred.

One drug used for treatment of SVT that is currently being introduced into the field deserves special mention. Adenosine is promising; the half-life is less than 10 seconds, making side effects transient and benign.[18] It is recommended as the initial drug of choice for hemodynamically stable SVT in the newest ACLS guidelines.[27] One hospital study reports successful use of adenosine in patients who previously would have been cardioverted because they were "unstable."[51]

Management of Trauma

The operational issue of "scoop-and-run" versus on-the-scene treatment for trauma has already been addressed in this chapter. Another major issue in the prehospital treatment of trauma patients concerns use of the PASG.[9,62,77] A controversy rages regarding the benefits of the PASG. Unfortunately the PASG became part of the EMS armamentarium without studies testing its efficacy. Later, it was introduced into the national EMT-A curriculum without data on its effects on patient outcome. Because it is already in general use, it is now difficult to remove the PASG. There is literature suggesting that it is detrimental in patients with penetrating chest wounds and hypo-volemia.[48,62] This effect may be caused by an increase in blood pressure leading to an increased rate of hemorrhage. One area in which PASG remains useful is the stabilization of pelvic fractures.

Prehospital fluid administration in trauma must be addressed. Although the efficacy of prehospital fluid resuscitation for patients with uncontrolled hemorrhage has been questioned, most systems still incorporate the use of one or two large-bore IV lines of lactated Ringer's or normal saline.[61] Lines should be established either en route or on-scene as long as this does not delay transport. A few systems carry other types of fluids such as hypertonic saline.[60] For cardiac patients, some systems use 5% dextrose in water solutions (D_5W). It is less cumbersome and more cost-effective, especially in systems with short transport times, to use a single fluid such as normal saline or lactated Ringer's. Another IV option is the saline or heparin lock. However, heparin is probably not necessary and may be dangerous, even in low doses.[31] With a saline lock, prehospital providers gain immediate IV access but save the expense and potential danger of fluid infusion.

The medical director may train prehospital personnel in the use of intraosseous (IO) lines.Pediatric patients often have difficult IV access, and this is an excellent alternative.[30,90,91] Glucose, epinephrine, atropine, valium, naloxone, fluids, and probably adenosine are therapies that can be administered through IO lines.

Fluid administration guidelines may be particularly difficult to develop in cases of head trauma. A trauma patient may require large volumes of fluids in spite of the risk of increasing intracranial pressure. In a system with long transport times, mannitol and furosemide should be considered for inclusion in treatment protocols for head trauma.

Although there is debate over what type of fluid is optimal for the hypovolemic trauma patient, normal saline may have advantages in some medical patients (for example, diabetics in ketoacidosis with huge intravascular volume deficits).[60] Also, when paramedics dilute medications, as in the case of 50%

dextrose in water ($D_{50}W$) for administration to children, normal saline is a better diluent.

One of the most important things field providers can do to alleviate patient suffering is provide analgesia. In the trauma setting this practice is generally discouraged. Especially in the presence of intraabdominal hemorrhage or head trauma, narcotic analgesia deleteriously affects vital signs, mental status, and accuracy of further evaluation. The medical director must decide if any type of analgesia will be allowed in the setting of trauma. For example, if a patient has an isolated long-bone fracture, should providers be permitted to administer morphine? Another potential pain-relieving medication, which is commonly used for trauma patients in Europe, is nitrous oxide.[80] Years ago and now again, nitrous oxide has been used in U.S. systems with generally positive results.[50]

In the management of trauma patients, even simple procedures are controversial. Aside from the use of the PASG, another classic area of controversy concerns the management of trauma that produces a pulseless extremity. Should the provider extricate and transport patients in the position in which they are found or should the extremity be immediately straightened? Similarly, should patients with a potential spine injury be transported in the position in which they are found or have their spine moved to a neutral position before immobilization? The medical director must clarify these issues and then specifically address them in the protocols.

The treatment of acute spinal cord injuries in the prehospital setting has until now involved spinal immobilization and fluids for the treatment of spinal shock. However, one study concludes that early use of methylprednisolone improves long-term outcomes.[13] Although this drug has rarely been used in the prehospital setting, it should be considered because these authors recommend administration as early as possible and within 8 hours of injury.

Management of Neurologic Emergencies

One of the most frequently encountered neurologic emergencies in the prehospital setting is the patient who presents with an altered level of consciousness (ALOC). The administration of IV dextrose to a hypoglycemic patient is straightforward. There is at least theoretical evidence that thiamine should be administered before glucose, especially in the alcoholic patient. The reason is that thiamine is a cofactor in glucose metabolism, and it is possible to precipitate an acute Wernicke's encephalopathy when administering glucose to a patient who is already thiamine depleted.[81] Thiamine is generally given intravenously in the hospital. Paramedics in New York City administer 100 mg of IV thiamine before IV dextrose to all patients with an ALOC.

Another common medication for patients with an ALOC is naloxone.[104] There is a trend toward using a 2 mg initial dose rather than the 0.8 mg dose used previously. However, in some patients this larger dose may precipitate withdrawal, which can be difficult to manage in the prehospital setting. On the other hand, there are some types of overdoses such as propoxyphene that require even higher doses of naloxone. In general, naloxone is probably most useful in the prehospital setting for patients with a depressed respiratory rate that might otherwise require ventilatory support. Based on the disease spectrum of a particular system the medical director must decide which dosage vial of naloxone the providers should carry. Naloxone may be given IM, sublingually, or via IV, IO or ET tube in patients with difficult access. As time progresses, other antidotes may become available and prove beneficial in the field such as flumazenil as a reversal agent for benzodiazepine overdose.[102]

A third prehospital emergency that requires immediate treatment is status epilepticus. Most systems use diazepam for treatment of this condition. However, there is a trend toward the use of lorazepam, which has not yet been studied in the field. A status epilepticus protocol is invoked in some systems simply because the patient is seizing when the providers arrive. Children presenting in status epilepticus can be especially difficult to treat. In addition to dextrose, many system directors have elected to use rectal diazepam, which has been effective in children in the prehospital setting and alleviates the need to start an IV line.[2,89] There are reports of apnea following rectal diazepam administration, but it is not yet clear whether this is directly related to the drug or the dose.[67] This raises the issue of whether it is beneficial to treat status epilepticus in the field at all. The provider may be doing more harm than good by creating an apneic patient in a moving ambulance. A group in San Francisco is currently studying this in adults by comparing diazepam with lorazepam and with placebo in a randomized, blinded fashion.[66]

Management of Childbirth

Management of prehospital childbirth is part of the EMT-A curriculum and therefore is not always addressed in the paramedic protocols. Because many systems are developing protocols for all levels of providers a childbirth protocol is appropriate and should specify when delivery should be prepared for and performed in the field as opposed to initiating transport of the patient to the hospital. Certainly, it is better to attempt to bring the patient to the hospital; yet delivery in a moving ambulance can be even more chaotic and dangerous than one prepared for in the field.

Management of Other Medical Emergencies

A controversial area is the prehospital management of poisonings or overdoses. Although it was once common to give ipecac in the field, this technique has fallen out of favor. The nature of the ingestion cannot always be reliably determined (especially in suicidal adults). Therefore it may be dangerous to give ipecac because the patient may develop, as in the case of a tricyclic antidepressant overdose, a decreased level of consciousness en route. This could lead to vomiting in a patient without a controlled airway. Even so the medical director may choose to stock ipecac either for children, when the type of ingestion is known, or for adults when there is a long transport time. Some systems such as Pittsburgh use activated charcoal in the field, which can be difficult and can delay transport times. Further studies are needed to determine if and when it is beneficial to administer charcoal during the prehospital phase. A few specific drugs can be lifesaving for certain types of overdoses (for example, glucagon for beta-blocker overdose), and the medical director may include a direct medical control option for these special cases.

Another medical emergency involves the treatment of an ALOC secondary to either hyperglycemia or hypoglycemia. Many systems include the use of a glucometer or dextrostick in the protocol of ALOC. It was previously thought that any patient with an ALOC should receive among other things a 25 to 50 ml of $D_{50}W$ IV push. In many cases patients felt to have strokes "recovered" after receiving $D_{50}W$, because they were actually hypoglycemic. Yet, there is evidence that the indiscriminate use of IV dextrose can worsen outcome in patients suffering from MI, stroke, or other conditions, placing them at risk for cerebral ischemia.[15,71] Others have concluded that the hyperglycemia seen in sicker stroke patients is a stress response, and measures to lower glucose are not beneficial. Another example of a potentially confusing presentation of ALOC is the patient who suffers an apparent head injury, but in reality suffers from hypoglycemia, which caused the accident. Until the controversy regarding the indiscriminate use of $D_{50}W$ is resolved, it is useful to be capable of determining a blood glucose level in the field and administering glucose based on the results. In patients with suspected or confirmed hypoglycemia but no IV access, IM or subcutaneous glucagon may be a protocol option.[95]

The administration of dextrose in children further complicates prehospital protocols. Most pediatric intensivists recommend $D_{10}W$ in infants and $D_{25}W$ in children rather than the $D_{50}W$ used in adults. The type of dextrose solution the prehospital provider should carry is therefore problematic. It would be costly and cumbersome to carry more than one type of solution. One option is to dilute $D_{50}W$ to $D_{25}W$ or $D_{10}W$ for those rare cases when it is required. An area that should be evaluated is whether $D_{25}W$ could be used safely and effectively in all age groups.

For patients who remain combative despite treatment of reversible causes of ALOC the medical director may consider chemical restraint in addition to traditional physical restraints. Benzodiazepenes or antipsychotic medications can be used for this purpose. For example, droperidol is used in the Portland system.

Anaphylaxis is one of the few medical emergencies that, in the absence of treatment, can proceed rapidly to death. Therefore EMT-A personnel can be taught to use epinephrine preparations specifically for this purpose. On the other hand, the medical director may adopt a protocol that allows EMT-As to administer the patient's own epinephrine. The issues need to be carefully examined if these protocols are used at the EMT-A or EMT-B level because state laws may not be permissive and these providers often do not make contact with direct medical control.

Summary

The medical director considers basic philosophical issues, tailors them to a particular system, devises specific interventions, and formally writes the protocols, ideally with the general support of the medical community. There must be a system to perform quality improvement on these protocols and to revise them as necessary. As new treatments are introduced into the hospital setting, they must also be considered for prehospital settings. There is a delicate balance between being the first and the last to introduce a new clinical intervention in the prehospital arena.

REFERENCES

1. Aijian P et al: Endotracheal intubation of pediatric patients by paramedics, *Ann Emerg Med* 18:489-494, 1989.
2. Albano A, Reisdorff EJ, and Wiegenstein JG: Rectal diazepam in pediatric status epilepticus, *Am J Emerg Med* 70:168-172, 1989.

3. American Heart Association: Standards and guidelines for cardiopulmonary resuscitation (CPR) and emergency cardiac care (ECC), *JAMA* 255:2905-2984, 1986.
4. American College of Emergency Physicians: Guidelines for 'do-not-resuscitate' orders in the prehospital setting, *Ann Emerg Med* 17:1106-1108, 1988.
5. Atherton GL and Johnson JC: Ability of paramedics to use the combitube in prehospital cardiac arrest, *Ann Emerg Med* 22:1263-1268, 1993.
6. Aufderheide TP et al: The diagnostic impact of prehospital 12-lead electrocardiography, *Ann Emerg Med* 19:1280-1287, 1990.
7. Barbash GI et al: Improved survival but not left ventricular function with early and prehospital treatment with tissue plasminogen activator in acute myocardial infarction, *Am J Cardiol* 66:262-266, 1990.
8. Barthell E et al: Prehospital external cardiac pacing: prospective, controlled clinical trial, *Ann Emerg Med* 17:1221-1226, 1988.
9. Bickell WH et al: Randomized trial of pneumatic antishock garments in the prehospital management of penetrating abdominal injuries, *Ann Emerg Med* 16:653-658, 1987.
10. Bonnin MJ and Swor RA: Outcomes in unsuccessful field resuscitation attempts, *Ann Emerg Med* 18:507-512, 1989.
11. Bonnin MJ and Swor RA: Prehospital cardiac arrest therapy, *Ann Emerg Med* 19:340, 1990 (letter).
12. Bonnin MJ et al: Distinct criteria for termination of resuscitation in the out-of-hospital setting, *JAMA* 270:1457-1462, 1993.
13. Bracken MB et al: A randomized, controlled trial of methylprednisolone or naloxone in the treatment of acute spinal cord injury, *N Engl J Med* 322:1405-1411, 1990.
14. Braun O, McCallion R, and Fazackerley J: Characteristics of mid-sized urban EMS systems, *Ann Emerg Med* 19:536-546, 1990.
15. Browning RG et al: Fifty percent dextrose: antidote or toxin? *Ann Emerg Med* 19:683-687, 1990.
16. Callaham ML: High-dose epinephrine therapy and other advances in treating cardiac arrest, *West J Med* 152:697-703, 1990.
17. Callaham M, Barton CW, and Kayser S: Potential complications of high-dose epinephrine therapy in patients resuscitated from cardiac arrest, *JAMA* 265:1117-1122, 1991.
18. Cairns CB and Niemann JT: Intravenous adenosine in the emergency department management of paroxysmal supraventricular tachycardia, *Ann Emerg Med* 20:717-721, 1991.
19. Castaigne AD et al: Prehospital use of APSAC: results of a placebo-controlled study, *Am J Cardiol* 64:30A-33A, 1989.
20. Cayten CG et al: The effect of telemetry on urban prehospital cardiac care, *Ann Emerg Med* 14:976-981, 1985.
21. Clawson J: *Principles of emergency medical dispatch,* Englewood Cliffs, NJ, 1988, Prentice Hall.
22. Cummins RO and Austin D: The frequency of 'occult' ventricular fibrillation masquerading as a flat line in prehospital cardiac arrest, *Ann Emerg Med* 17:813-817, 1988.
23. Cummins RO and Eisenberg MS: From pain to reperfusion: what role for the prehospital 12-lead ECG? *Ann Emerg Med* 19:1343-1346, 1990 (editorial).
24. Cwinn AA et al: Prehospital advanced trauma life support for critical blunt trauma victims, *Ann Emerg Med* 16:399-403 1987.
25. Eisenberg MS et al: Cardiac arrest and resuscitation: tale of 29 cities, *Ann Emerg Med* 19:179-186, 1990.
26. Eitel DR et al: Noninvasive transcutaneous cardiac pacing in prehospital cardiac arrest, *Ann Emerg Med* 16:531-534, 1987.
27. Emergency Cardiac Care Committee and Subcommittees, American Heart Association: Guidelines for cardiopulmonary resuscitation and emergency cardiac care, *JAMA* 286:2171-2302, 1992.
28. Erder MH and Davidson SJ: Telemetry in prehospital care, *Ann Emerg Med* 16:923, 1987 (letter).
29. Frank M: Should we terminate futile resuscitations in the field? Can we afford not to? *Ann Emerg Med* 18:594-596, 1989 (editorial).
30. Fuchs S, LaCovey D, and Paris P: A prehospital model of intraosseous infusion, *Ann Emerg Med* 20:371-374, 1991.
31. Garrelts JC: White clot syndrome and thrombocytopenia: reasons to abandon heparin IV lock flush solution, *Clin Pharm* 11:797, 1992.
32. Garza MA: Paramedics: the next generation, *JEMS* 8:89-96, 1993.
33. Ginsburg WH: When does a guideline become a standard? *Ann Emerg Med* 22:1891-1896, 1993.
34. Gold C: Prehospital advanced life support vs. "scoop-and-run" in trauma management, *Ann Emerg Med* 16:797-801, 1987.
35. Gray WA, Capone FJ, and Most AS: Unsuccessful emergency medical resuscitation: are continued efforts in the emergency department justified? *N Engl J Med* 325:1393-1398, 1991.
36. Greenberg H et al: Out-of-hospital, paramedic administered streptokinase for acute myocardial infarction, *Lancet* 2:1187, 1988 (letter).
37. Grim PS, Feldman T, and Childers RW: Evaluation of patients for the need of thrombolytic therapy in the prehospital setting, *Ann Emerg Med* 18:483-488, 1989.
38. Haft JI and Habbab MA: Treatment of atrial arrhythmias: effectiveness of verapamil when preceded by calcium infusion, *Arch Intern Med* 146:1085-1089, 1986.
39. Hargerten K et al: Prehospital prophylactic lidocaine does not favorably affect outcome in patients with chest pain, *Ann Emerg Med* 19:1274-1279, 1990.
40. Hargarten KM et al: Prehospital experience with defibrillation of coarse ventricular fibrillation: a 10-year review, *Ann Emerg Med* 19:157-162, 1990.
41. Hedges JR et al: Prehospital trial of emergency transcutaneous cardiac pacing, *Circulation* 76:1337-1343, 1987.
42. Hine LK et al: Meta-analytic evidence against prophylactic use of lidocaine in acute myocardial infarction, *Arch Intern Med* 149:2694-2698, 1989.
43. Hoffman JR and Reynolds S: Comparison of nitroglycerin, morphine, and furosemide in treatment of presumed prehospital pulmonary edema, *Chest* 92:586-593, 1987.
44. Hoffman JR et al: Does paramedic-base hospital contact result in beneficial deviations from standard prehospital protocols? *West J Med* 153:283-287, 1990.
45. Hoffman J et al: Effect of hypertonic sodium bicarbonate in the treatment of moderate-to-severe cyclic antidepressant overdose, *Am J Emerg Med* 11:336, 1993.
46. Holliman J, Wuerz RC, and Meador SA: Standing orders: does this system decrease the prehospital patient care error rate? *Prehospital and Disaster Medicine* 8:S57, 1993.
47. Holroyd B et al: Prehospital patients refusing care, *Ann Emerg Med* 17:957-963, 1988.
48. Honigman B et al: The role of the pneumatic antishock garment in penetrating cardiac wounds, *JAMA* 266:2398-2041, 1991.
49. Iverson KV: A simplified prehospital advance directive law: Arizona's approach, *Ann Emerg Med* 22:1703-1710, 1993.
50. Johnson JC and Atherton GL: Effectiveness of nitrous oxide in a rural EMS system, *J Emerg Med* 9:44-53, 1991.
51. Kargounis L et al: Impact of field-transmitted electrocardiography on time to in-hospital thrombolytic therapy in acute myocardial infarction, *Am J Cardiol* 66:786-791, 1990.

52. Keller RA and Forinash M: EMS in the United States: A survey of providers in the 200 most populous cities, *J Emerg Med* 15:79-100, 1990.
53. Kellermann AL, Hackman BB, and Somes G: Predicting the outcome of unsuccessful prehospital advanced cardiac life support, *JAMA* 270:1433-1436, 1993.
54. Kellerman AL, Stavew Dr, and Hackman BB: In-hospital resuscitation following unsuccessful prehospital advanced cardiac life support: 'Heroic efforts' or an exercise in futility? *Ann Emerg Med* 17:589-594, 1988.
55. Kellermann AL et al: Impact of First Responder defibrillation in an urban emergency medical services system, *JAMA* 270:1708-1713, 1993.
56. Koenig KL, Schultz CH, and Bade R: In-field extremity amputations, *Prehospital and Disaster Medicine* 8:205, 1993.
57. Koenig KL, Tamkin G, and Salness KA: Do-not-resuscitate orders: where are they in the prehospital setting?, *Prehospital and Disaster Med* 8(1), 1993.
58. Lavery RF et al: A survey of advanced life support practices in the United States, *Prehospital and Disaster Medicine* 7:144-150, 1992.
59. Losek JD et al: Prehospital care of the pulseless, nonbreathing pediatric patient, *Am J Emerg Med* 5:370-374, 1987.
60. Maningas PA and Bellamy RF: Hypertonic sodium chloride solutions for the prehospital management of traumatic hemorrhagic shock: a possible improvement in the standard of care? *Ann Emerg Med* 15:1411-1414, 1986.
61. Martin RR et al: Prospective evaluation of preoperative fluid resuscitation in hypotensive patients with penetrating truncal injury: a preliminary report, *J Trauma* 33:354-361, 1992.
62. Mattox KL et al: Prospective MAST study in 9-1-1 patients, *J Trauma* 29:1104-1112, 1989.
63. McGuire TJ and Pointer JE: Evaluation of a pulse oximeter in the prehospital setting, *Ann Emerg Med* 17:1058-1062, 1988.
64. McSwain NE: A thoracostomy tube for field and emergency department use, *JACEP* 6:324-327, 1977.
65. Melio FR, Mallon WK, and Newton E: Successful conversion of unstable supraventricular tachycardia to sinus rhythm with adenosine, *Ann Emerg Med* 21:589, 1992.
66. Minutes from the Emergency Medical Service Medical Directors Association of California (EMDAC) Scope of Practice Committee Meeting, San Diego, Sep 9, 1993.
67. Minutes from the Emergency Medical Service Medical Directors Association of California (EMDAC) meeting, Irvine, Calif., August 27, 1992.
68. Minutes of the Orange County Base Hospital Physicians Directors Committee meeting, Santa Ana, Calif., March 13, 1991.
69. Morris DL and Goldschlager N: Calcium infusion for reversal of adverse effects of intravenous verapamil, *JAMA* 249:3212-3213, 1983.
70. *National Association of Emergency Medical Service Physicians (NAEMSP) Newsletter*, Feb 1992.
71. Nielsen MM, Barsan WG, and Dimlich RVW: Effect of IV glucose on survival and neurologic outcome after cardiac arrest, *Ann Emerg Med* 20:454, 1991 (abstract).
72. Orange County Emergency Medical Service Agency Policies, Santa Ana, Calif., 1991.
73. Ornato JP: High-dose epinephrine during resuscitation, a word of caution, *JAMA* 265:1160-1161, 1991 (editorial).
74. Ornato JP and Peberdy MA: Prehospital end-tidal carbon dioxide monitoring, *JEMS* 3:140-147, 1993.
75. O'Toole KS et al: Intravenous verapamil in the prehospital treatment of paroxysmal supraventricular tachycardia, *Ann Emerg Med* 19:291-294, 1990.
76. Paradis NA et al: The effect of standard- and high-dose epinephrine on coronary perfusion pressure during prolonged cardiopulmonary resuscitation, *JAMA* 265:1139-1144, 1991.
77. Pepe PE, Bass RR, and Mattox KL: Clinical trials of the pneumatic antishock garment in the urban prehospital setting, *Ann Emerg Med* 15:1407-1410, 1986.
78. Phillips JA and Buchman TG: Optimizing prehospital triage criteria for trauma team alerts, *J Trauma* 34:127-132, 1993.
79. Pointer JE: Clinical characteristics of paramedics' performance of pediatric endotracheal intubation, *Am J Emerg Med* 7:364-366, 1989.
80. Pons PT: Nitrous oxide analgesia, *Emerg Med Clin North Am* 6:777-782, 1988.
81. Reuler JB, Girard DE, and Cooney TG: Wernicke's encephalopathy, *N Engl J Med* 312:1035-1039, 1985.
82. Rhee KJ and O'Malley RJ: Neuromuscular blockade-assisted oral intubation versus nasotracheal intubation in the prehospital care of injured patients, *Ann Emerg Med* 23:37-42, 1994.
83. Rice KL et al: Aminophylline for acute exacerbations of chronic obstructive pulmonary disease, a controlled trial, *Ann Int Med* 107:305-309, 1987.
84. Rosen P: The field airway controversy, J *Emerg Med* 2:305-306, 1985 (editorial).
85. Rubens AJ: Endotracheal intubation: the minimum for ACLS airway management training, (editorial). *Prehospital and Disaster Medicine* 6:491-492, 1991.
86. Salerno SM, Wrenn KD, and Slovis CM: Monitoring EMS protocol deviations: a useful quality assurance tool, *Ann Emerg Med* 20:1319-1324, 1991.
87. Salerno DM et al: Intravenous verapamil for treatment of multifocal atrial tachycardia with and without calcium pretreatment, *Ann Intern Med* 107:623-628, 1987.
88. San Francisco Emergency Medical Service Agency: *Policies*, San Francisco, 1992, The Agency.
89. Seigler RS: The administration of rectal diazepam for acute management of seizures, *J Emerg Med* 8:155-159, 1990.
90. Siegler RS, Teckleburt FW, and Shealy R: Prehospital intraosseous infusion by emergency medical services personnel: a prospective study, *Pediatrics* 84:173-177, 1989.
91. Smith RJ, Keseg DP, and Manley LK: Intraosseous infusions by prehospital personnel in critically ill pediatric patients, *Ann Emerg Med* 17:491-495, 1988.
92. Spaite DW and Joseph M: Prehospital cricothyrotomy: an investigation of indications, technique, complications, and patient outcome, *Ann Emerg Med* 19:279-285, 1990.
93. Stults KR et al: Prehospital defibrillation performed by emergency medical technicians in rural communities, *N Engl J Med* 310:219-223, 1984.
94. Tracey DF et al: Hyperglycemia and mortality from acute stroke, *Q J Med* 86:439, 1993.
95. Vukmir RB, Paris PM, and Yealy DM: Glucagon: prehospital therapy for hypoglycemia, *Ann Emerg Med* 20:375-379, 1991.
96. Vukov LF and White RD: External transcutaneous pacemakers in prehospital cardiac arrest, *Ann Emerg Med* 17:554-555, 1988 (letter).
97. Wasserberger J et al: Base station prehospital care: judgment errors and deviations from protocol, *Ann Emerg Med* 16:867-871, 1987.
98. Wears RL and Winton CN: Load-and-go versus stay-and-play: analysis of prehospital IV fluid therapy by computer simulation, *Ann Emerg Med* 19:163-168, 1990.
99. Weaver WD et al: Considerations for improving survival from out-of-hospital cardiac arrest, *Ann Emerg Med* 15:1181-1186, 1986.

100. Weaver WD et al: Factors influencing survival after out-of-hospital cardiac arrest, *JACC Coll Cardiol* 7:752-757, 1986.
101. Weaver WD et al: Use of automatic external defibrillator in the management of out-of-hospital cardiac arrest, *N Engl J Med* 319:661-666, 1988.
102. Weinbroum A, Halpern P, and Geller E: The use of flumazenil in the management of acute drug poisoning: a review. *Intensive Care Med* 1 (suppl 17): S32-38, 1991.
103. Weiss AT et al: The use of calcium with verapamil in the management of supraventricular tachyarrhythmias, *Int J Cardiol* 4:275-284, 1983.
104. Yealy DM et al: The safety of prehospital naloxone administration by paramedics, *Ann Emerg Med* 19:902-905, 1990.

13

Communications

James J. Augustine, B.A., M.D., FACEP

A woman calls 9-1-1 because her husband is ill. Later, he arrives in the emergency department and a record of the run appears on the emergency department chart. How much easier could it be? Unfortunately the EMS communications system is not that simple. Ideally the communications system integrates the various delivery components into the smooth, seamless operation described above that is desired by the public.

Prehospital medical care systems interact with numerous public groups in the provision of services. Therefore EMS communication systems must be efficient and coordinated with the following:

- Persons requesting assistance (systems access and dispatch)
- Fire, law enforcement, and other EMS units
- Medical oversight
- The general public
- Hospital personnel (medical records)
- EMS administration (administrative records)
- Disaster service providers

Rapid changes in communication needs and available equipment require continual monitoring by EMS medical directors. Each EMS system must consider the unique nature of its resources, geography, and funding to provide a functional and cost-efficient system. The system medical director is responsible for those elements that affect emergency medical care.

Objectives

The EMS communications system integrates the components, service providers, and administrators to provide quality emergency medical care. This establishes a pattern for day-to-day operations while allowing the flexibility and redundancy necessary for disasters and other special needs. The efficiency of the system must be measured locally; each system has unique geography, medical service providers, and public expectations. Common components of comprehensive systems are described in this and subsequent chapters on dispatch, data collection, and medical oversight.

Communication system priorities differ somewhat in rural and urban systems. Rural providers must compensate for large service areas, long prehospital response and transport times, in addition to variable response patterns. Communication hardware appropriate for the terrain and distances is necessary. Rural systems generally have lower service volumes and more volunteer providers. These factors increase the importance of skilled and available direct medical control. A 1988 survey of state EMS programs by the National Association of State EMS Directors (NAEMSD) revealed that 31 states and territories had inadequate EMS radio system coverage in some rural areas. Radio frequency congestion or interference was reported in 32 states, primarily in urban areas.[14]

Urban systems generally have higher call volumes and a propensity for radio congestion. These factors differentiate the most useful radio frequencies for each service and the modes for integrating dispatch and medical oversight. The importance of trained emergency medical dispatching is also greater in rural settings, allowing use of prearrival instructions and an appropriate response of personnel and equipment.

EMS medical directors are responsible for quality emergency medical care and prioritize those aspects of the communications system that promote such care. This begins with a public education program encouraging appropriate and timely use of EMS. Single number access provides timely activation and is easily taught and accepted. Prehospital care is supported by dispatch, communications protocols, and interagency linkages with fire, law enforcement, and other EMS units. Medical conversations with direct medical control physicians should be easily available, but evaluation and treatment protocols promote timely, standardized care. Medical records document that care and provide input for quality improvement and research activities.

Administrative information systems, which are not patient care related, keep the service available for patient care. Administrative information on nuts-and-bolts issues such as vehicle maintenance, equipment and supplies, personnel licensure and education, and facility upkeep are necessary. Human resource issues including due process, health surveillance, and employee recognition are also components of the management information system.

Components of an EMS Communications System

Access

In the last 10 years, researchers and providers identified a deficit in the public recognition of emergency medical situations and the activation of the EMS system.[15, 17] Activation is accomplished in a six-step process, (1) a need is detected, (2) a location is determined, (3) an appropriate method of transport and facility are chosen, (4) a provider is identified, (5) a communications device or telephone number is located to access, and (6) direct or indirect contact is made with the emergency service.* The EMS system must facilitate each of these steps and educate members of the general public about the proper process.[5] In its simplest form the system must provide a mechanism for citizens with an urgent medical need to easily and reliably access emergency providers. The public telephone, the most common access system, is supplemented with emergency call boxes, citizens and marine band radios, and cellular phones.

In the United States, emergency number 9-1-1 for access to all emergency providers is being implemented with federal, state, and local government support. Seven-digit numbers are difficult to remember and cause a delay in requesting emergency assistance. The enhanced 9-1-1 (or E9-1-1) system displays the caller's location and phone number at the dispatching site. This eliminates telephone queries about emergency location in many situations. This modification, although slightly more expensive, can reduce false alarms and assist callers unable to communicate because of age or nature of injury. This identification can be automatically tied to a system status computer that will immediately display the closest available emergency responders. However, E9-1-1 systems increase certain system demands: "hang up" calls must be responded to by emergency units. Many of these calls are made by curious citizens or youth testing the system to see how it works, but some originate from portable phones that dial random numbers when their batteries fade.

In areas without 9-1-1, access to the emergency system should be as easy as possible with a widely publicized single telephone number. In some areas, dialing 9-1-1 gets an operator who will manually relay the call to the appropriate emergency agency.

*References 10,13,14,19,20,25,27

Dispatch

The responsibility and function of the EMS dispatcher have evolved as demand for EMS services has grown and public expectations for a more sophisticated level of care have evolved. Just as the television show "Emergency" raised public awareness of highly trained and equipped prehospital care providers, "Rescue 9-1-1" has emphasized the role of the individual receiving the emergency call.

The Emergency Medical Dispatcher (EMD) receives calls, interrogates, determines response configuration and mode, and gives the caller appropriate prearrival instructions.[24] Following the initial response, the EMD supports field operations with information regarding scene location, the medical complaints, road conditions, potential hazards, special approaches, and simultaneous fire and police response. The dispatcher may designate which channel and hospital to use for medical control, and may also assist in linking field and hospital personnel. In some configurations, dispatch assists in research data collection, time-logging, and prompting for repeat drugs, procedures, or scene times. EMDs should know the entire emergency response system and be able to access all necessary support resources. EMDs in metropolitan areas shorten response times for urgent patients, decrease unnecessary use of backup resources, improve public perception of emergency services, and minimize inappropriate use of emergency resources.[24]

Many systems provide pre-arrival instructions to the caller until emergency medical personnel arrive. Cardiopulmonary resuscitation and first aid skills are taught or guided by telephone. In some localities the trained dispatcher operating under standing orders provides these instructions. In other areas the radio dispatcher is separate from the person performing the interrogation and giving telephone instructions.

Ideally, one dispatch center with trained EMDs should operate in an EMS region. Central dispatch usually saves money, manpower, and equipment when compared with individual dispatch centers for each community or service. It also minimizes delays in coordinating scene responses, particularly near jurisdictional borders. The dispatch center coordinates activities among responding vehicles including special rescue units, support services, and police, fire, and tow vehicles. Without timely coordination and communication the full lifesaving potential may not be realized.

Direct Medical Control Communications

Direct medical control is best provided by experienced physicians who are immediately available to guide field personnel. In some EMS systems this is provided by radio communications between the field and the receiving hospital. If there are a number of receiving hospitals, this arrangement may not be practical in terms of available radio frequencies, equipment, or personnel expenses. In these cases, direct medical control is provided by a single resource hospital. When the EMS system uses a nonreceiving hospital for direct medical control it is the hospital's responsibility to notify the receiving facility of the emergency situation, the patient's condition, the treatment, and the expected time of arrival. It is the responsibility of the regional EMS authority to determine system needs regarding the number of receiving hospitals and field units requiring communication channels. When voice communication is not used for direct medical control the dispatcher should notify the receiving hospital of the patient's condition, expected time of arrival, and other pertinent medical data that will help the receiving facility respond at the time of the patient's arrival.

Communications between physician and field provider may be by telephone, radio, or a combination of the two. Selection of equipment for hospital-to-ambulance communications must take into consideration transmission interference and distances, as previously outlined. In the early days, many EMS systems transmitted electrocardiograph (ECG) rhythm strips (telemetry) from field to hospital. Multiple studies suggest that in systems with paramedics well-trained in rhythm interpretation, telemetry does not improve patient care. However, 12-lead ECG transmission may evolve as a useful tool for minimizing the time until administration of thrombolytic therapy.[4,7]

Recent literature advocates use of evaluation and treatment protocols for standardization of care, training objectives, and improved standards for patient care.[11] Requirements for voice contact increase scene times and may actually increase the inappropriate use of drugs and intravenous lines.[18, 20] Medical contact rarely resulted in significant changes in therapy, and those patients who would benefit were easily identified through evaluation protocols.[9] Protocol errors were uncommon in another study, and about half the errors were made by direct medical control.[30] Standard treatment protocols also provide a backup system for patient care in the event of communications failure.

When field-to-hospital communication is advantageous the conversation should be standardized. The prehospital unit identifies itself and gives an estimated time of arrival. The patient's age, chief complaint, pertinent history, and physical exam should be conveyed. Vital signs should be identified as stable, or if not stable the values should be given. Interventions already performed should be reported, and further orders requested as necessary. Any orders given by direct medical control should be repeated to ensure a meeting of the minds. Detailed reports can wait until hospital arrival.[10]

Hardware

System hardware requirements are specific to the area's geography, budget, and communication goals. In all systems redundancy and flexibility should be engineered and available. Fixed-bases are established in the communications centers, medical facilities, and EMS vehicle stations. For large service areas, repeaters are necessary. These units may be ground-based or satellites. The mobile radio and portable ratio components are integrated. In metropolitan areas, cellular phone systems are another communication alternative, but require back-up systems. Air ambulance units, if a part of the system, must also be integrated into the communication system.

VHF Radio Systems

Many rural and suburban EMS systems use very high frequency (VHF) radios that have approximately a 15-mile range on flat terrain. VHF radio systems are simplex: messages can be sent only one-way at a time.

Under 1992 Federal Communications Commission (FCC) rules, EMS frequencies are licensed by the Special Emergency Radio Service (SERS), and repeaters are not allowed in the VHF band. Thus there are some range limitations in rural areas. Other factors affecting range include antenna height and power output.

UHF Radio Systems

Generally, more heavily populated areas rely on ultra high frequency (UHF) radio systems. UHF systems are usually duplex systems: messages can be sent and received simultaneously.

The FCC has designated 10 medical channels within the UHF spectrum in the SERS. Licensees are authorized to use all 10 channels. Although these frequencies usually do not have the range of VHF frequencies, they can better penetrate buildings. Also, mobile relays or repeaters may be added to extend range.

Coded Squelch

In both VHF and UHF radio systems, many EMS agencies have installed coded squelch systems to prevent monitoring or interference by unrelated agencies. Coded squelch systems prevent other agencies from hearing radio transmissions, but they do not prevent other transmissions on the same frequencies from interfering with or blocking messages.

Radio Telephone Switching Systems

A few areas have installed radio telephone switching systems (RTSS) enabling ambulance crews to talk to hospitals or dispatch centers beyond the normal ranges of radio systems. These systems enable mobile radios, usually UHF, to interface with telephone lines and extend radio system coverage to rural areas. RTSSs enable full duplex and, with appropriate equipment, accommodate ECG telemetry with physician-paramedic interrupt capabilities.

Microwave Relays

EMS radio systems can be interfaced with microwave relays extending along major highways. The ranges of the EMS radio system are extended hundreds of miles by converting radio frequencies into telephone-microwave frequencies and back to radio frequencies on the receiving end. Microwave systems accommodate a wide variety of radio systems for state and local emergency services and nonemergency services such as highway maintenance crews.

Mountaintop Relays

Some areas, especially in the western United States, interface EMS radios with mountaintop microwave base stations. Depending on the height of the mountains, EMS radio system coverage can be extended to large geographic areas.

800 MHz Public Safety Trunking Systems

The FCC has designated 800 MHz public safety radio frequencies (821 to 824 MHz and 866 to 869 MHz) for use in public safety trunking radio systems. As these systems develop, primarily in major urban areas, it is important that EMS agencies participate in the planning process with the local chapter of the Associated Public Safety Communications Officers (APCO).

Trunked systems, which are usually computerized, allow more efficient use of frequencies because a computer automatically searches for an open frequency when a call is made. Thus the caller does not have to manually select a frequency. This helps prevent radio frequency congestion and interference. Trunking is currently permitted by the FCC in the 800 MHz frequency band, but the technology exists for other frequency band trunking including the UHF bands. EMS agencies in busy systems should encourage the FCC to allow trunking of the 10 UHF medical frequencies.

One problem with 800 MHz systems is that vehicle repeaters are not allowed, posing problems for EMS responders caring for patients inside homes or other settings away from the ambulance.[17]

Another problem is that the FCC allowed different manufacturers to use different protocols or "architectures" for equipment design. This could cause problems in communication between service areas if different systems are used.

In some areas with 800 MHz trunked systems, EMS agencies have opted to stay on UHF frequencies, yet other public safety agencies have switched over to the 800 MHz frequencies. It is important for EMS entities to be involved in the planning process and have some mechanisms to communicate with other public safety responders.

A major drawback to 800 MHz radio systems in rural areas is the limited range. Usually, many more repeaters are needed to cover a geographic area than required with lower band frequencies. This can significantly increase the cost of 800 MHz radio systems in rural areas.

Cellular Telephones

Cellular telephone systems are common in urban areas throughout the United States, and they are spreading to rural areas as well. Advantages of cellular telephones for EMS communications include the following: they provide an alternate means of communicating in radio dead spot areas, they are easy to use, they provide easy access to the telephone systems, they provide duplex voice capabilities, and they provide mobile 9-1-1 emergency access.

Disadvantages of cellular systems include the following: dedicated lines usually are not available or are costly, they may become overloaded during disaster situations, and in multiunit or multiagency responses, it can be difficult to coordinate multiple cellular users in the field because users cannot monitor each others' transmissions. Cellular telephones can supplement EMS radio systems, but they should not be relied on exclusively.

Land Mobile Satellite Communications

In sparsely populated rural areas, EMS radio system coverage can be very expensive. In the near future, land mobile satellite communications may provide a cost-effective alternative to terrestrial radio systems. Several companies are developing this technology. Some plan to use satellites in fixed geostationary orbits, and others plan to use multiple low-orbit satellites. These systems will use omnidirectional antennas, which are more compact than the traditional satellite dishes that have to be pointed at a fixed-point in the sky.

Digital Technology

New digital technologies are being developed that will enable radios to use narrower frequency bands, thereby significantly increasing the number of frequencies available within each band. However, converting to this technology will require costly replacement of existing radio systems.

Integrating Fire, Law Enforcement, and EMS Response

There are three common organizational structures of EMS communication centers. A single center may house all staff communication equipment for dispatch and coordination of police, fire, and EMS.[18] The communication center may be located in and operated by a police or fire department responsible for EMS dispatch.[10] Each public service division police, fire, and EMS may have a separate communication center.[13] Despite recognizing local priorities the configuration of the center is not as important as the mechanism ensuring that vital functions of EMS are coordinated. It is desirable for EMS, police, and fire personnel to be capable of communicating directly with each other regarding needs for additional personnel or equipment, traffic or geographic problems, and coordination of activity in multiple response situations. Coordinated communications are essential in special circumstances such as hazardous material incidents, multiple casualty incidents, and disasters.

Public safety services are regulated by the FCC, as are all radio frequency users. Presently, EMS radio users are licensed under the SERS, competing with veterinarians, hospitals, school buses, rescue, and relief organizations for available frequencies. In some locations, severe radio congestion has occurred. The FCC has been petitioned to designate a separate emergency medical radio service included in the public safety radio service and overseen by groups familiar with the special needs of EMS. This should help alleviate congestion on current and future radio frequency bands. Detailed reference on radio frequency spectrum usage is available.[13]

EMS Communications Planning

In some states, a comprehensive EMS communications plan is available to assist local areas in developing emergency communications systems. States with structured plans include North Carolina, Florida, Tennessee, and Virginia. The 1988 communications system survey by the NASEMSD found that 34 states and territories had state EMS communications plans and 12 others had partial plans.[14] As technologies and frequency regulating requirements change, state EMS communications plans should be updated. To help address this need the NASEMSD developed a two-volume planning guide, "Planning Emergency Medical Communications." One volume deals with planning at the state level, and the other deals with planning at the local level. This guide can be obtained from the National Association of State EMS Directors, 1947 Camino Vida Roble, Suite 202, Carlsbad, CA 92008.

Disasters

Emergency service communication is the critical component of any disaster plan. Communication procedures for a disaster should be identified so resources can be coordinated under stress. Procedures should resemble day-to-day communication patterns as much as possible. The ability to override and block out nonessential components of the communications system must exist. Backup procedures and equipment should be available in the event of component failure. Disasters may render the public telephone system temporarily inoperable, thus emergency radios should be available and alternate radio frequencies designated for use if the usual channels become overloaded. To overcome the problem of incompatible radio frequencies among emergency response agencies working in a disaster situation, some systems have installed inexpensive radio scanners in response vehicles and dispatch centers. These scanners allow responders to listen to each other and to improve the communications net in spite of incompatible radios.

Hospital Communication Systems

Hospitals providing direct medical control should communicate with other hospitals in the system regarding the availability of beds and other resources. This is especially important during multiple casualty incidents when triage and transportation of many victims must occur in a timely manner. Hospital-to-hospital communication usually involves VHF and dedicated landlines, although microwave is another possibility. Hospital networks include dedicated air and ground ambulance units that supplement the EMS system.

Medical Records

Communications with other medical personnel and legal documentation of the patient interaction are provided by the Prehospital Care Report (PCR). Copies of this document should be kept in the patient's permanent hospital medical record, filed with the EMS service, and made available for reporting and auditing purposes. The record should represent a total picture of the EMS interaction. A minimum data set has been proposed, but the perfect PCR has yet to be designed.[8, 23] Because the PCR is often the only documentation of the field situation and care, medical directors should stress the importance of historical points and observations at the scene including environmental and situational factors.[3] Education should stress the importance of an accurate, precise, comprehensive, legible, objective, and time sequenced runsheet.[28] Proper documentation may prevent some lawsuits and dramatically improve the defense in others.[16] Documentation is particularly important for nontransport incidents that involve questions of informed consent and abandonment.

Several formats have been proposed for the PCR (see box below, left). The provider must select the appropriate memory cue that can be consistently applied with an audit and review system that reinforces documentation priorities. Medical director overview is a requirement. Medical documentation completed by the medical review and audit process provides quality improvement feedback to the provider.[18]

Key Components of Prehospital Care Reports

- Patient demographics
- Incident times
- Dispatch information and nature of call
- Vital signs recorded and timed
- Objective observations of patient, environment, and situation
- Assessment, treatment, and reassessment
- Direct medical control
- Pertinent oral statements made by the patient or bystanders
- Unusual circumstances arising during the incident

Administrative Records

Seemingly mundane and time-consuming, administrative records are necessary for the efficient operation of an EMS service and the provision of quality care. Certification and continuing education of personnel must be logged to ensure appropriate licensing. State licensure is required for drug dispensing. Vehicle, equipment, and supply purchase and maintenance are recorded. Documentation of equipment problems and their resolution are particularly critical, especially with equipment used directly in patient care. A final administrative concern is complaints from the public served by the system. These should be recognized as opportunities for service improvement, and respected for liability potential as well.

Communicating with the Public

The EMS system continually interacts with the general public, which ultimately funds the system. System administrators and providers should respect this relationship and acknowledge their responsibility. Informal and inexpensive public interaction programs such as school displays and blood pressure checks may be as effective as more formal and expensive demonstrations. The least expensive and most effective communication program is everyday interaction with patients, bystanders, and family. Each run has the potential for extensive public interaction, and serious or large incidents draw media coverage.[25] Media involvement should be positive and productive; tremendous damage can be inflicted to systems that ignore or antagonize these communications experts.[5] Many systems design programs that combine public and media interaction such as prevention education, open houses, and extrication or disaster drills. These foster good relationships with the public and facilitate an ongoing, productive partnership with the service community.

Setting up the Network

The communication system sets the stage for high-quality patient care. A needs assessment should be performed and objectives outlined for the various communication components. Respecting geographic, environmental, and operational factors, hardware and appropriate licenses are obtained. New configurations of system access, dispatch, and medical communications are becoming available. Smart radio systems integrate medical and administrative roles.[1] System status management is another efficient tool for facilitating medical care and providing critical management input.[27]

Medical and administrative protocols further improve operational efficiency. Medical standing orders based on patient complaint or problem guide the field provider through evaluation and decision-making. With regular quality assurance and medical review, protocols also guide the educational process, personnel evaluation, and recognition programs.[26]

Administrative protocols should guide system personnel in diverse areas such as needlestick management, restocking supplies, handling controlled substances, nontransports, "Do Not Resuscitate" requests, complaint management, and vehicle maintenance.

Summary

The EMS communication system is a tool facilitating the delivery of high quality emergency medical care. It can enable productive relationships with the general public and other emergency responders. It can bring the guidance of medical oversight to each patient interaction. It is the foundation for appropriate and timely response in multiple casualty and disaster incidents. It provides the input material for data collection, system evaluation, and quality improvement programs. With these ideals, communication is relegated a high priority in EMS system design and operation. Appropriate administrative dedication is crucial. The medical director should review and approve all components of the system that affect medical care.

REFERENCES

1. Adler S: Smart radio systems, *Emergency Medical Services* 17:37-38, 1988.
2. Ball R: Documentation: the overlooked aspect of emergency care, *JEMS* 31-32, May 1990.
3. Brown-Nixon C: Field documentation myths, *Emergency Medical Services* 19(8):18-21, Aug 1990.
4. Cayten CG et al: The effect of telemetry on urban prehospital cardiac care, *Ann Emerg Med* 14:976-981, 1985.
5. Edwards K: Emergency: when to call the squad, *Ohio Medicine* 12-13, Sept 1990.
6. Foosaner R: FCC regulation of EMS telecommunications, *Emergency Medical Services* 13:22-23, 1984.
7. Gustafson J et al: EMS telecommunications trends, *Emergency Medical Services* 17:36, 1988.
8. Hedges JR et al: Minimum data set for EMS report form: historical development and future implications, *Prehospital & Disaster Medicine* 383-384, Oct 1990.
9. Hoffman JR et al: Does pm-base hospital contact result in beneficial deviations from standard prehospital protocols? *West J Med* 153:282, 1990.
10. Holliman CJ: Maximizing prehospital radio communications, *JEMS* 5-9, May 1990.
11. Hunt RC et al: Standing orders vs. voice control, *JEMS* 26-31, Nov 1982.
12. Johnson M: Rural EMS communications, *Emergency Medical Services* 20:8, Aug 1991.
13. Johnson MS et al: Is EMS communicating with the FCC? *JEMS* 51-56, July 1989.
14. Johnson M: The states of EMS communications, National Association of State EMS Directors, Unpublished, Carlsbad, Calif, 1988.
15. Knolle LL et al: Knowledge of access to and use of the emergency medical services system in a rural Illinois county, *Am J Prev Med* 5:164-169, 1989.
16. Lazar RA et al: Presumed insufficient, *JEMS* 19(8):23-29, Aug 1990.
17. Mayron R et al: The 9-1-1 emergency telephone number, *Am J Emerg Med* 2:491-493, 1985.
18. Pointer JE: The ALS base hospital audit for medical control in an EMS system, *Ann Emerg Med* 16:557, 1987.
19. Pointer JE et al: Effect of standing orders on field times, *Ann Emerg Med* 18:1119, 1989.
20. Pointer JE et al: The impact of standing orders on meds and skill selection, paramedic assessment, and hospital outcome, *Prehospital & Disaster Medicine* 6:303, 1991.
21. Pozen MW et al: Cost and utility considerations in implementing ambulance telemetry, *Heart Lung* 9:866-872, 1980.
22. Shanaberger C: If it isn't written down..., *JEMS* 79-80, June 1990.
23. Shanaberger C: The unrefined art of documentation, *JEMS* 155-157, Jan 1992.
24. Slovis CM et al: A priority dispatch system for emergency medical services, *Ann Emerg Med* 14:1055-1060, 1985.
25. Stephens K: Effective news media handling critical at accident sites, *Emergency Medicine & Ambulatory Care News* 5, June 1989.
26. Stewart C: Communications with EMS providers, *Emergency Medicine & Ambulatory Care News* 8:103, 1990.
27. Stout J: System status management, *JEMS* 65-71, April 1989.
28. Strange J: Does your documentation reflect your care? *Emergency Medical Services* 19:8, Aug 1990.
29. Wasserbergen J: Base station prehospital care: judgment errors and deviations from protocols, *Ann Emerg Med* 16:867-71, 1987.
30. Yamamoto LG: Cellular telephone communications between hospitals and ambulances, *JEMS* 13:35-38, 1988.

14

Emergency Medical Dispatch

Jeffrey J. Clawson, M.D.

Surviving a life-threatening medical emergency is predicated by a series of actions that optimally occur within precisely defined periods of time. If all necessary actions occur within the prescribed time periods and are performed according to defined standards, the patient has a significantly increased chance of survival. The series of actions that must take place for one to survive a medical emergency has been called the "chain of survival." Survival is not the only issue. If the prescribed actions are performed late or inappropriately, the patient may survive, but impaired brain function or paralysis may result.

The first link in the chain of survival, the preresponse link, is the emergency medical dispatcher (EMD). Following recognition of an emergency, the caller must know who to call, how to call them, and be willing to perform basic lifesaving measures immediately if necessary. The caller must also avoid certain actions that may make the situation worse.

It is important to inform and educate the public in recognizing medical emergencies, notifying the emergency care system, instituting basic lifesaving measures, and refraining from doing further harm. The failure of the public to perform any one of these four tasks reduces the chance for survival, results in postincident impairment, or actually worsens the situation. Inappropriate action by the public can also render subsequent medical actions ineffective.

During the last 15 years it has become apparent that the public will access 9-1-1 for a range of medical problems from minor ailments to genuine life-threats. Properly trained 9-1-1 communications center staff can perform specific functions that enhance the efficiency and effectiveness of prehospital care. The dispatcher can rapidly elicit reasonably accurate symptom pictures from frightened callers, allowing more accurate medical categorization of victims. In addition the dispatcher can activate the configuration of responders optimally suited to deal with the specific emergency. It is not enough to mindlessly send paramedics on all cases; it is necessary to accurately determine the need for these highly trained individuals. If this is not done for all calls the number of available providers will be reduced because of their inappropriate use.

In 1979 this dilemma stimulated the development of emergency medical priority dispatching and its training process. The goals are sending the right thing, to the right person, at the right time, in the right way, and doing the right things until help arrives. Because the dispatcher is often the least medically trained provider in the chain of survival, these goals are accomplished through the careful use of a comprehensive protocol including the items in the box at the bottom of the page.

Unrestricted use of scarce medical resources gambles with the possibility of a concurrent need for those resources. Even in the best covered system, if a defibrillation-capable unit is used unnecessarily, precious minutes may be added to the arrival at the next call. In most systems those extra minutes are lethal. The value of dispatch prioritization in such situations, not to mention pre-arrival telephone

Items in the Emergency Medical Dispatch Protocol

- Systematized formal caller interrogation process
- Systematized scripted pre-arrival instructions
- Protocols that match the dispatcher's evaluation of the injury or illness type and severity with vehicle response mode and configuration
- Support and definitional reference information

interventions, is obvious. Even if the family and the media never know that the closest appropriate unit did not respond, the medical director still must endeavor to establish a system that balances all factors affecting appropriate medical dispatch.

The development and rapid growth of EMS have redefined the individual roles of prehospital providers and EMS physicians. Even the citizen has been identified as a potential key player in the evolving roster of the prehospital care team. However, the last in a long line of individuals identified as vital to the optimal functioning of the EMS system was the EMD. This key role for the dispatcher was accurately defined in 1978 when Salt Lake City EMS identified the medical dispatcher as the "weak link" in the chain of survival.[5] Until then the average medical dispatcher had less than 1 hour of formal medical training.

The emergence of structured EMD protocols and training as vital elements of appropriately functioning EMS systems was a phenomenon of the 1980s. A number of factors contributed to the delay in recognition. The dispatch function was rarely observed by early medical directors because for most emergency physicians a prehospital case begins when the telemetry radio announces a call. The dispatcher's function regarding the mechanics of dispatch and the decision-making process was unknown to the medical community. Whether the closest appropriate unit was sent, a paramedic unit was unavailable because of previous assignment to a "cat bite" call, or the first assigned vehicle never arrived because it was involved in an unnecessary lights-and-siren accident was hidden from most traditional EMS physicians.[7]

Myths of Medical Dispatch

1. The caller is too upset to respond accurately.
2. The caller does not know the required information.
3. The medical expertise of the dispatcher is not important.
4. The dispatcher is too busy to waste time asking questions, giving instructions, or flipping through card files.
5. Phone information from dispatchers cannot help victims and may even be dangerous.
6. More personnel and more units at the scene is always better.
7. It is dangerous not to maximally respond or not respond to lights-and-siren.

Myths

There are seven commonly held and virtually universal myths regarding medical dispatch that delay the development of sound programs; these are malignant myths rather than innocent misconceptions (see box above, right).

One by one these myths were proven false as medical dispatching was more carefully studied and better understood. They often are believed not only by police chiefs, fire chiefs, EMS administrators, politicians, and field personnel but also by medical directors and dispatchers themselves.

One of the more common myths is that most callers are hysterical. In 1986 Eisenberg compared the emotional levels of 640 callers reporting cardiac arrest with other complaints.[19] A standard emotional scale from 1 to 5 was used; 1 represents "normal conversational speech" and a 5 represents an individual "so emotionally distraught that information (for example, the address) could be obtained only with great difficulty." Of the 146 callers in noncardiac arrest cases the mean emotional score was 1.4. Contrary to popular belief the mean emotional quotient of the 494 callers reporting cardiac arrest was only 2.1. In 1990 a study of 160 random callers in Los Angeles revealed an average Emotional Content/Cooperation Score (ECCS modified) of 1.2. No callers were rated at 5.[15]

A second myth is that the callers do not know the required information. In dispatch, the common classifications for callers are first-, second-, and third-party. A first-party caller is the patient. A second-party caller is someone with the patient or intimately familiar with the patient's current condition. A third-party caller is someone who is neither with the patient nor knows the patient (for example, "I just saw a car accident out the window and it looks really bad!"). Sixty percent of callers can be classified as first- or second-parties; 40% are third-parties.[24] The high incidence of third-party callers is often the reason dispatchers fail to obtain significant information.

In reality this is the result of the dispatcher not asking the right questions rather than lack of knowledge on the part of the caller. This can be demonstrated by comparing interrogation sequences using formal protocols with those not using such protocols (Figure 14-1). Dispatchers left on their own usually invent questions to ask the caller, who routinely responds, "Look, I don't know." Rarely will an ad-libbing dispatcher ask the following structured series of questions:

1. Is the patient awake?
2. Did you ever hear the patient talk?
3. What was the patient doing (standing or sitting)?

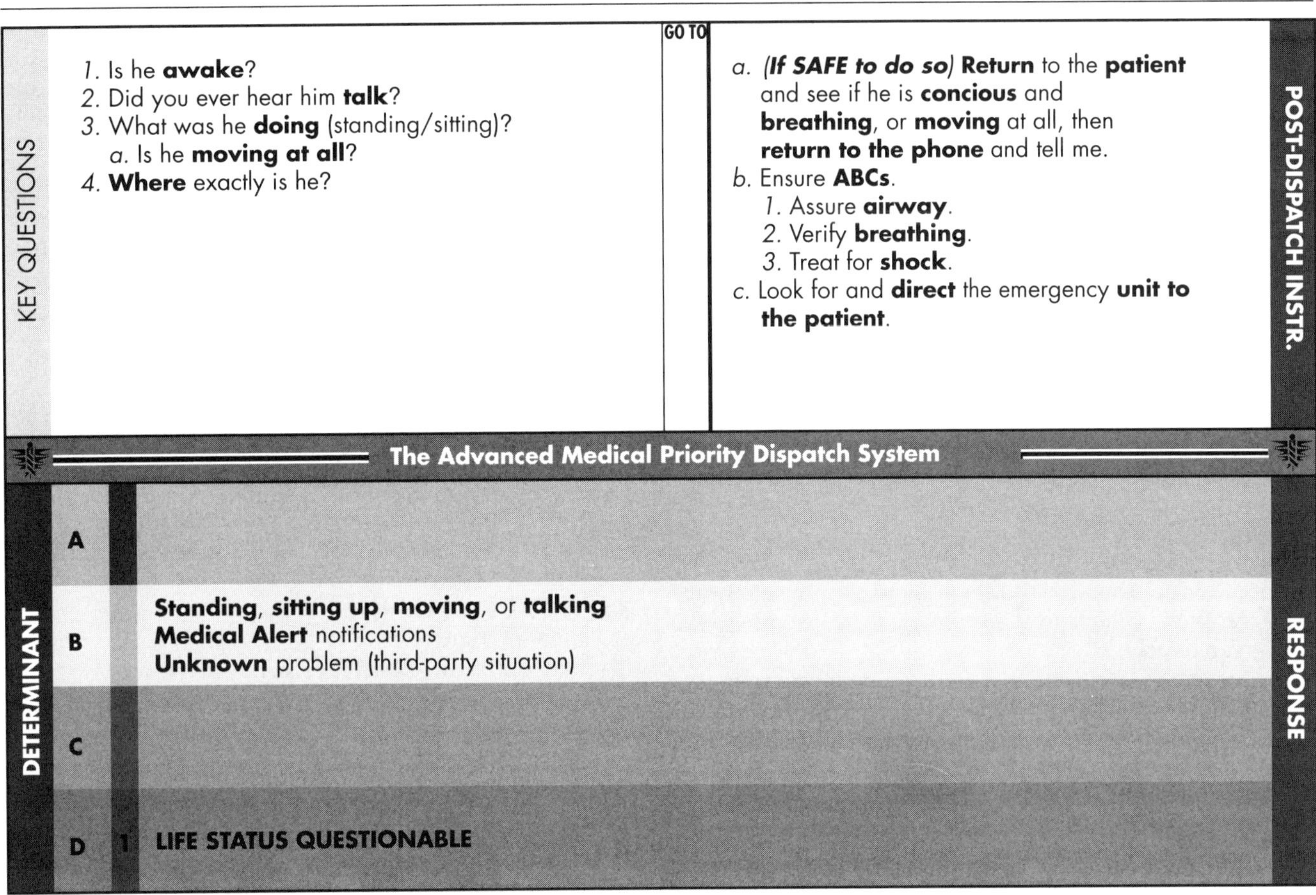

Figure 14-1. Example of formal protocol. (From AMPDS v 10.1, Medical Priority Inc., Salt Lake City.)

4. Is the patient moving at all?
5. Where exactly is the patient?

None of the questions in this series are medical in nature, rather they are situational. A caller may never have gotten any closer than 50 yards from the patient yet could easily answer the majority of the questions. A talking, moving, sitting patient is not in cardiac arrest and that is the major dispatch concern when dealing with "unknown problem" or "man down" situations.

The myths regarding the medical training of dispatchers and their use of protocols are disproved as EMS systems establish programs for EMD training and use medically approved protocols.[8] Hundreds of dispatch systems provide pre-arrival instructions with almost universal positive results medically, politically, and legally.[26] The National Association of EMS Physicians (NAEMSP) stated in its consensus document on EMD that "standard telephone instructions by trained EMDs are safe to give and in many instances [are] a morally necessity" (see Appendix I).

The myths that EMDs are "too busy" are usually coupled with the need to increase dispatcher coverage when implementing a medical priority dispatching system (MPDS). No dispatch center has ever been forced to increase the number of dispatchers as a result of using a MPDS. Once a complete MPDS is phased into dispatch operations the provision of patient-directed interrogations is not another time burden for the dispatchers. During the implementation phase of MPDS in Los Angeles, interrogation time actually decreased. The time to dispatch on critical cases (cardiac arrest and choking) shortens because the MPDS protocol identifies the most important items and addresses them first. An appropriate response is dispatched, followed by more questions or telephone treatment. The MPDS in Los Angeles did not affect the call waiting time before being answered by the dispatcher; it averaged 7 seconds before and after implementation.

Of the seven misconceptions, the last two are the result of the illogical extrapolation of lights-and-siren use by other public safety responders to EMS.[16] More attention is being focused on using lights-and-siren for all EMS responses.[13] Currently, there are neither data nor studies supporting the routine use of lights-and-siren. No published data establish the amount of time saved by lights-and-siren or by maximal response. The NAEMSP position paper, "Use of Lights-and-Siren in Emergency Medical Vehicle Response and Patient Transport," strongly supports the planned, medically controlled, deliberate use of lights-and-siren only when indicated from a patient care standpoint. The following three positions from that document relate to the impact of medical dispatching protocols on the use of lights-and-siren.

NAEMSP Position Paper

> The use of lights-and-siren during both response and transport must be based on sound patient problem assessment or on objective situational protocol. Written prospective protocol for the use of lights-and-siren during transport must be in place and approved by the medical director. In the absence of such protocol the paramedic or EMT on the scene should make contact with the base station hospital to clarify the vehicle Response Mode for transport of a given patient.
>
> Dispatch prioritization is an essential element in any EMS system for it establishes the appropriate level of care initially required including vehicle response configuration and mode of urgency. All medical dispatch centers must institute and monitor adherence to dispatch prioritization protocols that clearly delineate appropriate lights-and-siren use from those that do not.
>
> All jurisdictions allowing the use of lights-and-siren by emergency medical vehicles must require training and professional EMD certification of their emergency medical dispatchers and mandate the use of priority medical dispatch protocols approved by the local medical director that clearly delineate lights-and-siren use.

Emergency Medical Dispatcher

The role of the EMD in a modern EMS system is extensive and requires a detailed base of knowledge.[5] The typical role is multifaceted with at least six subroles. These include (1) interrogator, (2) radio dispatcher, (3) triager, (4) logistics coordinator, (5) resource provider, and (6) pre-arrival aid instructor. Specific training in each of these facets is essential. However, they represent only a portion of the skills requisite to the functioning of a public safety dispatcher.

A sound basis in generic telecommunication techniques is the first prerequisite for optimal emergency medical dispatching. Many high-volume EMS systems use computer aided dispatch (CAD) to divide responsibilities between the call-receiving operators (CROs) or call-takers (CTs) and the dispatchers. The following discussion applies to both groups of EMDs.

The EMD requires specific training in what is commonly referred to as the dispatch priorities.[5] It is an oblique cross section of prehospital medicine unique to dispatch appropriate interrogation, vehicle allocation, pre-arrival instructions (PAI) given to the caller, and concise information regarding the clinical situation and scene conditions given to the responding provider en route. The properly trained EMD must be a sophisticated health care professional because the fund of knowledge from which the dispatch priorities are gleaned is the same as that of the emergency physician, nurse, or paramedic; however, the types of treatments performed over the telephone are generally more elemental. The basic components of EMD are key question interrogation, PAI, and prehospital medical care dispatch. They are covered in more detail in subsequent sections of this chapter.

Medical Oversight

The inclusion of the dispatch process in EMS medical oversight lagged behind that of prehospital field care. For years, medical oversight was blissfully unaware of the pre-arrival phase of EMS. One reason for this was that fire services commonly were step-parents of EMS in the 1970s; for example, before 1990, no EMS physician had stepped inside the fire-EMS dispatch center for the District of Columbia. Resistance to medical oversight has been encountered when the practices of the medical dispatch center are first examined by the medical community. It is the medical director's responsibility to work with the EMS agency administration to establish appropriate, medically sound practices and quality management programs for EMDs.

The concept of EMD obviously encompasses more than training. In fact a practice standard has evolved that not only defines the role of the EMD but also the supervision, quality management, and risk management that must accompany it.[26] Medical oversight at dispatch is essential and is a key element of quality management for medical director.[1] The implementation process begins with training and certification. EMD courses average 24 hours.[5] Training is a critical basis for the rapid, precise decisions required. The NAEMSP described some of the difficulties in designing EMD training:

> In order to prioritize calls properly, the EMD must be well-versed in the medical conditions and incident types that constitute their daily routine. Training in these priorities must be detailed and dispatch-specific not EMT or paramedic training per se .... Since, much of the knowledge and many of the skills required by the EMD are dispatch-specific, a curriculum for their training differs substantially from those used in the preparation of EMTs or paramedics. Training as an

EMT or paramedic does not adequately prepare a person for the role of an EMD. Much of the required EMD curriculum cannot be found in standard EMS training curricula. It consists of content and emphasis which differ significantly from that used from the training of all other health professionals and public safety dispatchers (see Appendix I).

Quality Management

A quality management program is essential to the successful implementation and maintenance of an EMD program. To assure quality in practice there must be an understanding of how quality is defined. Inherent in the notion of EMD is the development of objective measurements of the performance of EMD activities. These measurement tools have four goals.

1. To assure that policy, practice, and protocol are correct and effective
2. To assure that EMDs understand policy, practice, and protocol
3. To assure that EMDs comply with policy, practice, and protocol
4. To correct or improve any deficiencies in EMD policy, practice, and protocol

The 11 components of a comprehensive quality management program for EMDs are listed below.[14]

1. Selection
2. Orientation
3. Initial training
4. Certification
5. Continuing dispatch education
6. Medical oversight
7. Data generation
8. Performance evaluation or case review
9. Recertification
10. Risk management
11. Decertification, suspension, and termination

Selection. If dispatchers are to be involved in the emergency medical care of patients the selection of new dispatchers must take that into account. Abilities to read written scripts, follow instructions, carry out multiple tasks, and exercise good judgment and self-control in stressful situations must be assessed. There are a number of attributes and predictors of success as an EMD that should be incorporated into selection criteria.

Orientation. EMDs must be inculcated from the start with the paradigm that EMS exists to help people, not just to save lives. Because the majority of callers do not have a time-critical or life-threatening medical emergency, unless EMDs are help-oriented they will view these callers as either undeserving of their assistance or a waste of time. Through proper orientation EMDs learn that although they cannot save the life of every caller, they can help everyone who calls. This orientation leads to enhanced self-esteem, higher morale, reduced frustration, and optimal customer relations.

Initial training. The training of EMDs must revolve around the use of medically appropriate and approved dispatch protocols. The difference between guidelines and protocols is profound; guidelines are permissive, protocols are not. EMDs use protocols to carry out their unique role in the chain of patient care. In the absence of medical dispatch protocols, dispatch quality management is simply not possible.

As the types of EMD training programs burgeoned over the years, two distinctly different methodologies have emerged. In one type the EMDs are trained without a significant or knowledgeable review of a specific protocol. In the other the protocol sets the practice standard because it defines the actions of the dispatcher throughout the call. A crucial element of any EMD curriculum is review by the teacher of each medical dispatch protocol; without review the EMD is left only with generalities. Understanding and practice of the protocols are essential to effective EMD training.

Certification. No informed patient prefers the care of a noncertified provider over that of a certified one. Formal certification of EMDs, whether by state or national bodies, is an essential component of medical dispatch.[2, 8] Certification attests that the EMD has been exposed to a defined body of medical dispatch knowledge and obligates the EMD to conform to a standard of care. There is a clear and growing trend toward the certification of EMDs, and medical directors must be involved. Minimum certification standards should include all of the items in the box on the following page.

The mission statement preceding the regulation rules for EMDs in Utah states, "The purpose of these rules is to provide for the establishment of minimum standards to be met by those providing medical dispatch services in the State of Utah so as to promote the health and safety of the people of this State."[14] In the 1990s there is no question of the dispatcher's ability to achieve these goals.

Continuing dispatch education. The half-life of medical knowledge is about 5 years. Much of what the EMD learns in initial training becomes obsolete as medicine moves forward. It is now technologically possible to defibrillate over the telephone and even view the person on the other end of the line.

EMD Certification Standards

- The use of a medical dispatch protocol system should be required and generically defined.
- A comprehensive quality management program should include significant performance evaluation through an ongoing medical case review process.
- A state or regionally approved training and certification program should include provision of medical oversight and a process for approval of individual agencies' written medical dispatch protocols.
- Appropriate wording should include a certified medical dispatcher program in existing EMS immunity clauses present in EMS enabling law.

Such developments will have profound implications for the future practice of EMD. Continuing education keeps EMDs abreast of the changes and progress in medical dispatching.

A formal continuing education program allows the EMD to share experiences with colleagues. Identified patterns in the medical dispatch practices of a given agency can be illuminated and discussed in an academic and nonthreatening forum. Positive behavior by EMDs is reinforced, and negative behavior is discouraged.

Continuing dispatch education (CDE) is essential to reinforce initial concepts and build on the science of dispatch priorities.[14] As the operational experience of new EMDs expands, CDE becomes their link with the changing aspects of medicine. Regular exposure to appropriate medical concepts as they relate to dispatch increases understanding and fosters application of medical principles at the point EMS actually begins—the dispatch center. Medical directors must take an active role in the quality management process by providing appropriate CDE for dispatchers. The fact that EMD is an emerging and changing field mandates an active CDE program to keep the dispatchers current.

Traditionally the major educational, occupational, and supervisory influences of dispatchers are related to public safety rather than medicine. A more equal balance of emphasis needs to emerge in combined dispatch centers; an active CDE program is required to keep EMDs current with medical standards and the ideas specific to their daily routine. A minimal CDE investment of 1 hour of education per month is becoming standard. As more experience is gained in the continuing education of EMDs the exact amount and type of training will be redefined. The physicians responsible for medical oversight must take an active role in the quality management process and providing sound CDE for dispatchers.

Oversight. All medical activities demand physician involvement and guidance. There should be physician involvement in the planning, organization, and clinical oversight of EMD activities. In reality, EMDs and other prehospital providers are physician extenders. Ultimately the EMS medical director is responsible and accountable for the performance, the personnel, and the adequacy of medical dispatch policy, practice, and protocol.

NAEMSP states, "Medical control for the EMD and the dispatch center is a part of the EMS physician's responsibilities" (see Appendix I). This responsibility includes initial training, CDE, medical dispatch case review, protocol review, and approval. The formal reviews should be performed on both the response assignments and the need for lights-and-siren responses. Although these activities are time consuming, they deserve adequate recognition. Once involved with dispatch the physician often becomes fascinated because medical dispatch lies at the core of EMS philosophy. Analogously, medical dispatch response protocols are the "messenger RNA" of the EMS system, putting planned desires of medical oversight into play for "replication" of the response system each time a call is processed. Thus sound medical input at dispatch influences the makeup and deployment of the system. The establishment of dispatch priorities often requires an unprecedented review of why the system does what it does.

To most medical directors the dispatch center is somewhat of an unknown because traditional direct medical control begins when the telemetry radio signals. Medical dispatch activities, because they occur before this event, are often excluded from the activities of the average medical director. Dispatch case review is the dispatch medical control equivalent to indirect medical control's prehospital care report (PCR) review. This review is accomplished through a medical management oversight committee process.

It is essential that the medical director attends an EMD training course taught by an instructor with EMD training experience. There is a 1-day, executive-level training program for dispatch and medical managers. Once physicians understand both the knowledge base required of a trained telecommunicator and the medical basis for dispatch priorities, they can provide adequate medical oversight for dispatchers.

Data generation. EMD managers and administrators must define what data are needed to objectively evaluate the effectiveness of an EMD program and the performance of the EMDs. Raw data must be analyzed and converted into useful information. A random sampling of roughly 10% of all cases should be reviewed for EMD protocol compliance. All dispatch life support (DLS) pre-arrival instruction cases should be reviewed for protocol compliance. Field responders' feedback, from obtained through the use of a formal reporting mechanism, is another means by which the efficacy of dispatch can be measured.[10] Other data that may be affected by EMD program performance are vehicle fuel consumption, maintenance requirements, and accidents.

Performance evaluation/case review. The fundamental issue in the evaluation of EMD performance is protocol compliance. Protocol was either followed or it was not. The goal of case review is to assist EMDs in improving performance and protocol compliance. However, case reviewers can listen to a case repeatedly; the EMD had only one chance.

The review of a case should begin with listening to the entire call to get an overall sense of the case. The call should then be successively reevaluated for compliance to case-entry and key question protocol, selection of appropriate unit response and mode, and adequacy of postdispatch and pre-arrival instructions.

Random review of cases assures that each dispatcher's actual state of practice (specifically compliance to protocol) is studied. In addition, review of smaller numbers of both exemplary and problem cases is useful. These cases are often identified by external sources. The involvement of EMS field personnel in reporting incidents that represent dispatch-related problems is beneficial to the performance and policy evaluation process.[29]

Careful review leads to the identification of the elements of success or the specific problems of compliance, understanding, policy, or protocol. Without adequate case review, dispatcher compliance to protocol generally falls well below 50% even when mandatory compliance is a formal policy requirement (Figure 14-2). The level of compliance of every dispatcher should be collected and cumulatively compared with established levels of acceptable practice.

Recertification. EMD recertification is the logical result of continuing EMD education. Without the condition that EMDs maintain certification, there is little incentive to stay current. More important, unless maintenance of certification is mandatory for EMDs, there is little incentive to participate in ongoing continuing EMD education.

Risk management. Risk management is the legal equivalent of preventive medicine. All the elements of EMD quality management contribute to a healthy EMD risk management environment and significantly reduce the chance of a dispatch disaster and subsequent litigation.

Decertification, suspension, and termination. Disciplinary actions involving EMDs should be progressive. Formal documentation of deficiencies and corrective actions are basic ingredients for successful remediation of individual EMD problems. The unnecessary loss of an employee who was recruited,

		CLEVELAND	MONTREAL	LOS ANGELES
Case entry	Key questions	Aug 1992 (%)	Sep 1992 (%)	1989 (%)
100	100	88	92	93
<100	100	83	86	82
100	<100	54	50	75
<100	<100	53	72	37

Figure 14-2. MPDS protocol compliance data.

selected, trained, and developed is costly. Therefore care must be taken to ensure that the employee has every reasonable opportunity to achieve acceptable levels of performance.

The preceding 11 components of medical dispatcher quality management are essential to maintain the type of employment environment that assures safe, effective patient evaluation and care initiate every EMS call.

Supervision

It is essential that effective and supportive operational supervision is available for these "air traffic controllers of the ground." Supervision should be delivered by individuals who have extensive training in EMD. To identify problems prospectively, the professional supervisor must have both EMS and EMD knowledge and be responsible for all quality and risk management processes.

It is essential that well-planned, active medical oversight exists to integrate all the components of a comprehensive quality management program. This medical management process usually follows a path separate from the regular chain of command; it consists of a linked set of quality management oversight committees. The medical dispatch review committee (MDRC) functions at the middle management level, initially reviewing and directing the activities of the quality management process. The second functional oversight group is the MPDS steering committee, whose membership is upper management and includes representatives of the chief administrative officer, the medical director, the dispatch supervisor, and the quality management unit leader. Based on quality management case review and other issues, the MDRC makes recommendations to the steering committee, which generally approves, disapproves, or sends suggestions back for further development. Dispatch personnel may sit on these committees.

Pre-arrival Instructions

Trained EMDs are the "first" First Responders. They provide the initial professional intervention, reducing the response time almost to zero for specific problems.[2, 12] There is no better justification for the provision of PAIs than landmark legal opinion delivered by James O. Page to the Aurora, Colorado, Fire Department in 1981[28]:

> After years of arriving 'too late' at the scenes of hundreds of life-threatening emergencies, it is difficult for me to offer a detached and unemotional opinion. Throughout the United States, we have spent billions of dollars constructing systems to respond to medical emergencies and we have done little to cure the deadly 4-minute gap at the front of the system. While we race through city traffic to get to the scene, a brain dies from lack of CPR (oxygen). Frankly, I don't understand how any public safety or health care worker can accept these recurring tragedies without actively seeking a solution to the 'response time' problem which proves fatal in so many cases.

There are many recurring and predictable situations that must be uniquely addressed and corrected before terminating a call at dispatch. To the field provider a cardiac arrest victim is a pulseless, motionless, nonbreathing patient; however, the same patient initially presents to the dispatcher in the following fashion:

> "Is he conscious?" . . . "No!"
> "Is he breathing?" . . . "Uh, I'm not sure. He's making funny noises."

In this case the funny noises, a common telephone description of the agonal respirations, must be correctly interpreted by the EMD.[4] To the trained EMD, until proven otherwise, this situation represents an unconscious victim with an uncontrolled airway that must be cleared. Just as the provider at the scene would immediately establish airway control rather than defer it to someone else later, the EMD must act appropriately and immediately.

Because the responsibility to provide initial care applies to EMDs, they must be trained to give PAIs. Some PAIs are simple commands such as "Don't move the patient," or "Call back if the patient's condition worsens," or "Turn on the porch lights, and flash them on and off when you hear the siren." Other PAIs are more detailed, for example, mouth-to-mouth breathing, the Heimlich maneuver, direct pressure hemorrhage control, and CPR. The more sophisticated or intricate PAIs are given through the use of DLS protocols (Figure 14-3). These protocols are algorithmic scripts using binary logic branching that the EMD reads to the caller. Dispatcher variation is reduced to a minimum. The protocol scripts encourage dispatcher intervention through the reduction of fear and anxiety as well as through the development of learned phrasing by repetitive use.

Pre-arrival instructions are an essential dispatcher practice. The failure to provide appropriate PAIs is described as negligent by a growing number of plaintiff attorneys. Although the notion that dispatch agencies will be successfully sued for providing PAIs has been a roadblock to the establishment of medical dispatch protocol systems, there has never been a dispatcher negligence lawsuit filed following the provision of PAIs. On the contrary, a significant number of recent lawsuits, com-

PRE-ARRIVAL INSTRUCTIONS

1 PATIENT TO PHONE	2 CHECK AIRWAY	3 CHECK BREATHING
Listen carefully. I'll tell you how to help her. **Get her as close to the phone as possible**. I'm going to tell you how to do CPR. **Don't hang up**. **Go do it now.** **Where is she now?**	Listen carefully. **Lay her flat on her back on the floor**. Remove any **pillows**. Now place one **hand** under the **neck**, the other on the **forehead**, and **tilt** the **head** back. Then **look** in the **mouth**. **Go do it now** and come right back to the phone. **Is there VOMIT in the mouth?**	I want you to see if she is **breathing**. Put your **ear** next to her **mouth**. See if you can **feel** or **hear** any breathing, or if you can **see** the **chest rise. Go do it now** and come right back to the phone. ***(If I'm not here, stay on the line.)*** **Can you FEEL or HEAR any breathing?**
→2	NO→3 YES→13	NO/UNCERTAIN→4 YES→16
4 START M-TO-M	**5 GIVE BREATHS**	**6 CHECK PULSE**
I'm going to tell you how to give mouth-to-mouth. Place one **hand** under the **neck**, the other on the **forehead**, and **tilt** the **head** back. **Pinch** the **nose** closed. Completely **cover** her **mouth** with **your mouth**.	Force **two deep breaths** of air into the lungs just like you were blowing up a big balloon. **Watch** for the **chest** to **rise** with each breath. When you have done this, come right back to the phone. **Don't hang up. Go do it now.** ***(If I'm not here, stay on the line.)*** **Can you FEEL the air going in? Did you SEE the chest rising?**	I want you to **check** her **pulse**. **Slide** your index and middle **fingers** into the groove next to the Adam's apple. **Feel carefully for a pulse**. Don't press too hard. Feel for **5 seconds. Go do it now** and come right back to the phone. ***(If I'm not here, stay on the line.)*** **Can you FEEL a PULSE?**
→5	NO→14 YES→6	NO→7 YES→17
7 RECHECK PULSE	**8 CPR LANDMARKS**	**9 COMPRESSIONS**
Try the **other side** of the neck. Feel for **5 seconds** again. **Go do it now** and come right back to the phone. ***(If I'm not here, stay on the line.)*** **Do you FEEL a PULSE now?**	Listen carefully. I'll tell you what to do next. Put the **heel** of your **hand** on the **breastbone** in the **center** of her **chest**, right between the **nipples**. Put your **other hand** on **top** of that hand.	Push down firmly **2 inches** with only the **heels** of your hands touching the chest. Do it **15 times**, just like you are "**pumping**" her chest **twice a second**. When you have done this come right back to the phone. **Don't hang up. Go do it now.**
NO→8 YES→17	→9	→10

DISPATCH LIFE SUPPORT

Figure 14-3. Dispatch life support protocols. (From AMPDS v 10.1, Medical Priority Inc., Salt Lake City.)

pleted or in progress, use the omission of PAIs (or dispatcher abandonment as legal terminology describes it) as either the primary or associated allegation.

The American Heart Association (AHA) states that[22]:

> EMDs have been identified as a vital but often neglected part of the EMS system. All communities should provide formal training in emergency medical dispatch and require the use of medical dispatch protocols, including pre-arrival instructions for airway control, foreign body airway obstruction, and CPR by telephone.

Dispatch Life Support

The concept of DLS provides the basis for establishing the actual content and application method of the special treatment protocols used by medical dispatchers.[17] In 1989 NAEMSP defined DLS as "the knowledge, procedures, and skills used by trained EMDs in providing care through pre-arrival instructions to callers. It consists of those life support principles that are appropriate to application by medical dispatchers" (see Appendix I). Because of the "blind" nature of the provision of PAIs and the need to rapidly teach the caller relatively intricate procedures in real-time (without practice tries or visual verifications), the protocols must be written succinctly and followed strictly.

The AHA life support procedures are based on the trainer's ability to teach in person the application of a physical procedure to a willing student, often over a significant period of time. Unfortunately, the EMD does not have such luxuries. The dispatcher (the instructor) must teach the caller (the unwilling student) a physical procedure (the PAIs) in real-time (seconds) without any visual aids or practice. There is verification neither of correct application nor of any follow through at all.

For example, although the chin lift is not a difficult psychomotor skill to teach in person, over the phone it is too difficult and time consuming. However, the head-tilt method of airway control can be easily taught to the caller as follows: "Put one hand on his forehead and your other under his neck. Lift up on the hand under his neck and push down on the hand on his forehead. This will open his airway." EMDs are instructed to be aware of hazards in neck manipulation if the patient has also incurred a significant mechanism of injury; this is rarely present in the PAI situations encountered by EMDs. DLS more realistically incorporates the fact that, although many treatments dispatchers provide are similar to basic life support, they simply must be different in content, process, and real-time instruction.

Unfortunately, a common problem for medical oversight during the initial review and adoption of DLS treatment sequence protocols is erroneous deviation from other current treatment standards such as those of the AHA.[17] In reality the dilemma is understanding the special limitations of the dispatch situation not the dispatch protocol itself. As NAEMSP stated in the Consensus Document, "Training and recertification in basic life support, *as is appropriate to application by medical dispatchers,* is necessary to maintain and improve this unique, and at times, lifesaving, nonvisual skill" (see Appendix I).

Dispatcher life support was formally defined to clearly establish the necessary functional differences between the dispatcher process and field care as legitimate. Medical dispatch training contains many dispatch-specific methods of description and caller application found in neither field provider training nor protocol.

Medical directors and others involved in the creation of CPR and ACLS standards are beginning to broaden their perspectives on how these standards should apply to PAIs. As the science of EMD evolves, medical dispatch experts and professional medical dispatcher organizations must be involved in the development of new standards that effect EMDs and their remote patients.

Compliance

Inherent in DLS is the necessity for medical dispatchers to adhere to written protocols for the provision of telephone treatment in a standard, reproducible way. Although there is growing interest and effort among public safety agencies to provide telephone instruction to callers, only about 5% of centers provide correct, nonarbitrary, medically approved PAIs read directly from detailed protocol scripts.

It is essential for the EMS medical director to understand the difference between PAIs and telephone aid; the two very different methods of patient care initiated by dispatchers are:

- *PAIs* are telephone-rendered, medically approved, written instructions given by trained EMDs to callers to aid the victim and control the situation before prehospital personnel arrive. These protocols are used word for word as is feasible.
- *Telephone aid* is ad lib advice provided by dispatchers based on their own experience and training in a procedure or treatment, but not following a written PAI protocol. This method exists in a system either because no protocols are used or because protocol adherence is not required.

There is a dramatic difference between the DLS process of PAIs and that of telephone aid. Telephone aid simply assures that the dispatcher has attempted to provide some sort of care to the patient through the caller, but does not assure that the care is necessary, correct, standard, or medically effective. Often, the use of telephone aid is sporadic and arbitrary.

Telephone aid provides the illusion of PAIs without consistently delivering high-quality and accurate advice. The following are common errors seen during medical dispatch case reviews in agencies providing telephone aid:

1. Failure to correctly identify conditions requiring telephone interventions, and therefore prearrival instructions, in the first place. For example, "saving" an infant having a febrile seizure who was incorrectly identified as needing CPR because of the failure to follow protocols designed to verify the absence of breathing before the initiation of potentially dangerous dispatcher invasive treatment such as chest compressions.
2. Failure to accurately identify the presence or lack of interim signs and symptoms during the provision of telephone intervention. For example, dispatchers who ad lib CPR sequences often fail to ask important nonvisual verifiers such as "Did you see the chest rise?" or "Did you feel the air go in?"
3. Failure to perform, describe, or teach multiple step procedures such as CPR care in a consistent and reproducible fashion. For example, quality management reviews often reveal that dispatchers in the same center (or even the same dispatcher) perform care differently on each occasion if they do not follow the scripted PAI protocols exactly.
4. Lack of medically approved protocols for use as a template for evaluating dispatcher performance during the case review and quality management processes. Nonmandatory guidelines cannot be quality assured.

The requirement of medical appropriateness within the EMS dispatch center through effective medical oversight is an essential element for assuring the correct, safe, and efficient application of dispatcher telephone intervention.

Psychological Components

Although it may seem to the casual observer that the emotional or hysterical behavior of callers is random or unpredictable, there are predictable, generic components present in most caller interrogation processes and PAI situations.[16] The following are the most common.

The hysteria threshold. All distraught callers have a threshold of hysteria control that can be reached through repetitive persistence. Bringing callers below the threshold is usually quite easy. Once below the hysteria threshold callers are often in complete emotional control and can repeat instructions word perfect.[9]

The Repetitive Persistence Methodology. The most successful method of crossing the hysteria threshold is repetitive persistence, which is performed by the EMD repeating in the same exact wording a request to calm down or perform any other desired act.[9] For example, "You're going to have to calm down, ma'am, if we're going to help your baby," should be repeated firmly to gain initial control of the caller. Usually this approach works after only two or three repetitions. Alterations in wording are perceived by callers as signs of indecision or lack of control on the part of the EMD.

The "bring the patient to the phone" problem. It is striking how many times PAIs are begun only to be interrupted by the caller yelling, "Bring him in here to the phone!"[11] Obviously this wastes time and interrupts the EMD's train of thought and provision of instructions. At the beginning of the telephone treatment sequence the EMD should always ask, "Where is the patient?"

The "refreak" event. There are three points at which callers may be reminded of the distressing state of the victim, "refreak," and cause the EMD to lose critical control.[9, 11] The first is when the victim is brought to the phone, and the caller is immediately reminded of how bad the victim appears. The second is when the EMD asks for verification of the absence of vital signs (breathing or pulse). The third is when the caller fails to revive the patient through the performance of CPR or the Heimlich maneuver, becomes frustrated, and may stop trying.

The "nothing's working" phenomenon. Average callers harbor the misconception that because they are following the EMD's instructions the victim will respond or immediately be revived. This belief results in a specific type of frustration refreak that can interrupt the treatment sequence. In despair, callers will commonly state that "nothing's working." The EMD can easily overcome this with appropriate encouragement, repetitive persistence, and by mentioning that they are "keeping the victim going until the paramedics get there."[11]

The paramedics "aren't coming" notion. During PAIs callers may often wonder fearfully if help is truly on the way and often repetitively ask "Are they coming?"[11] This may relate to the average citizen's skepticism regarding "the check's in the mail." The dispatcher need only confirm that the paramedics have left the station and are on their way. It is important that this be relayed in "lay terms" for easy comprehension because the distraught caller may not understand professional terms such as "en route."

The realization that these events will occur as predicted allows the dispatcher to prepare for them and then react appropriately. This "cause and effect" understanding is as valuable to the dispatcher as a road map would be to a traveler on an unknown journey.

Further study of the psychological aspects of PAIs and the interrogation of people in crisis will add significantly to the effectiveness of medical dispatching. Understanding the predictable actions and reactions of callers and those at the scene of a critical event increases the effectiveness and confidence of the EMD when dealing with these stressful and difficult situations.

Medical Dispatch Priorities

The development of dispatch priorities was a pivotal event in the evolution of EMD. These priorities lie at the heart of optimal medical dispatch functioning; they are the sum basis of the knowledge, decisions, and treatment of the dispatcher. Dispatch priorities are not a new concept to the emergency physician. In fact they are the subset of medical urgency science on which emergency department triage decisions are usually based (see Appendix II).

Because the EMD is often the least trained professional in the EMS chain of survival, the protocols should be fully understood and carefully adhered. An EMD protocol consists of the following three components: key questions, PAIs, and dispatch priorities including determinants and response (see Figures 14-1 and 14-4). An additional information dispatch card section should always be "in sight" and therefore "in mind," continually familiarizing the EMD with important medical information and axioms (Figure 14-5).

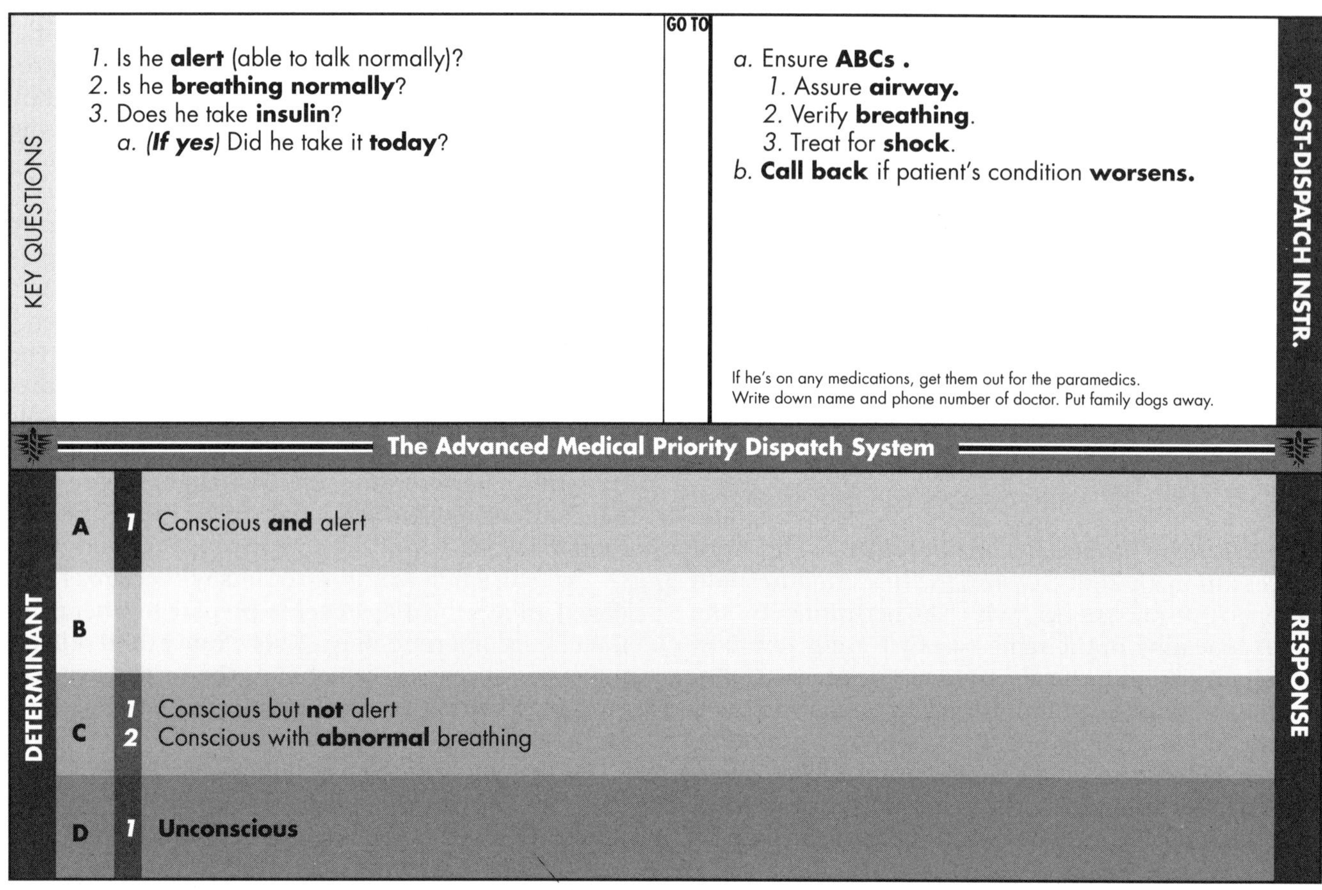

Figure 14-4. Protocol consists of key questions, pre-arrival instructions, and dispatch priorities including determinants and response. (From AMPDS v 10.1, Medical Priority Inc., Salt Lake City.)

Every key question asked on a dispatch priority card is included for one or more of the following reasons:

- It gleans information that is necessary to determine the appropriate response assignments.
- It identifies and verifies conditions that require pre-arrival instructions.
- It obtains information required by response personnel to preplan the call and address the patient (Figure 14-6).
- It identifies the presence at the scene of potential hazards and risks to patients, laypersons, and professional responders (Figure 14-5).

A key question group that leaves any of these necessary indications uncovered is defective and will result in an unsound interrogation. Often a system adopting a priority dispatch system is tempted to make preimplementation modification to existing key question sets, PAIs, and dispatch determinants. This common error is the equivalent of buying a new ambulance then changing the timing, wiring, and other sundry parts without road testing it first.

To a large extent the prime reason for the structure of the key questions is the identification of the most appropriate mobile response (that is, the dispatch priority) that reflects predetermined distinctions in response urgency. For example, the EMD's determination of the level of consciousness in a diabetic problem case results in one of three basic determinants, "conscious and alert," or "conscious but not alert," or "unconscious but breathing" (Figure 14-4). The clear division between these determinants makes dispatch response assignments relatively simple for this particular chief complaint. The "response" section of the dispatch protocol matches each of these determinants with the most appropriate mobile response available in the system.

In the past, many medical dispatchers were given lists of medical conditions considered in need of great urgency or a higher level of response. These lists were the "dispatch priorities" and might have included the following:

Appendicitis	Heat stroke
Anaphylactic shock	Pneumothorax
Heart attack	Pulmonary embolus

ADDITIONAL INFORMATION

DEFINITION OF LIFE STATUS QUESTIONABLE	DISPATCH DEFINITION OF LONG FALL
Existence of any information **suggesting** •Unconsciousness •Abnormal breathing •Cardiac arrest	The patient has **fallen** from a distance of **6 ft** or **higher** (that is, lowest part of the body is above 6ft).

AXIOM 1:	**Hidden exit wounds** and **internal injuries** may **complicate** the patient's status.
AXIOM 2:	**Electrocutions occuring above the ground** may result in **significant falls** causing injuries that may be **more serious** than those incurred from the electrical current itself. Answering all **key questions** should **ensure** this is **not overlooked**.
AXIOM 3:	It is not uncommon for **bystanders** and **rescuers** to also be **electrocuted** in attempting to help or treat the **initial** patient.
AXIOM 4:	A **bystander** can be **electrocuted** in just getting **close** to the patients, **without** even touching them, when **high voltage** is involved or the ground is **wet**.
Rule A:	All **electrocution** patients are **assumed** to be in **cardiac arrest** until breathing is **verified**. **Stay on the line** with caller **until** breathing can be safely **verified**.
Rule B:	Advise caller to beware of electrical **risks** and electrified **water**. **Do not** advise any **treatment** unless it is **safe** to do so.
FIRST LAW OF RESPONDERS:	**"Don't take more victims to the scene."**
SECOND LAW OF RESPONDERS:	**"Don't get it on you or even touch it."**

DEFINITIONS—AXIOMS—RULES

Figure 14-5. Additional information dispatch card. (From AMPDS v 10.1, Medical Priority Inc., Salt Lake City.)

Unfortunately the effectiveness of using such lists was severely limited because for the dispatcher to select the right response, the right problem had to be diagnosed first.[5] Each of the problems on this list could present with chest pain as the chief complaint or an associated symptom. To require the caller—the least medically trained person in the EMS system—to initially diagnose the problem (before interrogation or a scene evaluation) is flawed logic. Priority dispatch uses chief complaint indices that are symptom- or incident-rather than diagnosis-based. Because medical problems such as cardiac difficulties are usually reported by either the patient or a second-party caller, actual symptoms are more readily obtained than in traumatic situations. In those latter cases the determination of the type of incident or mechanism of injury is the basis of the initial response, because the calls are usually made by a third-party and access to individual patient symptoms is less available.

The answers to key questions lead to the second component of the protocol, the provision of appropriate PAIs. One reason that key questions are asked is to identify and verify conditions that require pre-arrival instructions. Before a problem can be treated over the telephone, it must be reasonably determined that it exists. Pre-arrival instructions cannot stand alone. They must follow as the result of proven interrogation scripts that identify those that need treatment and those that do not. Therefore PAIs are only one component, albeit an essential one, of a competent medical priority dispatch system.

In medicine, planning and knowledge aforethought are crucial to the effective functioning of medical providers. Emergency nurses, trauma surgeons, and aeromedical personnel clearly have a medical advantage if they have some idea of the emergency they are about to encounter; prehospital providers are no different. Postdispatch information that is succinct, yet contains scene situation essentials, is crucial to responders. Until someone actually arrives, no one knows more about the scene than the EMD. The EMD must determine the "big picture" and paint a verbal image for adequate en route preparation of the field providers.

Hazardous materials, the mentally disturbed, patients on drugs, and the "just plain mean and nasty armed to the teeth," pose significant risks to EMS responders, the caller, bystanders, and the patient.

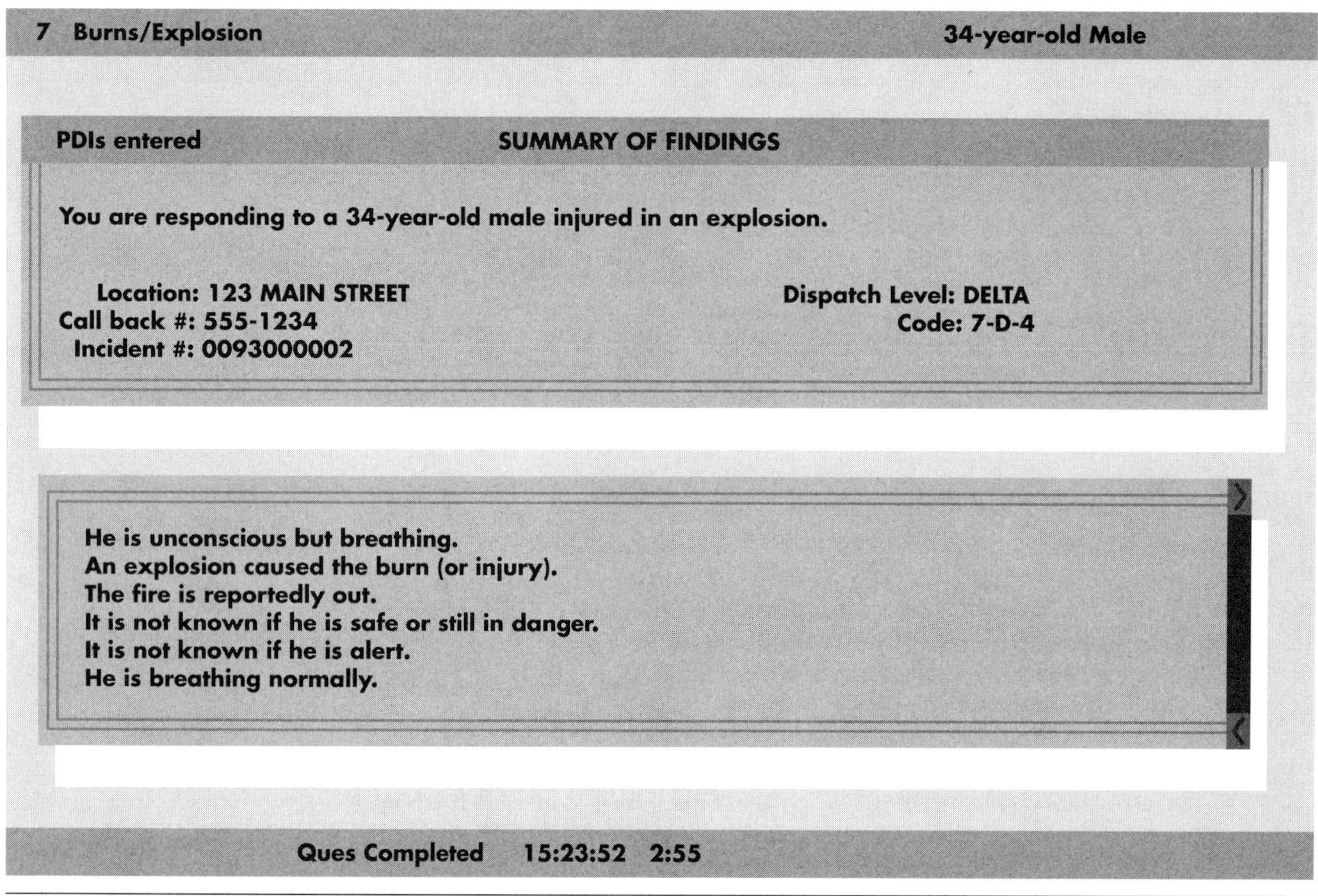

Figure 14-6. Information required by response personnel to preplan the call and address the patient. (From ProQA Software v 1.1, Medical Priority Inc., Salt Lake City.)

Obtaining and transmitting as a priority, information forewarning those that could benefit from such knowledge is within the role of the EMD (Figure 14-5). Failure to uncover essential information during an interrogation could cost the life of a responder.

Tiered Response

Before discussing the steps in assigning dispatch priorities, it is crucial to understand the concept of tiered response. A tiered response is one of the most common methods of response deployment. The availability of more than one type of either response vehicle or level of personnel is required. Usually, tiered responses are found in larger municipal systems, particularly those that are fire department based. The various types of response components may include First Response nontransporting units (fire engines or squads staffed with First Responder fire fighters), vehicles that do not transport (paramedic squads or paramedic fire engines), and transporting ambulances.

Tiered response systems make maximum use of dispatch priorities when the goal is to send "the right thing in the right mode to the right patient at the right time." The following is a generic example of possible dispatch response choices in a tiered system using Emergency Medical Technician-Basic (EMT-B) fire engines, EMT-B ambulances, and paramedic ambulances. HOT indicates lights-and-siren response; COLD indicates routine travel.

CODE	CONFIGURATION MODE
Omega	Referral to alternate (non-EMS) care
Alpha	Closest EMT-B Unit COLD
Bravo	Closest EMT-B Unit HOT
Charlie	Closest Paramedic Unit HOT
Delta	Closest EMT-B Unit HOT and closest Paramedic Unit HOT

A popular response configuration alternative to tiered response is the "all-paramedic ambulance" system in which all transporting vehicles are paramedic ambulances. Unfortunately, few all-paramedic systems, even with the benefit of excellent system status management, can provide initial response times of under 5 minutes without integration of more ubiquitously located units such as fire engines. These all-paramedic systems often use priority response determinations through the addition of First Responders when necessary and the determination of whether the initial ambulance response requires a HOT mode. When properly used through application of dispatch priorities and medical oversight the sometimes overlooked resource of public safety First Responders or EMT-B units can markedly reduce response times for specific life and time-priority cases.

Justification

Whereas the applicability of the key question and PAI components of the dispatch protocol varies little by system, choosing the appropriate local response assignments is greatly dependent on the specific model of the local system and the types of personnel and vehicles available. The development of local response configurations often requires an unprecedented and threatening review of why the system does things the way it does. There are a few basic questions to answer before formulating dispatch priorities (see box at the bottom of the page).[13]

The process of formulating response assignments based on the dispatch priorities is best begun by reviewing the generic response levels available. This will guide local development along well-established, tested paths that can be modified by formal interaction between the EMS administration and medical oversight. When multiple agencies are dispatched by a single central dispatch entity, it is important to adopt a single dispatch protocol agreed upon through joint development and consensus. If different protocols are required for each jurisdiction and dispatching is done centrally, often no protocol is followed. The frustrated dispatchers resort to using their own personal variation of available protocols in a "collage" format. This creates an extremely dangerous risk management situation.

Dispatch call prioritization had its early roots in the evolution of multiple levels of response vehicles and the system abuse that initially surfaced in larger municipalities.[29, 30] In addition, burgeoning numbers of response vehicles arriving at single patient scenes drew the attention of insightful system administrators, risk managers, and fiscal directors.

There are two common misconceptions regarding dispatch prioritization. The first is a misunderstanding of the 4-level determinant system (Alpha, Bravo, Charlie, and Delta). These levels are not related in an ascending linear order or urgency, A through D; the relationship is two-dimensional (Figure 14-7). The horizontal axis shows variations in the type of scene personnel required, and the vertical axis separates cases requiring immediate First Response from those needing only prompt but solitary secondary response by the appropriate vehicle and crew. Regardless of the type of system used in a given area the priority determinants assist in determining the optimal use of those resources.

The second misunderstanding lies in the false belief that one must have a tiered system to use priority dispatch protocols. The name priority was chosen because this methodology was first employed to prioritize the actions of the dispatcher, not just the response. The selection of response configuration and mode for each determinant code is always the discretion of the local agency. However, medical oversight should ultimately approve the process.

The benefits of medically approved dispatch response prioritization are many. By bringing more accurate information into the dispatch office through a more precise interrogation process, EMDs are better able to recognize and understand the true medical condition. Therefore, such protocols allow for planned, safer responses (fewer units responding in the dangerous lights-and-siren mode), fuel and energy savings, reduced personnel burnout, and conservation of scarce paramedic teams for appropriate emergencies.

Dispatch Priority Questions

- Will the time saved make a difference in the final outcome? Specifically, is the problem a true time-priority case requiring a response of less than 5 minutes? Such problems include cardiac or respiratory arrest, airway problems, unconsciousness, childbirth in progress, and severe trauma/hypovolemic shock.
- How much time leeway do you have? For example, what is the actual time frame of a safe response for a given determinant?
- How much time can actually be saved by going lights-and-siren (hot)? What are the other effects of lights-and-siren use?
- How much time can be saved by sending a closer but less sophisticated unit? What is the actual difference in arrival times for second arriving units? Does the patient need sophisticated care or immediate transport?
- When the victim gets to the hospital, will the time saved in the streets be significant compared with the time spent waiting for care in the Emergency Department?

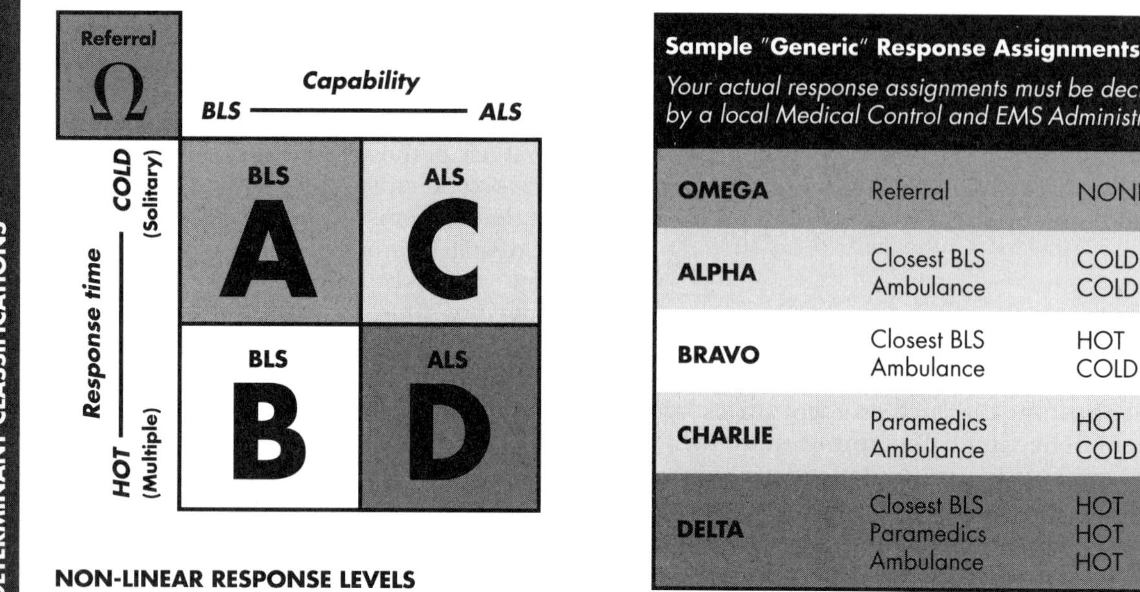

OMEGA	Referral	NONE
ALPHA	Closest BLS Ambulance	COLD COLD
BRAVO	Closest BLS Ambulance	HOT COLD
CHARLIE	Paramedics Ambulance	HOT COLD
DELTA	Closest BLS Paramedics Ambulance	HOT HOT HOT

In establishing routine vs. emergency response assignments to correspond to the **A**, **B**, **C**, and **D** determinant codes the following questions should be considered during any MPDS protocol implementation: (1) Will time make a difference in the outcome? (2) How much time-leeway do you have for that type of problem? (3) How much time can you save driving with red lights-and-sirens? (4) When the victim gets to the hospital, will the time saved be significant compared with the time spent waiting for care such as x-rays, lab tests, etc.? Response assignments and emergency mode should be carefully considered by local medical control based on a thorough review of call-volume history and available units.

Figure 14-7. Four-level determinant system. (From AMPDS v 10.1, Medical Priority Inc., Salt Lake City.)

Prioritization versus Screening

Unfortunately, there is a lack of distinction between call prioritization and call screening; these terms are often incorrectly used interchangeably. The distinction is the inclusion of the "no send" option as a dispatch choice in call screening; that is, some calls are actually "screened out."[16]

Callers have long been denied an EMS response by some large systems both with and without protocol; however, correct use of dispatch priority protocols does not include this option. Dispatch prioritization allows only for the decision of what to send, not whether to send. Screening out significantly increases the legal and media exposure of a system.[1, 21] A "low send," as opposed to a "no send," approach is legally, medically, and politically safer. Recently, attention has been given to the concept of alternative care rather than a traditional EMS response. For example, this has been done with ingestions in children under age 12 without clinical symptoms. Such an Omega response is accomplished by electronically transferring the caller to a regional poison control center (not ED-based systems) for further evaluation and possible home care.

The area of alternate care warrants considerable discussion and review. However, until significant progress is made regarding the modification of protocolized dispatch priorities to include routine alternative care tiers, as opposed to the "no send" choice, significant risks remain. Certainly, documentation of very high compliance to protocol is a necessary prerequisite to implementation of an alternative care option.

Dispatcher Configurations

In dispatch centers where several dispatchers are on duty, medical dispatching is best performed by dividing individual responsibilities between call interrogation and dispatch functions.[16] This team approach is called "horizontal" dispatching. The interrogator follows the entry-level and key question protocols while the radio dispatcher monitors the call (Figure 14-8). At predetermined points during questioning the dispatcher must send the appropriate response unit as indicated by the presenting information. This frees the interrogator to progress into PAIs without deciding which of the two functions, unit

CASE ENTRY PROTOCOL

THE ADVANCED MEDICAL PRIORITY DISPATCH SYSTEM

Location: ____________ (Verify location)

Call back #: ____________ (Verify call back #)

Chief complaint: ____________ (What's the problem? What happened?)

Age: ______ INFANT = <1 year; CHILD = 1-7 YEARS; ADULT = >8 YEARS

Number of patients: ______ (How many are hurt or sick?)

Conscious: ☐ ***Yes*** ☐ ***No*** ☐ ***Unknown*** → Try to verify breathing and respond accordingly.

Breathing: ☐ ***Yes*** → Ask ALL key questions then send appropriate units/mode. ☐ ***No*** ☐ ***Uncertain*** (Second-party caller) ☐ ***Unknown*** (Third-party caller)

Sex: ☐ *Male* ☐ *Female* (Ask only if not obvious)

- If patient is **not** breathing, a **maximal** response is sent immediately.
- If patient is **unconscious** and breathing **cannot** be verified (by second-party caller), a **maximal** response is sent immediately.
- **Verify** the need and prepare for **PAI-Treatment Sequence** intervention.

THE FOUR COMMANDMENTS

Figure 14-8. Case entry protocol. (From AMPDS v 10.1, Medical Priority Inc., Salt Lake City.)

dispatching or PAIs, is more important. When this team approach is used, usually the dispatcher has listened to the interrogation and therefore can give the prehospital responders accurate information regarding the situation. In large and busy horizontal dispatching systems, dispatchers and interrogators may operate at physically separate interactive computer terminals without the dispatcher monitoring the conversation between interrogator and caller.

"Vertical dispatching" holds each dispatcher responsible for a given geographic area and requires that one individual handles all functions for each call. The vertical dispatch configuration is less effective for EMDs using priority dispatch protocols because important choices must be made simultaneously, but it works well with a careful understanding of and adherence to protocols. Obviously, single dispatcher centers have no alternative other than to vertically dispatch.

The Maximal Response Dilemma

Millions of EMS responses occur every year. Before priority dispatch and call screening, virtually every response was run with lights-and-siren, not only to the scene, but often back to the hospital as well. This is an example of "maximal response" and is a combination of always responding with lights-and-siren or always sending multiple vehicles.[10, 13]

Maximal response takes root in three traditional myths. First, "It's an emergency; we've got to hurry!" Years ago when hurrying was all that was done for the victim, speed had some value because it got the victim to the hospital for treatment. Second, many systems have confused EMS response logic with that of fire response. A fire gets worse by the second, but a single cardiac arrest does not spread geometrically in the manner of fire. Although medical problems do progress, the vast majority involve a single patient, usually in a less than life-threatening crisis. Third and least acceptable, running lights-and-siren is fun and seems important. After the fire department management in Salt Lake City discussed sending First Response engines without lights-and-siren (cold), a paramedic captain remarked, "What are you guys going to do, take away the last thing on this job that's fun?" Fortunately, maximal response is a dinosaur in progressive EMS systems; medical priority dispatching is the route of its extinction.

Maximal response often has been touted as the method ensuring those in dire straits rapidly get help. But without medically appropriate guidelines for the dispatcher to follow, everyone will get help. In the recent past, maximum EMS response was always sent to avoid errors in judgment. Today, however, medical oversight may be unable to medically or legally defend a significant delay in arrival at a critical emergency because a paramedic team was sent to a minor "cat bite" call. Systems capable of tiered response or all-paramedic configurations that still send a "one of each" shotgun response rather than use their First Responder personnel or EMT-B ambulance crews efficiently are not functioning at an appropriate level of medical responsibility.

Fire and EMS dispatching are more similar to each other than either is to police dispatching. The majority of both fire and EMS calls are considered escalating emergencies, but that is true for only a small portion of police requests. However, there remains a subtle and less understood difference between fire and EMS dispatching that contributes to maximal response thinking.

Because combined fire and EMS dispatch is common, EMS medical directors must have a clear understanding of the difference between the two. The changing dispatch role during an incident can be thought of graphically as the variable width of a wedge (Figure 14-9). A report of a fire begins at the point of the wedge. The initial role of dispatchers is straightforward; they must get the location, discern what is burning, and then send the right resources based on those two factors. Varied interrogation sequences are usually not necessary. Once the first arriving crew sees the active fire scene, the process escalates and the wedge expands as on-scene command relays the specifics of the fire and requests additional responses. The dispatcher also gets busier with information relay as multiple command sectors are established and additional units stage. Move ups and mutual aid are often necessary, and other agencies such as police and EMS are notified if needed.

The small point at the beginning of the fire dispatch wedge represents the need to get suppression units on the road quickly without extensive questioning of the caller. Since the extent of the fire can rarely be determined initially, it is assumed that it is getting worse each second. In fire suspension, seconds count. But this pattern of response should not be extrapolated to EMS cases.

The greatest responsibility of the EMD occurs at the beginning of each call. The wedge is therefore reversed in EMS calls. The interrogation process should be the fulcrum on which the correct and efficient nature of the response rests. Medical priority dispatching is an effective and safe method to determine the nature of the emergency at the time the call is received, eliminating the need for the classical maximal response in most cases.

Moreover, the maximal response philosophy does not eliminate dispatch errors. It just replaces them with less apparent errors such as paramedic units

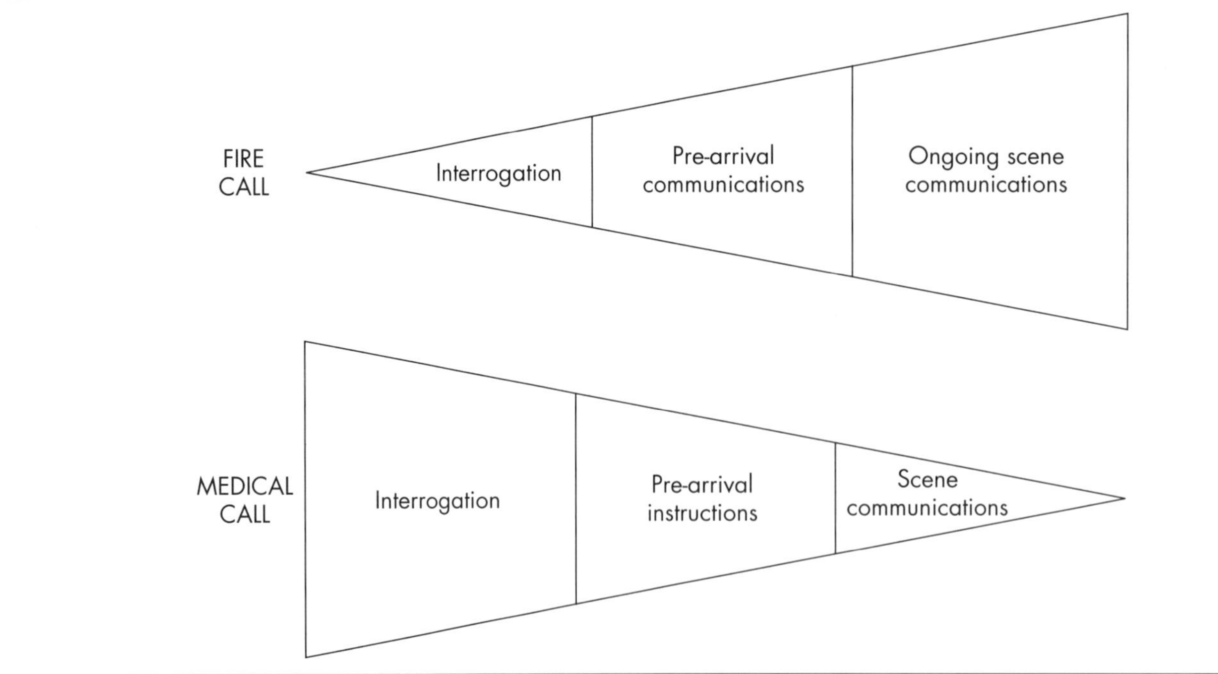

Figure 14-9. Fire and EMS dispatching comparison.

tied up on medically simple but administratively complex calls, First Responders used unnecessarily, and emergency vehicle accidents. As evaluation of EMS systems becomes more sophisticated, the inefficiencies and dangers of routine maximal response are more evident and incur a much greater liability than the occasional less than optimal result of a measured response. In 1991 the effectiveness of using priority dispatch methods to select calls for "only EMT-B initial responses" was studied. In 14,100 cases dispatched over a 90-day period a reasonable process was successfully used to determine response requirement, making paramedics units available more often. The negative effect on patient outcome as a result of paramedic delay was negligible.[18, 31] In EMS the maximal response should be reserved for only the highest level of actual or potential crisis.

Emergency Medical Vehicle Accidents

Thousands of emergency medical vehicle crashes occur every year in North America as a result of lights-and-siren and multiple unit responses. According to the U.S. Department of Transportation's national statistics, 50% of all reportable accidents involve an injury and 1% involve a fatality. In addition, hot responses cause many more crashes that involve other vehicles when the EMS unit slips safely by. Obviously, efforts made to appropriately limit hot responses and extraneous responding vehicles reduce the number of accidents. The original premise of medicine, "First to do no harm," still applies. The EMS philosopher Page asks:[27] "What is the likelihood you'll get sued? Let's start by putting things in proper perspective. By far the greatest legal hazards facing EMTs arise from ambulance vehicle accidents. For some reason or other, we don't like to talk about ambulance vehicle accidents. Even though most of them are preventable. Instead, we are fascinated—in a morbid kind of way—with the whole subject of 'medical malpractice'."

More recently, EMS literature has become replete with articles addressing emergency medical vehicle accident problems and various solutions to prevent and avoid them. Unfortunately, few of them suggest significantly reducing the use of lights-and-sirens. However, in 1992 the NAEMSP published its position paper, "Lights-and-Siren Use in Emergency Medical Vehicle Response and Patient Transport." Among its 14 wide-ranging positions are the following:

1. Quality assurance, loss control, safety risk management, and medical control and direction are essential elements in the management of emergency medical vehicle (EMV) response within the EMS system. The medical aspects of EMV operation and patient transport rationale are integral responsibilities of the medical director of an EMS system and lights-and-siren response and transport protocol must be ultimately approved by the medical director. Discretionary variation by EMS field personnel must be limited.
2. The use of lights-and-siren during both response and transport must be based on sound patient problem assessment or on objective situational protocol. Written prospective protocol for the use of lights-and-siren during transport must be in place and approved by the medical director. In the absence of such protocol the paramedic or EMT on the scene should make contact with the base station hospital to clarify the vehicle response mode for transport of a given patient.
3. The use of lights-and-siren must be restricted to only those situations of dire circumstance in which response time reduction has been proven to improve patient survival.
4. Other than in critical cases or multiple patient incidents the lights-and-siren response of more than one EMV is unnecessary and should be limited by medical dispatch center policy.

There exists no data that prove that lights-and-siren saves lives.

Medicolegal Issues

The fascination with legal aspects of EMS has also played a major role in retarding the development of EMD by perpetuating a myriad of inappropriate fears and supposed pitfalls awaiting this relatively new field. Specifically, there has been considerable concern about the potential liability dispatchers might incur when giving telephone instructions or prioritizing calls. With the exception of a 1984 dispatch incident in Dallas (related to a noncompliant call screener), there are no successful or unsuccessful suits addressing either area, even though hundreds of communities now perform both functions routinely.

The legal climate is getting warmer in all areas of medicine, and EMS is no exception. As the legal community learns more about the workings of the prehospital care system, it will discover the dispatch center as well; however, at this time failure to provide PAIs and "screening out" stand out as the major areas of risk.

The EMS medical director must understand the four essential components of negligence in a court of law. These are (1) duty, (2) breach of duty, (3) damages, and (4) causation. Most malpractice cases are won or lost in the area of causation by success or failure to show that acts of omission by the defendant were the "proximate cause" of the untoward result (damage). However, the concept of duty may play a more prominent role as medical dispatching evolves. Prosser states in regard to duty, "Changing social conditions lead constantly to the recognition of new duties. No better general statement can be made than that the courts will find a duty where in general reasonable men would recognize it and agree that it exists."[25]

In 1981 Page wrote[28]:

> I personally feel that the highly successful 'medical self-help' program introduced by the Phoenix Fire Department may have started a process, which will redefine a municipality's duty to its citizens. Similarly, the Emergency Medical Dispatch Priority Card System, created by Clawson in association with the Salt Lake City Fire Department, may have further advanced the municipality's duty. In other words, I can foresee a day when a citizen might allege that the municipality (which maintains a full-time public safety dispatching service) was negligent for failing to implement and operate such a service. In view of the fact that implementation of this new level of service does not constitute a major expenditure to the municipality—and thus is basically an organizational/management/training issue, rather than a funding/taxation issue—I feel the case for a legal obligation (duty) to provide it becomes stronger.

In 1993 the *Journal of Emergency Medical Services* reported that, on the basis of their annual 200-city survey, 94% of communication centers operated by EMS agencies were offering some sort of pre-arrival instructions to callers. However, only 70% of fire departments and 68% of police-operated centers offered pre-arrival instructions.[3] The courts must decide whether or when such a duty, therefore a standard of care, is actually created.

Legitimate concerns have been raised concerning pre-arrival instructions. The common expression is, "Doctors don't even give advice over the phone. Why should dispatchers?" However, in thousands of cases, trained EMDs have given excellent instructions via the telephone. Because the alternative is literally nothing, more intelligent concerns should focus on the questions listed in the box below.

The answers to each of these questions plays an important role in the risk management aspect of EMD. Because dispatchers are not any less accountable, just less accessible, than other EMS practitioners the answers to these questions should obviously be in the affirmative. In 1981 George stated in the *EMT Legal Bulletin*[21]:

> An 'upfront' clearly articulated written policy in support of telephone screening of emergency calls coupled with sound guidelines and protocols for use by dispatchers would provide a ray of legal light in an otherwise murky area of heavy potential liability. A reasonable system of call screening can provide a good legal defense for both the EMS dispatcher and his employer should a charge of negligent handling of emergency calls be raised by a plaintiff.

The less structure that is built into the interrogation the more questions are asked and the longer the interrogation lasts. Without structure, key elements are often omitted and unnecessary and anecdotal queries are interjected; the unfortunate result is that the four aspects of key questioning are not adequately or consistently covered. When a paramedic is shot because the dispatcher failed to ascertain the potential for violence at the scene, it becomes painfully apparent that "a hole" could exist in more than just the system.

The absence of standard protocols makes it difficult to reproduce the same sequence of interrogation or the same answers in relation to a given chief complaint. As George further warned[21]:

> EMS dispatchers must always avoid the appearance of responding to or categorizing emergency calls in a haphazard or arbitrary manner. A unified procedure will provide an excellent method of safeguarding against arbitrary decision making. Without a unified system, one dispatch may decide that a crucial situation exists primarily on the level of emotion he detects in the caller's voice, while another may depend on his own 'gut' reaction, without being able to articulate a clear reason for his decision.

Pre-arrival Instruction Concerns

1. Is there adequate identification of the problems requiring dispatcher "invasive" treatment?
2. Are dispatchers uniformly trained?
3. Do dispatchers use sound, medically approved algorithms that give more detailed instructions such as CPR?
4. Is there adequate quality management and medical oversight at dispatch including call review?

EMS resources are limited. This is increasingly evident as pressures to contain the costs of medical care rise. It is impractical for a community to have ambulances on each block; even if enough personnel could be trained, they would never get enough call volume to adequately retain their skills. Thus the use of the EMS system must be judicious and balanced. Prioritizing calls is one way to effectively and safely accomplish this. Prioritization provides a logical method to deal with apparent chaos. Instead of having the system whirl in a version of EMS roulette, paramedic units are sent to appropriate calls rather than those that come in first. The EMD must adhere to clearly established, medically controlled protocols. The science of medical dispatching requires nonarbitrary adherence to protocol.

Legal Immunity for the EMD

Some EMDs have limited protection from legal liability through a little known legal application discovered in 1983 when the rules and standards for EMDs were established in Utah.[20] These rules made the use of a "selective dispatch system" (the generic definition for a card file-protocol set) mandatory, but training and certification were standardized yet not required. The Utah EMS Systems Act stated that certified EMDs are:

> basic life support personnel who, during training or after certification,....in good faith provide emergency medical instructions or render emergency care authorized by this chapter shall not be liable for civil damages as a result of any acts or omissions, unless found guilty of gross negligence or willful misconduct.

This application of immunity to EMDs has resulted in widespread training and certification throughout Utah, especially in law enforcement-controlled dispatch centers.

Governmental immunity may not always protect an individual or their employer from liability damage recovery. However, in recent EMS court cases immunity has resulted in summary judgments or has been applied "at the beginning" of a case to define for jurors what measure of immunity must be proven. It is much better to have an immunity shield to take to battle rather than enter the fight without any immunity. However, immunity is not present unless the dispatcher is first adequately trained and then qualifies for certification as an EMS by a state that offers such legislated immunity. Immunity should never be provided to dispatchers without being clearly linked to appropriate training, use of protocol, compliance with protocol, measure of quality management mechanisms, and certification. If all these are not assured, then public safety dispatchers and their employers should be responsible for negligent actions.

Summary

At times, application of common sense seems impossible in a world of self-protectionism and "what if" mentality. Had EMS and EMD appeared in the 1930s the legal discussion would have been largely unnecessary. In those earlier times, actions themselves were considered more important than the imagined consequences. Today, however, this professional concern precludes more constructive activities by dispatchers in many systems. Optimal dispatching requires the courage to practice medicine at dispatch the same way it is done in the field. Many of the key decisions and diagnoses in medical practice are based on statistical predictability or the likelihood of finding a specific problem using standard evaluations and tests. Medical priority dispatching concepts were borne of this "physician-based" concept.

The EMD's role differs in major ways from that of the field provider. Street practitioners act as advocates for individual patients assumed to be dying until it is proven otherwise. EMDs are the advocate for the well-being of the entire system and they must constantly juggle the concepts of "allocate versus conserve" and "hurry versus wait." This requires a philosophy of training and protocol quite different from that of field personnel. The EMD's multiple roles of interrogator, prioritizer, and prearrival intervenor are analogous to the physician's tasks of history taking, evaluation, categorization, and treatment. It is no wonder that the modern EMS medical director feels comfortable with the philosophy of EMD and in providing medical oversight.

The advocacy of the system versus the individual patient is the dilemma faced in providing safe and efficient dispatch priorities. EMS physicians responsible for medical dispatch programs are repeatedly forced to deal with that dilemma.

Today, many EMS systems lack the money and human resources to respond maximally to every medical request. The improvements in patient care and survival and the appropriate tiering of response through structured call prioritization provide one answer to the specter of political or financial self-destruction in EMS.[21, 31, 32]

For the EMS physician, focusing on the system without paying appropriate attention to dispatch is analogous to picking up a deadly snake by the tail instead of just behind the head. The unexpected "bite" of medical dispatch has injured a number of unwary medical directors. Excellence at dispatch encourages excellence down the line. Nursing quality management expert Smith-Marker paraphrased it for medical dispatchers[33]:

> EMDs can function according to defined purposeful expectations or by intuition. A medical dispatching system can operate in a designated manner or haphazardly. Patient care by phone can be delivered by design or by impulse and habit. Standards either exist or they do not. If they exist, they must be detailed, consistent, and comprehensive or they will be shallow, irrelevant, and worthless.

In summary the core of emergency medical dispatching, as in most aspects of medical practice, is the provision of the correct medical interactions at the right time by appropriately trained practitioners. The critical functions of EMDs in prehospital medicine are unique and crucial parts of the responsibility of medical oversight.

REFERENCES

1. Adams R: Lessons learned from Dallas, *Firehouse* May 1984.
2. American Society for Testing and Materials: *Standard practice for emergency medical dispatch,* Pub No F1258-90, Philadelphia, Pa, 1990, The Society.
3. Cady G: EMS in the United States: a survey of providers in the 200 most populous cities, *JEMS* 18(1):71, 1993.
4. Clark J et al: Incidence of agonal respirations in sudden cardiac arrest, *Ann Emerg Med* 21:1464, 1992.
5. Clawson J: Dispatch priority training: strengthening the weak link, *JEMS* 6:2, 1981.
6. Clawson J: The red-light-and-siren response, *JEMS* 6:2, 1981.
7. Clawson J: Medical priority dispatch: It Works! 8:2/Feb 1993.
8. Clawson J: Regulations and standards for emergency medical dispatchers: a model for state or region, *Emergency Medical Services* 13:4, 1984.
9. Clawson J: The hysteria threshold: gaining control of the emergency caller, *JEMS* 11:8, 1986.
10. Clawson J: Medical dispatch review: "Run" review for the EMD, *JEMS* 11:10, 1986.
11. Clawson J: The Psychological components of prearrival instructing. In: *Emergency medical dispatcher training program manual,* Salt Lake City, 1986, Medical Priority Consultants.
12. Clawson J: Telephone treatment protocols: reach out and help someone, *JEMS* 11:6, 1986.
13. Clawson J: The maximal response disease-red lights and siren syndrome, *JEMS* 12:1, 1987.
14. Clawson J: Quality assurance: a priority for medical dispatch, *Emergency Medical Services* 18:7, 1989.
15. Clawson J: The value of protocol compliance, *Journal of the National Academy of EMD* 1:3, 1990.
16. Clawson J and Dernocoeur K: *Principles of emergency medical dispatch,* Englewood Cliffs, NJ, 1988, Brady/Prentice Hall.
17. Clawson J and Hauert S: Dispatch life support: establishing standards that work, *JEMS* 15:8, 1990.
18. Curka P, Pepe P, and Ginger V: Computer-aided EMS priority dispatch: ability of a computerized triage system to safely spare paramedics from response not requiring advanced life support, *Ann Emerg Med* 20:446, 1991 (abstract).
19. Eisenberg M et al: Identification of cardiac arrest by emergency dispatchers, *Am J Emerg Med* 4:4, 1986.
20. Emergency Medical Dispatcher Rules of the Utah Emergency Medical Services System and Standards Act, Title 26, Chapter 8.
21. George J: EMS triage, *Emergency Medical Technician Legal Bulletin* 5:4, 1981.
22. Guidelines for cardiopulmonary resuscitation and emergency cardiac care, *JAMA* 268:2172, 1992.
23. Kallsen G and Nabors M: The use of priority medical dispatch to distinguish between high- and low-risk patients, *Ann Emerg Med* 19:458-459, 1990.
24. Keene K: Promises, Promises: Does EMD really work? *Emergency Medical Services* 19:9, 1990.
25. Keeton P, editor: *The law of torts,* ed 5, St. Paul, Minn, 1984, West Publishing Co.
26. Keller R: EMD in the fire service, *Fire Chief* 36(5):46, 1992.
27. Page J: *EMT's legal primer,* Solana Beach, Calif, 1985, Jems Publishing Co.
28. Page JO: Personal correspondence, Sep 28, 1981. In: *Principles of emergency medical dispatch,* Englewood Cliffs, NJ, 1988, Brady/Prentice Hall.
29. Roberts B: EMS dispatching: its use and misuse, Dallas Fire Department internal report, 1978.
30. Robinson V: Call screening targets false emergencies, *International Fire Chief* 47:16, 1980.
31. Stratton S: Triage by emergency medical dispatchers, *Prehospital Disaster Medicine* 7:263, 1992.
32. Valenzuela T et al: Estimated cost-effectiveness of dispatcher CPR instruction via telephone to bystanders during out-of-hospital ventricular fibrillation, *Prehospital Disaster Medicine* 7:379, 1992.
33. Wheeler S: *Telephone triage: theory, practice and protocol development,* Albany, NY, 1993, Delmar Publishers Inc.

Appendix I

*Emergency Medical Dispatching**

The following document expresses the positions developed by the membership of the National Association of EMS Physicians (NAEMSP). This Position is based on the Consensus Document for Emergency Medical Dispatching, on file at the NAEMSP office.

Introduction

Medical Dispatching has been the last major area in the prehospital emergency medical services chain of care to be identified and developed. The "health" of many EMS systems can be gauged by the appropriateness of training, protocols, and medical control and direction of dispatchers. The involvement of prehospital EMS physicians in the world of dispatch is relatively new but unquestionably essential. For this reason, the National Association of EMS Physicians has taken the following position relative to Emergency Medical Dispatching.

Position

The trained Emergency Medical Dispatcher (EMD) is an essential part of a prehospital EMS system. Medical direction and control for the EMD and the dispatch center also constitutes part of the prescribed responsibilities of the Medical Director of the EMS system. The functions of emergency medical dispatching must include the use of predetermined questions, pre-arrival telephone instructions, and pre-assigned response levels and modes. The EMD must understand the philosophy and psychology of interrogation and telephone interventions, basic emergency medical priorities and interventions, and be expert in dispatch life support. Minimum training levels must be established, standardized, and all EMDs must be certified by governmental authority.

*National Association of Emergency Medical Services Physicians

Position Statements

1. The medical aspects of emergency medical dispatching and communications are an integral part of the responsibilities of the Medical Director of an EMS system.
2. Proven knowledge and skills in the area known as basic telecommunications are requisite for all public safety telecommunicators.
3. Understanding the philosophy of medical interrogation and the psychology of providing Pre-Arrival Instructions is integral to the training and functioning of EMDs.
4. Pre-arrival instructions are a mandatory function of each EMD in a medical dispatch center.
5. Dispatch prioritization is an essential element in any EMS system for it establishes the appropriate level of care including the urgency and type of response. Standard medically approved telephone instructions by trained EMDs are safe to give and in many instances are a moral necessity.
6. Training as EMDs is required for all dispatchers functioning in medical dispatch agencies and requires unprecedented cooperation between the diverse disciplines of telecommunications and emergency medicine necessary to provide this unique teaching forum. This training includes content and results in competence which differ substantially from that standardly provided for EMTs and paramedics. It must be taught by specially-trained instructors.
7. Quality Assurance, Risk Management, and Medical Control and Direction are essential elements to the management of medical dispatch operations within the EMS system.

8. Certification and authorization by government agencies in accordance with standards promulgated by NAEMSP in conjunction with other organizations must be required.

Definitions

Emergency Medical Dispatching: the reception and management of requests for emergency medical assistance in an EMS system.

Emergency Medical Dispatcher (EMD): a specially trained public safety telecommunicator with the specific emergency medical knowledge essential for the appropriate and efficient functioning of emergency medical dispatching.

Medical Dispatch Center: any agency that routinely accepts calls for EMD assistance from the public and/or that dispatches prehospital emergency medical personnel pursuant to such requests.

Public Safety Telecommunicator: an individual trained to communicate by electronic means with persons seeking emergency assistance and with agencies and individuals providing such assistance.

Basic Telecommunications Skills: the generic body of knowledge and skills necessary to function as a Public Safety Telecommunicator whether performing specifically in the role of medical, fire, law enforcement, aeromedical, park service dispatcher, or in any combination of these roles.

Medical Director:* the management and accountability for the medical care aspects of an EMD program including: (1) the direction and oversight of the training of the EMD; (2) development and monitoring of both the operational and the emergency medical priority dispatch protocol systems; (3) participation in EMD system evaluation; and (4) directing the medical care rendered by the EMDs.

Medical Control:* the EMS physician(s) responsible for the provision of education, training, protocols, critiques, leadership, testing, certification, decertification, standards, advice, and quality control through an official authoritative position within the prehospital EMS system.

Medical Priority Dispatch System: a medically approved system used by a medical dispatch center to dispatch appropriate aid to medical emergencies, which include: 1) systematized caller interrogation; 2) systematized Pre-Arrival Instructions; and 3) protocols which match the dispatcher's evaluation of the injury or illness type and severity with vehicle response mode and configuration.

Pre-Arrival Instructions: telephone-rendered, medically approved, written instructions given by trained EMDs through callers which help to provide aid to the victim and control of the situation prior to arrival of prehospital personnel.

Dispatch Life Support: the knowledge, procedures, and skills used by trained EMDs in providing care through Pre-Arrival Instructions to callers. It consists of those BLS and ALS principles that are appropriate to application by medical dispatchers.

Quality Assurance: the comprehensive program of setting standards and monitoring the performance of the clinical, operational, and personnel components of the medical dispatch center in relation to these accepted standards.

Risk Management: a sub-component of the Quality Assurance program designed to identify problematic situations and to assist EMS Medical Directors, dispatch supervisors, and EMDs in modifying practice behaviors found to be deficient by quality assessment procedures; to protect the public against incompetent practitioners; and to modify structural, resource, and protocol deficiencies that may exist in the emergency medical dispatch system.

Vehicle Response Configuration: the specific set of vehicle(s) in terms of types, capabilities, and numbers responding as the direct result of actions taken by the emergency medical dispatch system.

Vehicle Response Mode: the manner of response used by the personnel and vehicles dispatched which reflects the level of urgency of a particular required treatment or transport (e.g., use of emergency driving techniques such as red-lights-and-siren vs. routine driving).

*Relates specifically to Emergency Medical Dispatch.

Discussion

The Emergency Medical Dispatcher (EMD) is the principal link between the public in need of emergency medical assistance and the EMS system. As such, the EMD plays a key role in the ability of the EMS system to respond to a perceived medical emergency. Most often, all of the information obtained is through telephone communications with a caller who often is distressed and out of control. The EMD must have skills which allow him/her to match the personnel and equipment dispatched to the perceived emergency. Thus, the EMD must be able to discern the nature and the urgency of the illness(es) and/or injury(ies) in a manner which allows selection of the most appropriate response configuration and mode.

Therefore, the EMD must possess special knowledge and a set of medical and technological skills which are unique for the EMS system. They need to know sufficient medical knowledge in lay terminology to acquire an appropriate medical history and be cognizant of all of the characteristics inherent within the EMS system in which they function. Furthermore, recent studies indicate that EMDs may play an very important role in the provision of instructions by which a caller may initiate appropriate treatment and life support prior to the arrival of any of the EMS responding vehicles and personnel. The capable EMD provides "first responder" care through the surrogate caller. Such skills have been shown to help preserve lives, prevent further injuries, and even assist with the delivery of babies.

Without these specially trained, talented, dedicated, and skilled professionals, an EMS system cannot function optimally. Unfortunately, in most situations, persons performing the dispatch functions have had little more training than the average layperson. Inadequate personnel and equipment may be dispatched for major problems while too comprehensive a portion of the system may be mobilized for minor problems. This latter circumstance may result in depriving others in need of the committed services to be deprived of them. Any break in these important functions result in failure of the entire EMS system. An EMS system only can be as good as its EMDs.

Since emergency medical dispatching is key to the successful operation of any prehospital EMS system, the policies and procedures utilized by trained EMDs must conform to national standards and local capabilities. The history obtained by telephone and both the medical care dictated by the EMD and the responses initiated are functions of the type and level of medical care possible from the specific EMS system. The quality of all of the medical care delivered by a system is the responsibility of the medical director of that prehospital system. Therefore, all of the policies and procedures used by the Medical Dispatch Center in terms of medical care rendered are part of the responsibilities of the Medical Director and hence, must be approved by the Medical Director of the system. Key to the Medical Director's role in the management of medical dispatch centers is his or her detailed understanding of the concepts of EMD and its physical operation, involvement in all aspects of quality assurance of medical dispatch, and medical direction and accountability for the protocols, policies, and procedures relevant to the medical dispatch activities of the EMD. In summary, the medical aspects of emergency medical dispatching and communications are an integral part of the responsibilities of the Medical Director of each EMS system.

Certain skills are common to all public safety communicators. These include the theory and operation of complex communication equipments, troubleshooting the same, and basic radio and telephone communication skills. Serious liability for dispatch centers commonly results due to the lack of these essential skills. The training and certification of the EMD is built upon this baseline of knowledge and skills, which is generic for performing in the role of medical, fire, law enforcement, aeromedical, park service dispatcher, or any combination of these services.

The ability to interact with anxious, uncooperative, and, at times, hysterical callers rests on the ability of the EMD to anticipate the actions of the undirected caller, assist the caller in regaining control, and then, convert the caller into a calmer, first responder is a special one. Each is an essential step in the performance of the prescribed duties and contributes to the substantial responsibilities delegated to the EMD by the Medical Director and the Medical Dispatch Center. Each of these steps requires special training and the development of different skills. This knowledge and special set of skills are not part of the standardized EMT or paramedic curricula. Each is specific to medical dispatch training.

Since the value of EMDs providing Pre-Arrival Instructions to callers in attendance with victims of cardiopulmonary arrest was first demonstrated 14 years ago, Pre-Arrival Instructions have become a mandatory function of the EMD. In essence, the EMD is the first "first-responder" and through immediate action effectively can eliminate the often deadly gaps which may occur between receipt of the call and the beginning of treatment which is delayed until after the arrival of the responding vehicles and personnel. First response consists of telephone instructions provided by trained EMDs functioning from standard, medically approved protocols. Such instructions are safe and, in many instances, are a moral necessity. The telephone instructions are given through the caller to help another person or the caller protect the victim(s) from further harm or injury, to initiate life-impacting treatments, and to transform an undirected caller into a calmer scene "rescuer" who no longer needs to be helpless. Training, certification, and recertification in Dispatch Life Support (DLS), which includes that portion of BLS appropriate to application by medical dispatchers is necessary to maintain and continually upgrade this unique, and, at times, life-saving, nonvisual skill. Hence, it is essential that EMDs understand the philosophy of medical interrogation and the psychology associated with the provision of Pre-Arrival Instructions. This knowledge and the associated skills must be integral parts of the training, direction, and management of EMDs and any Medical Dispatch Center.

Dispatch Prioritization is an essential element in EMS and requires careful attention by both the EMD, his or her supervisor, and the EMS physician responsible for medical control. These priorities must reflect the level of appropriate response including types of personnel (ALS vs. BLS vs. first responder), response configuration (numbers and types of vehicles responding), and mode of response (red-lights-and-siren vs. routine). Haphazard or arbitrary dispatch decisions have been shown to place victims of serious illness or injury at unnecessary risk and have resulted in significant liability to systems lacking these essential protocols, procedures, and policies.

With the use of unified, standard protocols, the emergency medical dispatcher's conduct will be less vulnerable to charges of careless or reckless judgment. For example, without a unified system of standard protocols, one dispatcher may decide that a crucial situation exists primarily on the basis of the level of emotion he/she detects in the caller's voice, while another may depend on his or her own "gut" reaction without being able to articulate a clear reason for a decision. A unified procedure provides an excellent method of safeguarding against arbitrary decision-making. Similarly, EMS employers can point to such guidelines as a system of risk management in an area in which human error and its dire consequences clearly are foreseeable. The appropriate prioritization of the type, number, and manner of responses is essential to effect an appropriate reduction of responding vehicles traveling red-lights-and-siren, and therefore unnecessary vehicle accidents. This will assure that emergency crews will not be committed inappropriately to non-emergency cases, and that the right care will be sent in the right way to the right patient at the right time.

The necessity to prioritize responses is evident in the majority of EMS systems today. In order to prioritize calls properly, the EMD must be well-versed in the medical conditions and incident types that constitute their daily routine. Training in these priorities must be detailed and dispatch-specific (not EMT or paramedic training per se). The development of dispatch priorities for an agency or locality must be carefully thought out and ultimately approved by those physicians responsible for medical control.

Since much of the knowledge and many of the skills required by the EMD are dispatch-specific, a curriculum for their training differs substantially from those used in the preparation of EMTs or paramedics. Training as an EMT or paramedic does not adequately prepare a person for the role of an EMD. Much of the required EMD curriculum cannot be found in standard EMS training curricula. It consists of content and emphasis which differ significantly from that used for the training of all other health professionals and public safety dispatchers. The unique teaching forum necessary to provide this essential training requires unprecedented cooperation between the diverse disciplines of telecommunications and prehospital and emergency medicine. Instructor requirements should include line dispatch experience as a trained EMD for the Primary Dispatch Instructor and a minimum of advanced life support training and experience for the Medical Dispatch Instructor who is responsible for teaching the core course materials, specifically the medical dispatch priorities. All instructors should have successfully completed a credible EMD course prior to assuming a teaching role. Essentially, training of EMDs is required for all dispatchers functioning in medical dispatch agencies, and contains significant content and competence which differs substantially from that standardly provided to EMTs and paramedics.

Quality assurance, risk management, and medical direction and control are essential elements for the ongoing well-being of any EMS system. Routine medical reviews of the activities of EMDs and medical dispatch centers in general is vital to the health of all EMS systems. Dispatch review committees constitute one method of providing quality assurance for EMD activities and the medical aspects of the operation of a medical dispatch center. Such committees should be composed of prehospital EMS physicians and those responsible for the provision of medical control, dispatch supervision and management personnel, EMTs and/or paramedics, and EMDs. Each must be familiar with all aspects of EMS communications, specifically the medical dispatch process, and must be involved in an ongoing way with its function relative to medical issues, operations, and patient care.

Recognition of the important role of emergency medical dispatchers in the delivery of prehospital emergency medical services by responsible governmental agencies, and by the public in general, is important for the public health and protection. Without such recognition and action, it is unlikely that the training of these important professionals will be mandated. An ever-increasing number of states, regions, counties, and municipalities certify or at least require standard training of EMDs. This constitutes an essential prerequisite to the practice by EMDs. Minimum standards must be developed and promulgated for the training, certification, and or licensure of all public safety telecommunicators, specifically Emergency Medical Dispatchers.

Conclusion

In order to assure the professionalism of this key aspect of prehospital emergency medical care, EMS physicians should participate actively in the development, training, quality assurance, medical control and direction of EMDs and medical dispatch centers. The Emergency Medical Dispatcher provides an all-important professional link in the overall EMS chain of care and survival.

Appendix II

Example of Dispatch Categories with Priority and Unit Recommendation

This system was developed in the early 1980s in New York City for a three-tiered system that included EMT-Ds in ambulances (BLS), paramedics in ambulances (ALS), and paramedic nontransport units (PRU). It is primitive by modern standards.

TYPE	PRI	UNIT	PRU*	BACKUP	COMMENT
ABDPN	5	BLS			Abdominal Pain
ALTMEN	5	ALS			No history of EtOH, Drugs, Psych or Injury (CONSCIOUS)
AMPMAJ	3	BLS			Amputation (Leg, Foot, Hand, or Arm)
AMPMIN	5	BLS			Amputation (Finger or Toe) No other injuries
ANAPH	2	ALS	p	BLS	Anaphylaxtic reaction (drug, Food or Bite)
ARREST	1	ALS	p	BLS	Cardiac arrest (UNCONSCIOUS—No Breathing
BURNMA	3	ALS			Serious burn Adult >18% Child or Elderly >10%
BURNMI	7	BLS			Minor Burn Adult <18% Child or Elderly <10%
CHESTP	3	ALS	p		Chest pain
CHILDA	6	BLS			Child abuse (No Major Injuries)
CHOKE	1	ALS	p	BLS	Choking
CNS	3	BLS			Neck/Spinal injury or Paralysis
COLD	5	BLS			Cold/Hypothermia (CONSCIOUS)
CVA	5	BLS			C.V.A./Possible stroke (CONSCIOUS)
DIAB	6	BLS			Diabetic problem (No change in mental state)
DIFFBR	2	ALS	p		Difficulty breathing (ALL)
DOA	8	BLS			Confirmed death
DROWN	2	ALS		BLS	Drowning (Still in water or Conscious)
DRUG	6	BLS			Drug or Alcohol abuse (eg. PCP) (CONSCIOUS)
EDP	8	BLS			Psychiatric History (CONSCIOUS) No Injuries
ELECT	3	ALS	p		Electric shock (CONSCIOUS)
GYNMAJ	3	ALS		BLS	GYN/Severe Vaginal bleeding (No Pregnancy)
GYNMIN	5	BLS			GYN/Pain/Spotting (No Pregnancy)
HEAT	4	BLS			Heat exhaustion
INBLED	3	BLS			Internal hemorrhage (Vomiting Blood or Melena)
INGEST	4	BLS			Oral Ingestion of Poison (Lye, Corrosive)
INHALE	5	BLS			Smoke Inhalation (CONSCIOUS)
INJMAJ	3	BLS		ALS	Major injury (CONSC, Airway OK, Heavy bleed)
INJMIN	7	BLS			Minor injury (CONSC, Airway OK, Little bleed)
JUMPDN	1	ALS		BLS	Jumper down
JUMPUP	7	BLS			Jumper up

* ALS in nontransport vehicle to be *saved* for these cases and for ALS backup.

TYPE	PRI	UNIT	PRU*	BACKUP	COMMENT
MEDEVAC	5	BLS			Medical evacuation via helicopter
MVA	6	BLS			Auto accident (No confirmation of injuries)
MVAINJ	4	BLS			Auto accident (Confirmed injuries)
OBCOMP	2	ALS			OB Complication (5-9 Months Hemorrhage)
OBLAB	5	BLS			OB/Labor (1-4 Mos Hemorrhage or Routine Labor)
OBOUT	3	ALS	p	BLS	OB/Baby born or imminent
OD	4	ALS			Alcohol or Drug Overdose (Conscious)
OTHER	7	BLS			No Info Available (Choose priority and unit)
PEDSTR	3	BLS			Pedestrian, Motorcycle or Bicycle Struck
PRUNON	2	BLS			Confirmed back up of PRU required
PTS	8	BLS			Psychiatric transfer
RAPE	6	BLS			Rape (No injuries)
SEIZR	6	BLS			Seizures (SINGLE AND SHORT DURATION)
SHOT	2	BLS			Gun shot wound
SICK	6	BLS			Sick/Vomit, Fever, Headache (CONSCIOUS)
SICKPED	4	ALS	p		Sick/pediatrics (less than 1 year old)
SPEVNT	8	BLS			Special event
STAB	2	ALS		BLS	Stab wound
STATEP	2	ALS	p	BLS	Repeated or prolonged seizures
STNDBY	8	BLS			Standby assignment
STRANS	5	BLS			Stat Transfer
TRANS	8	BLS			Medical Transfer
TRAUMA	2	ALS	p	BLS	Severe Inj, Trapped, Shock or No Airway
UNC	2	ALS	p	BLS	Unconscious (ALL)
VENOM	2	BLS			Venomous bite (eg. snake bite)

15

Data Collection

Terence D. Valenzuela, M.D.
Elizabeth Criss, R.N., B.S.N.

Effectively and efficiently monitoring the resources of an EMS system is difficult. The task can be made less formidable through the use of a properly designed prehospital care report (PCR) system.

The EMS Systems Act of 1973 made recommendations for standardized recordkeeping including an outline for the basic data elements thought to be essential.[3,15,7,8] The legislation also emphasized the development of standardized patient recordkeeping as an important component of system evaluation. Early EMS planners realized that without comprehensive and standardized data collection the medical benefits of prehospital care could not be compared or evaluated. The basic data elements are listed in the box below.

These data elements resulted from cooperative efforts between relevant medical specialty representatives and state and federal agency officials. Early EMS planners felt that these elements provided the basic information necessary for EMS system evaluation and an adequate data base for research. Many states, regions, and agencies customized their reporting systems following input from the medical community.[9,11,17] A more recent and welcome development is the reporting formats defined by the results of scientifically valid clinical outcome studies, most notably in the area of out-of-hospital cardiac arrest.[6] Few provisions have been made for supraregional standardized recordkeeping; as a result, few jurisdictions can accurately compare system performance with similar jurisdictions around the country.

Basic Data Elements

Patient demographic data
EMS vehicle information (that is, level of care)
EMS response and transport intervals
Incident location
Patient complaint
Patient condition
Mechanism of injury
Therapy administered
Treatment outcome
Receiving medical facility

Needs Assessment

The development of a recordkeeping system for EMS requires consensus on the data elements and uniformity of system information and the physical format of the report. Each of these decisions affects all levels of system planners and the evaluation for performance needs.

The data that are available from the basic elements outlined by the EMS System Act in conjunction with any specialized modifications, allow system managers and medical directors to make informed decisions regarding EMS system expansion, provider training, vehicle base location, and the effect of out-of-hospital treatment on patient outcome.[13] Provision for ongoing, thorough EMS system evaluation and measurement of overall effectiveness should be the objective when determining needs. Care must be taken to work with all levels of providers in the EMS system when developing the reporting system. An effective, practical data collection process will be dictated in part by the structure of the EMS system. Basic information, necessary for the operation and evaluation of virtually every EMS system, is shown in the box at the top of the following page.

In addition, dispatch and transport decisions (such as, lights-and-siren used or normal traffic rules

Essential Items for Inclusion in Data Collection System

Emergency unit identifier	Patient gender
Crew identification	Vital signs
Date of incident	Glasgow Coma score
Time dispatched	Illness/Injury site
Time arrived at scene	Mechanism(s) of injury
Time departed scene	Basic Life Support procedures list
Incident location	Medications administered
Reason for dispatch	Outcome
Dispatch and transport code	
Receiving facility	
Patient name	
Patient age	

observed) should be included if not available from other sources. This information is critical to the implementation of dispatching protocols based on medical priority, a trend well advanced in leading EMS systems and destined to become standard of care.[2] An evaluation of the PCR currently used reveals how much of this information is already collected. Dispatching and government agencies must participate in the design process to ensure that items such as arrival and departure times and dispatch and transport information are available to personnel on responding units, as well as the system monitoring agency.

Once basic data elements for system operation and evaluation are incorporated into the report, specialized items can be added (see box above, right). These items allow medical control authorities to make decisions about transport frequency, medical appropriateness of dispatch, and public education on issues such as seat belt and helmet use. The local epidemiology of out-of-hospital cardiac arrest may be determined to promote citizen CPR campaigns, and different specialized data elements may be included in their reports. Input from provider agencies, the medical community, and system analysts is important for a complete system.

Planning

During PCR development, consideration should also be given to increasing the uniformity of data elements collected by different EMS agencies. This effort may be met with opposition by provider agencies because of their significantly different data requirements. Moreover, although the collection of common data elements by all EMS providers is desirable, the goal of a uniform reporting format used by all providers must not become a mindless exercise of authority. The purpose of data collection is improvement of medical care. Monitoring systems that only generate reports and are of no use to providers and physicians are a perverse misuse of scarce EMS resources.[16]

The lack of consensus regarding elements to include in a standard PCR presents a significant impediment to developing such a report (see box below). Proposed data elements should be discussed with participating EMS provider agencies, the medical community, and system planners and evaluators. Opposition to the inclusion of certain data must be thoroughly aired by all participants; the successful implementation of the project depends on agreement by all to the data points proposed for collection.

Suggested Items for Inclusion in Data Collection System

Type of unit responding and level of care provided at scene.
These data assist in evaluation of dispatching protocols.

Rationale for destination choice.
These data are used to evaluate prehospital triage and transport practices.

Residency status of patient.
These data are helpful in rural areas to demonstrate impact of interstate highways on local EMS needs.

A prehospital trauma severity scoring scale.
These data are useful for comprehensive trauma system planning.

Auto restraint and safety helmet use.
These data are used for public education programs in legislative initiatives.

Initiation of CPR by bystanders, witnessed versus unwitnessed cardiac arrest, and initial monitored cardiac rhythm.
These data allow medical directors to determine local EMS system performance in resuscitation of cardiac arrest and design interventions to increase survival.

Barriers to the Development and Implementation of a Uniform Reporting System

Lack of consensus on desired data elements
Business and political implications of collected data
Compliance monitoring
Public versus fee-for-service provider agencies
Quality control of data entry

Provider agencies, for competitive reasons, will be concerned with the collected data. Release of certain information can strain the working relationships among agencies in a community. Hospitals, other medical facilities, and physicians may harbor similar concerns. Before the system begins operation, good faith attempts must be made to achieve consensus regarding data analysis and access.

EMS systems, regardless of size, need a method to monitor compliance with the data collection system procedures. If the EMS data base is to reflect the actual status of the community, as many providers as possible must participate in the data collection. Thus an essential component of the call reporting services is designation of a monitoring agency.

Public safety agencies and for-profit EMS providers will have different needs regarding the type and method of data collection. Once these needs are identified, provisions can be made to accommodate each participating agency. This may require development of parallel data collection systems with different formats and methods of data entry. For example, when a statewide PCR was implemented in New York State, New York City EMS, with half the state's PCR's, was allowed to continue using its existing PCR and transmit the data elements tape-to-tape; however, the rest of the providers transmitted hard copy for keypunching.[9]

Quality control is a necessary component of any EMS data collection system.[13] Problems of poor quality control regarding entries on the report form result in the "garbage in–garbage out syndrome." Without adequate screening of report forms before data entry, inaccurate or incomplete data can be entered into the data base. Interpretations based on such data may be misleading or impossible. For example, attempts to use data from a variety of states as a needs assessment for the new EMT-B curriculum were unsuccessful.[1]

Once consensus has been reached on data elements and the entry format has been standardized, the program is ready for implementation. The considerations outlined thus far are important when creating a new data collection system or altering an existing one. Program implementation includes detailed instruction of agency personnel that use the form daily. These in-service programs can be handled by the individual provider agencies.

The physical method of data collection must also be determined during the needs assessment phase. To accomplish this one must examine the current or proposed EMS operation. What is the extent of EMS demand? Is the service area of low population density or in a rural setting? What level of prehospital medical care is contemplated in the jurisdiction? Will only EMT-Bs operate, only paramedics, or a combination? For example, an area with high acuity and high volume must consider data collection methods that provide receiving hospitals essential information concerning the prehospital care rendered and still allow the emergency unit to return to service as quickly as possible.

The resources available for maintenance of a data reporting system may dictate the method chosen. Are sufficient personnel available to manipulate the forms? Is a computer of adequate capacity available? The demand placed on a computer is determined by the call volume, the type and complexity of the report, and the sophistication of the software used for data analysis. The answers to the foregoing questions are the basis for PCR design and data storage method.

Data Entry

After identifying call volume, call type, and available resources, delineating essential data points, and listing specialty items developed, the medical director must decide on a data entry method. Presently, the following two alternatives exist: 1) optical scanning and 2) manual entry (Figure 15-1). There are advantages and disadvantages to each. To a large extent, resource availability and the degree of detail in the data to be collected determine which method is selected.

Optically Scanned

Optically scanned reports represent the easiest method of data entry.[1] Forms are marked by field personnel, forwarded to a central processing facility, and then fed into an optical scanner that "reads" the marks on the page. This method is less costly and more rapid in terms of labor than the manual alternative.[12] Current optical scanners can read forms completed in ink and pencil. This innovation has made such forms more acceptable to field personnel. In areas of low-to-moderate volume a part-time position would be needed to review and process the forms. In high-volume EMS systems or if the data base is used for formal scientific research, a full-time person would be required. Responsibilities of such a position include quality control, form processing, and report generation.

The optically scanned data entry method is limited to the number of data elements that may be collected in a one-or two-page report form. Because every possible response must be preselected and listed on the form, it is impossible to create a form containing great clinical detail unless one is willing

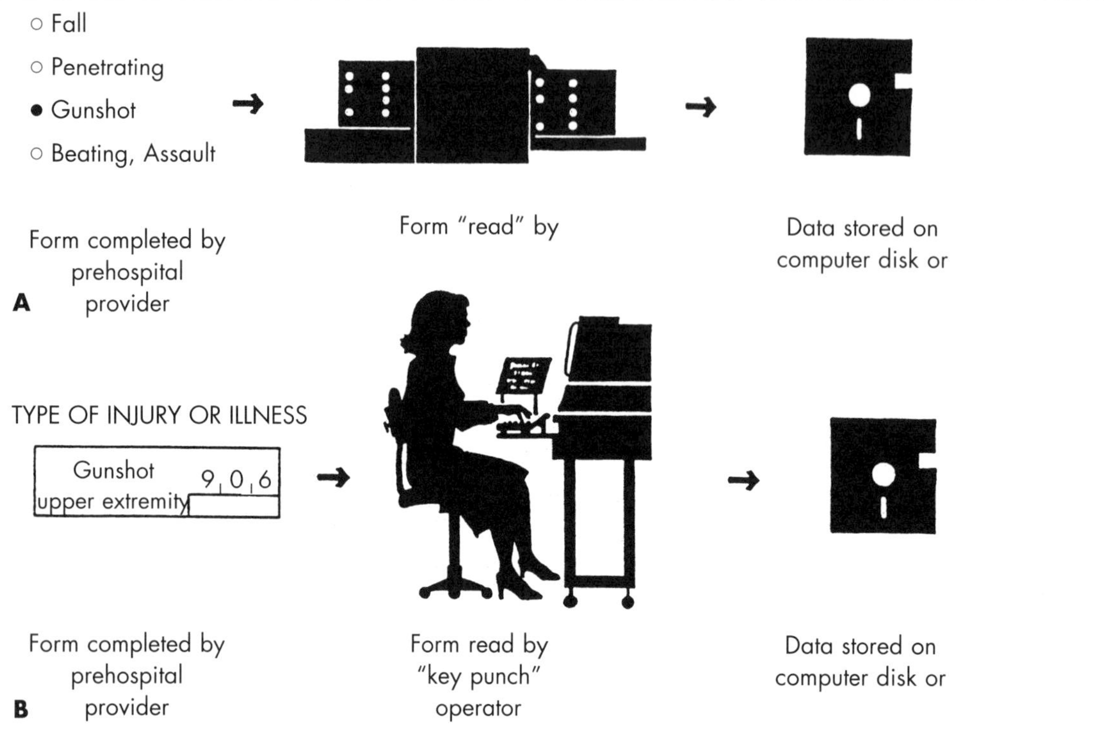

Figure 15-1. **A,** Data collection by optically scanned form. **B,** Data collection by manually processed form.

to contemplate a PCR of several pages. Also, optically scanned forms must be examined before processing for completeness, stray marks, and errors. Recently, software that can "kick out" incomplete or erroneous forms has been developed.[10] An optically scanned system is an excellent choice for low-volume EMS systems or individual EMS agencies to computerize basic data at reasonable costs.

Manual Entry

Manual data entry is an established technology that allows better quality control on the data entered in the system and more detailed descriptions of physiologic status, injury, illness, and mechanisms of injury. This enhanced flexibility results from coding systems based on ICD-9 classifications of illnesses and injuries.[14] Similar coding specificity and flexibility are possible for data elements such as unit identification and receiving facility designation. Because the data points are not preselected as in the optically scanned format and all choices are not listed on the PCR, more data can be assembled on a single page. Visual inspection at the time of data entry allows for identification of mistakes or incomplete entries; these PCRs may then be returned to providers for correction and completion. Manual data entry is a more expensive method, because more personnel resources must be invested. In addition to the "keypunch" personnel, responsibility must be assigned for review and completion of erroneous report forms. Unlike the optically scanned form, successful use of a keypunch form requires careful education of the EMS providers that use it daily. Instruction books containing data entry codes, must be developed and distributed to each prehospital provider completing the PCR.

Despite the significant costs, this type of reporting system works well in an environment that is familiar with tight quality control and willing to commit resources to meticulous system management. Some agencies already have uniform data-gathering systems; many fire departments use the Uniform Fire Incident Reporting System (UFIRS).[14] UFIRS is a data collection format for manual entry that employs a comprehensive coding system to describe fire and medical emergencies. When a system containing some of the basic necessary data elements is already in place, it is simple to create additional computer files containing expanded clinical data and then program the computer to link these together. Such a modification of the UFIRS has been used by the Tucson Fire Department for several years.[17] Departments already using the UFIRS format have committed the necessary resources to develop a state-of-the-art data collection system.

Implementation

Careful planning of a reporting system by EMS system managers and medical control physicians enhances the final implementation process. Plans should include provisions for program introduction to system managers and medical directors and a comprehensive training program for field personnel. Such a training program should include a historical perspective of the design process and complete guidelines for form completion. Obviously, field provider input throughout the process is helpful.

Summary

The final configuration of a PCR and data collection format is related to the structure of the EMS system for which it is intended. PCRs must be designed by managers in conjunction with potential system users. Above all, the collected data must be directly and easily accessible to EMS physicians and providers for rapid use in patient care and EMS system function.

REFERENCES

1. Bell JM et al: Computer management of prehospital information, 7:33-38, 1982.
2. Clawson JJ and Dernocouer KB: *Principles of emergency medical dispatch,* Englewood Cliffs, NJ, 1988, Prentice Hall.
3. Cobb LA, Alvarez H III, and Copass MK: A rapid response system for out-of-hospital cardiac emergencies, *Med Clin North Am* 60:283-290, 1976.
4. Commission on Professional and Hospital Activities: *The international classification of diseases,* ed 9, 3 vols, Oct, Ann Arbor, Mich, 1987, The Commission.
5. Cowley RA et al: An economical and proved helicopter program for transporting the emergency ill and injured patient in Maryland, *J Trauma* 13:1029-1038, 1973.
6. Cummins RO et al: Recommended guidelines for uniform reporting of data from out-of-hospital cardiac arrest: the Utstein style, *Ann Emerg Med* 20:861-874, 1991.
7. DHEW: *Program guidelines: emergency medical services systems,* Bull No (HSA) 75-2013, revised Feb 1975.
8. *Emergency Medical Services Act of 1973,* Public Law 93-154, Washington, DC, Nov 14 1973.
9. Gilbertson M, Stern A, and Elling R: Getting the facts: a progress report from New York State, *JEMS* 11:35-39, 1986.
10. Joyce SM and Brown DE: An optically scanned EMS reporting form and analysis system for statewide use: development and five years' experience, *Ann Emerg Med* 1991 (in press).
11. Joyce SM and Criss EA: Guidelines for development of EMS reporting forms: nationwide survey, *Ann Emerg Med* 16:508, 1987.
12. Joyce SM et al: Development of an optically-scanned EMS reporting form and database for statewide use, *Ann Emerg Med* 16:508, 1987.
13. Kresky B and Henry MC: Responsibilities for quality assurance in prehospital care, *QRB* 12:230-235, 1986.
14. National Fire Protection Association: *Uniform fire incident reporting system (UFIRS)* Boston, 1977, The Association.
15. Samuels D: *EMT-B curriculum panel,* WAEMSP National Meeting, Pittsburgh Pa, June 19, 1992.
16. Valenzuela, TD: Optically scanned ambulance report forms and uniform data collection, *Ann Emerg Med* 1991 (in press).
17. Valenzuela TD et al: Implementation of a computerized management information system in an urban fire department, *Ann Emerg Med* 18:573-578, 1989.

16

Evaluation

C. Gene Cayten, M.D.

The evaluation of EMS systems is a difficult but critical task of the medical director. Yet in many EMS agencies, evaluation is a low priority; it should not be. Evaluation is necessary to ascertain whether the system is fulfilling its goals. Without evaluation, expenditures cannot be objectively prioritized. To make the most of limited resources it is critical that evaluation efforts be sharply focused. Evaluation must provide periodic data relating to EMS operations and quality of care and data for future planning. This chapter discusses an EMS systems model, an overall evaluation model, a strategic evaluation model, and methodologic issues.

EMS Systems Model

More than many other aspects of medical care the handling of emergency cases depends on the harmonious coordination of community resources. Past neglect, however, has caused emergency care in many communities to rely on a fragmented assortment of transportation, communication, hospital, and physician services. Hospitals frequently have been concerned only with the operation of their own emergency departments. Ambulance organizations and police and fire departments have set up their own procedures for responding to requests for emergency assistance; little emphasis has been given to coordination among emergency transportation services and hospital emergency departments.[29]

Figure 16-1 illustrates the multiple aspects of an EMS care continuum. The phases of care include prevention, prehospital, hospital, and rehabilitation.

Evaluation of a system is only possible if the goals and objectives define the desired results. In defining the goals, the limits of the program are also defined. Program designers structuring the system must appropriately balance the resources available for each aspect of emergency health care. Furthermore, they must determine how resources should be organized and operated to coordinate the various system elements. This involves two key concepts, goal orientation and feedback loop. Goal orientation is a set of realistic, general goals for the system that must be agreed on and prioritized. The feedback loop ensures that as old goals are achieved new goals are set. As experience indicates needed modifications, goals and programs are changed appropriately.[7]

As illustrated in Figure 16-2 the general planning process involves the following activities[7]:

1. Evaluating program progress with consequent modification of goals and alternative approaches
2. Setting general goals
3. Describing the status of the system under consideration
4. Developing specific objectives consistent with the general goals
5. Devising alternate strategies for achieving objectives
6. Selecting alternatives and structuring the programs
7. Implementing the program

General goals for EMS systems often are set by political government agencies. EMS staff is then responsible for turning these broad objectives into specific programming actions. A systematic description of the system being planned is essential for the development of such actions. A description should include the current demand for services, the nature of services provided by the system, and the resources currently employed within the system and any constraints on their use. Together these data indicate where improvements are needed, and they provide a yardstick against which future progress

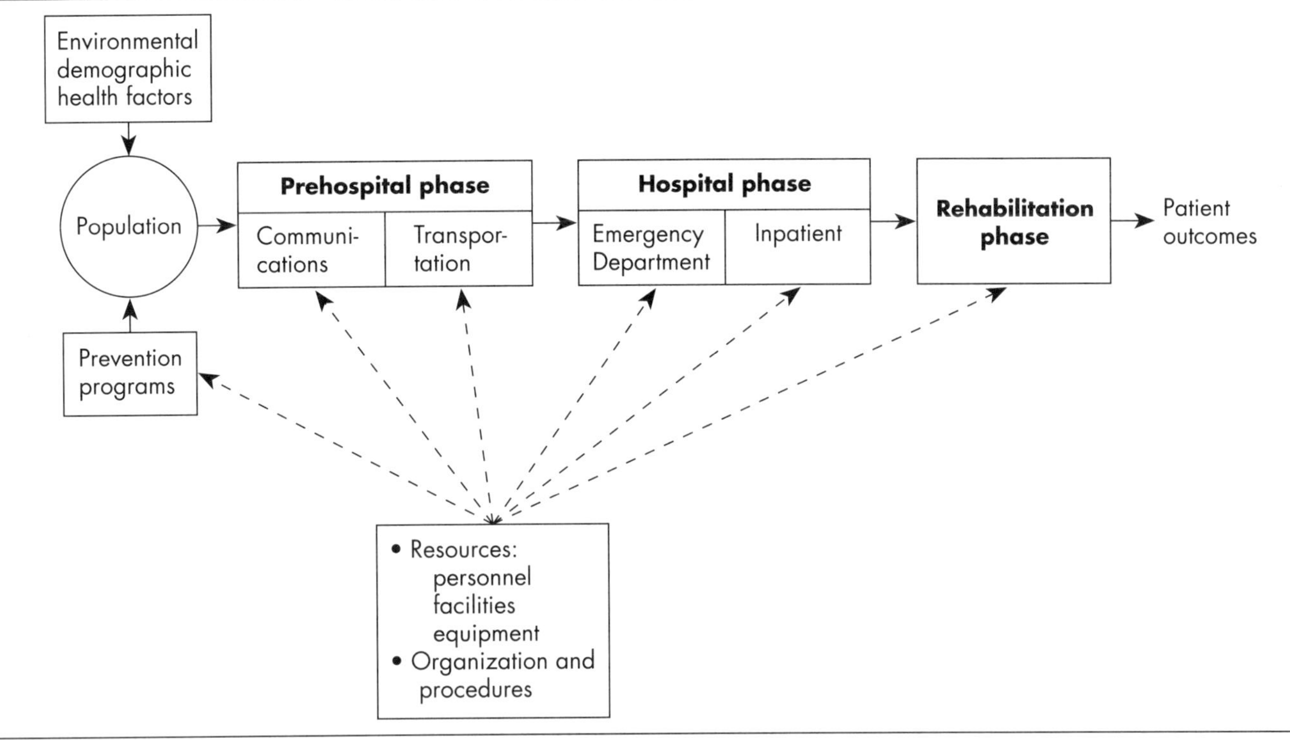

16-1. Aspects of EMS planning.

can be measured. A chronologic issue of actions taken on behalf of a typical emergency patient is also a valuable part of the system description.

Specific objectives are necessary for the planning and evaluation process to maintain continuity relative to indicators of system performance. Comparison of system structure and performance with available standards or EMS systems developed in other communities may aid in identifying inadequacies and further defining objectives. At this level, each objective should be stated in terms of the difference between the current value of the system performance measure and its desired value. Each objective should also include a target time for its achievement. For example, a specific 1-year objective might be to decrease to less than 5% the proportion of ambulance responses taking longer than 10 minutes.

Associated with each objective should be several viable courses of action that could be taken to satisfy the objective. These alternatives may be devised by local system managers and planning experts or they may be suggested from the experiences of other communities.

Having gathered data and set objectives, EMS personnel next select strategies and implement programs. Evaluation techniques for selecting among alterna-

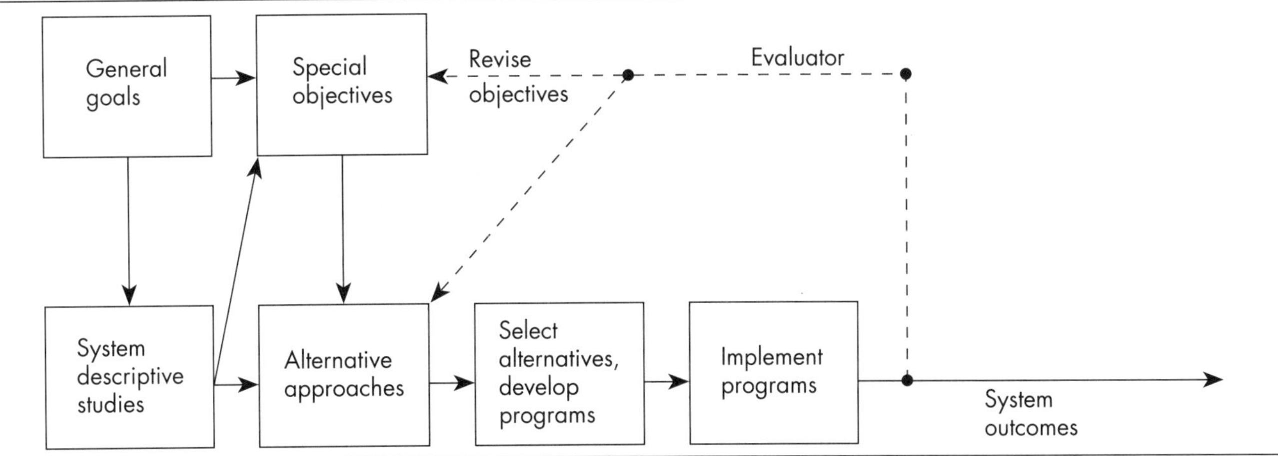

Figure 16-2. The EMS planning process.

tives differ with the type of decision being made. In some cases a simple cost analysis might be used. In others, sophisticated statistical and operations research methods such as queuing analysis, computer simulation, or optimization techniques might be required. When the needed resources or expected outcomes are difficult to quantify, subjective assessments by local experts or trained consultants using a consensus technique may be the basis for decisions.

In selecting particular approaches for accomplishing objectives, EMS managers should first specify the criteria alternatives will be compared with. Cost and the time period required before results will be observed usually must be considered, is another. Potential problems that may be encountered when implementing a prospective approach should also be addressed.

The final step in the process is ongoing evaluation. Such evaluation is a key aspect of system management and planning, but it also serves other significant functions. For example, information on system performance helps answer questions asked by public officials, the general public, and other agencies about EMS provided to the community. Evaluation also indicates where changes in the system structure or medical procedures are most needed.

Thus EMS system evaluation is considered broadly as covering an assessment of the total system, and quality improvement is considered more narrowly as process evaluation focusing on the performance of personnel in the EMS system. For example, if a community has a high percentage of cardiac patients that are not successfully resuscitated in the field, despite adequate numbers of well-trained paramedics compared with other communities, the EMS agency should compare response times as well. If not, the following planning options should be considered: 1) increase the number of paramedic squads, 2) develop an emergency medical technician-dispatcher (EMT-D) program, 3) train fire department personnel as First Responders and 4) develop a program of public cardiopulmonary resuscitation (CPR) training. In deciding on an alternative or combination of alternatives cost, implementation time, and special problems such as dealing with unions or specific agencies must be considered. Once the new program is defined and implemented, it must be monitored and evaluated to determine whether the prehospital cardiac resuscitation rate has improved. If not, the program may need to be modified or supplemented by others.

In summary, planning, management, and evaluation as described in the aforementioned steps are aspects of an ongoing process, not isolated or one-time activities. They are an integral part of system management and control, providing the objectives to be pursued by the system and feedback on the effectiveness of programs already undertaken.

Overall Evaluation Model

During the past 25 years many publications have been devoted to the development and implementation of evaluation models. In the field of medical care evaluation, Donabedian proposed a basic framework of structure, process, and outcome that has been effectively adapted to EMS system evaluations.[13]

Structure evaluation (or input evaluation) measures the credentials and level of personnel training, the adequacy of facilities and equipment, and the method of organizing resources in the EMS system. Gibson compiled an extensive list of structural criteria for EMS system evaluation.[15] Although system inputs may be measured easily and statistically, the validity of structural standards remains uncertain. Unfortunately, research has not demonstrated that fulfilling the input standards, that is, meeting all available standards for facilities, equipment, and personnel of a "model" EMS system, has any impact on patient health. In many cases input standards are considered "necessary but not sufficient" for achieving the optimal outcome.

Process evaluation assesses the performance elements of medical care. Process assessment techniques include analysis of the appropriateness of care, the patterns of care, case reviews using implicit or explicit criteria, and the data used for clinical decision-making. Currently, most process evaluation methods consist of record audits to establish compliance with protocols. Validity and reliability problems have been noted when explicit process criteria are employed in medical record audits. For example, the degree to which prehospital care reports (PCR) reflect the care provided is frequently questioned. Although research has indicated somewhat stronger correlations between process indicators and patient outcome measures, process-outcome relationships are considered weak for most medical conditions.

Because outcome measures are the most important indicators of overall system success, they should be incorporated in all system evaluation efforts.[7] However, patient outcome measures reflecting mortality and morbidity are insensitive to the individual phases of emergency care; thus other indicators must be employed as well. Also, ultimate-outcome measures are not sensitive measures of the early phases of emergency care. The further one moves toward measuring ultimate or long-term outcome, the less can be said regarding the quality of the initial emergency care.

To study the results of care, intermediate-outcome measures have a closer temporal relationship to the care being rendered, and are more relevant than long-term measures.[7,24] Figure 16-3 indicates where intermediate-outcome measures may be useful indicators of system status and effectiveness. For each phase of the EMS program, measures selected should reflect the specific objective pursued. For instance, to monitor the effectiveness of care provided at the scene intermediate-outcome measures (outcome III) might include the number or proportion of patients suffering cardiac arrest that is successfully resuscitated in the field. Prehospital trauma care could be assessed by change in trauma score (TS) or revised trauma score (RTS) from initial field status to initial emergency department status.[18] Potter et al used the intermediate-outcome measures of survival to ICU admission, and 24-hour survival and morbidity measures, and survival to discharge.[2]

Strategic Evaluation Model

Because any attempt to evaluate an entire EMS system on a day-to-day basis is a costly and time-consuming process, the medical director must focus evaluation efforts on several specific "tracer" medical conditions using structure, process, and outcome measures selectively. The following represents a possible approach:

1. Use intermediate-outcome measures (that is, choose a set of outcome measures that reflect care given at a selected phase along the EMS system continuum) (see Figure 16-3).
2. Use structural (or input) measures to supplement the intermediate-outcome measures.
3. Use process measures to supplement the intermediate-outcome measures.

As defined by Kessner and Kalk, a "tracer" condition should meet the following criteria: it should have a significant functional impact on those affected, be well-defined and easy to diagnose in field and practice settings, be sufficiently prevalent to permit the collection of adequate data, have a natural history that varies with use and effectiveness of medical care, have a well-defined medical management approach, and be well understood in terms of its socioeconomic affects.[19]

Although other medical conditions and outcome methods can be used, evaluation systems usually begin with cardiac and trauma tracers. Cardiac arrest and major trauma deaths often are used as tracers for medical care evaluation of an EMS system's outcome. For cardiac arrest, ventricular fibrillation survival to the hospital and survival until discharged are good measures of a system's impact because there are good comparative data available. Attempts to study prehospital cardiac-care outcomes have been limited because of a lack of consistency in the type of sample studied. The literature identifies the following four sampling strategies for prehospital cardiac-care evaluation: 1) patients with out-of-hos-

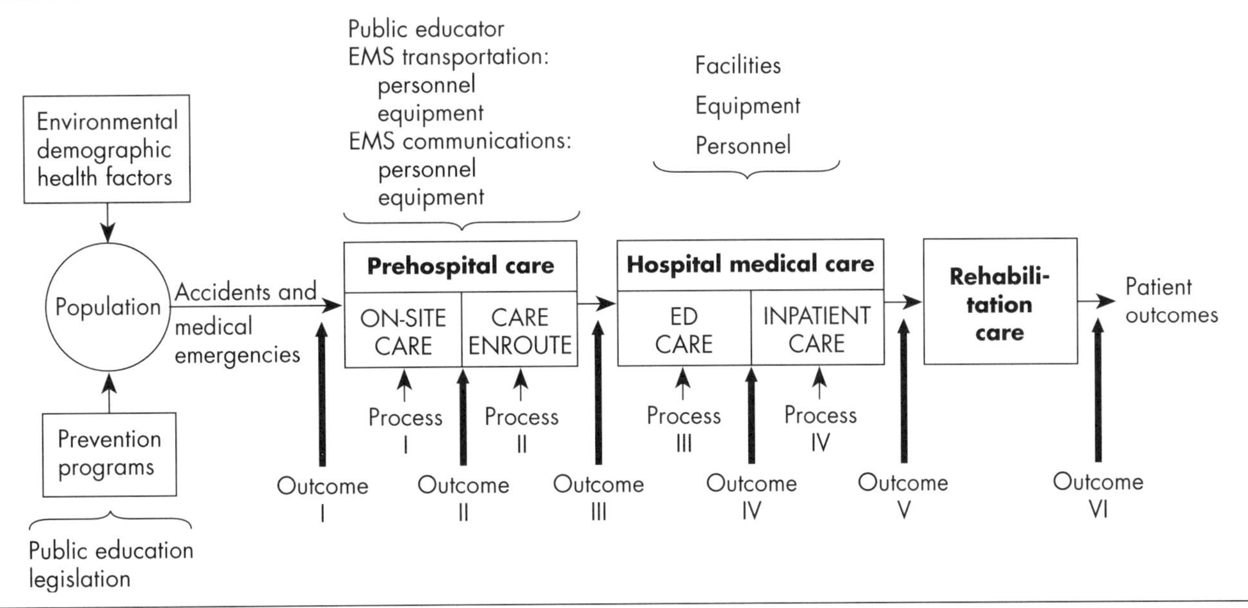

Figure 16-3. Aspects of EMS evaluation.

pital cardiac arrests, 2) patients with a final diagnosis of myocardial infarction in hospital discharge records, 3) patients with an emergency room diagnosis of rule out myocardial infarction, and 4) those identified by prehospital providers as suspected heart attack patients. Each of these samples has its own potential biases that must be considered when interpreting results. Hearne compiled a comprehensive analysis of cardiac arrest outcome studies including case definitions, methodologic characteristics, and summary outcome data.[16] Because of the great variation in definitions of outcome measures, Eisenburg et al proposed a uniform reporting system.[14]

For major trauma, actual survival is often compared with the probability of survival using the injury severity score (ISS) alone or in combination with the TS or RTS (that is, the TRISS method).[2] The American College of Surgeons Committee on Trauma's Major Trauma Outcome Study (MTOS) provides data for comparison purposes.[4]

To evaluate trauma care systematically trauma patient data must be collected on a regional basis. One such example is the organized approach described by Shackford et al for San Diego County.[26] It is a multidisciplinary, concurrent audit of the quality of medical care in a trauma system; a committee of physicians, nurses, and health officials representing trauma centers, nontrauma hospitals, the public agency administering the trauma system, and a computerized trauma registry are the primary tools. Prehospital cardiac arrest registries (for example, Seattle) have also been developed.[14]

Another approach to outcome assessment for trauma patients is a preventable death study, which can be done by an autopsy method using 500 consecutive deaths caused by motor vehicle accidents. Patients that died from central nervous system or prehospital cardiac arrest injuries are not included; they cannot be effectively studied by this method.[30,31] Each record is assessed by a group of surgeons and emergency physicians according to a set of criteria focused on whether death was preventable. Although this technique is relatively inexpensive, its reliability in different settings is questionable. The clinical method requires only 250 consecutive deaths from motor vehicle accidents obtained by reviewing death certificates.[6] In such a study prehospital, hospital, and medical examiner reports are used. Even though the team used criteria-based worksheets, the degree of subjectivity inherent in these judgments precludes comparing results among geographic areas.

If the proportion of observed deaths is higher than predicted by data from other sources, the medical director should focus evaluation efforts on a basic structural evaluation. Structural evaluations are relatively easy and inexpensive. For example, if the ventricular fibrillation survival rate is low, the evaluator should determine variables such as how many advanced life support units per 100,000 population the community provides relative to areas reporting better survival rates, the number of paramedics on each run, and the presence or absence of an accompanying basic life support (BLS) response.

Once readily available input standards have been used, attention should be turned to process evaluation. System process measures such as response time for trauma and cardiac cases and time from injury to operating room in penetrating abdominal cases are especially useful.[15,26] These simple measures should indicate the system's efficiency in dealing with critical patients. If any of these measures are grossly out of line with national standards or recommendations, action must be taken to improve them.

Assessing individual provider performance is an important part of the ongoing evaluation of prehospital care. Specific analysis formats should be designed for this purpose. Data coded for performance evaluation should also be used for system evaluation. Care must be taken to focus such ambulance run report analysis to complement the outcome and structural (input) components of the EMS system evaluation approach. Wading through reams of PCR cross-table analyses is an extremely time-consuming and costly approach to evaluation. If carefully planned, review of PCRs can identify areas of strength and weakness in an EMS system.[1] Considerable experience and data processing sophistication should be used in designing an EMS report form and analysis scheme.[23]

Methodological Issues

In EMS systems there are distinct methodologic issues that must be considered in any evaluation effort. These issues are severity indices, difficulties in developing process criteria, and the reliability and validity of the data.

Severity Indices

To perform acceptable medical outcome evaluation it is essential that the status of the ill or injured patient be adequately quantified and controlled. Unless control patients for case mix are provided, the results of outcome studies are difficult to interpret and impossible to reproduce.

Although numerous indices quantify the status of injured patients, indices for medical patients remain largely untested. Injury status indices have been designed for a number of purposes including triage, epidemiologic studies, clinical studies, and system studies. An index should be selected with care as many were not developed with the necessary methodologic rigor to ensure that valid interpretations can be made. Injury indices developed primarily along two lines, anatomic and physiologic. Presently the abbreviated injury score (AIS) and the ISS that derived from it are the most widely used anatomic severity scores.[28] The RTS is the most widely used physiologic severity score; the TRISS method, derived from the RTS, the ISS, and age, is gaining acceptance.[8]

Abbreviated Injury Score

The AIS was first published in 1971 to scale injuries caused by motor vehicle accidents.[11] It grades each of six anatomic regions on a scale of 1 through 5, with 1 considered minor and 5 considered fatal. The AIS was revised in 1976, 1980, 1985, and 1990; the revisions increased the specificity of the coding and assured that the AIS is useful in assessing patients with penetrating injuries.[10] Studies show that the AIS can be reliably abstracted, particularly by physicians and nurses. The average time required per medical record is 10 to 30 minutes depending on the complexity of the case and the clinical skills of the abstractor.[22]

The values and limitations of the AIS must be taken into consideration. Because it was initially designed for motor vehicle injuries, recent versions attempted to improve it for scaling penetrating injuries. The AIS is not a linear progression; the difference between an AIS 1 and 2 may not be the same as the difference between an AIS 4 and 5.[11] Also, a 3 in a given body area may not be the same as a 3 in another area, although an effort was made to make them roughly comparable. The AIS contains injury codes, and does not code the results of injuries such as blindness. The AIS cannot be determined directly from codes.[28] According to McKenzie only 67% of the International Classification of Disease (ICDA) codes can be translated directly into AIS codes. However, many of the noncompatible ICD-9 CM codes are infrequently used. McKenzie also found that intrarater abstracting reliability is higher for patients with blunt injuries than patients with penetrating injuries. An AIS cannot be reliably coded from emergency department records, as it requires the complete hospital record.[9] This is particularly true for patients with penetrating injuries. Because hospital record face sheets and computerized hospital data sets do not provide a comprehensive list of all injuries, conversion tables based on current versions of the AIS and ICD-9 CM should be used only for statistical analyses of large data sets looking at trends as areas for further investigation.[28]

Injury Severity Score

The ISS was developed by Baker et al based on the AIS.[25] The ISS combines the patient's injuries in a single score representing the overall severity of injury. The score is the sum of the squares of the highest AIS value in each of the three most severely injured regions of the body. If there is a score of 6 in any one body system, the maximum overall score of 75, indicating a fatal injury, is given. Injury severity scores range from 1 to 75. Bull et al and Stoner et al studied the validity of the ISS and found that it is correlated with such outcomes as length of hospital stay, time of death, disability, necessity for surgery, and plasma cortisol concentrations, but correlated less firmly with mortality and morbidity rates. By itself the ISS explains only 49% of the variance in mortality.[28] Also, a small error in AIS (for example, scoring a 4 instead of a 3) results in a large ISS difference because the AIS is squared.

Trauma Score

The TS is a physiologic index derived from the Champion and Sacco's Triangle Score, which was developed using logistic regression to determine the physiologic variables that best predict mortality.[27] It is not designed for small children. The TS is based on systolic blood pressure, respiratory rate, respiratory effort, capillary refill, and the Glasgow Coma Scale (GCS). The TS explains 73% of the variance in trauma mortality.[17]

The dates to calculate TS are frequently not available for retrospective studies. Many field providers do not routinely collect GCS scores or capillary refill.[20] The TS has a sensitivity rate of approximately 80%.[28] Thus 20% of patients with severe injuries will not be identifiable by the TS because they physiologically compensated or because response time is so fast that decompensation did not take place. The specificity rate for the TS is approximately 75%; it overestimates severity of injury when physiologic changes are related to factors other than hypovolemia, cerebral edema, or hypoxia.[28]

The RTS was developed from the 1986 MTOS analysis following insights gained from an audit of patients with "unexpected outcomes." It includes only the GCS, systolic blood pressure, and respiratory rate.

TRISS

The TRISS method combines the anatomic ISS, the physiologic TS, and age.[5] Age was added because the MTOS found that a patient age greater than 55 years significantly increased mortality. When ISS is used alone, the score would be identical for a patient with a gunshot wound to the abdomen who was brought promptly to the operating room and a patient who has spent many hours in the field bleeding into an irreversible shock state. On the other hand, patients with identical TS scores could have vastly different ISS scores, depending on the amount of time following the injury when the TS is measured and on the physiologic response of the patient. Using ISS, TS, age, and coefficient based on whether the injuries were blunt or penetrating, a probability of survival (PS) for a group of patients can be calculated and compared with a large date base such as the MTOS.[10,11] Such a comparison uses the Z statistic to relate the observed to the predicted survival rates in two populations. The M statistic assures that different ranges of trauma scores between the two populations does not distort the comparison. The M statistic comparison prevents the bias that results when a population with fewer injured patients and a high percentage of survival is compared with a population with more severely injured patients and a lower percentage of survival. Recently, the RTS replaced the TS in the TRISS method for developing outcome norms.[4]

Difficulties of Developing Process Criteria

Explicit criteria are specific, written criteria used to evaluate care, and implicit criteria are in the minds of evaluators when judging the quality of care. The use of explicit criteria is more objective and reliable. There are several different methods by which explicit process criteria can be developed. All methods attempt to achieve some degree of consensus either by reference to textbooks, expert panels, small group discussions, questionnaires to larger groups, or statistical summaries.[25]

It is often difficult to establish process criteria, particularly if they need to be detailed and specify the sequencing of treatments.[12] Once process criteria are established, they are usually employed in a checklist format to score prehospital, direct medical control, and emergency department forms. Generally, such criteria are used to screen for cases that should be reviewed in more depth. Few attempts have been made to weigh process criteria for EMS evaluation, though this has been attempted for other types of medical audit.

One of the most sophisticated approaches to the use of process criteria for EMS system evaluation has been developed by Wolfe.[32] The criteria are algorithms that are weighted and programmed allowing PCR data to be computer scored. The computer compares recommended treatment with the treatment actually recorded, and the appropriateness of each step is scored. Cases in which the treatment provided varies significantly from that specified by the algorithm are screened out by the computer for in-depth medical review. Although the criteria require that certain actions are taken within specified periods of time, the scoring system does not take into account sequences of actions when multiple actions are required during the same period of time. An in-depth discussion on using process criteria is in the chapter on quality management (see Chapter 21).

Reliability and Validity

The satisfactory quality of data used for evaluation should not be taken for granted. Both the reliability and validity of the data should be considered. Reliability is the extent to which measurement results are free from experimental error and are therefore reproducible. Reliability depends on the consistency of the characteristic being measured from individual to individual (homogeneity across individuals) and its stability over time. A measurement can be reliable without being valid. Reliability, however, establishes the upper boundary of validity because an unreliable scale cannot be a valid one. Validity is the extent to which the data are unbiased and relevant to the characteristic being measured. In this sense, data measurement should be free of systematic error caused by the measuring instrument itself, the user of the instrument, the subject, or the environment in which the scaling procedure is administered.

In terms of the overall design of evaluation efforts, Sherman et al presented a case study describing their evaluation of mobile intensive care units; 18 threats to the validity of the evaluation and methods used to control the threats were discussed.[27] These authors conclude that the major threats to validity are the effects of history, maturation, instrumentation, regression, and the potential interaction of selection and experimental unit composition. A list of these potential parameters and the methods to control them might be a useful guide to EMS evaluators in the planning stage. Through identifying and documenting potential threats to validity, the overall quality and credibility of EMS evaluations should improve.

There are two additional concerns. The first is the validity with which the care providers make the observations or measurements, and the second is the reliability of the data abstracting and recording processes. Cayten et al conducted a study assessing the validity of EMS data.[8] Emergency department nurses and EMT-As took simultaneous vital sign measurements with nurses who were specially trained and standardized against measuring devices. Tolerance limits were developed for the quantitative variables. Table 16-1 shows that emergency care personnel did better assessing qualitative variables than quantitative. Among quantitative variables, diastolic blood pressure was the least accurately assessed. Certain participants had a tendency to "err" in the sense that they disagreed with the standard on several of the variables.

In terms of research and evaluation this study indicates that users of basic clinical data must establish their level of validity before interpreting the results based on them. When it is essential that all the data are of high quality or critical medical decisions will be based on the data, multiple measurements may be necessary as well as an ongoing emphasis on carefully obtaining accurate data.

Hermann et al investigated the interobserver reliability in the collection of EMS data.[17] In this study, charts were selected from five hospitals to test the interobserver reliability of nurse abstractors. Different nurses reabstracted the charts. The results show that there is considerable variability in the accuracy with which the different variables were abstracted. Intraobserver abstracting reliability was consistently better than interobserver abstracting reliability. For the 26 variables studied, intraobserver values ranged from 0.62 to 0.99 with most falling above 0.80. This means vital signs had interobserver agreement of 0.95 or better; however, final diagnosis, emergency department diagnosis, condition on arrival, and elapsed time since onset had interobserver values of less than 0.60.[17]

Linn has similarly found that the accuracy with which data are abstracted from medical records leaves a great deal to be desired.[20] He found that when nurse clinicians abstracted medical record data using 33 data elements, there were discrepancies in 16% of the cases. In coding the patient's major diag-

Table 16-1. Vital Sign Observations within the Tolerance Limits

Variable	Group*	Observations within limits (No.)	Total observations (No.)	Proportion within tolerance limits
Systolic BP	ED Nurses[†]	66	80	.825
	EMT-As[‡]	91	115	.791
Pulse rate	ED Nurses	65	80	.813
	EMT-As	86	116	.741
Respiration rate	ED Nurses	56	80	.700
	EMT-As	84	116	.724
Diastolic BP	ED Nurses	51	80	.638
	EMT-As	61	114	.535

*Four observations per nurse of EMT-A.
†20 emergency department nurses.
‡20 EMTs.

Qualitative Variables: EMT Observations in Agreement with Standard

Variable	Observations with agreements (No.)	Total observations (No.)	Proportion with agreement
Age	116	116	1.00
Neck vein distention	114	116	.983
Pupil size equality	113	116	.974
Level of consciousness	112	116	.966
Pupil reactivity	112	116	.966
Pupil size	110	116	.948
Obesity	108	116	.931
Pulse character	104	116	.929
Respiration character	99	115	.861
Pulse regularity	98	116	.845

nosis there was a 46% discrepancy. Therefore, when system evaluation requires abstraction of data from records, periodic review of both intraobserver and interobserver reliability testing must be performed.

Summary

EMS system evaluation should be viewed as an ongoing process; the general goals of the system and each of its components provide a framework for planning, management, and evaluation. Initially the adequacy of the various components of the EMS system must be assessed. Objectives then give rise to alternative courses of action, and from these alternatives specific programs are selected for implementation. Thereafter, system and subsystem performance are monitored continually to evaluate effectiveness of programs and determine whether objectives have been achieved.

Evaluation is a key aspect of the EMS planning process. Its purposes are to indicate whether EMS systems are effective in diminishing death and reducing disability, and more important, they demonstrate where improvements are needed. Techniques for evaluating EMS systems include assessments of system structure, medical care process, and patient outcomes. System evaluation studies the results of system and subsystem function, regardless of specific programs designed for each area.

In EMS system evaluation the case mix must be precisely described and reliable. In addition, valid process criteria and outcome measures must be developed. In general, two techniques have been employed to define case mix, specifying tracer medical conditions by diagnostic codes and using severity indices. It is also essential to develop explicit criteria for assessing the quality of care when process evaluation is used. The limitations of severity scales must be fully understood.

Care must be taken to assure that the data used for EMS evaluation are valid and reliably collected. Specialized data collections for evaluation and research purposes alone are expensive and often do not provide sufficient sample size for statistical significance. Because in many situations EMS system evaluators will be interested in using data that are collected on an ongoing basis, it is essential for EMS medical directors to develop quality controls in the data collection process.

REFERENCES

1. American Association for Automotive Medicine: *The abbreviated injury scale,* 1985 revision, Arlington Heights, Ill, The Association.
2. American College of Surgeons Committee on Trauma: Quality assessment and assurance in trauma care, *Bull Am Coll Surgeons* 71:4-23, 1986.
3. Baker SP et al: The injury severity score: a method for describing patients with multiple injuries and evaluating emergency care, *J Trauma* 14:187-196, 1974.
4. Boyd CR, Tolson MA, and Copes WS: Evaluating trauma care: the TRISS method, *J Trauma* 27:370-378, 1987.
5. Bull JP: The injury severity score of road traffic casualties in relation to mortality, time of death, hospital treatment time and disability, *Accid Anal Prev* 7:249, 1978.
6. Cales R: Medical evaluation in trauma care systems, Rockville, Md, 1986, Aspen Publications.
7. Cayten CG and Evans WJ: *EMS systems evaluation.* In Boyd D, Edlich R, Mycik S, editors: Systems approach to emergency medical care, 1983, Appleton-Century-Crofts.
8. Cayten CG et al: Assessing the validity of EMS data, *J Am Coll Emerg Physicians* 7:390-396, 1978.
9. Champion HR: Major trauma outcome study: bulletin to participants, Feb 1986.
10. Champion HR, Frey CF, and Sacco WJ: Determination of national normative outcomes for trauma, *J Trauma* 24:651, 1984.
11. Champion HR, Sacco WJ, and Hung TK: Trauma severity scoring to predict mortality, *World J Surg* 7:4-11, 1983.
12. Cole L et al: Prehospital cardiac care: illusion of consensus, *J Am Coll Emerg Physicians* 6:552-555, 1977.
13. Donabedian A: *A guide to medical care administration,* vol 2, *Medical care appraisal-quality and utilization,* New York, 1969, American Public Health Association.
14. Eisenberg MS, Bergner L, and Hearne T: Out of hospital cardiac arrest: a review of major studies and a prospered uniform reporting system, *Am J Public Health* 70:236-240, 1980.
15. Gibson G: Guidelines for research and evaluation of emergency medical services, *Health Serv Res* 89:99, 1974.
16. Hearne: *The development of emergency medical services.* In Eisenberg MS, Bergner T, and Hallstrom AP, editors: *Sudden cardiac death in the community,* New York, 1984, Praeger Publishers.
17. Hermann N et al: Interobserver and intraobserver reliability in the collection of emergency medical services, data, *Health Serv Res* 15:127-143, 1980.
18. Jacobs LM et al: Prehospital advanced life support: benefits in trauma, *J Trauma* 24:8-13, 1984.
19. Kessner DM, Kalk CE, and Siner J: Assessing health quality: the case for tracers, *N Engl J Med* 288:1891-1894, 1973.
20. Linn BS: Effort of burn education on quality of emergency care, National Center for Health Services Research Management Series, 1975-1978.
21. MacKenzie EJ: Injury severity scales: overview and directions for future research, *Am J Emerg Med* 2:537-548, 1984.
22. Moreau M et al: Application of trauma score in the prehospital setting, *Ann Emerg Med* 14:1049-1054, 1985.
23. Petrucelli E, States JD, and Homes LN: The abbreviated injury scale: evaluation, usage and future adaptability, *Accid Anal Prev* 13:29-35, 1981.
24. Pozen M: Confirmation parameters for assessing prehospital care, final report, Hyattsville, Md, 1980, National Center for Health Services Research.
25. Romm FJ and Hulka BS: Developing criteria for quality of care assessment: effect of the delphi technique, *Health Serv Res* 14:309-312, 1979.
26. Shackford SR et al: The effect of regionalization upon the quality of trauma care as assessed by concurrent audit before and after institution of a trauma system: a preliminary report, *J Trauma* 26:812-820, 1986.
27. Sherman M et al: Threats to the validity of emergency medical services evaluation: a case study of mobile intensive care units. *Care* 17:127-138, 1979.

28. Stoner HB et al: Measuring the severity of injury, *BMJ* 2:1247-1249, 1977.
29. Thomas W and Cayten CG: *Emergency medical services planning and evaluation.* In Schwartz GR, editor: *Principles and practice of emergency medicine,* Philadelphia, 1986, WB Saunders Co.
30. West JG: An autopsy method of evaluating trauma care, *J Trauma* 21:32-34, 1981.
31. West JG: Validation of autopsy method for evaluating trauma care, *Arch Surg* 117:1033-1035, 1982.
32. Wolfe H: *Computerized model for EMS performance, PHS 80-3271, 1980,* Department of Health and Human Services.

17

Research

Donald M. Yealy, M.D., FACEP

Prehospital care experienced a "honeymoon" from the early 1970s until recently. Therapeutic interventions and system configurations were employed based on limited scientific data. Treatments usually were extrapolated directly from the hospital setting, even though the prehospital environment is markedly different. The honeymoon is now over, and EMS providers must prove what is beneficial. Additionally, academic prehospital care physicians interested in professional advancement must show the same ability to expand the knowledge base of their chosen field as more traditional medical academicians.

This chapter highlights the basic features and identifies the potential benefits and pitfalls of prehospital research. This chapter is not a cookbook for EMS research, nor does it obviate the need for accessing other sources on research design. The following section helps medical directors start or better supervise research and avoid certain traps.

Benefits of Prehospital Research

The first benefit of prehospital research is that data obtained can help improve the care of those treated in the future. In addition, the current quality of care is usually improved. This fact contrasts the perception that care is variable in a randomized research trial and some patients will have a worse outcome. Patients treated within a well-designed protocol generally receive high-level, homogeneous care. The knowledgeable investigator tries to control all outside influences and optimize ancillary treatments and actions to detect the effect of the study intervention. Data from inpatient research suggest that many patients in an experimental trial demonstrate greater subjective and objective improvement than those with similar diseases treated outside a study protocol.[10] These benefits may occur even when subjects are randomized to an intervention that eventually proves less effective. This result is due to a well-defined, consistent treatment plan (including ancillary treatments) coupled with vigilant monitoring for benefit or harm. To reap these advantages the investigator must carefully plan the trial so the study intervention and ancillary care are practical, medically sound, clearly defined, and monitored.

When a trial is well-designed, closely monitored, and successful in answering a question, others aside from current and future patients benefit. All involved gain insight in the pathophysiology of the problem studied. Additionally the authors and the system gain academic recognition. The field providers derive satisfaction from seeing "science in the field" impact care. The people within the system learn that medical practice is dynamic and gain better understanding about the natural evolution of care. Thus clinical skills, judgment, and *esprit de corp* are positively influenced.

Basic Research Design

Although cellular and animal experiments are common in biomedical research, EMS research largely focuses on the investigation of humans including both patients and providers. The interventions studied range from a drug or device to a more efficient method of managing resources.

Research trials can be performed using a variety of formats. The researcher and medical director must choose between less sophisticated but more "doable" designs and more detailed but difficult designs. The reader is referred to other works for a more nuts-and-bolts approach to research design and implementation.[2-4,9,10]

Research designs can be broadly divided into the following two categories: observational and experimental studies. In observational designs, events are monitored and analyzed without attempts to manipulate or alter the outcome. Traditional quality improvement (QI) often follows this format. For example, the administration of a specific drug by paramedics can be monitored and analyzed to discover the patterns that govern its use. Although this design is simple, it cannot define cause-and-effect relationships. Qualitative studies are a variant of observational designs in which events are analyzed without attempts to measure outcomes.

Experimental designs introduce an intervention and then monitor its effect on outcome. Most experimental designs in human research are *quasi-experiments.* The latter term reflects the lack of absolute control over all events and characteristics (termed variables) needed to create a true experiment.[2,3] Although animal and human trials seek to control all interventions and treatments, in practice this is impossible. Particularly in prehospital investigations, we may not recognize every factor that can influence outcome and therefore fail to control these factors. This lack of control can cloud or magnify any difference noted after treatment. True experiments occur only when all variables influencing outcome are identified and controlled. For convenience, we use the term *experiment* in this chapter to denote both true and quasi-experiments.

In general, observational studies are easier to perform than experimental studies; however, experimental studies afford the investigator an improved ability to define any cause-and-effect relationship. Prehospital research, especially disaster medicine, lends itself to observational studies because the events studied are sporadic, beyond control, and unpredictable. In these specific investigations, meticulous attention to obtaining data in a detailed and structured format produces information better able to define causality. Events that occur more frequently or predictably are studied better using an experimental design once the problem is well-defined.

The next factor in choosing a specific research design hinges on the length of time subjects will be studied. Cross-sectional designs measure all variables at one time; the traditional survey is an example of a cross-sectional design. The trials are easy to perform and provide data on the prevalence of an outcome or other measured variable in a population. However, cross-sectional designs cannot prove a cause-and-effect relationship between variables or events.

Longitudinal studies follow a group of subjects over time and can better determine a cause-and-effect relationship. This benefit is not without cost; longitudinal studies usually require more time and effort than cross-sectional designs. Longitudinal designs can be further categorized based on the timing of outcome measurement relative to patient identification and enrollment. Retrospective (or case-control) studies identify a specific outcome and then find what past actions or characteristics could account for the outcome. Prospective (or cohort) designs identify potential enrollees without the desired outcome and follow them over time to detect differences in outcomes or measured variables. For example, a retrospective study of cardiac arrest could identify survivors and then compare their treatments and characteristics with those of non-survivors. A prospective design could enroll patients in arrest and then observe or manipulate therapies and measure outcomes.

Although both types of longitudinal studies enhance the ability to define causal relationships compared with cross-sectional designs, well-designed prospective trials are less prone to biases and error than retrospective trials. The researcher can specify when and what interventions, measurements, and ancillary treatments are to be performed during a prospective trial. In the retrospective design the investigator is "at the mercy" of what was done and recorded. Again the benefits of a prospective trial are often at the cost of time, effort, and finances.

Because of these limitations, observational and cross-sectional designs are useful to generate and refine questions rather than solve problems. A retrospective study can further refine the question and provide preliminary data regarding the answer. When an event or outcome is rare (for example, survival from asystole), a retrospective design may be the most practical method of evaluating a problem. Prospective experimental designs are best used for mature research questions (that is, those questions well-refined by previous studies) pertaining to common or predictable events. Thus an investigator with a question in previously "uncharted waters" creates the basis for a series of works, beginning with cross-sectional and observational studies and culminating in a prospective experiment.

Two features can further limit the biases that creep into prospective experimental designs; randomization and blinding. Random enrollment of subjects is ideal to ensure that the characteristics of each group are similar at entry into a trial. Randomization does not obliterate all inequalities between groups in a comparative trial, but it does lessen the potential of this occurrence. *True randomization* means that each subject has an equal chance of being assigned to any of the treatment groups.

This is usually done with a text or computer-generated table of random numbers, although the time-honored "coin flip" is equally valid. Alternatives to true randomization including "every other" patterns (for example, every other patient, every other day or week) or assignment based on seemingly haphazard variables (for example, birthdate, social security number) ease the perceived logistic difficulties with in-field randomization. These alternatives should be used sparingly, because the benefits are slight and the protection from initial group inequalities are less than those provided by randomization.

Blinding refers to actions that prevent participants from knowing which specific intervention is being used during the trial. If only the study subject is unaware, the design is single-blinded. If the study subjects, care providers, and data collectors are unaware, the design is double-blinded. Blinding limits the natural biases the patient or care providers have about the utility of any interventions. Some interventions cannot be blinded, especially device applications (for example, PASG, airway products). Even when blinding appears simple the researcher must vigilantly ensure it occurs. Curiosity can spur patients and care providers to devise ingenious methods to unblind a trial. For example, a prehospital trial comparing outcomes in patients with electromechanical dissociation treated with dexamethasone or a saline placebo fell prey to this ingenuity.[12] Some of the field providers tasted the study solution before administering it; a salty taste identified the placebo thus unblinding the trial. The effect of this knowledge on the other events occurring during resuscitation is unclear; a potential bias existed that could not be resolved with posttrial data analysis.

Experimental designs often compare a new intervention to the current standard therapy; this is termed a *controlled* trial. A "no treatment" control also helps identify the natural course of events in the trial. In the absence of this the experimental effect may be overestimated. Both the experimental (new) and control (standard or absent) treatments may be amenable to blinding, especially in drug trials. Although intended to be pharmacologically inactive, placebos may produce a subjective and objective benefit. This fact justifies their use in trials involving nonlife-threatening diseases. When a scientifically proven standard of care exists, it should be used as the control agent in an experiment.[13,19]

A prospective, randomized controlled (PRC) experiment, particularly when coupled with blinding procedures, is best able to provide data to define a cause-and-effect relationship. These trials are the "gold standard" in biomedical research, but are not the most common design in current published *EMS* literature.[21] This is because of the prodigious effort and finances required to complete such trials.

Data Analysis

The basic goal of statistical analysis is to help organize and compare information from research trials. Descriptive statistics allow a large body of data to be summarized; this paints a picture of what happened during the observational or experimental period in a compact and organized form. Often a measurement of the central tendency (the average) such as the mean, median, or mode is helpful, as well as a measurement of the variability of the individual scores (the standard deviation and range).[9,11] When reporting on exclusive events such as survived or died, male or female, improved, worsened or no change, frequency tables and cumulative totals organize the results. Some data are easier to interpret if grouped in more meaningful sets such as percentiles or confidence intervals.[4,15]

Analytic statistics compare groups by determining whether a difference truly exists or can be excluded.[1,4,9,14] Because many trials intend to prove that a different outcome occurs after an intervention, the major goal of analytic evaluation is to provide a mathematic estimate of the probability that any observed difference could have been the result of chance alone. This estimate is communicated as the familiar p value. The p value answers for an investigator, "How likely is it that my data are fooling me and chance alone could account for any differences?" When a chance event is erroneously thought to be due to a treatment effect, a Type I (or alpha) error is committed. One can never eliminate the possibility of a Type I error, but before data are collected and analyzed the probability of error acceptable should be set. By convention, if p is less than or equal to 1 in 20, results are considered significant.

If no mathematic difference is seen between two or more groups, analytic statistics can define the Type II (or beta) error. A type II error occurs when a true treatment effect was not detected. This usually results from inadequate sample size or excessive variability among individual observations. Analogous to the p value is the power calculation, which estimates the likelihood that a difference could have been detected given the study population and variability. Thus it answers for us, "How hard did we look for a difference?" The power estimation is related to the Type II error and is equal to 1-beta. The conventionally acceptable Type II error is 1 in 5 (0.20) or less. This value correlates to a power of 0.80 or higher.

Contrary to popular belief, analytic testing does *not* evaluate the clinical importance of the observations.[1,14] Low p values and high power estimates do not mean more important observations, but merely estimate the mathematic likelihood of error. There are a multitude of analytic tests to compare data, and the choice is driven by the type of data collected and the specific comparison sought. The reader is referred to a more exhaustive work for further details.[2-4,9-11]

Pearls and Pitfalls in EMS Research

Well-designed prehospital research provides many benefits, but certain pitfalls must be avoided. Identifying these traps before and during a study creates research that improves patient care.

Ask a Question

The conclusions reached from a study depend on why the data were obtained. A common reason trials fail to get off the ground or are rejected for publication is the absence of a clear question. Without a question an answer cannot follow. Information from an unfocused investigation will produce data that are difficult to interpret.

The question asked should be important to the researcher and the field. Embarking on the project simply because it has "never been investigated" may waste resources.[5,6,9,10] Many problems that arise during data collection, analysis, and publication can be corrected, but an unimportant question is irreparable. Ask colleagues and other experts for advice before investing resources in an idea.

Although useful information may be gleaned from a trial intended to answer a question on an unrelated topic, this is the exception rather than the rule. Good research is focused; ask a specific question then design a trial that answers that question.[5,6,9,10] One helpful exercise is to write in one or two succinct sentences the questions that are important before starting any research endeavor. After generating a list, set priorities and focus the first trial on the most important question or questions. The question may be modified later, but starting with a clear focus improves the quality of the design and data collected. If a long list of questions is created, focus on the top two initially; the rest will serve as incentive for later trials.

Write a Hypothesis

Not only must a question be asked, it must be as specific as possible. In research jargon, a hypothesis is generated based on the question. The hypothesis is a declarative thought to be proven or disproven; the null hypothesis states that no difference will exist between two or more groups after treatment. The research (or alternated) hypothesis states that a difference or change will be seen between groups. The research hypothesis can be either directional (that is, states whether improvement or worsening in an outcome will be noted) or nondirectional (that is, does not indicate which therapy is better or worse). A study of adenosine use in the prehospital treatment of narrow complex tachycardia could test any one of the following hypotheses:

Null—Heart rate and blood pressure will be unaltered after treatment with adenosine.

Research (nondirectional)—Heart rate and blood pressure after adenosine therapy will differ from pretreatment values.

Research (directional)—Heart rate will be significantly lower and blood pressure higher after adenosine therapy compared with pretreatment values.

Each hypothesis differs slightly, although all are acceptable and overlap. Usually the null hypothesis is chosen in formal research design because comparative statistics reject or fail to reject this statement. The use of a null hypothesis is not mandatory; the key is choosing a clear, concise hypothesis.

Invest Time "Up Front"

After a specific research question is created, the current literature must be reviewed in at least two computerized searches followed by a manual review of the cited references. Sometimes the question will be answered and validated by previously published works, obviating the need for a trial. More commonly, information about unanticipated problems or useful methods to measure outcomes is discovered. Then the question can be refined or the design adjusted to avoid potential traps. The search may eliminate the need to "reinvent the wheel" during protocol development. When the search is complete, the investigator should be an expert on the topic.

Before a prospective trial is conducted, the available data should suggest that each treatment including a placebo has an equal chance of benefitting the subjects. Although final analysis may demonstrate that one treatment is better than another, knowledge of this before the trial obviates the need for an investigation. Usually, investigators believe one treatment will be more beneficial before designing a trial; however, this belief does not constitute scientific knowledge.

Decide What to Measure

Once the hypothesis is generated and refined the next step is deciding what measurements are needed. The characteristics and responses quantified are variables; these range from age, sex, weight, and height to blood pressure, survival rates, and neurologic function scores. Three types of variables are seen in research trials; often, events that are one type of variable in a particular design serve a different function in another design.

Dependent (or response) variables are measured to define the outcomes of a study and the effect portion (for example, blood pressure, peak flow rate, or survival after treatment) of any cause-and-effect relationship. Independent (or classification-treatment) variables defining the cause are factors brought into a study (for example, age, sex, weight) or imposed by the investigator (for example, dose of drug). Extraneous variables are also called noise or confounding variables; as the names suggest, these events or characteristics are beyond control or not recognized, yet still influence observations.

Bias is a distortion of any relationship between cause-and-effect; it occurs when extraneous variables alter results or when the dependent or independent variables are not properly controlled or measured. The investigator must anticipate all sources of bias and seek to reduce them. This is best done through careful thought and "bouncing" the idea around with colleagues.

Define the Population

Before enrolling subjects, the researcher must ask, "What is my target universe?" and "Do I have access to that or a similar group?" The target universe is all people who could be studied (for example, all patients with out-of-hospital arrest or all patients with severe pulmonary edema). Once they have defined the universe, investigators must determine if they have access to part of it; in practice, no one has access to the entire target universe. If a group that is similar to the target universe is accessible, a research trial is feasible. If only a dissimilar group or a very small number of subjects similar to the target universe are accessible, a study will not be meaningful.

Seek Help with Statistics

Before writing a protocol, an investigator who is unfamiliar with this area should seek the help of a statistician, especially in an experimental comparative trial. In addition to formulating a strategy for data tabulation and analysis, the statistician can determine the size of the study population needed. Sometimes, it is obvious that the question asked requires such large numbers of subjects that it cannot be done in a timely or economic fashion. This consult prevents the investigator from performing a study that cannot provide the information desired or worse provides misleading information. It also prevents unnecessarily enrolling too many subjects.

Before approaching the statistician, the investigator decides what measurements are the most important and how much difference between groups is clinically important. These two factors guide the sample size determination; often, investigators decide on these after the trial is complete based on the results of mathematic manipulations. The latter produces data with statistical significance but without clinical significance.

Create a Protocol

The key to protocol development is precise identification of the actions taken and information collected. It must be clear who is eligible for enrollment, what measurements are to be made by whom, and what interventions will occur. Measurements as simple as weight (estimated, in metric or English units) and blood pressure (palpated, auscultated, by whom and with what technique) are a source of confusion and error if not specifically defined.

Unless similar trials have been completed previously, research protocols require multiple drafts to refine. These drafts are circulated among colleagues and local or national experts to improve the quality of data collected. It is wise to involve those responsible for data collection and subject treatment at this point. The actual providers are often ignored in this stage of research. Often a "street smart" prehospital provider provides practical tips to streamline the protocol.[20]

Whenever economically feasible and practical, those collecting data should not be responsible for providing clinical care. Having a research assistant with medical knowledge ride along to ensure protocol adherence improves the quality of the data collected. This approach, although costly, reduces the perception of "extra work" by the field providers. Often, students, off duty medics, or others perform this task on a voluntary or stipend arrangement.

Regardless of who treats subjects and collects data, each action should be as simple as possible. It is tempting to collect mountains of data. Although data uncollected are lost forever, there is a diminishing return to recording more information in the field. Clinical experience suggests that the accuracy of data collection is inversely proportional to the complexity and number of data points. Use the specific hypothesis as a reference point—actions interfering with attaining an answer should be eliminated.

The ideal data form is simple and differs from the prehospital care report (PCR). Organizing the study form so information is recorded at the time of each intervention or measurement and using a "checklist" or electronic bar coding system whenever possible, improves the quality and consistency of the information. A cumbersome form that requires redundant information or lengthy prose produces inconsistent data that are often incomplete and hard to interpret.

When planning a trial, the researcher must outline other specific steps in the protocol. The handling of any experimental drug or device must be defined and criteria to terminate treatment must be specified. If blinding procedures are used, the indications and methods for unblinding must be clear and practical. These steps ensure that the clinical care of each patient can be tailored if a problem arises. Finally the data accumulated are analyzed at defined intervals by individuals not directly involved with patient enrollment. This identifies any inappropriate enrollment of subjects or unexpected harm. If compelling, these preliminary data may require the trial to be modified or terminated.

Get IRB Approval

Institutional review boards (IRBs) evaluate research protocols to ensure that the cost-benefit ratio is acceptable and patient autonomy and safety are maintained. IRBs are based on federal guidelines that mandate inclusion of lay and professional members. Any institution can create an IRB by contacting the Department of Health and Human Services (DHHS) for guidance and approval. Most IRBs are university-or hospital-based, although pharmaceutical companies and other research-oriented organizations also develop IRBs.

Until recently, most published EMS research trials did not receive the same IRB evaluation required of in-hospital trials.[21] EMS research is not exempt from this process, but identifying the appropriate IRB can be problematic. Non-hospital affiliated providers or those affiliated with multiple hospitals often scramble to access established IRBs. Usually the institution most closely related to the EMS system or the principal investigator reviews the proposal. In certain circumstances a separate IRB is created to serve the needs of prehospital researchers unable to access more traditional, established boards. The latter approach is time consuming, labor intensive, and associated with certain administrative costs and therefore is best reserved for organizations performing research frequently.

Not all trials must have IRB approval; EMS researchers should consult their local IRB or review the published DHHS guidelines for the exemption criteria. Any EMS study that requires approval when done in the hospital should be submitted to an IRB. Additionally, most prospective human trials should be reviewed, particularly if any interventions are planned. Often an abridged review is possible for low-risk protocols.

Once an IRB chooses to review a proposal, the investigator may encounter difficulties. Prehospital care is foreign to hospital-based physicians and nurses or laypersons. Researchers should educate members about EMS. This may be done through the protocol, cover letter, or personal contact if permitted. In the absence of this, gaining approval is slow and difficult. The wise investigator approaches the IRB's concerns as opportunities to improve the protocol or educate the members. Treating the IRB as a barrier to overcome impedes progress and approval.

Time can be an ally in gaining IRB approval. The first proposals submitted to an IRB unfamiliar with EMS are often closely scrutinized. As more high quality protocols are submitted, members of the IRB become familiar with and accepting of prehospital research. Another mechanism that aids the process is becoming involved. Physicians can volunteer to serve on the IRB and become an educator "from within"; in the author's experience, this is the most useful way to ease the process over time.

Obtain Informed Consent in Field Research

Obtaining and documenting informed consent for prehospital research presents special challenges.[22] By definition, informed consent is voluntarily obtained from a competent patient who is aware of the alternatives, risks, and benefits. This process ensures that the patient maintains autonomy and control throughout the study. The tradition of reading and signing a document that outlines the trial design and patient rights is cumbersome in the field, and the physician investigator is rarely present at the time of enrollment. As a solution, consent can be gained by proxy through field providers or by distant contact such as over a radio or telephone. This consent is obtained after a brief oral description of the design, and it is documented by initialing a smaller document or recording radio or telephone communications. In certain groups of patients known to frequently access the EMS system (for example, asthma, sickle cell disease), consent is obtained before any acute exacerbations; this is termed *prospective consent.*

The DHHS allows an IRB to waive the requirement for informed consent in selected designs. This can be done only if the following four conditions are met:

1. The research could not be practicably carried out without the waiver.
2. When appropriate, subjects are provided with additional pertinent information after participation.
3. The research involves no more than minimal risk.
4. The waiver does not adversely affect the rights and welfare of the subjects.

Failure to meet and document any of the conditions removes the potential waiver of consent. Of these conditions the issue of research risk is the most vexing in prehospital research. Although many prehospital trials study diseases with poor outcomes (for example, cardiac arrest), the true risk is based on the relative difference in outcome expected between the standard and the experimental interventions. Thus the differential risk must be minimal to satisfy this criterion.

The Food and Drug Administration also has four criteria that must be met to waive consent when studying a new or unapproved drug.

1. The subject is confronted by a life-threatening situation requiring the drug.
2. Informed consent cannot be obtained because of impaired communication or inability to obtain legally effective consent.
3. Time does not permit obtaining consent from the subject's legal representative.
4. There is no other reliable alternative therapy that provides an equal or greater likelihood of saving the patient's life.

Different than the DHHS guidelines, these criteria deal with drug use in life-threatening diseases. The fourth condition poses the greatest difficulty when studying field interventions. However, if no data support the clear utility of one treatment over another (for example, standard versus high-dose epinephrine), this criterion is met. As noted earlier, suspicion of a benefit is not proof.

Alternatives to obtaining formal consent in all subjects or waiving consent have been developed. Stepped and deferred consent allow enrollment of subjects with little or no initial information. Later, full disclosure and options for withdrawal are presented to the subject or representative. This approach is used in resuscitation research and other trials where the effectiveness of an intervention is highly time dependent. Some ethicists argue that this is not truly informed consent and offers little advantage to waivers. Another alternative is surrogate consent, which is usually obtained from a panel of laypersons. Again, although this provides safeguards with respect to the safety of the subjects as a group, it does not facilitate individual patient autonomy.

When faced with consent issues in prehospital research contact the IRB and other local and national experts. No one rule solves all problems, and the EMS physician should expect some ambiguity and negotiating. The entire process involves balancing the needs of the individual and society, a task formidable for seasoned ethicists as well as the investigator.

Interact with the Providers

Before and during a field trial, all personnel should be educated about the goals.[20] Emphasizing the importance of each EMS provider's role and the practical and scientific benefits increases enthusiasm for the project. This is done through continuing education or mandatory conferences with the field teams. Although large meetings make the task easier for investigators, it is best to follow them with smaller group sessions to further educate the teams. The use of other adult education techniques such as videotape or public service television stations also helps.

Questions and potential problems should be solicited from the field teams. If the investigator does not seek these, the problems and concerns can undermine the field teams' confidence in the trial. This negatively impacts enrollment and data collection, and fosters a feeling of distance from the investigator.[20]

For example, in a randomized controlled experiment the field providers must administer a specific treatment based in part on a factor outside their control (the randomization table or a coin flip). If blinded, the provider does not know which therapy is used at the time of treatment. Specific measurements must be taken at set intervals even if inconvenient. These actions are a source of confusion and concern for the provider accustomed to treating each patient individually. Also troublesome to field personnel is the possibility that one group of patients receives inferior or less optimal treatment (although a harmful treatment is never investigated). These conflicts are mitigated by close attention to proper design and implementation and communication of the scientific benefits of the PRC-blinded design.

Use Pilot Trials

Often a smaller group of subjects is studied initially to detect any problems with the protocol. This is particularly true when studying an area new to the investigator or the EMS system. These pilot trials may not produce "usable" data, especially if significant changes are required based on the initial evaluation. Thus the focus of the pilot phase differs from the actual trial; problem identification and resolution assume more important roles. If minimal or no changes are needed, pilot data are incorporated with those of the actual trial.

Keep the Ball Rolling

The major reason a field trial hits obstacles such as missed enrollment or protocol nonadherence is that the field teams lose faith or enthusiasm in the usefulness of the trial. As they did in the preparatory phases, investigators must continually seek input from field providers and answer any concerns raised during the trial. Scheduled frequent meetings with the supervisors and field providers identify concerns or problems before they mushroom.[20] Without this contact, research is often perceived as increased work with no benefit. A recent trial of nebulized albuterol for the field treatment of wheezing suffered from this problem.[7] The investigators planned to collect objective data concerning the severity of symptoms before and after treatment, using a miniature computerized pulmonary function testing device. The field teams were educated about the importance of these data before the trial started. When the trial was complete, compliance with the protocol was found to be poor. The field teams felt that the pulmonary testing did not influence decisions of the command physicians and the data were unimportant. As a result the study failed to answer the intended question.

The inclusion of one or more field providers in the design and implementation of a trial builds support from within the system. These colleagues aid the principal investigator in "keeping the ball rolling" after data collection begins, especially if any difficulties arise. Studies without this involvement may have problems with perceived or real shortcomings in the protocol identified by the field providers. The medical director and researcher should be sure that the field teams and system are always recognized during professional and lay dissemination of the study intent or results. This again fosters a "team approach."

Pitfalls in Interpreting Data

Observational, cross-sectional, and retrospective designs uncover shortcomings in patient care and resource allocation and identify areas for prospective research. These designs do not interfere with clinical care; thus the diligence of the investigator is the major stumbling block in completing the trial. In addition to the cause-and-effect shortcomings outlined previously, these designs face challenges based on the validity of the data recorded and conclusions reached.

Internal validity refers to the truth within a study. Simply put, *internal validity* means investigators measured what they thought they were measuring. For example, if using a change in the Glasgow Coma Score (GCS) to assess the effect of a treatment in trauma care, it should be calculated by the same observer or observers with similar training. Comparing GCS at the scene (estimated from the prehospital record or calculated by the field provider) with those judged by an attending emergency department physician is invalid; any change may be the result of a treatment effect, different observers, charting anomalies, or a combination. Problems with internal validity are best sought and addressed before data collection.

External validity refers to the ability to generalize results and conclusions from a study population to other systems or geographic areas. Some data are system specific, and others reflect features shared by many systems. Quality management projects crafted into research trials after the fact are prone to problems of limited external validity. For example, poor outcome in out-of-hospital cardiac arrest may reflect problems within that system alone (such as faulty defibrillators, long response times, a skewed population). Although this information is a useful quality tool within the system, it has a limited external validity. There are no rules to determine the external validity of collected data and conclusions; the investigator merely asks before and after the trial, "What do my observations mean to others?"

Finally, data from all patients enrolled in a trial are analyzed. This analysis is based on "an intention to treat," and it uncovers benefits or harm that might have been missed if only those who completed the protocol were examined. For example, a trial investigating the effect of inhaled nitrous oxide/oxygen for pain that analyzes only those who completed a minimum 5-minute course of treatment may overlook side effects experienced by those who refused further participation after 1 to 2 minutes.

What to Do with Research Data

Not all investigations deserve to be published, and the choice of where to publish or present is perplexing. If the data collected have limited external validity or utility, they should not be submitted just "to get something published." Editors and reviewers are knowledgeable, and it is not often that this process results in publication. In these cases the information is used for individual system refinement.

Sometimes, data obtained from a quality management investigation is useful to others, and therefore submitted for publication.[15,16] These trials along with well-designed prehospital experiments or observational studies should be matched to the right audience. Not all EMS research needs to appear in the *New England Journal of Medicine, JAMA, Annals of Emergency Medicine,* or *Prehospital and Disaster Medicine.* Each journal or meeting focuses on different audiences and themes; the author should ask "Who do I want to impact and how do I access that group best?" This guides the choice of venue both written and oral. For example, dispatch-related studies are better suited to EMS administrators and medical directors; the audience reading a general medical journal may not include these key people. Conversely a breakthrough intervention that dramatically affects a disease encountered by a broad group of providers (for example, cardiac arrest or trauma) is better presented in a meeting or journal that attracts a wide audience.

Summary

Prehospital research is rewarding for the investigator, field teams, system, and patients. The choice of a specific design is based on the question asked and resources available. By investing time during the preparatory phases and preventing common pitfalls in design and implementation, data collection and analysis are eased. Finally, the people involved in the daily aspects of a field trial—the care providers and supervisors—must be included in the process.

REFERENCES

1. Browner WS and Newman TB: Are all significant p values created equal? *JAMA* 257:2459-2463, 1987.
2. Campbell DT and Stanley JC: *Experimental and quasi-experimental designs for research,* Boston, 1963, Houghton Mifflin Co.
3. Cook TD and Campbell DT: *Quasi-experimentation: design and analysis issues for field settings,* Boston, 1979, Houghton Mifflin Co.
4. Elston RC and Johnson WD: *Essentials of biostatistics,* Philadelphia, 1987, FA Davis Co.
5. Gibson G: Emergency medical services: the research gaps, *Health Serv Res* 9:6-21, 1974.
6. Gibson G: EMS evaluation: criteria for standards and research designs, *Health Serv Res* 11:105-111, 1976.
7. Heller MB et al: Data collection by paramedics for prehospital research, *Ann Emerg Med* 17:414-415, 1988.
8. Holyrod B, Knopp R, and Kallsen G: Medical control, quality assurance in prehospital care, *JAMA* 256:1027-1031, 1985.
9. Hulley SB and Cummings SR, editors: *Designing clinical research,* Baltimore, 1988, Williams & Wilkins.
10. Iber FL, Riley WA, and Murray PJ: *Conducting clinical trials,* New York, 1987, Plenum Publishing Corp.
11. Menegazzi JJ and Yealy DM: Method of data analysis in the emergency medicine literature, *Am J Emerg Med* 9:225-227, 1991.
12. Paris PM, Stewart RD, and Deggler F: Prehospital use of dexamethasone in pulseless idioventricular rhythm, *Ann Emerg Med* 13:1008-1010, 1984.
13. Pasternak SJ and Paris PM: *Placebo therapy.* In Paris PM, Stewart RD editors: *Pain management in emergency medicine,* Norwalk, Conn, 1988, Appleton & Lange.
14. Riegelman R: The importance of significance and the significance of importance, *Postgrad Med* 66:119-124, 1979.
15. Simon R: Confidence intervals for reporting results of clinical trials, *Ann Intern Med* 105:429-435, 1986.
16. Spaite DW et al: A prospective evaluation of prehospital patient assessment by direct in-field observation: failure of ALS personnel to measure vital signs, *Prehosp Disast Med* 5:325-334, 1990.
17. Swor RA and Hoelzer MH: A computer-assisted quality assurance audit in a multi-provider EMS system, *Ann Emerg Med* 19:286-290, 1990.
18. Swor RA, Bocka JJ, and Maio RF: A paramedic peer-review quality assurance audit, *Prehosp Disast Med* 6:321-326, 1991.
19. The Coronary Drug Project Research Group: Influence on adherence to treatment and response of cholesterol on mortality in the coronary drug project, *N Engl J Med* 303:1038-1041, 1980.
20. Warnke WJ and Bonnin MJ: Direction and motivation of prehospital personnel to do research: how to do it better, *Prehosp Disast Med* 7:79-83, 1992.
21. Yealy DM and Scruggs KS: Study design and pre-trial peer review in EMS research, *Prehosp and Disaster Med* 5:113-118, 1990.
22. Yealy DM, Scruggs KS, and Weiss LD: Informed consent in prehospital research, *Am J Emerg Med* 5:560, 1989.

Section Two

Medical Oversight Elements

Section Two focuses specifically on medical oversight, which is the most important and historically the most commonly neglected EMS component. The initial chapter summarizes the historical and philosophic development of medical oversight and then describes several approaches.

The second chapter addresses indirect (off-line) medical control, which is that portion of medical oversight traditionally assigned to the administrative system physician or project medical director. Although indirect medical control often includes the overall design and implementation of an organizational framework, other significant aspects such as teaching and improving quality, both of which are often performed by delegated physicians, are emphasized.

The third chapter of Section Two examines the structure and operations of direct (on-line) medical control, which is delivered concurrent with the provision of prehospital patient care. The concept of direct medical control has expanded beyond providing simple radio and telemetric direction to include actual physician involvement in patient care at the scene; however, the ultimate responsibility for direct medical control remains with the system medical director. The provision of direct medical control is only one of many responsibilities of the physician charged with EMS medical oversight.

Although quality management and risk management are often considered subsets of indirect medical control, these two elements have grown in importance as EMS has matured; therefore they are subjects of separate chapters that stress the critical need to close information and evaluation loops. The education and empowerment chapters expand the scope of awareness into critical areas where most physicians have little formal experience and, unfortunately, less interest.

In sum, the medical oversight of prehospital and disaster medicine continues to evolve; in many jurisdictions medical oversight remains somewhat confused. What follows is a 1987 policy statement from the New York State Department of Health that attempts an explanation of "medical control." Although other states have more specific and formal definitions, this particular one captures the flavor of the political, philosophical, and medical evolution of the unique practice of prehospital medicine. Read it carefully, and then compare this 1987 policy with the subsequent 1991 EMS amendments to the New York State Public Health Law concerning medical oversight.

New York State Health Department Policy Statement (1987)

What is Medical Control?

Medical control is the physician-provided medical responsibility for emergency medical services.

All aspects of the organization and provision of emergency medical services (EMS), including both basic and advanced life support, require the active involvement and participation. To optimize medical control of all prehospital emergency medical services, these services should be managed by physicians who meet the following requirements:

1. Familiarity with the design and operation of prehospital EMS systems;
2. Experience in prehospital emergency care of the acutely ill or injured patient;
3. Routine participation in base-station radio control of prehospital emergency units;
4. Experience in emergency department management of the acutely ill or injured patient;
5. Routine active participation in emergency department management of the acutely ill or injured patient;
6. Active involvement in the training of basic and advanced life support prehospital personnel;
7. Active involvement in the medical audit, review and critique of basic life support and advanced life support prehospital; and
8. Participation in the administration and legislative process affecting the regional and/or state prehospital EMS system.

Medical control should be implemented by a statewide emergency medical services medical control board comprised of physician representatives from each emergency medical services region, appointed by the commissioner of health. The board shall advise the commissioner on:

1. Statewide minimum standards for medical control;
2. Treatment and triage protocols including invasive procedures;
3. Hospital categorization and specialty center designation;
4. Use by emergency medical technicians of regulated medical devices and drugs;
5. Quality review of prehospital and interhospital care; and
6. Matters relative to the training of emergency medical technicians relative to standards of patient care.

There should also be local and regional emergency medical services medical control boards responsible for the provision of medical control within their respective areas. These boards should be structured to include the medical directors or their physicians' designees from each of the hospital emergency departments and services in the area covered by the board, as well as such other physicians whose participation may be of value. The structure of the local and regional emergency medical services medical control boards should be approved by the statewide emergency medical control board.

It is the recommendation of the state emergency medical services council that the issue of medical control is not that of its physical location but that of its provision by properly qualified physicians as described above, operating within the guidelines outlined.

The New York Public Health Law (1991) Emergency Medical Services

Sec.3001.Definitions

11. "Advanced life support" means definitive acute medical care provided, under medical control, by advanced emergency medical technicians within an advanced life support system.
12. "Advanced life support system" means an organized acute medical care system to provide advanced life support care on site or en route to and from, or between general hospitals or other health care facilities.
13. "Medical control" means advice and direction provided by a physician or under the direction of a physician to certified First Responders, emergency medical technicians or advanced emergency medical technicians who are providing medical care at the scene of an emergency or en route to a health care facility. Medical control shall also include the written policies, procedures, and protocols for prehospital emergency medical care and transportation developed by the state emergency medical advisory committee, approved by the state emergency medical services council and the commissioner, and implemented by regional medical advisory committees.

Sec.3002-a. New York State Emergency Medical Services Council

1. There shall be a state emergency medical advisory committee of the state emergency medical services council of twenty-nine members.
2. The committee shall develop and recommend to the state council statewide minimum standards for: (a) medical control; (b) treatment, transportation and triage protocols, including protocols for invasive procedures and infection control; and (c) the use of regulated medical devices and drugs by emergency medical services personnel certified pursuant to this article. The state emergency medical advisory committee, with the consent of the commissioner, may issue advisory guidelines in any of these areas, which shall not have the force and effect of law unless adopted as rules and reg-

ulations by the state emergency medical services council. The state emergency medical advisory committee shall advise the state emergency medical services council prior to the issuance of any guidelines. The Committee shall also review protocols developed by regional emergency medical advisory committees for consistency with statewide standards.

Sec.3004-a. Regional emergency medical advisory committees.

1. Regional emergency medical advisory committees shall develop policies, procedures, and triage, treatment, and transportation protocols which are consistent with the standards of the state emergency medical advisory committee and which address specific local conditions. Regional emergency medical advisory committees may also approve physicians to provide on-line medical control, coordinate the development of regional medical control systems, and participate in quality improvement activities addressing system-wide concerns. Hospitals and prehospital medical care services shall be authorized to release patient outcome information to regional emergency medical advisory committees for purposes of assessing prehospital care concerns. Regional quality improvement programs shall be presumed to be an extension of the quality improvement program set forth in Section 3006 of this article, and the provisions of subdivisions two and three of such Section 3006 shall apply to such programs.
2. The committee shall nominate to the commissioner a physician with demonstrated knowledge and experience in emergency medical services to serve on the state emergency medical advisory committee.

Sec.3030. Advanced life support services.

(1) Advanced life support services provided by an advanced emergency medical technician shall be provided under the direction of qualified medical and health personnel utilizing patient information and data transmitted by voice or telemetry.

Sec.3031. Advanced life support system.

Advanced life support system must
(1) be under the overall supervision and direction of a qualified physician with respect to the advanced life support services provided,
(2) be staffed by qualified medical and health personnel.

The philosophical evolution from 1987 to 1991 is subtle yet real. In 1987 a physician "assumed responsibility" for "all prehospital medical care," and it was recognized that regional EMS medical control boards would "include the medical directors (of all the EMS) services in the area" and "were responsible for the provision of medical control." The legislation in 1991 defines medical control as "advice and direction" plus written material "developed by the committee," "approved by council and commissioner" and "implemented by

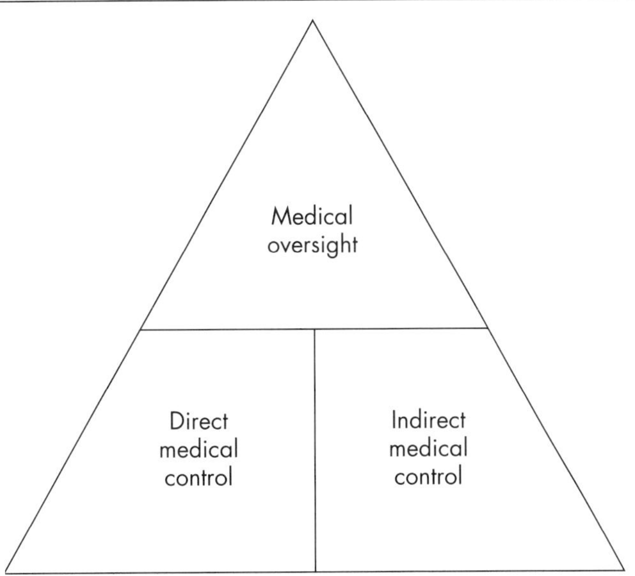

regional medical advisory committees." Nowhere does the law speak of the responsibility or authority of the service medical directors; and nowhere are the service medical directors assured a position on the regional medical advisory committees.

Medical oversight is the legal, moral, and medical authority responsible for the provision of prehospital medicine. It varies somewhat in extent and structure from state to state. The physician or organization responsible for medical oversight may choose to deliver all aspects of direct and indirect medical control or may delegate them to others. Nonetheless, the ultimate responsibility for prehospital medical care cannot be delegated away. Direct medical control activities are those wherein a physician makes contemporaneous decisions about patient care or personally delivers care. Indirect medical control activities are all other activities performed prospective, concurrent, and retrospective to the prehospital care of the patient.

18

Medical Oversight

Edward M. Racht, M.D.
Howard David Reines, M.D.

Most prehospital medical emergencies occur in locations that are removed from a medical facility. In some countries a mobile response team brings a physician to the scene of the medical emergency to provide care. In the United States, however, because most physicians are hospital-based, the acutely ill or injured patient is transported to the physician. Patient outcome is influenced by early medical intervention, and therefore contemporary prehospital care systems are a well-defined practice of medicine. As such, one of the most important aspects of prehospital medicine is the oversight provided by the medically and legally responsible physician.

Provider as a Physician Extender

Prehospital care in the United States is effected through the use of providers who assess patients and deliver defined care based on medical criteria. Before 1970, emergent patient care was provided in separate, independent segments. The care provided in the prehospital phase was often not coordinated with that provided in the hospital phase. The physician treated the patient only after arrival at the emergency facility with little or no input in the initial scene management. As understanding of the pathophysiology of emergent illnesses and injury advanced, it became clear that the ideal care progressed in a coordinated fashion from initial field contact through emergency department treatment and further inpatient definitive care. It is the responsibility of a physician to direct the prehospital system and prehospital providers in the overall clinical management of patients. This responsibility and authority is EMS medical oversight.

The application of sophisticated medical interventions including manual defibrillation, intravenous access, medication administration, and invasive airway management necessitated physician participation in the supervision of prehospital care. After 1974, many states, localities, and medical societies required a licensed physician to be accountable for prehospital care provided at the paramedic level. As physician input increased, it became clear that the provision of quality prehospital medical care required medical oversight not only for paramedics, but also for First Responders, EMT-As, system operations, call reception, and dispatch.

In some states the legal requirement for medical oversight rests on the American Law Institute's Restatement of the Law of Agency, which defines the doctrine of "borrowed servant" as follows: "A servant directed or permitted to perform services for another may become the servant of such other in performing the services. He may become the other's servant as to some acts and not as to others." In prehospital care this concept means that the medical oversight physician is the borrower of another's servants or employees. The paramedic employee of the ambulance service is borrowed to perform certain acts sanctioned by the responsible physician. Furthermore the concept of *respondeat superior* states that the borrower of the servant is ultimately liable for the acts and omissions of the surrogate as long as the surrogate is under the borrower's supervision. In the prehospital arena the medical oversight physician bears legal responsibility for the acts of the providers.[4] Despite these legal dictums, it has taken a number of years for physicians to become leaders in the development of systems and the training of personnel.

Ultimately the only real authority for medical oversight is based in law. Numerous states mandate medical oversight for paramedic systems, and a few others such as Virginia and New York mandate medical directors for all prehospital providers. As physician involvement is further encouraged and required for the entire scope of prehospital care, the confusing and unnecessary differentiation between basic and advanced providers becomes moot. In California, each local EMS agency must have a physician medical director "to provide medical control and ensure medical accountability throughout the planning, implementation, and evaluation of the EMS system."[2] In 1991 the Emergency Medical Services Act of Alabama provided for implementation of medical oversight and accountability for all prehospital care. Physician responsibility for the management of patient care including the issuance of physician orders, patient treatment, and transportation requirements were enumerated. Each region is required to appoint "a medical director who shall be a physician with experience and knowledge of EMS."[3] Unfortunately, a few states still do not address medical oversight responsibility in state law.[2] Others such as New York recently included medical oversight responsibility in state law.

Models of Medical Oversight

For an EMS system to function effectively, there must be a seamless combination and coordination of the direct and indirect medical control, functioning under the authority of medical oversight. Together the aspects of medical oversight facilitate the delivery of clinical care in a unique fashion. By analyzing the available prehospital and hospital resources in a particular community, the medical oversight system can be structured to meet the needs of the prehospital providers, the emergency department physicians, the hospitals, and ultimately the public who relies on a clinically sophisticated EMS system. Obviously, as technology, hospital capabilities, and patient populations change, the relative balance of indirect and direct medical control may shift. For example, if a community originally required direct medical control approval for a procedure such as thoracic decompression, an enhanced educational program driven by the quality management (QM) process allows the procedure to be performed under standing orders without any direct medical control. Ideally the medical oversight structure nurtures the system's educational and QM components.

An EMS agency medical director seldom acts alone. Most commonly the medical director seeks the advice and often the approval of a group of physicians familiar with the management of acutely ill or injured patients. The formal relationship between the medical director and the individual agency, the providers, and the participating physician groups varies greatly from system to system. The relationship is often defined by state law, local ordinance, or medical society regulations.

In its simplest form, medical oversight is the authority and responsibility of a single physician charged with making independent decisions regarding all the medical aspects of the system. The physician may provide both indirect medical control and direct medical control, and does not need approval from other physicians or organizations before taking action.

Occasionally a system or jurisdiction appoints or elects a single medical director who functions more or less at the pleasure of a medical oversight or advisory board. The physicians on the board are area physicians charged as a group with medical oversight; they attempt to reach consensus regarding system issues, and assist or direct the medical director in decision-making. A medical oversight board model has the advantages of involving many physicians in the decision-making process and providing peer support. Under the New York State EMS amendments that went into effect in July 1993, the regional EMS board, rather than the New York City EMS medical director or any other individual agency medical director, has the ultimate authority and responsibility for medical oversight.

A medical oversight physician or committee may be responsible for an individual provider, a group of providers, an agency, a group of agencies, a geographic region, or an entire state. Logically a given provider can have only one physician or one physician group as medical oversight; however, there are undoubtedly many ambiguous situations. The oversight physician may delegate specific medical control responsibilities to other physicians, especially in large systems. Indeed, only medical oversight itself cannot be delegated.

Medical oversight structures are as varied as the systems served. A particular model may function well in one locality yet not at all in another. Indeed, some functional models may not be allowed under local law. If a system's medical oversight relationship does not serve the interests of its patients, the medical director must seek change.

Components of Medical Oversight

For the physician community to positively impact provision of patient care in any prehospital system, a formal relationship must be established between the prehospital providers and the responsible physician. Given the nature of prehospital illness and injury, this relationship or medical oversight must provide consistent clinical guidance under a variety of circumstances. The terms used to describe EMS medical oversight both structurally and operationally are still evolving. Although one physician (or in some states a group of physicians) should retain responsibility and ultimate authority, many aspects of medical oversight may be delegated to other physicians. There are two basic subsets of medical oversight activities—direct medical control and indirect medical control.

Direct Medical Control

Direct medical control is also called "on-line," "base station" or "immediate" medical control. Simplistically, direct medical control is the contemporaneous physician direction of a field provider. This communication may be via radio, telephone, or actual contact with a physician on-scene. The advantage of direct medical control is the ability of the physician to order or withhold a direct patient intervention based on an assessment or report given by the on-scene provider. This activity requires the establishment of communication between the provider and either the responsible oversight physician or a delegated medical control surrogate. Although this traditional approach epitomizes the concept of the field provider being the "eyes and ears" of the physician, there remains ongoing debate regarding the impact of direct medical control on comprehensive patient care.[5-7]

The specific form of direct medical control in any EMS system is based on the specific characteristics of the prehospital community and receiving hospital structure. When direct medical control is required, it may be accomplished via communications with the delegated receiving facility staff, the EMS system medical director, or a delegated regional medical control physician. In some systems a physician medical director or surrogate responds to the scene to provide direct medical control and assist with patient care.

Indirect Medical Control

In the early 1970s an "off-line" or "project" medical director was defined as a "physician directing the lead EMS agency in the overall system design, implementation and evaluation; and (who) is responsible for the ultimate medical accountability and appropriateness of the entire regional system."[9] Within the scope of medical oversight, everything that is not direct medical control is indirect. In the early 1970s, such an off-line medical director had ultimate medical responsibility and accountability; however, today the provision of prehospital care by a field provider is an extension of the practice of medicine of a physician located much closer to the provider. Although the physician may not be immediately available to provide direct prehospital patient care, protocols and standards are established and accepted by that responsible physician for use by the prehospital care provider. The oversight physician under whose license the provider functions may delegate large aspects of indirect medical control to others. However, to be effective the indirect aspects of medical control must guide all participants in the EMS system on patient care issues. Indirect medical control must also interface with and guide many of the system's operational and administrative issues to assure an effective patient care process. Therefore the physician accepting medical oversight must oversee those tasks that are delegated to others.

Of all the clinical components of an EMS system, indirect medical control activities require the most physician energy and provide the essential base for clinical excellence. They also require that the physicians are knowledgeable of operational, financial, and political issues that affect the ultimate delivery of clinical care; few physicians have formal training in those disciplines. Indirect medical control is in part a dynamic, prospective, planning process that enables the system to design and evolve the optimal patient care "provider."

As EMS systems become more sophisticated, it is clear that the delivery of quality clinical care results not only from strong medical oversight, but also from collaborative efforts among physicians, operations managers, field providers, administrators, public officials, and community leaders. For example, medical directors often must either justify the cost-effectiveness of a specific field intervention or prioritize program development based on available resources. A solid understanding of the complex forces involved in such decision processes helps the physician maximize abilities to improve overall patient care. The most astute, innovative EMS physician cannot impact prehospital patient care if the system will not give financial and political support.

Many elements of indirect medical control that impact the provision of patient care may be delegated by the physician responsible for medical oversight to other physicians. They include system design, protocol development, education and quality improvement. Each is intimately related to the others. The development of the elements in a vacuum leads to a fragmented and defective system of prehospital care.

System Design. Few physicians ever have the opportunity to design an EMS system from scratch; rather, most are charged with creating change in response to the evolving environment of prehospital care. One of the most important aspects of system design is the choice of provider levels of care. This decision is based on the availability of resources, the geographic characteristics of the service area, the annual call volume, the amount of available physician support, and the clinical philosophy of the medical director.

Because the pathophysiology of acute illnessand injury begins at the time of insult not provider arrival, the physician must assure that patient care begins with system access and that the system is accessible by 9-1-1 or enhanced 9-1-1. Communication access and dispatch procedures provide pre-arrival instructions in an effort to minimize morbidity while the ambulance is en route. The sequence and content of caller interrogation should allow dispatchers to reliably send the appropriate resources to the patient in a timely fashion. Similarly the system should predetermine ambulance and personnel placement to maximally decrease the interval from call receipt to arrival at the patient. Emergent patient management is as dependent on a timely response as it is on adequately trained and equipped providers.

Protocol development. A protocol is a preauthorized course of care for use by prehospital providers in managing patients. Protocols are developed by the responsible physician with input from providers and other physicians so that a consensus is established. In addition to clinical protocols, the physician is responsible for developing appropriate triage protocols such as those used during a multiple casualty incident or for determining the level of response in a tiered response system. Transport protocols must be developed to route patients to appropriate centers based on clinical criteria. A thoughtful, objective, collaborative approach to patient destination protocols minimizes the financial and political pressures on and from the hospitals participating in the system. The physician responsible for medical oversight should be actively involved in designating specialty referral centers such as trauma centers, burn centers, cardiac specialty centers, hazardous materials receiving facilities, and pediatric emergency and critical care centers.

As in all of medicine, responsible EMS physicians rely on scientific literature to establish the foundation of all protocols. Individualizing protocols to fit a particular system is the art of prehospital medicine. Protocols, especially of a clinical nature, require a significant degree of local medical consensus and should never be transferred verbatim from one system to another.

Education. The indirect medical control activity of education is an investment in quality. The medical director establishes the standards for entry level and continuing medical education, course content, and educational performance. A comprehensive educational program provides the necessary assessment, diagnostic, and therapeutic skills to adequately carry out the clinical mandates of medical oversight as well as the requirements of the state certifying agency. In some systems the physician responsible for medical oversight never meets the physician educators who are delegated to provide that aspect of indirect medical control.

Quality management. Webster's dictionary defines quality as " a degree of excellence."[11] QM in prehospital care provides continuous feedback to the medical director about the effectiveness of the entire system. It allows the medical director to shape the educational program and provides data supporting change or reevaluation of one or more segments of the system. The overall responsibility for QM rests with the medical director.[8] By involving providers in the quality review process, auditors demonstrate an improvement in quality of care, or identify logistical issues that impede improvement.[10]

A substantial difficulty in prehospital QM is outcome analysis. Because patients are delivered to a multitude of institutions with varying access to hospital records, it is often difficult to collect follow-up data for QM purposes. Nevertheless this data is essential not only to monitor system performance, but to assess the impact of various treatment modalities on prehospital morbidity and mortality.[1]

Summary

The physician responsible for medical oversight is the cornerstone of every EMS system. Through the use and delegation of the tools of direct and indirect medical control, the system can be designed and operated to optimize prehospital patient outcomes. A successful collaborative relationship among the medical director and delegated medical control physicians, receiving facilities, field providers, administrators, and operations personnel enhances the medical oversight physician's ability to influence patient care decision-making. That physician is constantly learning from the collective experience of the system to effectively build and contribute to his or her expertise. Rapidly emerging scientific literature, newly developed technologies, and constantly changing political and financial climates all coalesce to require constant evaluation and modification of contemporary EMS systems.

REFERENCES

1. Bonnin MJ and Swor RA: Outcomes in unsuccessful field resuscitation attempts, *Ann Emerg Med* 18:507-512, 1989.
2. Boyd DR et al: Medical control and accountability of emergency medical services (EMS) systems *IEEE Transactions on Vehicular Technology* T-28:249-262, 1979.
3. Emergency Medical Services Act of Alabama, Section 132, 1991.
4. EMS Medical Services in South Carolina: *A guide for medical control physicians division of EMS,* Columbia, SC, Department of Health and Environmental Control.
5. Erder MH, Davidson SJ, and Cheney RA: On-line medical command in theory and practice, *Ann Emerg Med* 18:261-268, 1989.
6. Gatton MC et al: Effect of standing orders on paramedic scene time for trauma patients, *Ann Emerg Med* 20:1306-1309, 1991.
7. Pointer JE et al: The impact on standing orders on medication and skill selection, paramedic assessment, and hospital outcome: a follow-up report, *Prehospital and Disaster Medicine* 6(3):303-308, 1991.
8. Stout JL: Organizing quality control in EMS, *JEMS* 13:67-74, 1988.
9. Subcommittee on Medical Control: *Medical control in emergency medical services: subcommittee report, conclusions and recommendations,* Washington, DC, 1981, National Academy Press.
10. Swor RA, Bocka JJ, and Maio RF: A paramedic peer review quality assurance audit, *Prehospital and Disaster Medicine* 6(3): 321-326, 1991.
11. *Webster's new collegiate dictionary,* Springfield, Mass, 1975, Merriam-Webster Inc.

19

Indirect Medical Control

Norman E. McSwain, Jr., M.D., FACS

Medical care in the United States must be provided under the direction of a physician. No state allows prehospital providers to function as totally independent practitioners. Although a few states allow the emergency medical technician-basic (EMT-B) to function independently, most have specific legislation requiring the provider functioning beyond the EMT-B level to work under the direct supervision of a physician via radio or telemetry communications. The new EMT-B curriculum being developed requires medical direction at that level also. Although a few communities allow the use of standing orders alone, prior medical approval is required. It is the individual physician's license that allows advanced EMTs to function in this special fashion. In communities using standing orders in association with electronic communications, prehospital providers usually establish direct communication with a physician after initiating the standing orders. This chapter uses *prehospital provider* as a generic term referring to all levels of personnel. Specific levels are referred to by the United States Department of Transportation (DOT) designation. The terminology that follows is used by the DOT, the National Registry of Emergency Medical Technicians (NREMT), the National Association of Emergency Medical Technicians (NAEMT), and most other major national EMS organizations:

EMT-BASIC—EMT-B is the initial level of prehospital care. Using the current and proposed DOT program, 110 hours are required. Until recently this level was called EMT-Ambulance (EMT-A). In theory the new DOT EMT-B is educated to use the automated external defibrillator and requires medical oversight.

EMT-INTERMEDIATE—EMT-I includes additional training to manage shock, use advanced airway maneuvers (EOA and ET), and start and maintain intravenous fluid replacement. The current DOT curriculum does not state an hour requirement. The specific educational objectives of the curriculum must be met.

EMT-PARAMEDIC—EMT-P includes a full-range of medication and procedures to initiate and complete definitive care. The current DOT document does not have an hour requirement. The specific educational objectives of the curriculum must be met.

Additionally, some states have legislation that authorizes the local medical groups to develop and approve protocols for prehospital care. Other areas have voluntarily established protocols; in those cases regional medical consensus is important. Protocols are total patient care, and standing orders are only a part of protocols. The protocols describe the limits of prehospital function and outline any standing orders that may be used within them.

Medical oversight has the ultimate authority over and responsibility for the medical aspects of the entire EMS system and its impact on patient care. For convenience this discussion of medical oversight is in three temporal phases initially described in 1978 as part of a definition of medical control.[13]

PROSPECTIVE—The steps taken before the call is received that assure adequate training, equipment, and personnel to meet the needs of the patient are prospective.

IMMEDIATE—The supervision of the prehospital provider during the call is immediate; this includes providing or supervising the patient care given while assuring that the assessment and therapeutic skills used are performed correctly. This requires frequent physician observation of the provider in the field.

RETROSPECTIVE—The review of calls is done both collectively for the entire EMS service and individually for each prehospital provider. This assures that patient care is correct and that the knowledge and the skills of the provider person are not deteriorated.

To perform these three temporal phases of medical oversight, two general types of physician involvement are necessary: administrative and clinical. Administrative involvement includes setting up protocols and reviewing what has been accomplished. Sufficient administrative involvement requires at least 2 hours of physician time per week per EMS unit. Clinical involvement includes giving on-scene patient care, observing prehospital provider performance, overseeing training, and directing patient care via the telecommunications system.

Medicolegal considerations must be kept in mind. Because prehospital providers function either under the license of the medical director or under the "borrowed servant" or "respondent-superior doctrines," it is imperative that appropriate quality management (QM) steps are taken so the physician's license is not jeopardized. In some states the EMT-B does not function as a physician extender; however, in other states the EMT-B, EMT-I, and EMT-P all work under physician-approved protocols.

Two types of EMS physician positions have developed. Direct medical control physicians provide medical instructions while the prehospital provider is on-scene. This is medical oversight in the immediate phase. Indirect medical control physicians are administrative, clinical, and medicine quality control physicians that work in all three phases. In the early days of EMS development the direct medical control physician was the most pro-minent person on the EMS team. As EMS has matured the indirect medical control physician has become a much more important member of the team. A 1989 study by Erder et al describes an 8-minute increase in scene time and no significantly different medical outcome when direct medical control was used rather than protocol.[6] Improvement in health care status was 5.5% with physician-directed scene care and 3.2% by protocol. Deterioration in health care status was 1.3% versus 1.1%. The benefits of direct medical control certainly did not justify the time and cost of such physician involvement. An informal survey in March 1992 found that fewer systems relied on 100% mandatory radio communication than 5 years ago. Although the increasing independence of EMT-P personnel may or may not be a wave of the future, it is certainly a major force at present. Systems allowing greater use of standing orders require even more indirect medical control and surveillance to provide the type of quality assurance that the medical community has come to expect in EMS systems.

In a position paper adapted in 1982 the American College of Emergency Physicians (ACEP) provides a definition of medical oversight and the requirements of the physicians providing such care[1]:

> All aspects of the organization and provision of EMS require the active involvement and participation of physicians. These aspects should incorporate design of the EMS system prior to its implementation; continual revision of the system; and operation of the system from initial access, to prehospital contact with the patient, through stabilization in the emergency department. All prehospital medical care may be considered to have been provided by one or more agents of the physician who controls the prehospital system, for this physician has assumed responsibility for such care.
>
> Physician control of prehospital emergency care may be accomplished through direct voice communication with prehospital emergency medical personnel (direct control) or through provision of care according to patient care protocols developed and promulgated by physicians (indirect control). All training of emergency prehospital personnel, including course design, supervision of training, retraining, continuing education, ongoing performance evaluation through audit, review and critique sessions, and other appropriate components, must be under the direction of a physician.
>
> To optimize medical control of all prehospital emergency medical services, these services should be managed by physicians who meet the following requirements:
>
> 1. Familiarity with the design and operation of prehospital EMS systems,
> 2. Experience in prehospital emergency care of the acutely ill or injured patient,
> 3. Routine participation in base-station radio control of prehospital emergency units,
> 4. Experience in emergency department management of the acutely ill or injured patient,
> 5. Routine active participation in emergency department management of the acutely ill or injured patient,
> 6. Active involvement in the training of basic and advanced life support prehospital personnel,
> 7. Active involvement in the medical audit, review, and critique of basic life support and advanced life support prehospital personnel, and
> 8. Participation in the administrative and legislation process affecting the regional and/or state prehospital EMS system.

Notice how this 1982 philosophy was the basis of the definition used by New York State in 1987 (see p. 178). The acceptance of EMS systems as part of the total medical team and the coordination of transportation to the appropriate medical facility have been hampered by a lack of positive physician involvement in medical oversight and by those who have spoken negatively about EMS rather than becoming actively involved in the provision of optimal care. As Pons pointed out in 1984, physicians are eager to implement a prehospital care system, but often unwilling to maintain an interest, monitor the performance of the system, and institute the necessary change or discipline.[16] Unfortunately, this "head in the sand" attitude has led to serious abuses of prehospital decision-making, for example, patients with chest pain or penetrating thoracic trauma and stable vital signs sent to the hospital by automobile after evaluation by paramedics. Although this sort of behavior by prehospital personnel cannot be tolerated or condoned, it is the failure of physicians to maintain control that bears the greatest responsibility for such a sorry state of affairs.

In 1984 McSwain noted that many physicians, especially surgeons, complained that prehospital providers worked too slowly, performed needless procedures, and took patients to the wrong hospital; yet these physicians neither became involved in the EMS system nor taught the prehospital providers better methods. Today, in many cities and communities there are physicians interested enough in EMS to get in the trenches and make an impact.

The QM mechanism for EMS evolved early and was constructed to be the tightest. When done correctly, the EMS QM system is far more stringent than that used by hospitals for physicians and nurses. QM is a part of all three phases of medical oversight, but is most evident in the retrospective review of care and the prospective changes instituted as a result of such retrospective oversight.[10,12]

In 1986, Holroyd et al gave the following description of quality assurance[8]:

> Medical control is a system of physician-directed quality assurance that provides professional and public accountability for medical care provided in the prehospital setting. In an EMS system, medical control provides the operational framework and authorization for paramedics and other physician extenders to provide emergency treatment outside the hospital.

The same article also describes the qualifications of an "off-line (indirect) medical director"[8]:

> Knowledge and demonstrated ability in planning and operation of prehospital EMS systems, experience in the prehospital provision of emergency care for acutely ill or injured patients, experience in the training and ongoing evaluation of all levels of participants in the prehospital care system, knowledge and experience in the application of medical control to an EMS system, and a knowledge of the administrative and legislative processes affecting regional and/or state prehospital EMS systems.

For the medical director ultimately responsible for all medical oversight or the physician delegated to perform the indirect aspects of medical control to function properly, the job must be an official position duly appointed by the responsible political entity with authority to make decisions involving any and all medical conditions that impact on patient care.

Prospective Indirect Medical Control

The prospective phase of medical oversight is entirely indirect. It begins when the community first decides to provide EMS. The initial action is the identification of the level of prehospital service required to provide the desired patient care for the community. After this decision is made, protocols are written, training programs are designed, ambulance equipment is chosen, supplies are purchased, mechanisms for retrospective review are implemented, and an appropriate prehospital care report (PCR) is designed. Each step must be compatible with applicable local, state, and federal legislation. The physician responsible for medical oversight has significant input at each step. Although the administrative entity that provides financial support for the service also has concerns and responsibilities, the factors that impact the quality of medical care are ultimately the responsibility of the physician. The administrative entity cannot have veto power over medical or QM requirements that could compromise patient care.

Protocols

Protocols have been erroneously considered synonymous with standing orders. Protocols are the overall steps in patient care management undertaken by the prehospital provider at every patient contact. Standing orders are those components of prehospital care that the prehospital provider initiates before establishing communications with the physician. The statement that "Voice communication should be established after initiation of the standing orders; only radio failure should prevent such communication" was made in the first edition of this book. It represents a strong bias by this author that subsequently has been questioned and perhaps proven false. Several research studies demonstrate that (1) there is no difference in survival with or without direct medical control, (2) less time is spent in the field without the requirement to call a direct medical control physician, and (3) the prehospital providers are not threatened by making decisions without reporting before providing patient care.[4,9] The findings of these studies apply not only to voice communication but also to telemetered electrocardiograms (ECGs). These studies were done in systems with tight indirect medical control including complete review of all PCRs and comparisons of patient outcome to the prehospital care provided.

There are two instances in which standing order field medical care requires communication. One is when the provider feels the need to transmit an ECG for assistance in interpretation of difficult rhythms; the other is when some component of patient evaluation, treatment, or response is not done "by the book." In addition, there is always communication alerting the hospital of the arrival of certain patients so proper preparations for immediate patient care can be made. No emergent or critical patient should ever present to a hospital without prior notification. The protocols must address each step of prehospital patient care management and include the medical conditions most likely to be encountered. Several textbooks provide specific protocols for almost every condition seen in prehospital care. The protocol for management of the trauma patient developed by the American College of Surgeons Committee on Trauma (ACS/COT) is an example of such a protocol. A protocol can address general patient conditions or symptoms such as coma, chest pain, seizure, and impending delivery, or it can address diagnoses such as diabetes, myocardial infarction, epilepsy, and pregnancy.

Using the assessment-based condition or symptom approach is desirable because an accurate prehospital diagnosis is often difficult to establish. Because patients demonstrate complaints, conditions, and symptoms, a stepwise protocol for the management of these presentations is easy to develop. The primary emphasis of prehospital care is not to make a diagnosis but rather to evaluate and manage the patient's emergent condition while the patient is being transported to the appropriate hospital for definitive care. Emergent condition management is necessary; obtaining an accurate diagnosis is not.

During the development of prehospital care in the early 1960s, the initial thrust was toward the management of the trauma patient; in the early 1970s, it shifted to the management of the cardiac patient; and in the 1980s the thrust focused on redefining trauma management. These changes caused confusion regarding the specific role of the prehospital provider and how protocols are developed. It is the prehospital provider's responsibility to provide definitive care for the patient's condition as rapidly as possible. Some definitive care is best provided in the field by the prehospital personnel, but other components can only be provided in the hospital. The differences must be understood by the providers, those who write the protocols, the medical director, and the medical community at large.

An example of definitive care that is best provided in the field is that required by the cardiac patient. The First Responder can provide definitive care in the field by initiating CPR, which is only a holding pattern while definitive care is set up. If advanced personnel are on the scene, then the definitive care is defibrillation and stabilizing drugs followed by transport of the patient to the closest appropriate hospital. Frequently this is the closest emergency department staffed by well-trained emergency physicians. On the other end of the spectrum is the hypovolemic trauma patient; definitive care can be provided only in the operating room as hemorrhage control. Therefore it is the prehospital provider's responsibility to immobilize the patient for transport, assure adequate oxygenation, and initiate shock therapy while transporting the patient to the closest appropriate facility. In this situation the closest appropriate facility is a hospital that not only has an emergency department staffed by emergency physicians, but also has in-house capabilities to immediately place the patient in the operating room.

In a rural community with only one hospital a prehospital transport decision is not required unless air transport response is available. In an urban center with multiple hospitals, usually one or two facilities are committed to the specialized needs of the trauma patient by having appropriate personnel and equipment immediately available. All hospitals without in-house surgical capability should be bypassed and the patient transported to the trauma facility. Such decisions are part of the system of protocols developed by indirect medical control.

Protocol Approval Process

After protocols are developed, the next step is consensus approval by the appropriate entity. This entity can be the system medical director, the county medical society's EMS committee, a regional medical board, or a state medical board. Approval of the protocols is necessary to (1) assure community agreement on the level of care, (2) assure the standards of care, and (3) provide a medical basis for communitywide prehospital care that addresses the needs of patients in concert with all physicians and all hospitals in the community. Even in those jurisdictions where a designated medical director drafts and implements protocols without outside approval, achieving medical consensus is valuable. After the protocols have been approved, the receiving hospitals, the provider personnel, the ambulance service, the administrative directors, and the physicians providing direct and indirect medical control each receive a copy.

In collaboration with medical oversight the training officer then plans educational sessions addressing any differences between the protocols and the initial prehospital provider training program. Because protocols are the principles of medical care, the choice of the exact methods by which they are carried out remains the preference of the medical director. Discussions among the physicians providing direct medical control and the field providers encourage mutual familiarity. The terminology should be standard, and there should be specific understanding of exactly what the protocols mean. A review process that converges the PCR, the emergency department record, and the protocols must then be established so continuous QM can be performed.

Training

As both medical science and available prehospital medical interventions change the protocols must be modified. Potential protocol changes will be identified by the ACS in the *Advanced Trauma Life Support* (ATLS) course, the NAEMT in the *Pre Hospital Trauma Life Support* (PHTLS) course, the BTLS Foundation in the *Basic Trauma Life Support* (BTLS) course, and the American Heart Association in the *Advanced Cardiac Life Support* (ACLS) course, the *Pediatric Trauma Life Support* (PTLS) course and the *Pediatric Advanced Life Support* (PALS) course. The responsible physician or medical advisory committee uses these and other standard updates to formulate protocol changes and curriculum alterations.

Standardized training programs using the National Standard Teaching Curriculum have been developed by the DOT, and they have been adopted by many states as the accepted teaching program for the various EMT certification levels. Some states and regions, because of peculiarities in environment and industry, add to the minimal curriculum to address specialized problems; local medical input is required in developing such additions.

Both the initial and subsequent training programs must educate the prehospital provider to the appropriate level of expertise for each community. This level is based on the predicted needs of the community and then validated by experience. Of the predicted one emergent EMS call per 10,000 population each 24 hours, one third will be trauma, one third will be non-cardiac medical, and one third will be cardiac. Although 30 to 40% will require some type of advanced evaluation, less than 20% will actually require advanced treatment. Less than 5% of all patients will require any drug intervention other than intravenous (IV) fluids and oxygen, and approximately 10% of the trauma patients will have hypotension as one of the presenting problems.[3,15]

An EMS program serving a population of less than 10,000 people obviously has less absolute demand for advanced interventions than a large urban system. This creates a complex problem in rural areas where a provider may see only one cardiac arrest every year. Maintaining proficiency in ECG interpretation and drug skills at such a low level of exposure is difficult. Thus a low-volume EMS system may elect to use an automated external defibrillator (AED) for cardiac resuscitation; to maintain IV proficiency by having prehospital providers work in the emergency department; to use frequent mannequin training for intubation skills; and to run weekly "hands-on" psychomotor skill training. Such varied approaches allow a typical low-volume system to provide quality care to almost every patient; fewer than ten patients per year would require care beyond the system's capabilities. Maintaining the advanced skills necessary for prehospital providers to provide sophisticated care once or twice yearly is not impossible, but it is extremely expensive and time-consuming. More than 90% of all prehospital patient care encounters can be effectively handled by an EMT-I with IV skills, intubation skills, and AED capability.

In communities with a large number of patients with cardiac, diabetic, or other problems in which acute intervention includes medications the training and the skill maintenance necessary to keep the prehospital providers proficient at the paramedic level is easily justified. However, the cost-per-patient-encounter to advance and maintain paramedic competence is high. Such advancement should not be undertaken without understanding the long-range difficulties of skill maintenance.

Ambulance Equipment and Supplies

The equipment and supplies necessary on an ambulance are outlined in the essential equipment list published by the ACS/COT.[5] That document identifies the standard equipment necessary to provide adequate patient care at the basic, intermediate, and advanced EMT levels.[3,14] Deviations from these minimal levels of equipment and supplies are indicated if dictated by either local community need or changes in prehospital care standards. ACEP developed a position paper defining the optimal advanced level prehospital skills, medication, and equipment.[2] Both the ACS/COT and ACEP documents provide a valuable reference for the medical director and physicians responsible for indirect medical control.

Local variations in response time, transport time, and vehicle use dictate the actual stock of materials necessary. Although it is the responsibility of the administrative entity to keep supplies available on the unit, it is the responsibility of the indirect medical control physician to identify what is required and how many of each are necessary.

Ambulance Operations

Determining the number and location of properly equipped and staffed ambulances necessary to provide appropriate response times that meet the specific needs of the system requires analysis not only of population density, but also of the peculiarities of the patients being served. For example, certain geographic areas have a high rate of drug-related or penetrating trauma calls; other areas have a high density of blunt trauma calls; still other areas have high rates of calls concerning problems of the elderly. Therefore identification of areas with young suburban families, high crime rates, elderly residents, or busy roadways must be considered in planning the placement of vehicles. Ongoing modifications of vehicle placement are based on a statistical analysis of the calls, the time out of service while responding to a particular type call, the location of the hospitals to which patients are transported, and the amount of additional support required to cover an area while an ambulance is on a call. Although many of these tasks are administrative, indirect medical control input is necessary to assure that response times are appropriate and to predict the individual characteristics of the various service areas.

Communications

Although addressed in another section of this text (see Chapter 13), the importance of medical oversight of EMS communications must not be overlooked. It is the key to ambulance placement, dispatch, hospital communication, and immediate review of the current status of the system by the indirect medical control physician.

The indirect aspect of medical oversight includes prioritizing individual calls so emergencies that require immediate care have quick responses, and those that require less rapid care do not take precedence. There are various acceptable approaches; however, calls must be prioritized.

Slovis et al point out that a protocol-driven priority dispatch system improves the response time by 4 minutes to the 30% of patients in the most urgent category and increases the use of advanced medical procedures for the group of patients in a multi-tiered system.[20] There is only a 0.3% dispatch error when using a protocol-assisted dispatch system. This type of protocol assistance is of less benefit to a system using a single level of care.

A second benefit of a priority dispatch system is a reduction in non-emergent calls for ambulance transportation. Several studies confirm that more than 50% of the calls that come into dispatch require emergent transportation.[7,17,18] Reduction in overall call volume improves response time on other calls and reduces public cost.

Immediate Medical Oversight

Medical oversight of patient care during the call has the following two components: direct and indirect. Direct medical control is discussed in the following chapter. An important use of mandatory direct medical control is in all "do not transport" and "do not resuscitate" decisions; every decision should be contemporaneously made by direct medical control. System protocols define the limitations and guidelines for such decisions.

The medical director is responsible in the immediate phase for periodic "on-site" observation of prehospital providers including patient assessment and treatment. Such observation should be performed by both the medical director and the training officers reporting to the medical director.

As part of this contemporaneous component, the medical director must regularly monitor communications between the prehospital providers and the physicians providing direct medical control to assure that the information transmitted is concise, accurate, and complete. Communication between the physicians and the providers should reflect the relative urgency of the particular case. The direct medical control physicians should not order inappropriate evaluation procedures, delay transport, or deviate from protocol unless permitted by the protocols.

When the patient is delivered to the hospital the emergency department physician should evaluate the adequacy of the PCR, checking for correctness and completeness including the patient's condition and prehospital diagnosis. The mandated management steps should have been carried out completely and rapidly within the confines of the specific prehospital emergency. Unnecessary or unauthorized diagnostic steps or procedures should be noted. The medical director, the designated indirect medical control physician, physician, and the training officer also should retrospectively perform such reviews.

Other aspects of indirect medical control such as reviewing the ambulance response and scene times, assuring transport to the appropriate hospitals, and completing retrospective analyses of the individual runs and the overall system are performed during the retrospective phase. However, the medical director and his delegated assistants also have the responsibility to be in the field observing the actions of the individual prehospital providers and the overall functioning of the EMS system. Because such observations cannot be made on a retrospective basis and many of the problems of a system are not visible on the PCR, the physician responsible for these aspects of indirect medical control must spend time in the field.

Retrospective Indirect Medical Oversight

The retrospective component of medical oversight occurs after the case is completed and involves the medical director, delegated training officers, and the EMS committee. This is an indirect medical control component. It is the medical director's responsibility to assure that the data are gathered and appropriately reviewed. An oversight committee then reviews the medical director's actions and, based on the analysis, agrees or disagrees with the steps taken. Formal modifications in the protocols can then be made when indicated.

Such an oversight committee may also be responsible for taking political steps to improve the fiscal aspects of the system. A formal medical process should be developed to designate receiving hospitals and specialty referral centers and to change facilities if they are not functioning appropriately.

Prehospital Care Report Review

PCR design and data analysis are addressed in another chapter of this text (see Chapter 15). Medical oversight should review and act on issues such as (1) systemwide response time, scene time, and transport time for various types of calls, (2) percentage of runs using drugs, IVs, endotracheal intubation, and other procedures broken down by medical category and the individual provider, (3) the individual provider's success rates at the various skills, (4) aborted transfers, (5) patient refusals, and (6) any other information that provides insight in the quality of care provided. An individual PCR critique must ask the following five crucial questions:

1. Was the prehospital diagnosis the same as the emergency department diagnosis?
2. Was anything done in the field that should *not* have been done?
3. Was anything *not* done in the field that should have been done?
4. Was there an inappropriate delay in transporting the patient to the hospital?
5. Was the patient transported to the appropriate hospital?

Computer-assisted QM systems are available that greatly ease the workloads of the medical director and the training officer. Although expensive to design and implement, the computer programs reduce the hours required for review resulting in long-term savings and improved reviews. Stewart et al report that when such a system was implemented in Pittsburgh the number of patient care errors identified increased 700% and documentation errors identified increased 250%.[21] Computer-assisted evaluation of field performance, as judged by PCRs, ensures compliance with standards in patient care and EMS recordkeeping.

A far less sophisticated system was introduced by the New Orleans EMS system in the early 1980s to identify skill deterioration or poor skill application. It identified paramedics to be moved from less busy stations to busier ones and stimulated in-service training and skill review. The system detected an unusually high incidence of "patient refusals" by one paramedic; appropriate counseling sessions changed the individual's attitude toward patient needs.

Counseling

If inappropriate care is rendered by a specific individual, the medical director should formally counsel the provider and follow-up with targeted instruction to eliminate the problem. The counseling is best done one-on-one.

Counseling can be supplemented by changing the provider's shift or ambulance station; thus performance is improved by putting the provider in a more appropriate work environment. Another method to improve care is requiring rotations through clinical areas of the hospital. If structured appropriately, rotations will help the individual regain deteriorated skills.

Retention

The retention of knowledge and psychomotor skills is extremely important in the rapidly advancing field of medicine. The rapid advancement in the types and levels of patient care provided since the late 1950s when the first prehospital provider training program was developed in Chicago, through the development of the EMT-A National Standard

Training Curriculum in 1968, to the current expansion of provider curricula is representative of the major changes in EMS philosophy, skills, and knowledge. Changes in information and knowledge continue, unfortunately, skills and knowledge are simultaneously lost because of misuse and bad habits. Nothing remains stable; change is the ultimate constant. To remain static is to fall behind. The extent and rapidity of skill and knowledge deterioration in the EMS community is thought to be significant, but this has never been verified. Only one study was done in the late 1970s.[19] Other authors have stated that "skill deterioration is EMS' number one enemy in the streets."[11]

Education

Frequent, formal educational sessions promote satisfactory field performance. These sessions are focused by both the initial educational objectives and the subsequent additions such as protocol changes, new drugs, different equipment, and QI reviews. Continuing education sessions can be presented in the form of didactic lectures, interactive discussions based on individual PCRs, interactive computer learning programs, and sound-slide tapes or video cassette tapes with discussion periods afterward. Sound-slide programs or video cassette tapes without immediate feedback in the form of discussion periods are ineffective because there is a minimal stimulus to absorb the information. Skill laboratory sessions to learn and master extrication, cardiopulmonary resuscitation, intubation, and other psychomotor skills are extremely useful.

Continuing education is divided into two components (1) refreshing previously learned material, specifically that in the initial training program, and (2) adding new information developed since the initial training program. Some well-organized standard refresher training programs are available. The most notable are the DOT EMT-B refresher course, ACLS, PHTLS, and BTLS. Typically they are mandated for each provider every 2 years. In their specific clinical areas these courses provide excellent, but limited, refresher education. Because these national courses only cover specific subjects or are aimed at particular audiences, most EMS continuing education is best developed locally.

The medical director of the individual service is responsible for assuring that within each educational cycle the entire curriculum for the specific provider level has been covered. This goal is best achieved by working from an outline of the behavioral objectives in the curriculum. The objectives are then the targets of periodic training sessions. Over a 1- or 2-year cycle, depending on the requirements of the particular program, all the objectives are covered with each individual. The medical director maintains an attendance log to assure that each provider receives all the necessary information.

Because learning is a type of behavioral modification, simply exposing a person to information does not result in learning. It is one thing for a student to daydream through a lecture, and an entirely different process to seriously consider the information presented and then ultimately modify patient care. The continuing education process must assure that the student gains appropriate information from the training sessions. Postinstructional examinations are one method of identifying how much information is retained. Periodic examinations are important to assure that the teaching objectives are not only mastered, but mastered satisfactorily. Another method to gauge the success of learning is observing the performance of the providers in the field before and after the educational process. This feedback allows additional emphasis to be placed on the components of the refresher program that appear the least effective.

Specific areas determined to be weak can be covered individually. This feedback process requires significant time and effort on the part of the medical director. Observing field performance, reviewing PCRs, reassessing the curriculum, developing objectives, preparing lectures, setting up educational objectives, and giving lectures are all important components of the medical director's job. The medical director usually has one or several individuals working that assist with such day-to-day activities. Those individuals can be nurses, supervisors, or training officers. Each service is organized differently, but these jobs must be carried out.

Subsequent evaluations of performance identify what has been learned. The following questions should be asked of the training program: If the trainees did not learn, why not? Are there deficiencies in the education process that prevent the providers from learning or are they not motivated to learn? If the trainees are not motivated, is it a problem of a specific provider or of a specific service? Steps must then be taken by the medical director to solve educational problems.

Another effective teaching mechanism is critique of individual runs. This is best achieved when the medical director is on-site during the emergency run and reviews the job performed from both the operational and medical standpoints. The emergency department (ED) physician who sees the patient also performs a critique, but such an activity cannot substitute that done by the medical director. Unfortunately, the ED physician often does not know what went on in the field and therefore cannot discuss specifically any errors made as medical care was provided. Obviously, the physician can discuss what should have taken place, confirm with the prehospital providers that it occurred, and review the PCR for completeness.

The medical director must remain current with prehospital and emergency medicine literature to identify areas in protocol and patient care that need to be changed. It is obvious throughout this process that medical directors infrequently in the field cannot perform their jobs competently. In very large systems, several associate medical directors may be required.

Definitions

There continues to be confusion regarding the following terms; they are often incorrectly and interchangeably used. Strict adherence to the philosophy of each is necessary to prevent confusion in their application to prehospital patient care.

- **CERTIFICATION**—the process whereby individuals qualify to practice their particular profession, skill, or art. *Recertification* is the process of reevaluation by an agency to ensure that the necessary skills and knowledge to continue their practice have been maintained and changed to keep abreast of new ideas and skills.
- **REGISTRATION**—the process whereby an organization verifies that individuals have completed a system of qualification in a particular profession by meeting and maintaining national standards.
- **LICENSURE**—the process whereby a state allows qualified persons to practice their profession within its borders.

Of all the fields of medicine the first to require a stringent continuing education and recertification process was prehospital care. The recertification process for prehospital providers is required every 2 or 3 years; some states require annual recertification. Few states do not include this most important component. Even though other providers of medical care have not been as diligent in requiring recertification, prehospital care should not give up the advances that have been made.

The length and mechanism of recertification programs prompt controversy because no definitive studies identify how recertification is best accomplished. Because of this lack of data, the standard approach is to select an arbitrary certification period and require completion of a prescribed number of continuing education hours within that period. Currently, one state requires 1 year; thirty-one states require 2 years; fifteen states require 3 years; and three states require 4 years.

The NREMT is the national registration agency. The standards set by the NREMT require a prescribed number of hours covering the primary curriculum including either BCLS or ACLS and additional subjects as dictated by specific provider level and individual local needs. The trauma component is satisfied by either the PHTLS or BTLS course. Other components of prehospital care are also included to reach the required number of hours over the 2-year NREMT registration period. Significantly the medical director must attest to satisfactory maintenance of the required psychomotor skills for the particular level of prehospital care. Most states require recertification by either a state agency or the NREMT to maintain certification. The current NREMT standards of all three levels (EMT-B, EMT-I, EMT-P) for both certification and recertification are set by a panel of nationally recognized EMS authorities with additional input from the National Association of State EMS Directors, the National Association of State EMS Training Coordinators, NAEMSP, ACEP, NAEMT, and individual representatives from many states.

An additional option for recertification is to test successfully at the conclusion of each recertification period. Passing the examination results in automatic recertification; failure precludes recertification and mandates additional training directed at reestablishing the provider's level of competence. Completion of either a targeted refresher course or an entire initial training course are acceptable options for individuals who fail the exam; however, passing a retest is eventually required.

Both skill and knowledge maintenance are critical to recertification. Currently there is no proven answer regarding what is the best way to assure that the ability to care for the patient has been maintained. However, the EMS community set a precedence from a medicolegal standpoint, if not from a scientific standpoint. Recertification and continuing education similar to that promulgated by NREMT in its reregistration process should be used until formal studies identify a better approach. In reality, medical directors decide about each provider on an individual basis because their licenses are essentially on the line each time an EMS unit rolls.

Summary

Indirect medical control is the key to establishing and maintaining a high quality EMS system; knowledgeable and dedicated physicians are necessary to provide this aspect of medical oversight. Indirect medical control is provided through the medical director, delegated assistants, and training officers representing the local EMS community. Indirect medical control is the channel for the medical community to both input and appraise the functioning of the prehospital medical care system. The bottom line of the system is to assure excellent medical care for every patient.

REFERENCES

1. American College of Emergency Physicians: Medical control of prehospital emergency medical services, *Ann Emerg Med* 11(7):68, Jul 1982.
2. American College of Emergency Physicians position paper.
3. Blum J: *Ambulance placement strategy,* Research Study, 1974, Georgia Institute of Technology.
4. Cayten CG et al: The effect of telemetry on urban prehospital cardiac care, *Ann Emerg Med* 14:976-981, 1985.
5. Committee on Trauma, American College of Surgeons: Essential equipment for ambulances. *ACS Bulletin* 68(8), 36-38, revised, May 1983.
6. Erder MH, Davidson SJ, & Cheney RA: On-line medical command in theory and practice, *Ann Emerg Med* 18(3):261-268, Mar 1989.
7. Gibson G: Measures of emergency ambulance effectiveness: unmet need and inappropriate uses, *JACEP* 6:389, 1977.
8. Holroyd BR, Knopp R, & Kallsen G: Medical control: quality assurance in prehospital care, *JAMA* 256(8):1027-1031, Aug 1986.
9. Hunt RC et al: Standing orders versus voice control, *JEMS* 26-31, Nov 1982.
10. Krentz MJ and Wainscott MP: Medical accountability, *Emerg Med Clin North Am* 8(1):17-32, Feb 1990.
11. Latessa EM: The physician medical director: a guideline for the roles and responsibilities in a prehospital advanced life support service, *J Emerg Med Serv* 6(4):46-47, Apr 1981.
12. Maio RF and Bronken T: Quality assurance in emergency medical service systems in Michigan: report of a survey, *Qual Rev Bull* 17(12):392-395, Dec 1991.
13. McSwain NE Jr: Medical control: what is it? *JACEP* 7:(3):114-116, Mar 1978.
14. McSwain NE Jr: Medical control of prehospital care, *J Trauma* 24:172, 1984 (editorial).
15. McSwain NE Jr: *Prehospital emergency medical systems and cardiopulmonary resuscitation.* In: Moore EE, Mattox KL, and Feliciano DV: *Trauma,* ed 2, Norwalk, Conn, 1991, Appleton & Lange.
16. Pons P: Medical control of prehospital care, *J Emerg Med* 1:449-450, 1984 (editorial).
17. Robinson V: Call screening targets false emergencies, *The International Chief* 47:16-18, 1981.
18. Scalice B: Abuse of EMS: is there a remedy? *Emergency* 10:51-56, 1978.
19. Skelton MB and McSwain NE Jr: A study of cognitivie and technical skill deterioration among trained paramedics, *JACEP* 6(11):436-438, Oct 1977.
20. Slovis CM et al: A priority dispatch system for emergency medical services, *Ann Emerg Med* 14:1055-1060, 1985.
21. Stewart RD et al: A computer-assisted quality assurance system for an emergency medical service, *Ann Emerg Med* 14:25-29, 1985.
22. Subcommittee on Medical Control, Committee on Emergency Medical Services: Medical control in emergency medical services systems, Washington, DC, 1981, National Academy Press.

20

Direct Medical Control

Odelia Braun, M.D., FACEP

What is direct medical control? Who does it? How much control is necessary? For which kinds of calls and whose benefit is it? These are simple questions with no clear answers. Before attempting to answer such questions, one should demonstrate whether direct medical control improves prehospital care services. Because of the difficulties inherent in data collection during prehospital care, it is difficult to define and evaluate the effectiveness of direct medical control. In addition to myriad care-related variables, prehospital care integrates multiple services and factions (that is, health and fire departments, individual hospitals, multiple levels of providers, and provider agencies), which makes it difficult to achieve the cooperation essential for good data collection. Consequently, defining and evaluating the effectiveness of direct medical control requires that EMS physicians overcome potential obstacles while embarking on controlled, scientifically rigorous analysis and evaluation of the principles and systems involved in direct control.

Origins of Direct Medical Control

Prehospital care is the provision of medical care in the field by nonphysicians who, in many states, function under the extension of a physician's license. *Direct medical control* is defined as the "direction via radio or telephone of field personnel at the scene of an emergency and en route to an emergency department."[8] The stated advantages of direct medical control include (1) formal acceptance of legal responsibility by a physician, (2) close supervision and education of prehospital care providers through prompt feedback, (3) transmission of information regarding patient condition, treatment, and progress in a uniform manner, and (4) ability to deviate (with permission) from standing orders or protocols if within the scope of the EMS system's authorized capabilities.[29] In current prehospital practice, direct medical control varies greatly among EMS systems; some mandate that field personnel contact direct medical control for every patient, and others require limited or no direct medical control.

The definition of the need for direct medical control fluctuates over time. In 1976 Boyd defined advanced life support (ALS) measures as requiring absolute physician-directed medical control (citing clinical tradition and EMS program experience as evidence), allowing that basic life support (BLS) measures represent emergency first aid that does not require strict medical supervision (physicians often remained responsible for field personnel training and actions).[4,5] Today, all medical care should be subject to direct medical control and managed by qualified and experienced EMS physicians. Therefore differentiating between BLS and ALS is now impossible. However, it is still rare for emergency medical technician-Basics (EMT-Bs) to have immediate access to physician input.

Paramedic training initially was designed to develop accurate patient assessment skills including history-taking and physical examination, and then relay the assessment to a physician to diagnose and define treatment to be provided. Because physicians could not see, hear, or examine the patient, they felt confident when the on-scene condition of the patient was described using "bedside-rounds" terminology; thus the ability to intervene immediately in patient diagnosis and treatment was retained. Direct medical control ensured that physicians assimilated field data to initiate appropriate treatment. Whether field personnel were capable of diagnosing the patient and initiating appropriate treatment was not evaluated until the late 1970s.

Prehospital care services developed in response to acute cardiac events because 50% of all patients with out-of-hospital acute myocardial infarction (MI) died during the first hour, before reaching the hospital.

Cardiologists postulated that preventing fatal dysrhythmias with early prehospital intervention might significantly impact this high early mortality rate.

In the United States the decision to staff ambulances with paraprofessionals rather than field physicians was practical; ensuring physician availability to respond quickly to all cardiac calls was neither feasible nor cost-efficient. Physicians gradually moved from direct care to supervisory and training roles. Physician-designed protocols permitted training paramedics to treat by protocol. Task-oriented competency could thus be measured and tested, and rapid training could be provided in essential skills for managing specific, common emergency problems. Protocols including clinical algorithms allowed uniformity of approach and provided a mechanism ensuring that paramedic care maintained a specified level regardless of the level of training or experience. However, algorithms are limiting because they make no provision for subtle differences in patients or diagnostic and decision-making skills of paramedics.[21]

The development of a nationwide (EMS) system in the United States was due largely to the success of these early systems. Federal funding was provided for development of EMS services, giving different local constituencies (some medical, many political) the authority to organize and control the new systems. Physician input in the implementation of the new EMS programs varied by locale as did physician control. Most EMS systems in the United States still struggle with the legacy of this history and its bureaucracy.

Initially the need for direct medical control of EMS personnel was clear, because most EMS patient care contacts were individuals with cardiac disease experiencing critical events and most field personnel were minimally trained via nonstandardized curricula. As public awareness of prehospital and emergency department services developed, their use dramatically increased. Prehospital personnel began to encounter the full spectrum of disease, and EMS was used for transportation and care of relatively minor illnesses up to 60% of the time; critical cases ultimately contributed as little as 17% of all calls.[9] By 1990 only 12% of all paramedic patient contacts had chest pain of presumed cardiac etiology, and only 7% of all chest pain calls had an acute MI.[25,49] As the severity of the illnesses declined, the value and cost-effectiveness of direct medical control became questionable.

The Base Hospital Concept

In 1979 Boyd recommended that all EMS systems develop physician-directed, hospital-based direct medical control teams responsible for remote management of patients in their jurisdiction who required direct medical control, as well as effective processes for patient care, audit, and review.[5] At the core was a base hospital responsible through its medical director for system implementation, operations, monitoring, and evaluation activities (see box on following page). The local or regional EMS agency designated the base hospital.

Boyd recommended two models for providing direct medical control via the base hospital (Figure 20-1). In the "centralized model" (Model X), medical control is provided through a single base hospital that is the sole communication link for patient care and referral in the prehospital treatment phase. In the "satellite model" (Model Y) the central base hospital is augmented by a radial configuration of associate hospitals to provide service for a larger geographic area or handle a greater workload. The satellite model is the most suitable for rural systems.[5] In both models the base or associated hospital operates by uniform policies and protocols and is responsible for referring patients to appropriate hospitals. Boyd used ALS to describe any unit that needed direct medical control; an ALS patient was one who received an advanced clinical intervention.

The following were attributes of two models:

Model X	Model Y
Centralized control	Satellite control
One hospital-based ALS team	Involvement of participating hospital-based ALS teams
Greater continuity and more consistent orders	Community is more aware and more involved in the EMS system
Potentially greater ALS team training because fewer require training	
Significant direct medical control experience	Potential for insufficient experience at directing calls
Nonresource hospital providers not involved with EMS system	Potential enhancement and support by multiple associate or receiving hospital providers
Direction may be more consistent with fewer providers	Direction more subject to interpretation of multiple providers
Potential loss of identification with greater number of ALS units	Better identification of associate or receiving hospital with respective ALS units
Better research laboratory for systems and clinical effects	
Lower requirement for communication systems designs and equipment	

Base Hospital Responsibilities

- Designate medical director
- Designate MICN coordinator if applicable
- Orient base hospital staff to the EMS system
- Coordinate network of receiving hospitals
- Provide direct medical control for treatment, triage, and transfer of all ALS patients
- Transfer all ALS patient care information to receiving facility
- Daily review of all ALS encounters
- Weekly case review sessions for prehospital and hospital teams
- Maintain system records including patient care records
- Maintain competency and certification records for physician, MICN, and paramedic personnel
- Train new EMS personnel
- Monitor paramedic field performance
- Directly observe paramedics via regular ambulance ride-alongs

From Boyd D: Emergency medical services systems development: a national initiative. *IEEE Transaction on Vehicular Technology*, VT-25(4): 104-115, 1976.

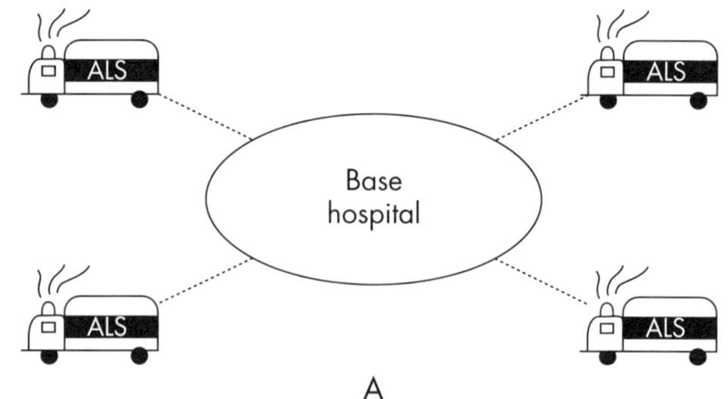

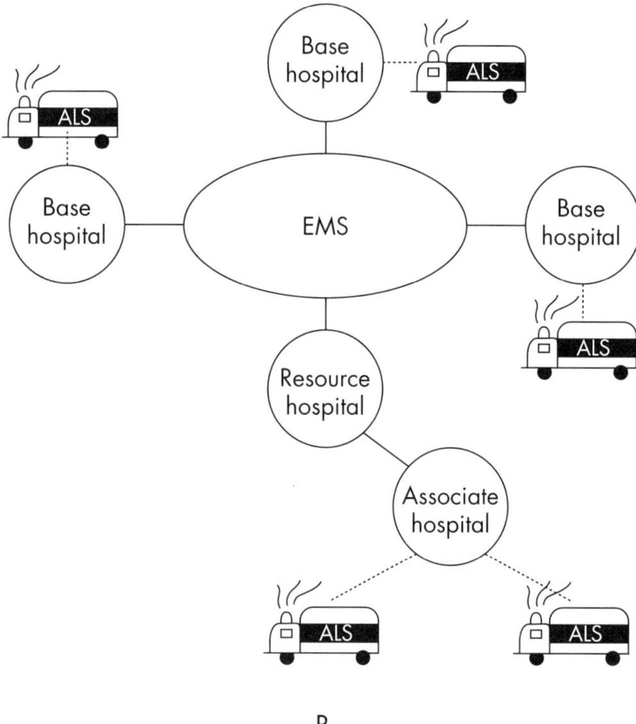

Figure 20-1. **A,** Model X: Centralized control. **B,** Model Y: Satellite control.

Direct medical control traditionally was provided from the hospital setting, but the quality of the control was determined by the provider not the setting. Because qualified physicians were not always available 24 hours a day in hospitals, alternative modes of communication were established. In some areas, remote radios were used to communicate to the field from the hospital; in others, direct medical control was established in separate communication centers external to the hospital; in still others, physician surrogates, mobile intensive care nurses (MICNs), and paramedic communicators directed field care because there were too few physicians. Thus the evolution of prehospital care first removed physicians from direct field care, and then distanced them from direct medical control.

The American College of Emergency Physicians (ACEP) first recommended guidelines for the provision of direct medical control in 1984[29]:

1. Base hospital supplies, equipment, and personnel for medical control should be located within the emergency department.
2. All requests by rescue personnel for medical direction should be promptly accommodated with an attitude of participation, responsibility, and cooperation while following established protocols.
3. Cooperation with the regional EMS system in collecting and analyzing the data necessary for evaluation will be assured.
4. Patient confidentiality will be maintained.
5. The direct physician will issue transportation instructions and hospital assignments based entirely on objective analysis of patients needs and the facilities capabilities and proximity. No effort will be made to obtain institutional or commercial advantage through the use of such transportation instructions and hospital assignments.
6. When the base hospital is acting as an agent for another hospital, information regarding the patient shall be given to that hospital in an accurate and timely manner.
7. Physicians at base hospitals should conduct regular case conferences involving the medical control physicians and EMS personnel. This identifies

problems involving both groups and provides continuing education to correct them.

Interestingly these ACEP standards were markedly less strict and specific than Boyd's, reflecting both the recognition of the various modalities for providing direct medical control and the slow progress toward a clear definition of direct medical control.

For many EMS systems the base hospital model of control is a source of concern and controversy based in part on the fear that base hospital personnel influence ambulance destination. In a study conducted in Multnomah County, Oregon, Neely et al found that the proportion of calls received by the base hospital did not differ significantly with or without direct medical control. Excluding critical cases, which were diverted to outlying community hospitals rather than the base hospital, the institution of a base hospital in that EMS system had no significant impact on ambulance destination. However, base hospitals can divert traffic; thus ensuring appropriate ambulance destination flow requires both establishing clear destination policies and monitoring these policies.

Use of Standing Orders

Whether direct medical control confers an additional benefit to the use of well-designed, conscientiously implemented protocols is controversial. Some physicians suggest that direct medical control is not necessary when well-defined medical protocols are established and followed; the physician is replaced by a physician surrogate or paramedics trained to implement standing orders without physician contact. Historically, east coast EMS systems use standing orders often; physician communication is required in few cases. West coast EMS systems typically demand extensive direct medical control, even for EMT-Bs in some areas.

The controversy is understandable. Evaluating the benefits of direct medical control is difficult because prehospital care involves multiple variable factors and most prehospital care systems perform little or no statistical analysis of outcomes. Morbidity and mortality for cardiac arrest and trauma victims are used most often to evaluate EMS system function. However, neither of these acute states benefit from direct medical control, which may actually cause harm by prolonging time to definitive therapy. To evaluate direct medical control adequately requires studies defining the types of calls likely to benefit. Such studies are scant and those available have serious limitations (see box above, right).

In 1979 Hunt et al evaluated the effect of direct medical control on a group of cardiac arrest patients in North Carolina.[23] The paramedics involved had 450 hours of training. The study included retrospective review of 100 cardiac arrest cases, in which direct medical control was established before institution of airway control with a bag-valve mask, defibrillation, or intravenous drug therapy. The review group was compared with a prospective group of 100 consecutive cardiac arrest patients for whom therapy was similar except for the addition of esophageal gastric tube airway (EGTA) for airway control and the ability to perform the advanced procedures before initiating radio contact. The resuscitation rate (defined as restoration of blood pressure and pulse on arrival at the emergency department) and hospital admission rate did not differ statistically for the two patient groups. In addition, there were improved hospital admission rates in both EMS-witnessed trauma and cardiac arrests for the paramedic group operating only under standing orders, but this was not statistically significant. Finally, although the average time on-scene remained almost identical for the two paramedic groups, these investigators postulated that advanced therapy in the standing orders group was delivered an average of 1 to 4 minutes faster than radio contact with a physician permitted.[40]

One might expect the standing orders group to perform better based on the current understanding of the need for immediate definitive therapy in cardiac and traumatic arrest. However, the magnitude of beta or Type II error in this comparison was not examined, and would in fact be large. In addition, Hunt et al did not evaluate discharge from hospital because hospital mortality might not be an appropriate measure of EMS system function; this stance differs from that of most other cardiac arrest literature. Finally, direct medical control in the EMS system studied often was provided by a physician unfamiliar with the system and paramedic capabilities. The authors therefore concluded that direct medical

Uses of Direct Medical Control

- Critical medical cases (for example, acute myocardial infarction, pulmonary edema, severe respiratory distress, hypotension of various etiologies, dysrhythmia recognition)
- Large and varied differential diagnosis (for example, chest pain, abdominal pain, allergic reaction)
- Maximization of resources (for example, pronouncing death in the field, paramedic refusal of transport)
- Medicolegal assistance (for example, patient refusal of transport, physician on scene)
- Assist in determining appropriate destination

control provided by an uninformed physician may not serve the patient as effectively as appropriate standing orders created by a knowledgeable physician dedicated to the system.

In 1983 investigators in Multnomah County, Oregon, which previously ran on standing orders, conducted a 6-month trial of direct medical control. During the study period, paramedics were required to make radio contact with the base hospital physician for all calls that required intravenous catheterization or electrocardiogram (ECG) monitoring. Direct medical control was provided 24 hours a day by physicians, but their level of expertise in prehospital care and degree of orientation to the EMS system were not stated.

During the study period the base hospital responded to 2072 calls, an average of 11.5 calls per day. Paramedics and physicians reviewed all calls in which radio contact was made and ranked the benefits and disadvantages of the contact (Table 20-1). Eighty-three percent of contacts were simple notification in compliance with the trial format; 16% involved medical consultation between paramedic and physician; 1% reflected paramedic contact to provide information, resulting in physician initiated advice. Most often this advice was simply a reminder to comply with existing standing orders, for example, to administer intravenous (IV) glucose to patients with altered mental status. Other physician-initiated orders included direction to use third line drugs in cardiac arrest cases, repeat administration of nitroglycerin or lidocaine in patients with chest pain, inject additional doses of naloxone in narcotic overdose cases, or conduct field cardioversion of conscious patients with symptomatic supraventricular tachydysrhythmias.

Physician directed instructions resulting in patient improvement were documented in two cases. (1) Respiratory and mental status improved in a case of suspected narcotic overdose when the physician ordered injection of additional doses of naloxone, and (2) cardiovascular status improved after the physician ordered cardioversion of a conscious patient with a symptomatic supraventricular tachycardia. Paramedics considered direct medical control detrimental when there was a delay in getting a physician to a radio, but such delays did not cause deterioration of the patient's clinical status during prehospital care. However, in general both paramedics and physicians felt that direct medical control is beneficial in selected cases. In addition, direct medical control was useful for teaching and quality assurance of prehospital care management, for example, (1) the written and taped documentation of advanced events provided an excellent source of teaching material for both medical issues and communications techniques, (2) the taped communications provided a useful medicolegal record, and (3) both forms of documentation reflected a central means of collecting medical care data and conducting prehospital quality assurance audits.[47]

Table 20-1 Evaluation of Benefits of Communication

	Physician Calls*		Paramedic Calls†	
	(No.)	(%)	(No.)	(%)
Call made during treatment or transport				
Of critical importance	8	0.4	8	0.9
Medically helpful	354	17	115	12
Of no immediate medical significance	707	34	257	27
Inappropriate	4	0.2	16	2
Detrimental	1	0.1	8	0.9
No evaluation	—	—	150	16
Call made after treatment or transport	998	48	391	41

Of critical importance, physician's orders had a definitive impact on patient outcome, significantly decreasing morbidity or mortality;
Medically helpful or supportive, physician indicated treatment that was not yet given, (provided triage support [DOAs, patient refusals, information on hospital facilities] or provided support for paramedic's choice of treatment, as sought by paramedic);
Of no immediate medical significance, report notification only, no physician advice was given or requested (simple hospital notification request);
Inappropriate, paramedic could have better used other sources for services (unwieldy paramedic-physician interaction caused avoidable delay in patient transport to hospital);
Detrimental, use of medical resource delayed patient's emergency care, causing notable harm to patient, (inappropriate physician's orders caused notable harm to patient).

*From 2072 physician reports.
†From 945 paramedic reviews.

One limitation of this study is that the investigators did not report the results for the early months of the trial when physicians were inexperienced at radio medical control separately.

In an editorial accompanying publication of this study the editors of the *Journal of Emergency Medicine* reflected that those who favor extensive standing orders "have much agreement in the paramedic community." They observed that in many cases the physician contact did not help the paramedic or the patient, because many physicians who provided voice control were inconsistent, ill-prepared, or poor communicators. The editors suggested that prehospital patients would be better served by use of clear, consistent, written protocols thoughtfully prepared by competent emergency medicine specialists.[19] Many physicians who provide voice control fit the editors' description. In addition, very few localities mandate the minimal training, experience, or certification required to provide direct medical control.

Physician consistency in providing direct medical control was studied in a single base hospital system in Oregon. Hedges et al reviewed all calls in which paramedics requested the use of morphine for a patient with chest pain and evaluated whether physician refusals followed consistent guidelines. They found that physicians generally approved the request, but reasons for refusal such as medical history, current medications, age, blood pressure, pulse, respiratory rate, and breath sounds were inconsistent.

In response to such findings and observations the "voice control" advocates suggested that no paramedic training program sufficiently covers every medical contingency, and the use of protocols alone risks that important symptoms will be overlooked or misread by paramedics. Furthermore, they feel that the requirement for voice control reminds paramedics that they are not free agents.[42] In fact in poorly organized systems with inadequate training and supervision of paramedics and little quality assurance or outcome measurement, direct medical control provides a monitoring mechanism that is not necessary in systems that achieve quality performance in other ways.

The controversy over concurrent direct medical control versus extensive standing orders relates to other problems encountered by EMS systems and cannot be assessed independently of the whole EMS system. Well-designed and implemented standing orders serve both paramedics and patients better than physicians inadequately trained to provide voice control. However, does direct medical control provided by knowledgeable physicians confer an additional benefit over standing orders alone? How knowledgeable must physicians be? How do they acquire the requisite knowledge when even residency trained emergency physicians often receive no formal training in direct medical control and EMS?

In a study of direct medical control in a Philadelphia EMS system, Erder and Davidson found that patient health status improved in 5.5% of those treated via direct medical control compared with 3.2% treated without direct control.[14] Similarly, paramedic compliance with prehospital protocols significantly improved (r=4.92; p=0.001) with direct medical control; only 35.8% of cases were diverted to medical investigation compared with 64% of cases without direct medical control. However, 1.3% of patients treated by direct medical control deteriorated compared with 1.1% treated without direct medical control, and both cardiac and trauma patients treated via direct medical control remained on-scene an average of 8 minutes longer. Accordingly there is a trade-off between the benefit derived from direct physician guidance and the impact of a prolonged prehospital phase. In the management of trauma patients as we presently understand it this trade-off favors reducing scene times over the potential benefits of physician guidance. In the management of medical patients, particularly those with complicated or unclear diagnoses, additional minutes on-scene might be outweighed by physician expertise in assessment and diagnosis (assuming the physician is knowledgable and familiar with direct medical control and prehospital care management).

One limitation of this study acknowledged by Erder and Davidson is that the number of critical patients was small, making it difficult to assess the impact of direct medical control on the health status of patients most likely to benefit. Their system required broad patient inclusion rules with minimal paramedic discretion. They suggested that limiting patient inclusion rules would shorten scene times and assign direct medical control to the patients most likely to benefit from physician intervention, thereby optimizing the potential benefits of direct medical control. However, this leaves the determination of the need for direct medical control to paramedics.

Hoffman et al studied the incidence of deviation from protocol among paramedics and base hospital personnel, postulating that radio contact would be unnecessary if patients received standard therapy based exclusively on algorithms.[20] They studied patients with four common prehospital complaints—abdominal pain, syncope, seizure, and altered mental status—based on the belief that treatment of each group would be similar. Of 659 patients only 13 required unanticipated therapy, and all 13 had abnormal vital signs, diaphoresis, respiratory distress, or a second prominent symptom. The investigators did not evaluate whether paramedic interventions were appropriate to the patient presentation or whether the intervention impacted outcome with and without protocols being followed. Their finding of interest was that reducing the number of radio contacts significantly curtails the costs of running a base hospital.

In a review of the field records for all paramedic responses from 1974 to 1975, Diamond et al found that 56% of all patients were noncritical (normal vital signs and minor complaints requiring minimal or no treatment), and 13% reflected serious but non life-threatening medical problems. Although most of the latter required little or no intervention, certain diagnoses proved difficult for paramedics. In patients with hypovolemic symptoms who presented with cardiorespiratory symptoms such as shortness of breath, dizziness, weakness, and tachydysrythmias, paramedics focused on the cardiac evaluation rather than providing volume expansion and rapid transport. Similarly, patients who presented with the combination of hypovolemic symptoms and abdominal pain typically were not recognized as having a potential aortic aneurysm.[9] Advocates of direct medical control say that such difficult diagnoses are more readily recognized by experienced physicians who then intervene appropriately. Proponents of standing orders say that paramedic diagnostic abilities can be cultivated and honed via education, skills assessment, and various forms of feedback and continuing education.

Peacock et al reviewed 263 consecutive patients in cardiac arrest to determine (1) the accuracy of diagnosis of presenting rhythm by paramedics and medical control physicians and (2) the appropriateness of the treatment rendered. Treatment errors by paramedics were identified in 46% of cases. Errors were attributed to misdiagnosis of rhythm (6%), failure to establish an IV (18%), failure to secure an airway (6.4%), equipment failure (n=2), minor deviation from protocol (14%), provision of the wrong treatment (6%), unrecognized ventricular fibrillation not treated with defibrillation (n=9), ventricular tachycardia (n=3), and bradycardia not treated in accordance with appropriate protocol (n=3).[34]

In the Alameda County, California, EMS system the institution of standing orders for advanced calls decreased scene time by an average of 3.5 minutes when compared with base hospital contact. Paramedic compliance with protocols remained high (97%) during a period when only standing orders were required.[37] However, Gausche et al found that when base hospital contact was made, vital signs were more likely to be taken in all age groups.[16]

More research is required to resolve this question. A key failure of existing studies is that the potential effectiveness of direct voice control cannot be adequately tested without assuring that it is provided by experienced, well-trained physicians or physician surrogates. No one would be surprised that an uninformed, inexperienced, untrained physician adds nothing, yet such voice control is commonplace in many systems. To adequately test the hypothesis that direct voice control is beneficial a study must be conducted in an EMS system that guarantees and documents quality direct medical control. Then "critical medical cases" that are most likely to benefit from direct medical control can be carefully studied. Ideally the study design would be prospective and the runs randomized to direct or no direct medical control. A large study population also would be required, because the number of patients in which a change in outcome is expected is small under even the best of conditions. Conclusions about lack of impact (beta or Type II error) cannot be safely made from small numbers.

Telemetry

Telemetry is the "transmission of an ECG strip over one of eight dedicated ultra-high frequency (UHF) pairs from a paramedic-staffed ambulance to a medically staffed operation center."[38] Because the initial goal of prehospital care was to prevent sudden death in patients dying of MI, the focus was to treat the dysrhythmias that occurred early in the course of an MI. Telemetry was the mechanism by which physicians diagnosed dysrhythmias so field personnel could treat them; the assumption being that dysrhythmias could not be accurately diagnosed by field personnel. In 1971 this assumption was tested in Brighton, England, where the only procedures allowed for the mobile coronary unit were defibrillation and oxygenation. "Ambulance men" received approximately 40 hours of lectures on acute coronary care from cardiologists. On review of the telemetry tapes the ambulance men were found to have correctly diagnosed 91% of 620 dysrhythmias, and, excluding sinus rhythm, they correctly diagnosed 86% of all dysrhythmias. Eight cases of ventricular fibrillation occurred with the ambulance men on-scene; all such patients were resuscitated, and five lived to be discharged. This is the earliest report on the ability of field personnel to diagnose and treat dysrhythmias. These field personnel had the fewest hours of training of all subsequent reports and were the most successful in diagnosing dysrhythmias.

In 1969, Nagel et al in Dade County, Florida, believed prehospital diagnosis and medical control was the responsibility of the in-house physician. Once again the focus was almost entirely on the prehospital patient with acute myocardial ischemia and infarction. Nagel perceived the ambulance unit as analogous to the coronary care unit (CCU), in which nurses perform procedures previously conducted only by physicians; that is, paramedics in the field were providing treatment previously administered only by physicians. Later, CCU nurses began to diagnose and treat acute, life-threatening dysrhythmias without physician contact. This development is paralleled in field care; the paramedic needs to operate independently of ECG or voice control in an acute emergency.

Telemetry and direct medical control evolved early as mandatory functions and were relatively efficient because field teams were fairly unsophisticated and minimally trained. Now, some EMS systems have field personnel with up to 2200 hours of training, that operate in systems in which acute cardiac patients are a distinct minority. In systems using physician surrogates, direct medical control often is provided by individuals with levels of expertise no greater than that of the paramedics in the field. In such situations, direct medical control provides no more benefit than the opinion of another paramedic on-scene; this scenario renders telemetry optional, and useful only in selected cases. Initially, telemetry was designed for and applied to populations having a relatively high incidence of significant dysrhythmias; it is currently applied to large populations with noncardiac disease. This practice may result in a higher incidence of dysrhythmias that are clinically insignificant, which may increase the incidence of unnecessary and potentially harmful interventions.

Providing telemetry capability is expensive, raising the question of whether it provides a clinically and financially justifiable benefit. This question, like many others in EMS, has not been satisfactorily studied. Pozen felt that routine telemetry transmission improves patient care in a paramedic system by (1) improving diagnostic skill in recognizing patients with possible acute ischemic heart disease, (2) increasing paramedic accuracy in interpreting ECG rhythms, particularly the life-threatening dysrhythmias (LTAs), and (3) broadening the scope of enforcing paramedic compliance with medical oversight.[38]

Early studies that showed a low rate of diagnostic accuracy by EMT-Bs in New Haven, Connecticut, suggested that telemetric medical control would have considerable impact on the process of care.[6] However, as paramedic programs became more sophisticated the diagnostic skills of paramedics and EMT-Bs improved. Two studies, one from Boston using only EMT-Bs and the other from Cape Cod using EMT-Bs and paramedics, demonstrated 60% diagnostic accuracy in determining heart disease; high false positive rates were 40% and false negative rates were less than 5%, which is excellent.[30] Paramedics erred in diagnosing cardiac disease when it was not present 40% of the time (similar to physicians' false positive rate when admitting potential MIs to a CCU); however, less than 5% of patients who truly had cardiac disease were incorrectly diagnosed (similar to physicians' false negative rate). Whether telemetry improves these rates is questionable.

Pozen also stated that sufficient evidence showed that the paramedic who correctly recognized and appropriately provided treatment for LTAs increased the probability of a good outcome.[2] He defined LTAs as ventricular fibrillation, ventricular tachycardia, premature ventricular contractions exceeding four per minute, bradycardia (fewer than 40 beats per minute), hemodynamically significant bradycardia at 40 to 70 beats per minute, and second degree or greater heart block.

The incidence of LTAs in an EMS system varies. Early in EMS, when ambulances were sent only to suspected cardiac patients, the incidence of LTAs was high; in 1977 80% were reported in Belfast.[33] Later the incidence of LTAs in prehospital patients varied from 12.9% in routinely-monitored patients to 21% of patients with chest pain in Nassau County and 32% of patients with chest pain in Baltimore.[26,41] The latter study found the incidence of LTAs in patients with ischemia but without infarction was the same as that observed in patients with documented MIs. The incidence of LTAs has not been reported recently, but because the volume of EMS use is steadily increasing and the incidence of heart disease is declining, it is expected that the current figures are even lower. Unexamined factors include whether LTAs are truly life-threatening and whether patients benefit from treatment. For example, premature ventricular contractions (PVC) often are perceived and treated as LTAs; however, in the absence of ischemic heart disease, PVCs are benign. Treatment could conceivably increase rather than decrease morbidity.

Deciding if a particular EMS system would benefit from using telemetry to enhance management of LTAs requires considerable statistical information. Telemetry can be analyzed for sensitivity, specificity, and positive and negative predictive value as can any other diagnostic test. Because the usefulness of the test depends on the incidence of significant dysrhythmias and the skills of prehospital personnel and direct medical control physicians, analysis must be performed separately for each EMS system. The number of cases in the system of true possible ischemic heart disease including MI and angina is determined. Paramedics should correctly suspect that 95% of these patients have ischemia and treat them accordingly. A 5% false negative rate is equal to emergency physician performance. Then the numbers of all dysrhythmias and LTAs occurring in transported patients with suspected ischemic disease are also determined. This requires that all patients with ischemic heart disease be continuously monitored by telemetry. The paramedic records any diagnosis or dysrhythmia and the treatment. The direct medical control provider does the same. Later an objective, blinded, emergency physician or cardiologist reviews all tapes and records the diagnosis and recommended therapy. Paramedics and their direct medical control decide on an acceptable error rate. Based on a consensus of the local medical community, telemetry is indicated if the paramedic error rate in diagnosis and therapy exceeded a predetermined rate. Similarly the adequacy of direct medical control is determined by an acceptable error rate for the physician. The false positive rate of diagnosis should be analyzed and evaluated, because erroneous treatment of dysrhythmias is not benign. Such a study would provide conclusions about the benefits conferred by direct medical control with and without telemetry (see box below).

A serious question arose in Pozen's study of the interaction between direct medical control physicians and paramedics during ambulance transport of 288 "seriously ill" cardiac patients. His disturbing results suggest that physician consultation on telemetry strips may not be beneficial because of inaccurate diagnosis by the direct medical control physician. Although the participating physicians had backgrounds ranging from emergency medicine to general surgery to internal medicine, all had extensive experience in emergency departments. All telemetry strips taken during each patient encounter were reviewed independently by a board certified cardiologist unaware of the diagnosis or treatment. Of the rhythms, 35% were incorrectly classified by both the paramedic and the telemetry physician. Also, 35% of potentially life-threatening dysrhythmias (PVCs, ventricular tachycardias (VT), ventricular fibrillation (VF), agonal rhythm) were misclassified. Patients with potential LTAs were diagnosed and treated correctly in only 39% of cases, whereas 64% of those without LTAs were correctly diagnosed and treated. This difference is highly significant. Potential explanations for the poor performance of the direct medical control physicians include (1) the cardiologist read a telemetry strip that may or may not have correlated with the monitor or strip read by the control physician and (2) although the authors state that "persistent artifact for any specific patient was not a problem," the frequency with which sinus rhythm was misdiagnosed by medical control as VT/VF (4 of 72 cases) and the frequent discrepancy on reading PVCs (18 of 44 cases read by medical control as having PVCs were diagnosed as "something else" by the cardiologist) are significant. The basis of most errors was artifact, which is endemic to telemetry. However, these errors demonstrate the need to have experienced physicians reviewing telemetry. Telemetry cannot confer an additional benefit to the system if those providing direct medical control do not have competent telemetry interpretation skills.

Cayton and associates in Philadelphia performed a 3-year controlled trial evaluating the efficacy of direct medical control provided with and without telemetry. Medical radio contact was initiated after immediate emergency measures (CPR, defibrillation, extrication) were instituted. The direct medical control physicians were second year, internal medicine residents; full-time emergency department attending staff provided back-up. Overall, telemetry did not affect the paramedics' ability to interpret rhythm strips in the test or field situations. Paramedics using telemetry spent more time in the field with patients than paramedics not using telemetry. The survival rate of patients in ventricular fibrillation was not significantly affected by the use of telemetry. However, using matched telemetry strips, direct medical control physicians were significantly more accurate than paramedics. This is the first paper to establish that direct medical control physicians are more accurate in rhythm strip interpretation; after Pozen's earlier reports this was a welcome finding. Cayton's conclusion is particularly important because the results involved "less significant" rhythms. There were not enough "more difficult" rhythm strips to analyze, but the difference in

Factors Affecting Volume of Direct Medical Control

- Demographics of EMS call volume
- Incidence of critical disease seen in the system
- Incidence of significant arrhythmias
- Incidence of misdiagnosis or incorrect treatment of critical cases
- Expertise offered by those providing direct medical control
- Requirements for contact mandated by medical director

performance would be even greater if the rhythms were more complex. The authors recommended that EMS medical directors test paramedics to determine which life-threatening dysrhythmias are the most difficult to interpret. If special education sessions in recognition and detection of these dysrhythmias do not improve interpretation, then telemetry can be used.[7]

In an accompanying editorial, Stewart stated that the small number of telemetry strips (214 in the 2-year study) made it difficult to rule out telemetry as a learning tool.[45] He further stated that he did not expect use of telemetry to affect the survival of patients in ventricular fibrillation, but that telemetry would affect patients with rapid supraventricular or ventricular dysrhythmias because identification of the rhythm may influence therapy. The value of telemetry might be more apparent if these specific rhythm disturbances were studied selectively.

Erder and Davidson of Philadelphia suggested that the incidence of telemetry use may determine its potential efficacy.[13] In the study by Cayton and in one by Hitt the use rates for telemetry were low. To assess the efficacy of equipment, an acceptable level of technical ability must either be assumed or specified. For example, if the telemetry equipment in Philadelphia had been easier to carry, more reliable, or faster to operate, the incidence of its use could have been higher, and its effectiveness in improving the quality of care could have been more apparent. Hitt felt that the technical efficacy of the equipment was so low that underuse precluded evaluation of the impact on survival.[12]

In the early 1980s the cost of telemetry was estimated to be $9000 per base hospital for equipment and $7500 per ambulance.[10,19,27,38] An appropriate use rate must be determined before cost per strip can be determined and the impact of telemetry on outcome must be determined before a cost-benefit analysis is performed. To date, such an analysis has not been performed for EMS systems.

The discussion of telemetry focuses on whether well-trained but unsupervised paramedics can correctly diagnose and initiate therapy for significant dysrhythmias in the field. In 1979 Berezin et al[4] found that paramedics incorrectly diagnosed dysrhythmias (40% of which were life-threatening) in 24% of patients and incorrectly treated 42% of patients. The training of these paramedics was not stated.[3] Studies evaluating the ability of field personnel to select patients for monitoring and to diagnose a patient's condition or dysrhythmias still have not been conducted. Consequently a vital piece of information in the evaluation of telemetry use for direct medical control is missing. In 1981 Jacobs reported disagreement between physicians and EMT-Bs in the diagnosis of 33% of potential cardiac patients, 32% of poison patients, and 35% of psychiatric patients. The overall congruence between the physicians' and EMT-Bs' assessments was 81.1%.[24]

The discussion of telemetry also focuses on the ability of paramedics to select patients for monitoring. In 1977 Pozen found that providers with 171 hours of training poorly selected patients for cardiac monitoring. He found that 47 of 71 patients later diagnosed with acute ischemic disease received ECG monitoring, and 24 did not. A subsequent, similar study showed that EMT-Bs trained for 81 hours underdiagnosed MI patients at a rate of 41%, acute ischemia 63%, and pulmonary edema 52%.[41] In a later study, Pozen showed that EMT-Bs reduced their false negative rate to less than 5% by using telemetry in patients with suspected ischemic heart disease.[38]

In 1978 Pozen showed that EMT-Bs failed to follow through with correct treatment of patients with suspected MIs in 41% of cases, suggesting a need for greater direct medical control.[39] In 1987 Wasserberger et al documented that overall paramedic compliance to protocol was 94%.[48] Similarly, Peacock et al found that paramedics correctly identified the presenting rhythm in cardiac arrest in 84% of cases, and their direct medical control physicians were correct in 89% of cases.[34]

Provision of Direct Medical Control

Medical oversight is provided with varying expertise and directness. The continuum includes care provided with standing orders only, direct medical control from non-physicians, direct medical control from non-physicians for noncritical cases, with eventual physician assistance, direct medical control from physicians after standing orders are applied up to a specified point, and direct medical control by physicians for all procedures. Few systems require the latter. The most common form is direct medical control provided by a physician after field personnel implement a set of standing orders, including some advanced interventions. All forms of direct medical control evolved through historical precedent, and they are vigorously defended by local special interests and bureaucracies that often have little or no scientific basis to substantiate them (see box on p. 206).

Prehospital care began with direct medical control by physicians for all care. However, as systems grew, many could not or would not find physicians to continue providing supervision. As a result the search began for direct medical control personnel

Continuum of Direct Medical Control

- Standing orders only, no direct medical control
- Direct medical control by non-physicians
- Direct medical control by non-physicians, physician assistance on critical calls
- Direct medical control by physicians, after standing orders
- Direct medical control by physicians on all calls

that were more available and less costly, but also less trained than physicians.

In 14 states it is legal for individuals other than physicians to provide direct medical control. Non-physician direct medical control usually is conducted by either MICNs trained to direct prehospital field personnel or paramedic communicators. Typically, MICNs are not required to obtain immediate physician agreement before issuing orders, whereas paramedic communicators are. MICNs may or may not be required to obtain a physician signature on orders. Paramedic communicators are rarely permitted to operate independently; rather, they act as screeners, calling for physician assistance when field care beyond standing orders is needed. In most areas, paramedic communicators function primarily in other capacities such as quality control officers.

A crucial question is whether non-physician personnel provide effective direct medical control. Typically, they are used where direct medical control is mandatory for all sophisticated interventions, and sophisticated physicians need not be involved for simple procedures. Rather than use standing orders, such systems believe that this method decreases errors made by selected groups (for example, "new," "minimally trained," "poorly trained," or "poorly functioning" personnel).

Some fail to see how a non-physician operating from a set of protocols provides any benefit to another non-physician using the same protocols. Prehospital field personnel commonly complain that when MICNs or other non-physicians are used, physicians abdicate their responsibilities. Physicians consequently become inexperienced and uncomfortable with providing field direction; when asked to intervene, they are unfamiliar with the process, as well as the capabilities of field personnel.

Qualifications of Personnel

The qualifications of physicians providing direct medical control are another issue addressed. In 1981 Dinerman et al stated that physicians providing direct medical control should be at least (1) experienced in emergency medicine, (2) appropriately trained in prehospital protocols, (3) familiar with EMS personnel capabilities, and (4) aware of regional critical care centers.[11] Holroyd et al echoed these criteria and added that the direct control physician should possess "knowledge of the local EMS system design, goals, and operation." California ACEP, the state of South Carolina, and groups from other parts of the country developed their own "base hospital physician" courses that emphasize the scenario approach and the legal aspects of prehospital care. To be useful in a particular jurisdiction these generic courses require the addition of material relative to local and state EMS laws, policies, procedures, and protocols (see box below).

Certain locales instituted specific education requirements for initial and continuing education of the physicians providing direct medical control. In Alameda County, California, direct medical control must be initiated before most sophisticated procedures, and a defined course of training is mandated for all direct medical control physicians. All emergency department physicians employed by a base hospital must complete certification requirements for providing direct medical control within 90 days of employment. Prerequisites for certification include current certification in ACLS, completion of a 16-hour base hospital physician course, 8 hours of field observation experience, a review of the physician's first 10 calls, and the successful completion of both a skill and a written exam. The 2-day base hospital physician course includes a 4-hour lecture introducing the physician to the system. Experienced paramedics provide a field perspective for two hours. The skills test (consisting of six simulated runs) is the backbone of the course. On the second day the physician completes the skills test and a written exam that

Criteria for Providing Direct Medical Control

Background

- Understand EMS system design and operation
- Experience in prehospital emergency care
- Understand administrative and legislative arenas of EMS

Routine active participation in

- Base station radio control
- Emergency department patient management
- Prehospital personnel training
- Medical audit of prehospital personnel

covers six broad clinical areas. Physicians are required to recertify biannually by completing an 8-hour course. To retain their certification, physicians also must complete 10 calls and attend two formal tape review sessions per year.[35]

Few EMS systems demand such stringent and specific requirements for direct medical control physicians; most make no demands at all. One of the strongest recommendations made at the 1987 National Association of EMS Physicians (NAEMSP) conference was the development of a generic course of training for direct medical control. Also recommended was required training for advanced cardiac life support (ACLS) and advanced trauma life support (ATLS) including an expanded prehospital component. However, making such courses mandatory may be beyond the jurisdiction of the local EMS medical director, and they do not assure any particular level of competence. The lack of an objective oversight agency to supervise conflicting special interests is a common woe of EMS. Another problem with mandatory requirements is that interested physicians are so scarce in many areas that it is impractical to require any qualifications at all.

In areas where nurses legally serve as "medical radio operators" and provide direction to field personnel the requirements typically include a 100-hour course in the medical, legal, and procedural aspects of prehospital care. The nurse must achieve ACLS certification and participate in a certain number of appropriate ambulance ride-alongs. These MICNs are usually audited on initial calls (10 to 20); to maintain certification they must participate in a given number of calls per month. Additionally there are formal tape review and continuing education requirements. Systems with strict and specific criteria for MICNs often have no physician requirements, as if the ability to provide adequate direct medical control is innate in physicians.

Legal Issues

In Illinois the emergency physicians rendering direct medical control generally functions under the medical oversight and delegated authority of the project medical director. They are subject to the hospital's agreement to participate in the EMS system and must follow the protocols, policies, and procedures established by the system. Emergency physicians rendering direct medical control are generally bound by administrative and medical treatment policies and procedures established by the system. When their judgment differs from the established policies and procedures, emergency physicians face the dilemma; they can either assert independent medical judgment (and be potentially liable for violating the standards of the system) or follow established policies and procedures (and be potentially liable for medical misjudgment). Systems should have policies and procedures that address the need for uniform application of the system protocols, as well as provide an "escape clause" for use when compelling circumstances of the case require independent medical judgment.[15]

Direct medical control physicians may be held liable for prehospital care rendered by EMS personnel through "vicarious liability," because a master-servant relationship exists.[15]

Minors or patients impaired by alcohol, drugs, psychiatric disorders, trauma, or a medical condition that affects reasonable judgment may not validly refuse care. The direct control physician can assist. Emergency physicians for their own benefit and that of the emergency providers, should extensively document all efforts made on behalf of the patient by thoroughly describing them over the radio, presuming such communication is recorded, to preserve evidence.[15]

When a person accesses the EMS system and requests treatment, a decision by the direct medical control physician to deny treatment may be a violation of federal law. The law indicates that the examination conducted by providers is not sufficient to meet the obligation for a screening examination. Violation of the law (COBRA 9121) carries a fine of up to $50,000 for both the physician and the hospital.[15]

Physicians and their surrogates providing direct medical control must be cautious about confidentiality. Patient names or other identifying information should not be transmitted over radio channels, because of scanners tuned to emergency frequencies.[15]

Because policies and protocols are evidence of standards of care, direct medical control physicians and surrogates should be updated often regarding changes in the EMS system; they should have a policy manual immediately available for consultation if requested to provide advice or direction.

Providers and Patients Requiring Direct Medical Control

As the public's use of EMS has grown the proportion of truly life-threatening calls has declined. Increasing costs and financial pressures make it desirable to spend resources and professional time only on calls that actually require direct medical control.

Boyd et al estimated that 80% of calls EMS units respond to are nonemergent, 15% are truly emergent, and 5% are critical.[5] In their review of 2152 consecutive paramedic responses, Diamond found that 56% of all runs were not critical (that is, with normal vital signs, minor complaints, and minimal treatment) and an additional 27% had non life-threatening but serious medical problems that required minimal intervention. A breakdown of the diagnoses in this latter group included overdose (7%), syncope (6.4%), seizures (5%), CVAs (2%), pregnancy (1.7%), psychiatric episode or disorder (1.1%), hypoglycemia (1.1%), and coma (1%). The remaining 17% were critical including possible MI (9.2%), cardiac arrest (5.6%), major trauma (2.6%), DOA (1%), and nontraumatic hemorrhage (0.4%).[9]

Many EMS physicians agree that direct medical control is indicated for critical cases, which comprise 17 to 25% of all calls; however, they disagree about the degree and timing, especially in cases of cardiac arrest and major trauma. The 56 to 80% of patients in the noncritical realm may not require direct medical control, depending on the training level of the prehospital personnel. Whether direct control is necessary or beneficial for the 15 to 27% of patients considered to have serious but non life-threatening disorders is a source of ongoing debate.

There is general agreement that direct medical control be initiated when (1) there is need to deviate from established protocols, (2) optional drugs or procedures are being contemplated, (3) field care personnel need physician assistance, (4) a physician surrogate needs physician assistance, (5) field personnel feel that the patient requires intervention, but the patient is refusing transport, or (6) there is disagreement between field care personnel and the physician surrogate. Additionally there is debate that direct medical control is indicated for the following types of calls: (1) resuscitation calls, (2) pronouncement of death in the field, (3) multivictim incidents requiring triage, (4) interference from other public safety officers or physician on-scene, (5) childbirth, (6) patients in shock with blood pressure less than 90 mm Hg, and (7) patients in severe respiratory distress. Some physicians also believe that direct medical control should be initiated when chest pain or possible MI presents. Others add to this list pediatric cases, falls from heights greater than 10 feet, certain types of serious overdoses such as tricyclic antidepressants, and certain types of trauma. Additionally, direct medical control sometimes assists with calls that do not result in transport of the patient, because the paramedic does not deem the call worthy or the patient refuses transport. In some states and locales, direct medical control must be initiated at any time certain procedures or treatments are contemplated. Those procedures often include minor interventions such as establishing an IV line or cardiac monitoring, thereby resulting in high-volume radio traffic.

Evolving roles for direct medical control include (1) assisting with diagnosis of ischemic chest pain (to determine candidacy for 12-lead ECG), (2) assisting with the interpretation of 12-lead ECG data, (3) defining candidacy for thrombolytic therapy and initiating it, and (4) initiating prehospital use of neuromuscular blocking agents.[1, 17,46]

Before deciding the extent of direct control necessary in a particular system, the volume of each type of call is evaluated. A review of the field personnel's ability to diagnose critical disease correctly dictates how much direct medical control is required. These decisions require good data and good indirect medical control. If those administering the system have accurate and detailed information about field activity and act to maintain high quality care, then direct medical control is less essential and thus used less often. Because most systems in this country do not have such information and quality assurance, direct medical control including physician observation in the field serves as a primary mechanism of quality control (see Table 20-1).

Direct medical control is useful in assessing patients who wish to be left at the scene against the advice of the providers. In one study an additional 33% of patients agreed to be transported following physician consultation.[44] In this system, 10.2% of direct medical control calls or 1.5% of system calls were for such patients.

There is an inverse correlation between how frequently physicians actually provide direct medical control and how frequently radio contact is required; that is, systems that use physician surrogates require more radio contact. This is particularly ironic because, in these systems, prehospital personnel often consult a person with expertise no greater than their own. The premise is that the quantity of contact compensates for its lack of quality or depth.

Recently, concern has increased that EMT-Bs have been neglected in the whole medical oversight discussion. Medical oversight at the EMT-B level is as desirable as at the paramedic level, although it is rarely legally required. It may be even more essential, because EMT-Bs transport large numbers of patients and have minimal skills in recognizing the seriously ill. Because of trends toward developing new levels of training and skills for prehospital care providers, the need for comprehensive, stringent medical oversight is crucial.[22] This is particularly true when minimally trained personnel use powerful modalities such as defibrillation. Indeed the new DOT EMT-B curriculum assumes that the providers will be subject to medical oversight and have access to direct medical control.

In California, medical oversight is mandatory for all services that provide automated external defibrillation. At question is whether direct medical control should be available for the following type of transport. EMT-Bs are transporting a stable patient, but during transport, the patient becomes severely diaphoretic and clutches his or her chest. Proponents of direct medical control suggest that a physician should expedite the appropriate course of action and choose the correct course of action. Others counter that "for any emergency the EMT-Bs should divert to the nearest hospital." However, prehospital care personnel unfamiliar with critical situations may not have adequate skills to recognize the emergency and decide to divert. What is obvious in retrospect often is not in obvious mid-crisis, when the decision to divert from a predesignated plan is crucial. First Responders and other prehospital providers obviously require medical oversight; they may also require direct medical control.

Sample Systems

There are many systems for the provision of direct medical control. Those that follow appear to be highly effective.

New York City

MDs only, single communication center (Figure 20-2). Since 1984 most direct medical control in the New York City 9-1-1 EMS system has been conducted from a centralized communication center at EMS headquarters. The communication center is staffed by a 24-hour attending physician who provides direct medical control and advises all prehospital units. Attending physicians have significant emergency medicine experience, most are board-certified in emergency medicine. Following initial orientation and examination, each physician works an 8-hour shift. Experienced paramedics who manage the communications equipment and assist with quality assurance work with the physician. Approximately 100 calls are processed each day. In New York City, paramedics operate with extensive standing orders; only two out of ten paramedic calls require phone or radio contact. A medical director of the telemetry center oversees the physicians providing direct medical control. Of the 30 to 40 calls received during every 8 hours, approximately 50% are paramedic requests to surpass the standing orders. The other 50% involve transport decisions, triage, and pronouncement. The communication center handles several calls at once, but if too many calls come in, they may be patched out to "base hospitals" that provide a secondary source for direct medical control. Radio contact is mandatory in calls such as nontransports involving patients less than 5 or more than 70 years of age, calls that keep units on-scene longer than 20 minutes, and implementation of optional standing orders. The receiving hospitals are notified by direct medical control of incoming patients only in specific cases such as cardiac arrest or major trauma or if the crew requests notification. Several private hospital-based units receive direct medical control from their individual hospital-based medical directors.

Seattle, Washington

MDs only, single base hospital (Figure 20-3). In Seattle, direct medical control is provided by physicians through a single base hospital. These "Medic 1

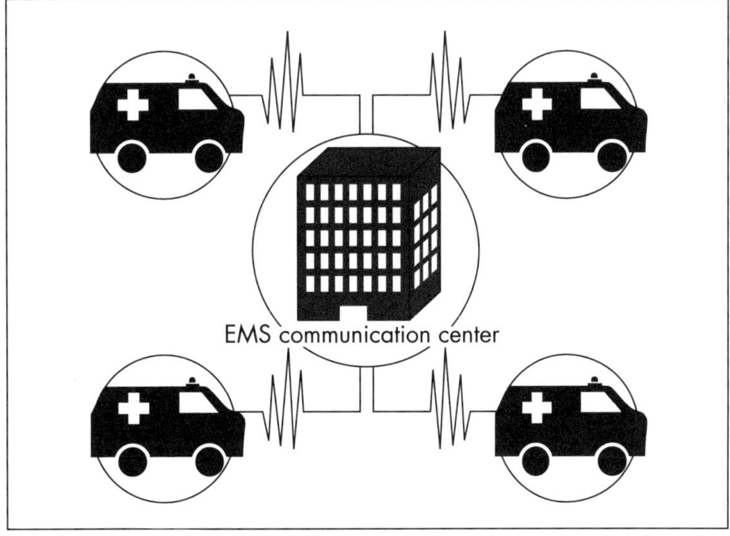

Figure 20-2. New York: Physician-directed medical control only. Centralized communication center at EMS headquarters.

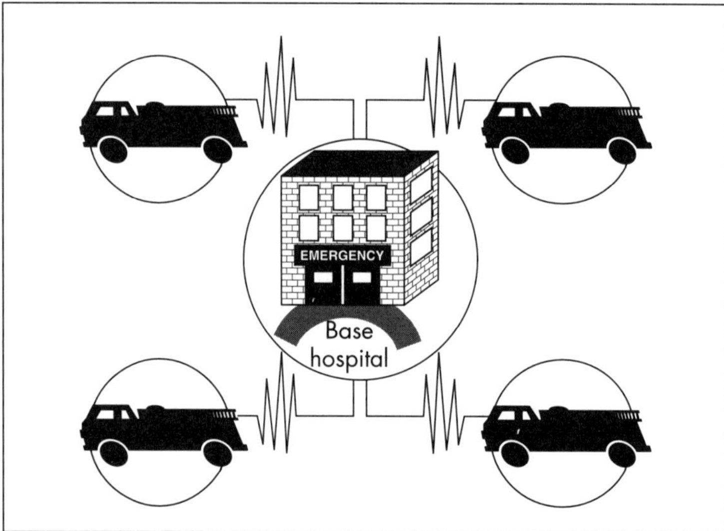

Figure 20-3. Seattle: Physician-directed medical control only, through a single base hospital.

Docs" are rotating medical and surgical residents, and the deputy medical director of the Medic 1 Program provides radio backup 24 hours a day. The base hospital receives approximately 35 calls each day. Medic 1 physicians undergo a 4-hour orientation to general protocols and ride-along with paramedics for two, 4-hour shifts before initiation of their duties. The three sets of standing orders in Seattle include ventricular fibrillation, asystole, and hypovolemic shock. All other advanced procedures are initiated through communication with direct medical control. Unsuccessful cardiac resuscitations are pronounced by direct medical control physicians. All patients refusing care and all patients experiencing chest pain require direct medical control contact. The physician notifies the receiving facility of incoming ambulance traffic. The deputy medical director obtains follow-up information on all contacts. This follow-up information is provided to the paramedics and direct medical control physicians on a 24-hour basis.

Pittsburgh, Pennsylvania

MDs only, single communication center, MD field supervision (Figure 20-4). In Pittsburgh, direct medical control is provided by physicians carrying portable radios; communications are centralized in the Center for Emergency Medicine. The physicians are emergency medicine residents with a curriculum on direct medical control, and they have faculty backup on all calls. The Center handles 25 to 30 calls a day. Any advanced procedure necessitates physician contact. Physicians often provide additional direct medical control by going to the scene of calls such as cardiac arrests, multiple alarm fires, gunshots, stab wounds, hypotension, respiratory failure, ethical dilemmas, and disasters. Such events occur approximately 4 times a day, and attending physicians travel to the scene in specially marked vehicles with lights-and-sirens. Physicians carry additional drugs and equipment, and they can provide additional emergency interventions including the use of ketamine, magnesium, and succinylcholine. Receiving hospitals are notified of all transports.

Milwaukee, Wisconsin

MDs and paramedic communicators, single base hospital (Figure 20-5). Direct medical control in Milwaukee is provided by physicians from a single base hospital, although paramedic communicators act as screening and quality assurance mechanisms. The use of standing orders is limited to cases of cardiac arrest, hypoglycemia, and major trauma (call for notification only). Paramedics initiate IV fluids, airway management, and PASG via standing orders for trauma. For calls that require IV fluids, oxygen, telemetry, dextrose or naloxone, paramedics call the base hospital and give this information to the paramedic communicator, then the paramedic communicator calls the receiving hospital with the patient information. For more critical calls the paramedic communicator notifies the physician, then the physician initiates orders and calls the receiving facility. Direct medical control is provided by junior or senior emergency medicine residents with the backup of an

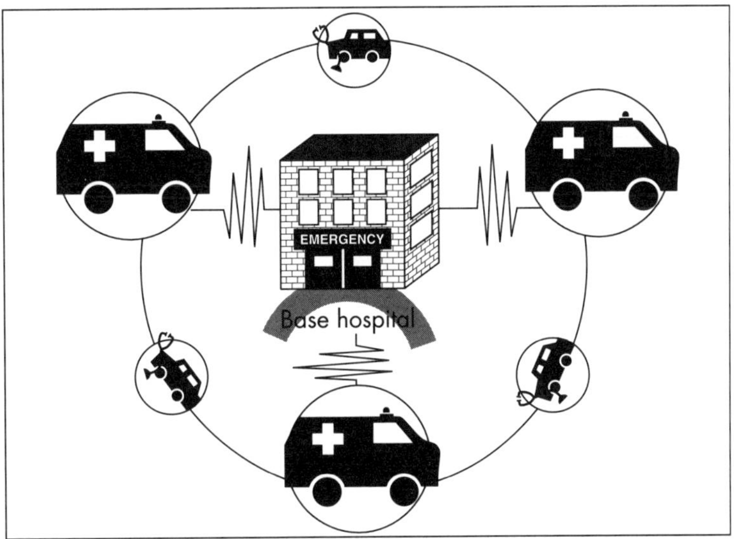

Figure 20-4. Pittsburgh: Physician-directed medical control. Communications centralized in the Center for Emergency Medicine.

attending physician. The residents receive direct medical control and EMS orientation lectures, and are required to go on three or four ride-alongs. Physicians attend to approximately 10 calls each day. Paramedic communicators are notified any time an ambulance is sent and they provide information to the medical director on both paramedic and base hospital physician function. Follow-up information on all calls involving physicians is obtained by the paramedic communicator. The receiving facility is called 2 hours after the patient arrived and diagnosis, disposition, and medical record number are obtained. A follow-up record is created and attached to the direct medical control record to permit further follow-up as necessary.

Chicago, Illinois

MDs and MICNs, central and associate base hospitals (Figure 20-6). In Chicago, direct medical control is provided by physicians and MICNs from four central base hospitals. Because the call volume is extremely large, each base hospital appoints two or three asso-

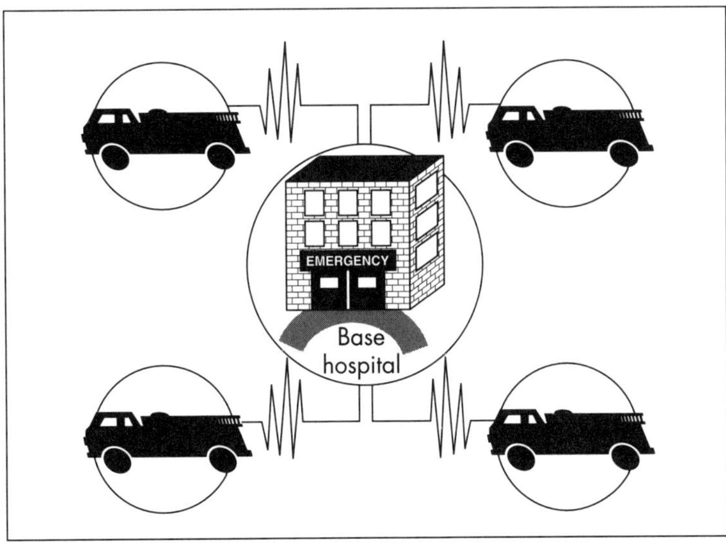

Figure 20-5. Milwaukee: Physician-directed medical control only, paramedic communicators provide quality assurance.

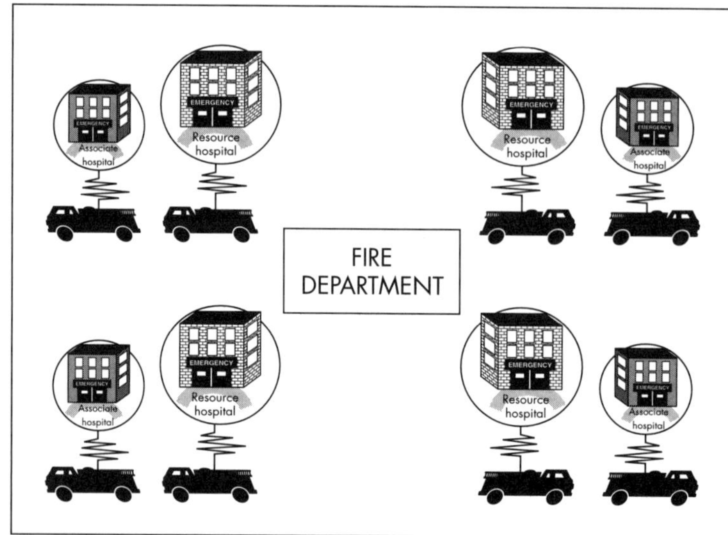

Figure 20-6. Chicago: Half MICN-directed medical control, half physician-directed medical control only.

ciate base hospitals to handle a portion of the calls and assist with quality assurance. Although the standards and requirements of these hospitals vary, MICNs generally handle 40 to 50% of all calls. When physicians are used, they are emergency medicine residents with attending physician backup. Resident training includes EMS lectures, an 8-hour direct medical control physician course for orientation, and a required 8-hour ride-along. The following continuing education requirements for MICNs are strict: attendance at monthly tape review, a specified volume of calls handled per month, and a yearly ride-along, as well as initial certification. All cases in which advanced interventions are initiated are communicated to the base hospital, and receiving facilities are notified of all such patients. All pronouncements must be made by a direct medical control physician, because there are no criteria for death in the field.

San Diego, California

Predominantly MICNs, multiple base hospitals (Figure 20-7). Direct medical control in San Diego County is provided primarily by MICNs via radio, and attending physicians are available for consultation 24 hours a day. Eight base hospitals provide direct medical control. All paramedic calls require base hospital contact, and EMT-B calls can contact the base hospital to give a report. The base hospitals handle 700 to 900 calls per month. Each base hospital has its own medical director, a MICN coordinator, and a dedicated MICN. Dedicated MICNs' sole responsibility is to provide direct medical control; they have no primary responsibility in the emergency department. MICNs have completed a 100-hour course on the principles of prehospital care as described in the section of qualifications of direct medical control personnel. Each direct medical control physician must pass a policy and protocol test. Physicians are involved in fewer than 10% of calls and sign direct medical control forms only if a variation of a standing order is used. In some base hospitals, MICNs contact receiving facilities 2 to 8 hours after the call to obtain the diagnosis and disposition of critical patients. Critical patients include those with trauma, cardiac arrest, hypotension, potential lethal arrhythmias, and respiratory arrests.

Columbus, Ohio

Paramedic and MD field supervision (Figure 20-8). Columbus does not require direct medical control contact. Paramedics provide care entirely through standing orders; however, there is a significant degree of field supervision. Each unit has 3 paramedics and during each 24-hour shift one paramedic is charged with supervision. In addition, the EMS medical director is frequently at the scene to provide direct medical control.

Direct Medical Control: Field Supervision

Most of this chapter centers on the provision of direct medical control by remote means such as radio or telephone. However, in the early days of prehospital care, direct medical control was provided by physicians in

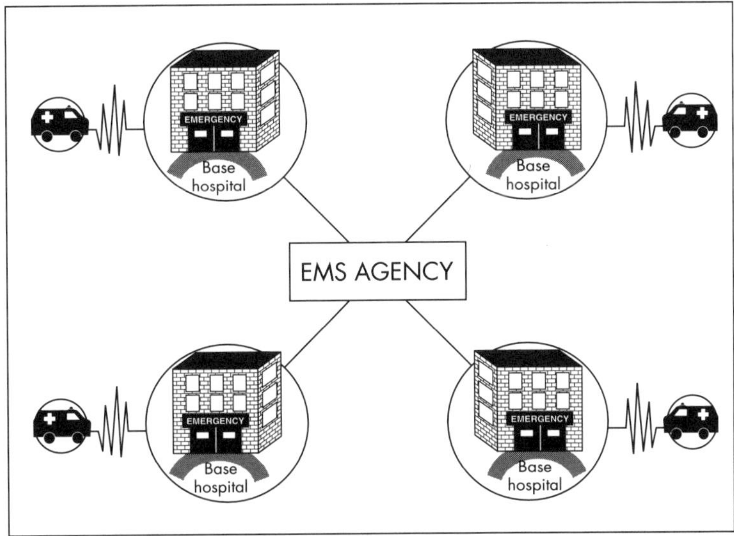

Figure 20-7. San Diego: Predominantly MICN-directed medical control with physician backup.

the field. Field supervision by physicians and clinically selected paramedic supervisors still may be the single best mechanism to provide direct medical control and effective quality assurance. To optimize the benefits of field supervision, paramedic supervisors must be carefully selected by the medical director for both clinical and teaching skills, and they must routinely respond to the scene of major resuscitations to supervise, assist, and teach. Paramedic supervisors should meet regularly with their physician supervisor to solve problems such as paramedic providers requiring remedial strengthening of certain skills. In the most refined form of such meetings, paramedic supervisors and the EMS physician have a daily "morning bedside rounds" conference, discussing serious cases, complaints, and problems of the previous 24 hours. Much of this activity is actually indirect medical control.

Quality Management of Direct Medical Control

Simply providing direct medical control is no assurance of either good medical control or good outcome.

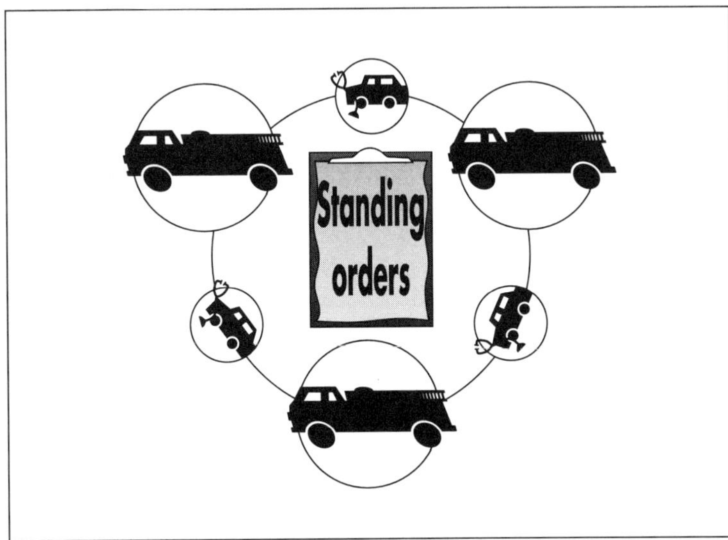

Figure 20-8. Columbus: No direct radio medical control, physician on-scene medical control.

Not surprisingly the process of evaluating the mechanism rather than the mechanism itself matters most in providing quality care. No system is better than its quality assurance. Many providers of direct medical control are not monitored and assessed, and therefore the quality of direct medical control in many systems is poor.

Review of communication tapes is useful in assessing the performance of the field team and those providing direct medical control. Tape review is most useful when conducted in association with the prehospital care report (PCR), direct medical control record, and the follow-up form. The focus on field personnel evaluates communication skills, initial field assessment, sense of urgency regarding the patient's stability, and completeness of the PCR. The direct medical control provider's accuracy of interpretation of the reported findings, appropriateness of recommended therapy, and communication skills should also be considered. Copies of the tape review can be sent to field personnel and direct medical control personnel to provide feedback. In addition, the prehospital care profile resulting from tape reviews and patient records can identify specific educational values or problems requiring the attention of the physicians responsible for direct medical control.[43]

Tape review conferences attended by the field providers and direct medical control personnel are very successful. In a nonstressful situation, retrospectively evaluating the care provided by the field team and the direct medical control physician is a useful springboard for discussion. Typically a tape review conference is 1 to 2 hours long and includes a review of several calls chosen for their educational value. These calls may center on one topic, thus suggesting an associated didactic lecture as part of the tape review. Alternatively the calls may span several topics, but they have educational value either because of the problems encountered or the high quality of the communication team's effort. This conference format provides feedback for both field personnel and those providing direct medical control; it is an opportunity for each part of the team to understand the perspective of the other. Providing patient outcome information affirms the continuum of care that exists among the various parts of the system. Perspective on patient care improves if outcome information is available to prehospital personnel.

A communication log that records all incoming calls daily including type of call and hospital destination can track the volume of calls, identify specific calls, and specify types of calls for further analysis. Ideally this log is maintained by computer to ease case selection and compilation of statistics.

A mechanism of immediate follow-up that requires direct medical control personnel to obtain diagnosis and disposition soon after ambulance transport is used in Milwaukee, Seattle, and San Diego. It enables field and direct medical control personnel to gather statistical data and incorporate constructive information. This information on the appropriateness and effectiveness of field care is gathered from the receiving clinicians and relayed to other personnel involved in the case while their memories are fresh. The most effective method of collecting follow-up information is a call made by the direct medical control provider to the receiving hospital. Patient diagnosis, disposition, medical record number, and any problems are discussed during this call. The receiving emergency department usually has the requested information within 4 hours. In some cases a second call is necessary if the diagnosis or disposition of the patient were not yet determined. However, the medical record number makes further follow-up achievable, and any initial patient presentation problems are identified early. This rapid and effective follow-up system is most successful in systems that have personnel dedicated exclusively to providing direct medical control.

A small number of highly trained personnel providing direct medical control have the best opportunity to provide effective direct medical control. With smaller numbers of providers, there is a greater potential for more intensive training and quality assurance. However, just as having physicians provide direct medical control does not guarantee expertise and quality, neither does having a small number of any level of personnel providing direct medical control. Direct medical control provided by a small number of poorly trained and overworked personnel is as low in quality as that provided by a large number of unqualified, inexperienced personnel. Quality relates to both the adequacy of training and the relative workload.

The base hospital audit is used by some EMS agencies to evaluate direct medical control. Those providing direct medical control are subject to the same performance scrutiny as field personnel. Since hospitals providing direct medical control, like other organizations, are capable of narrow self-interest, they cannot evaluate their own performance objectively. Evaluation must be done periodically by an impartial source, using objective criteria. In Alameda County, California, there are four hospitals providing direct medical control, each of these hospitals receives approximately 600 calls per month. The EMS agency conducts an audit every 6 months. The audit primarily evaluates direct medical control; it takes 3 to 5 hours to complete and includes five components. However, the EMS agency believes that hospitals should set an example of good overall patient care for other hospitals in the community, and the audit therefore includes components of the emergency department. The objectives of the audit include (1) to assure compliance with the EMS agency-base hospital contract, (2) to assure compliance with county EMS policies and procedures, (3) to assess direct medical control, (4) to ensure due process if subsequent action is taken against the hospital, (5) to provide documentation, (6) to assess recordkeeping and organization of the hospital, (7) to meet and discuss problems and concerns with liaison personnel, and (8) to collect and recommend ideas and suggestions for system improvement.[36]

The base hospital contract with the EMS agency is another method of quality assurance. EMS systems should develop direct medical control standards that are specific for mechanisms of quality assurance and staffing criteria and can become a legal contract or memorandum of understanding. Such a contract establishes specific expectations of base hospital personnel and any subsequent audit, and it provides a documented basis for revocation of designation if the performance standards are not met. Unfortunately, in many EMS systems, neither contract nor standards exist or they are extraordinarily nonspecific and undemanding.

EMS-base hospital contracts can include the following specifics, some of which are not direct medical control functions:

Education—the extent of the hospital's participation in educational activities including tape reviews and didactic seminars for both field and direct medical control personnel;

Field supervision—who participates in direct field supervision and to what extent;

Liaison with receiving hospitals—the hospital's role as a liaison with receiving hospitals including quarterly liaison meetings to discuss problems and receive input;

Direct medical control—the direct medical control providers, their requirements for initial training and continuing education, and the supervisory personnel who evaluate the performance of direct medical control providers;

Notification and communication of medical information to receiving hospitals—personnel responsible for notifying the receiving hospitals of incoming traffic and the required time of notification;

Obtain follow-up information—personnel responsible for obtaining follow-up information, the types of calls requiring follow-up information, and the schedule for providing follow-up information to field personnel and direct medical control providers;

Assist with provision of quality assurance for system—the hospital's requirements to assist with the quality assurance of the system;

Conduct and direct research studies—whether the base hospital participates in prehospital research projects and the requirements for such participation;

Provide detailed information on hospital performance—information regarding hospital performance to be reported to EMS and the personnel responsible for reporting;

Physicians—those who provide direct medical control, their qualifications, initial training, ongoing field experience, and educational requirements including attendance or presentations of tape critiques and participation in continuing education for field personnel, as well as the methods of monitoring direct medical control personnel performance; and

Physician surrogates—adequate surrogate staff to provide direct medical control, the qualifications, initial training, and ongoing educational requirements, and the methods of evaluating their performance. In California, it is predominantly physician surrogates who provide direct medical control, and the average staffing pattern is one physician surrogate (MICN) for each 600 radio calls handled per month. A minimum of 400 calls per month are necessary to provide an appropriate experiential level, but the maximum workload is 900 calls per month.

Summary

Because of the 24-hour nature of direct medical control, it is the portion of EMS medical oversight most often delegated to others. In some parts of the country, direct medical control is delegated to non-physicians who, like physicians, may advise and direct either remotely or on-scene. Whether responsibility for EMS direct medical control is delegated to an individual practitioner or to an institution, the obligation to assure quality direct medical control remains with the physician charged with EMS medical oversight. Although telemetric data transmission from the scene has waned and the use of standing orders has waxed, the most significant recent trends are the shifts toward contemporaneous on-scene direct medical control and required contact in problem situations such as refusal of care.

REFERENCES

1. Aufderheide T and Hendley GE: The diagnostic impact of prehospital 12-lead electrocardiography, *Ann Emerg Med* 19:1287-1380, 1990.
2. Alvarez H, Wills R, and Cobb L: Sudden cardiac death: physiologic observations and therapeutic implications, *Am J Cardiol* 31(116):1973.
3. Berezin M et al: Implications of paramedics' diagnostic and therapeutic accuracy, 276A, 1979.
4. Boyd D: Emergency medical services systems development: a national initiative, *IEEE Transactions on Vehicular Technology* VT-25(4):104-115, 1976.
5. Boyd D et al: Medical control and accountability of emergency medical services (EMS) systems, *IEEE Transactions on Vehicular Technology* VT-28(4):249-262, 1979.
6. Cannon J: Emergency medical technician performance: a clinical trial, 1974.
7. Cayten C et al: The effect of telemetry on urban prehospital cardiac care, *Ann Emerg Med* 14(10):976-981, 1985.
8. Subcommittee on Medical Control in EMS Systems: Medical control in emergency medical services systems: Subcommittee report, 1981.
9. Diamond N, Schofferman J, and Elliott J: Factors in successful resuscitation by paramedics, *JACEP* 6(2):42-46, 1977.
10. Dillon J et al: Task force III: diagnostic procedures, *Am J Cardiol* 50:382-392, 1982.
11. Dinerman N, Rosen P, and Pons P: Medical control in prehospital care, *Current Topics II in Emergency Medicine* 7, 1981.
12. Erder H: Prehospital care telemetry: how essential? (review). In: Wagner, editor: *The year book of emergency medicine,* Chicago, 1986, Year Book Medical Publishers Inc.
13. Erder M and Davidon S: Editorial, *Ann Emerg Med* 16:923, 1987.
14. Erder MH, Davidson SJ, and Cheney RA: On-line medical command in theory and practice, *Ann Emerg Med* 18:261-268, 1989.
15. Frew SA: Emergency medical services legal issues for the emergency physician, *Emerg Med Clin North Am* 8(1), Feb 1990.
16. Gausche M, Henderson D, and Seidel J: Vital signs as part of the prehospital assessment of the pediatric patient: a survey of paramedics. *Ann Emerg Med* 19:173-178, 1990.
17. Hargarten KM, Aprahamian C, and Steuven H: Limitations of prehospital predictors of acute myocardial infarction and unstable angina.
18. Hedges JR et al: Analysis of base station morphine orders: assessment of supervising physician consistency, *J Emerg Med* 8:587-590, 1990.
19. Hitt J and Sanders A: Prehospital care telemetry: how essential? *J Emerg Med* 1:417-420, 1984.
20. Hoffman JR et al: Does paramedic-base hospital contact result in beneficial deviation from standard prehospital protocols, *West J Med* 153:283-287, 1990.
21. Hoffman JR, O'Neill N, and Luo J: Algorithm use in the treatment of prehospital ventricular fibrillation: an analysis of 160 cases, *Resuscitation* 17:131-141, 1989.
22. Holroyd B, Knopp R, and Kallsen G: Medical control: quality assurance in prehospital care, *JAMA* 256(8):1027-1031, 1986.
23. Hunt R et al: Standing order versus voice control, *JEMS* 26-31, Nov 1982.
24. Jacobs L, Luise J, and Eisenscher J: Congruency in physician-EMT assessment, *Ann Emerg Med* 10(4):205-208, 1981.
25. Karagounis L et al: Impact of field transmitted electrocardiography on time to in-hospital thrombolytic therapy on acute myocardial infarction, *Am J Cardiol* 66:786-791, 1990.
26. Lambrew C: The experience in telemetry of the electrocardiogram to a base hospital, *Heart Lung* 3(5):756-764, 1974.
27. Lambrew C, Schuchman W, and Cannon T: Emergency medical transport systems: use of ECG telemetry, *Chest* 63(4):477-482, 1973.
28. Lewis R et al: Effectiveness of advanced paramedics in a mobile coronary care system, *JAMA* 241(18:1902-1904, 1979.
29. Medical control of emergency medical services: an overview for emergency physicians, *Physicians* 1984 (editorial).
30. Mitchell J, Pozen M, and D'Agostino R: Acute cardiovascular condition recognition: emergency medical technicians versus paramedics, Presented to American Public Health Association, 1978.
31. Nagel E et al: Telemetry-medical command in coronary and other mobile emergency care systems, *JAMA* 214(2):332-338, 1970.
32. Neely KW et al: The effect of base station contact on ambulance destination, *Ann Emerg Med* 19:906-909, 1990.
33. Pantridge J and Adgey A: Prehospital coronary care: the mobile coronary care unit, *Am J Cardiol* 24:666-673, 1969.
34. Peacock JP, Blackwell VH, and Wainscott M: Medical reliability of advanced prehospital cardiac life support, *Ann Emerg Med* 14:407-409, 1985.
35. Pointer J: The emergency physician and medical control in advanced life support, *J Emerg Med* 3:31-35, 1985.
36. Pointer J: The advanced life support base hospital audit for medical control in an emergency medical services system, *Ann Emerg Med* 16(5):557-560, 1987.
37. Pointer JE and Osur MA: Effect of standing orders on field times, *Ann Emerg Med* 18:1119-1121, 1989.
38. Pozen M, Berezin M, and Kulp R: Cost and utility considerations in implementing ambulance telemetry, *Heart Lung* 9(5):866-872, 1980.
39. Pozen M et al: An assessment of emergency medical technicians' performance as related to seasonal population influx, *J Comm Health* 3(3):227-235, 1978.
40. Pozen M et al: Effectiveness of a prehospital medical control system: an analysis of the interaction between emergency room physician and paramedic, *Circulation* 63(2):442-447, 1981.
41. Pozen M, Fried D, and Voigt G: Studies of ambulance patients with ischemic heart disease: II, *Selection of Patients for Ambulance Telemetry* 67(6):532-535, 1977.
42. Question of control, *JEMS* 7, Nov 1982.
43. Rottman S and Fitzgerald-Westby K: A method for reviewing radio-telemetry paramedic calls, *Ann Emerg Med* 10(1):36-38, 1981.
44. Stark G and Hedges J: Patients who initially refuse prehospital evaluation and/or therapy, *Am J Emerg Med* 8:509-511, 1990.
45. Stewart R: When less is more: teflon and telemetry in the space age, *Ann Emerg Med* 14(10):992-994, 1985.
46. Syverud SA et al: Prehospital use of neuromuscular blocking agents in a helicopter ambulance program, *Ann Emerg Med* 17:236-242, 1988.
47. Thompson S and Schriver J: A survey of prehospital care paramedic/physician communication for Multnomah County (Portland), Oregon, *J Emerg Med* 1:421-428, 1984.
48. Wasserberger J et al: Base station prehospital care: judgment errors and deviations from protocol, *Ann Emerg Med* 16(8):867-871, 1987.
49. Weaver D et al: Myocardial infarction triage and intervention project-phase I: patient characteristics and feasibility of prehospital initiation of thrombolytic therapy, *Jam Coll Cardiol* 15:925-31, 1990.

21

Quality Management

Joseph L. Ryan, M.D., FACEP

Quality Assessment to Quality Assurance

The challenge of quality of care is inherent in scientific medicine. To a great extent, the advancement of medical science results from the rigorous application of structured thinking and its principles to investigation. The physician scientist is well-acquainted with this "scientific method," and the practitioner struggles to integrate "medical fact" into the vagaries of clinical encounters with patients.

Ensuring that medical care provided in the field by physician surrogates is safe, compassionate, timely, consistent, appropriate, cost-effective, and positively influences patient outcome is a responsibility of the first order for the EMS medical director. This quality assessment and monitoring is basic to the successful provision of prehospital health care.

Structured thinking in medical quality assessment is well-developed. The significant work of Donabedian articulated a conceptual framework for quality of care.[9] In *Explorations in Quality Assessment and Monitoring,* Donabedian describes the definitions of quality and approaches to its assessment, the criteria and standards of quality, and the methods and findings of quality assessment and monitoring. These principles form the basis for understanding the dimensions of quality in health care.

However, quality assurance (QA) in the sense of a warranty of quality (and therefore having to do with its causation) is a far more complex and difficult goal. The costs of poor quality in any dimension are enormous. Although extended effort has been applied to "assure" quality in medical practice, a crisis of credibility contests the ability to produce quality that is recognizable to patients, communities, and the nation. "Quality assurance" as health care policy has largely backfired in enabling good care, and it is a major cause of the crisis facing organized medicine in the United States.

QA functions of the health care system largely developed to retrospectively police the quality of medical care. Influenced by the increasing spectre of societal expectation and government oversight, QA as defined by American health care and others evolved almost exclusively into utilization review and "terminal inspection" (the autopsy being the ultimate in terminal inspection). QA processes became mechanisms motivated to identify "offenders" failing to adhere to normative values for hospital stay, frequency of laboratory tests, and consultations. Physicians equated QA with trouble and responded with a practice of "defensive" medicine that has become a preponderant influence in health care and resulted in an increasingly estranged patient and paranoid practitioner. The QA analysts maintained that the root cause of poor quality in health care was the problem of flawed people.

In 1989 Berwick characterized the sad state of affairs in health care quality assurance as the "Theory of Bad Apples"[1]:

> . . . because those who subscribe to it believe that quality is best achieved by discovering bad apples and removing them from the lot. The experts call this mode "quality by inspection," and, in the thinking of activists for quality in health care, it predominates under the guise of "buying right," "recertification," or "deterrence" through litigation. Such an outlook implies or establishes thresholds for acceptability, just as the inspector at the end of an assembly line decides whether to accept or reject finished goods. They search for outliers—statistics far enough from the average that chance alone is unlikely to provide a good excuse. Bad Apple theorists publish mortality data, invest heavily in systems of case-mix

adjustment, and fund vigilant regulators. Some measure their successes by counting heads on platters.

In this landmark article, Berwick presented the arguments for a different way of doing business.

Quality Assurance to Continuous Quality Improvement

In the early 1980s, many American industrialists recognized that the competitive edge the United States once enjoyed in world markets had been eroded by the Japanese. "Made in Japan," once a synonym for poor quality, was rapidly becoming the benchmark for comparison, and American products were not measuring up. The study of this phenomenal turnabout in Japanese industry led to a shocking realization; the manufacturing and production strategies that revolutionized Japan were invented by American industrialists in the early twentieth century and were generally ignored or forgotten at home.

The rediscovery of these *industrial* quality management (QM) strategies has been a focus of the vanguard of American manufacturing and service industries in the latter 1980s and is becoming the pervasive feature of a new philosophy of management. The ideas of Shewhart, Deming, Juran, Fiegenbaum, Crosby, Drucker, Peters, Ishikawa, Taguchi, and Imai, are gaining new recognition. Their philosophies have a wide variety of names including statistical process control (SPC), statistical quality control (SQC), total quality control (TQC), companywide quality control (CWQC), total quality management (TQM), and continuous quality improvement (CQI), and each has conceptual nuances and disciples. The precise taxonomy of these terms is complex and unsettled. For purposes of this discussion the broad group of these industrial concepts will be referred to as QM. CQI is the predominant term adopted by authors to refer to the adaptations of these concepts to medical practice.

The general principles of QM are best expressed in the works of Deming and Juran.[14] In Deming's "Fourteen Points," the fundamentally different way of doing business is described (see the box below, left).

The Fourteen Points

Point One:	Create constancy of purpose for the improvement of product and service
Point Two:	Adopt the new philosophy
Point Three:	Cease dependence on mass inspection
Point Four:	End the practice of awarding business on price tag alone
Point Five:	Improve constantly and forever the system of production and service
Point Six:	Institute training and retraining
Point Seven:	Institute leadership
Point Eight:	Drive out fear
Point Nine:	Break down barriers between staff areas
Point Ten:	Eliminate slogans, exhortations, and targets for the workforce
Point Eleven:	Eliminate numerical quotas
Point Twelve:	Remove barriers to pride of workmanship
Point Thirteen:	Institute a vigorous program of education and retraining
Point Fourteen:	Take action to accomplish the transformation

The Red Beads

The relevance of Deming's work to medicine is readily seen in an experiment he uses to illustrate the flaws in our thinking about producing quality.[40] Although certainly the experiment was not originally designed to describe health care delivery, the message applied is bitterly diagnostic of the ills of medicine. The parable of the red beads can be viewed as the plight of the health care industry with the physician as producer (the industrial worker) of health (the product).

A group of workers is given a box of beads; 80% are white and 20% are red (good and impaired health status). The workers' job is to make white beads (good health). They are given a paddle with 50 holes arranged in five rows of ten (the tools of medical care). Each is told at length of the importance of making white beads, the elaborate and rigid procedures to be followed, and the severe consequences for failing to produce the quota of white beads required. The workers then in turn dip into the box, return a paddle filled with beads, and are inspected (by the Utilization Review Committee) for the percentage of white beads produced. The workers are variously praised, exhorted, threatened, retrained, suspended, or dismissed for their production of red beads despite objections that the raw materials (health status) and the imperfect processes (medical care) by which they are forced to work are flawed.

The fundamental flaws of our current strategies of QA for health care are plainly evident from this analogy.

Although workers are held responsible, exhorted, intimidated, and coerced to produce white beads (health), they are ultimately unable to effectively influence the quality of raw materials or the processes on the line, which are designed to mitigate illness rather than produce health.

Industrial Quality Management Models Applied to Medicine

In 1987 the Harvard Community Health Plan hosted the first meeting of 21 health care agencies and an equal number of industrial QM experts to launch the National Demonstration Project on Quality Improvement in Health Care (NDP). As a reference point for the mainstream of the medical care establishment, this project can be considered the point of departure from traditional medical models of QA to the application of industrial QM concepts to health care delivery systems.

This experiment, funded by the John A. Hartford Foundation, was designed to answer the question, "Can the tools of modern quality improvement with which other industries have achieved breakthroughs in performance, help in health care as well?"[2] The answer was a clear if qualified yes. Although the problems of health delivery systems are somewhat unique, the principles of QM hold great promise for revolutionizing and humanizing the pursuit of quality in health care.

EMS Quality Management

Quite significantly, in 1987 a number of EMS systems had been using concepts of QM to measure and improve clinical service provision for about 8 years.[33,35] System status management (SSM), developed in 1979 by Stout, remains the most highly evolved and successfully implemented example of the concepts of QM in EMS.[34] This anticipatory ambulance deployment strategy based on the pathophysiology of cardiac arrest and the mandate of equal access to care is archtypical of patient-oriented service delivery.

In the Public Utility Model of EMS, Stout's concepts of EMS system design and operation were developed independent of influence from contemporary industrial quality theorists and represent a parallel evolution of customer-centered QM for EMS systems.[36,37] The Advanced SSM Workshops sponsored by The Fourth Party characterize the vanguard of current thought in QM in EMS for system managers.*

*The Advanced SSM Workshops, The Fourth Party, Inc, 760 Crandell Rd,. West River, MD 20778, (619) 492-4283.

Leadership for Quality

It is unfortunate that rare opportunities exist for medical directors to define a priori the structure of the system they oversee. Typically, configurations of systems are inherited, having been designed by well-intended but medically näive government committees with little input from prehospital practitioners. The genesis of the system is often tangential to the provision of emergency medical care. It may have been motivated to capture funding opportunities, extend power bases, or stunt free-market competition. Understanding the sometimes Byzantine political realities of a given system is paramount to the success of the medical director. The "system" at its worst lacks definition altogether. Definition and refinement of system configuration, however, are the foundations of effective quality planning.

The ability of the medical director to plan for quality is a prerequisite for effective system medical control. In general, state law and local ordinance grant authority to direct. This authority is further defined in the contract between the medical director and the system. This contract should include a detailed description of the medical director's role in defining, monitoring, and modifying the configuration of the system and its attributes. It should describe the humanpower, equipment, and funding necessary to fulfill the medical oversight requirements of the system.

These elements are fundamentally lacking in most current systems. For example, the information management tools that enable any meaningful retrospective, let alone real-time, monitoring of quality of care remain primitive. The computerized information systems in the dispatch center (except for emergency medical dispatching systems) remain provider rather than patient oriented in their data collection. For example, the prevailing definition of response time ends on the scene, not at the patient.

Davidson distinguishes authority from power in characterizing the ability of the medical director to be effective in his or her role.[4]

> Power comes to the medical director through the careful exercise of authority and through the expertise that the medical director brings to the activity of EMS and through his/her ability to negotiate the interests of all while serving as a consultant to everybody, thereby enhancing everyone else's ownership of issues and solutions. In this fashion, rather than serving as a single voice on high whose opinion is delivered, as if *ex cathedra,* the medical director serves at every opportunity in the role of the physician expert, consultant, and educator, thereby facilitating and bridging the multiplicity of political interests into consensus.

Physicians have traditionally been recognized as "knowing what's best for their patients." In the development of EMS systems, however, this expertise has been inconsistently provided, recognized, and integrated into the processes of care. In many ways the mandates of medical authority have been seen as näive and unrealistic when applied to the prehospital environment and rightly so, because much proposed has no basis in scientific fact or is extrapolated from fundamentally different and controlled environments. There will be less acceptance of this paternalistic perspective in future medical care systems.

In their experience, the NDP recognized that involving doctors in QI is difficult. Underlying barriers include availability, skepticism regarding appropriateness, relevance and helpfulness of these groups, and reluctance to share authority over aspects of care for which they viewed themselves as disproportionately accountable. "For doctors in the past decade or more, the word 'quality' has meant 'trouble.'"[2]

Industrial quality theory acknowledges that the key to creating a successful QM program lies in the consensus support and substantive commitment of leadership to the mission of quality. Deming recommends, ". . . create constancy of purpose for the improvement of product and service, . . . adopt the new philosophy, . . . improve constantly and forever the system of production and service, . . . institute leadership, . . . and take action to accomplish the transformation."[6] Because of the unique and diverse relationships in the hierarchies of EMS systems, accomplishing these goals is quite difficult. The medical director has a pivotal role in articulating an inarguable mission of quality in patient care for the system capable of catalyzing consensus among leadership in support of these goals.

The Juran Trilogy

Juran identifies three universal processes of management for quality. These are interrelated as shown in the Juran Trilogy diagram. Figure 21-1 shows graphically the relationship of time on the horizontal axis and quality deficiencies (cost of poor quality) on the vertical axis. The initial activity of QM involves quality planning. After processes are designed and tested to meet customer needs, they are implemented on the production line. Quality control monitors in real-time the conformance of production processes in relation to product goals. The results of these monitoring functions are evaluated continuously by quality teams to discover production breakthroughs and reduce quality deficiencies quality improvement (QI).

Structure and Quality Planning

Donabedian defines structure as[8]:

> the relatively stable characteristics of the providers of care, of the tools and resources they have at their disposal, and of the physical and organizational settings in which they work. . . . But the concept also goes

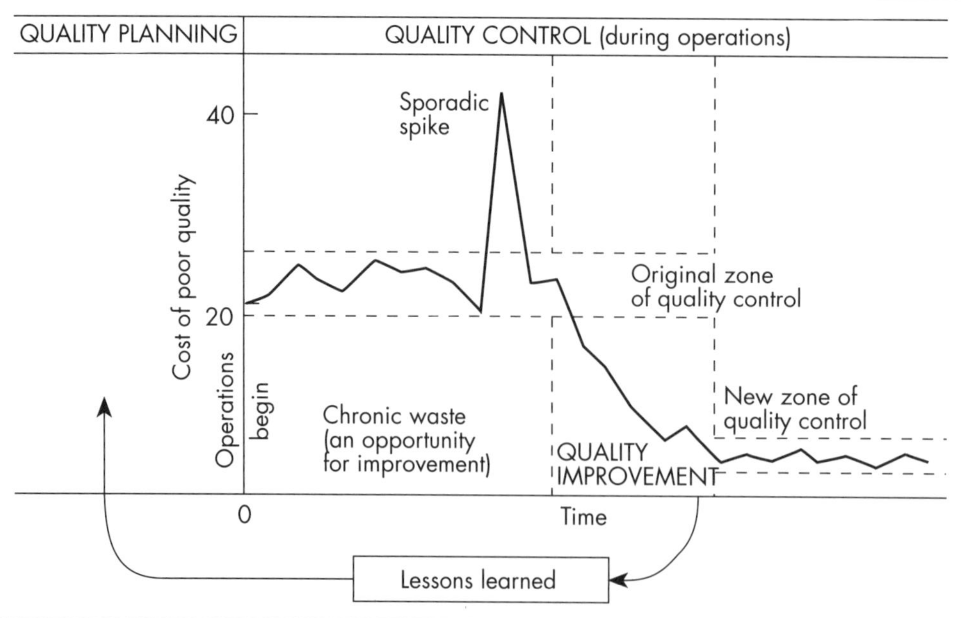

Figure 21-1. The Juran Trilogy. (From Juran Institute, Inc., Wilton, Conn.)

> beyond the factors of production to include the ways in which financing and delivery of care are organized, . . . The basic characteristics of structure are that it is relatively stable, that it functions to produce care or is a feature of the 'environment' of care, and that it influences the kind of care that is provided. . . . Structure, therefore, is relevant to quality in that it increases or decreases the probability of good performance.

He further notes that[24]:

> . . . as a means for assessing the quality of care, structure is a rather blunt instrument; it can only indicate general tendencies. The usefulness of structure as an indicator of the quality of care is also limited because of our insufficient knowledge about the relationships between structure and performance. It remains to be seen what improvement in specificity and sensitivity can be achieved by the development of more detailed, more condition-specific structural requirements.

This concept illustrates a telling difference between the medical and industrial philosophies of quality. Structure in an industrial sense (that is, the design of products that meet customers needs and the organizations and mechanisms that produce them) is of paramount importance to the company. Through quality planning the problems in reliability and efficiency are recognized and eliminated from the production line before they ever appear. The effects of "getting it right the first time" in eliminating product failure and rework are monumental in industry and have literally saved many companies from doom. The reader can speculate why this has not been more widely recognized in medical care. Perhaps it relates to the virtual monopoly allopathic medicine enjoys in western society vis-à-vis alternative health care philosophies. Or perhaps it is the refusal of medical organizations to recognize the "85/15 rule" that is well proven in industry, ". . . the potential to eliminate mistakes and errors lies mostly (85%) in improving the *systems* through which work is done, not in changing the workers (15%)." The systems being the responsibility of management.[28]

Quality Planning

- Determine who the customers are
- Determine the needs of the customers
- Develop product features that respond to customer needs
- Develop processes that are able to produce the features
- Transfer the resulting plans to the operating forces

Juran on Quality Planning

Joseph M. Juran, in his book on leadership for quality, identifies a series of requirements for the transformation of companies into quality driven organizations. These benchmarks serve as a guide to the application of QM to EMS (see box below, left).

Engineering Quality by Design

Stout noted, "Of all the forces influencing an EMS system's ability to convert available dollars into clinical performance and response time reliability, system design is by far the most powerful."[38]

Quality planning for EMS derives from a fundamental principle. It is the standard of care that defines the system; the system does not define the standard of care. The transformation of EMS systems into quality-driven organizations (after Deming) requires the commitment of leadership and management to this constancy of purpose. There are no "sacred cows" that escape scrutiny in the planning process.

Determine Who the Customers Are

The "customers" of EMS are patients. Despite any sense among clinicians that regarding patient as customer inadequately expresses or even denigrates the unique relationship with the patient, considerations of the industrial concepts of customer are enlightening.

Parallel to our concept of patients, industrialists recognize the consumers of their products as customers. However, the industrialist considers that the company has many more types of customers both external and internal than simply buyers of goods and services. Quality management defines my customer as anyone who depends on me.[18]

Therefore the customers of EMS services are not only patients but also their families, their physicians, their hospitals, the medical community, other public safety agencies, the community at large, and the governments of the geopolitical units in which the systems operate. These are referred to in QM jargon as "external customers."

A wide variety of interdependent processes exist within organizations, and each has its own internal suppliers and customers. The quality of any intermediate product in the manufacturing assembly line depends on the quality input of the up-line suppliers, the workers' own processes of production, and their output as supplier to their down-line internal customers.

Industrial QM views each person in an organization as part of one or more processes. Each worker, through a number of individual tasks, receives the work of others, adds value to that work, and supplies it to other workers in the process. Therefore, each individual has a triple role—customer, processor, and supplier (Figure 21-2).[21]

It is worthwhile to extrapolate these views to problems in prehospital medicine. For example, the application of these concepts to the "chain of survival" from cardiac arrest yield striking insights. For example, the product of poor dispatch—failure in early notification and mobilization of resources—irrevocably impairs even the best on-scene automatic defibrillation.

The methods to determine the customers of an EMS system are recognizably complex. Juran recommends developing flow charts for the important processes of an organization to enable management to clearly identify the range of customers. This is useful for the following reasons:

1. Flow charts provide the team with an understanding of the whole. Frequently, individuals understand their own parts of the puzzle but have little understanding of the interrelation of process elements.
2. Flow charts often identify customers previously neglected. The discipline necessary to prepare the chart reveals internal customers with overlooked needs.
3. Most flow charts reveal subprocesses or "loops" that are evidence of the rework of previous elements of the process. These are often chronic deficiencies in systems and are the targets of improvement planning.[22]

The flow chart is one of a number of basic tools used to clarify elements of QM. An example of a flow chart for an EMS system response to a cardiac arrest is illustrated in Figure 21-3.

Determine the Needs of the Customers

In medicine there exists a confounding and destructive arrogance regarding the customer's needs. Patients are almost never consulted to express their perspectives on the characteristics of quality health care. The current liability crisis in medicine is the result in great part of our failure to recognize and appreciate this aspect of care. Patients can accept mistakes made in good faith; they are unable to accept being treated in a callous, dehumanizing, and discompassionate manner.

These problems have parallels in industry. The manager's or engineer's view of a product often varies substantially from the consumer's. Ishikawa distinguishes the concepts of true quality characteristics from substitute quality characteristics.[17] The patient may perceive the answering of the 9-1-1 call within 2 rings or the lack of need to repeat their complaint as attributes of quality. The system recognizes these as aspects of a streamlined process to triage and respond in a timely and appropriate manner to the entire community. The reliability of this process in an individual encounter is a substitute quality characteristic for the consistency of call processing that matches demand to supply in the most timely and efficient manner for the needs of the public. Future QM in EMS will require leadership to seek out and incorporate these customers' perspectives. The role of the medical director is in part that of a "quality engineer." Detailed understanding of the scientific basis of medical practice is key in integrating the substitute and true quality characteristics of system goals into the quality planning process.

Cardiac arrest is the ultimate personal emergency. Although the paramedic's scope of practice is certainly broad based, it is fundamentally directed toward a knowledge base and psychomotor skills that resuscitate the patient in arrest. Understanding the pathophysiology of sudden cardiac death resolves to a small number of basic facts. Patients survive, practically speaking, only ventricular fibrillation. The key factors influencing their survival are early provision of bystander CPR and defibrillatory shock. This is illustrated graphically by Eisenberg et al (Figure 21-4).[12]

For the individual patient the definition of customer need in this worst case scenario is straightforward and is extensively addressed in medical literature. The requirement of a high level of reliability for the provision of equal access to definitive care for

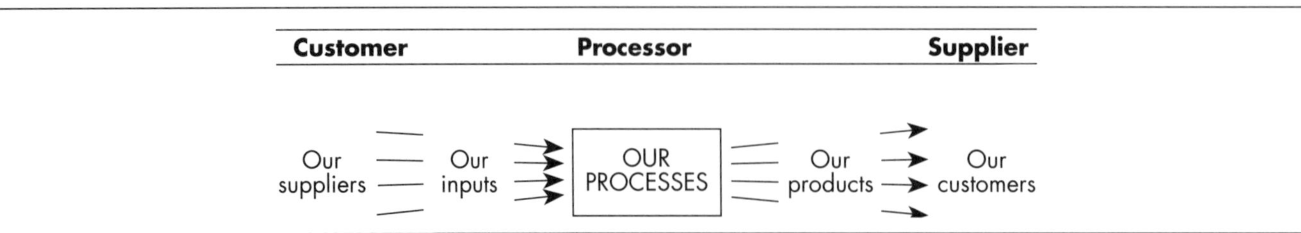

Figure 21-2. Juran's Triprol diagram. (From Juran Institute, Inc., Wilton, Conn.)

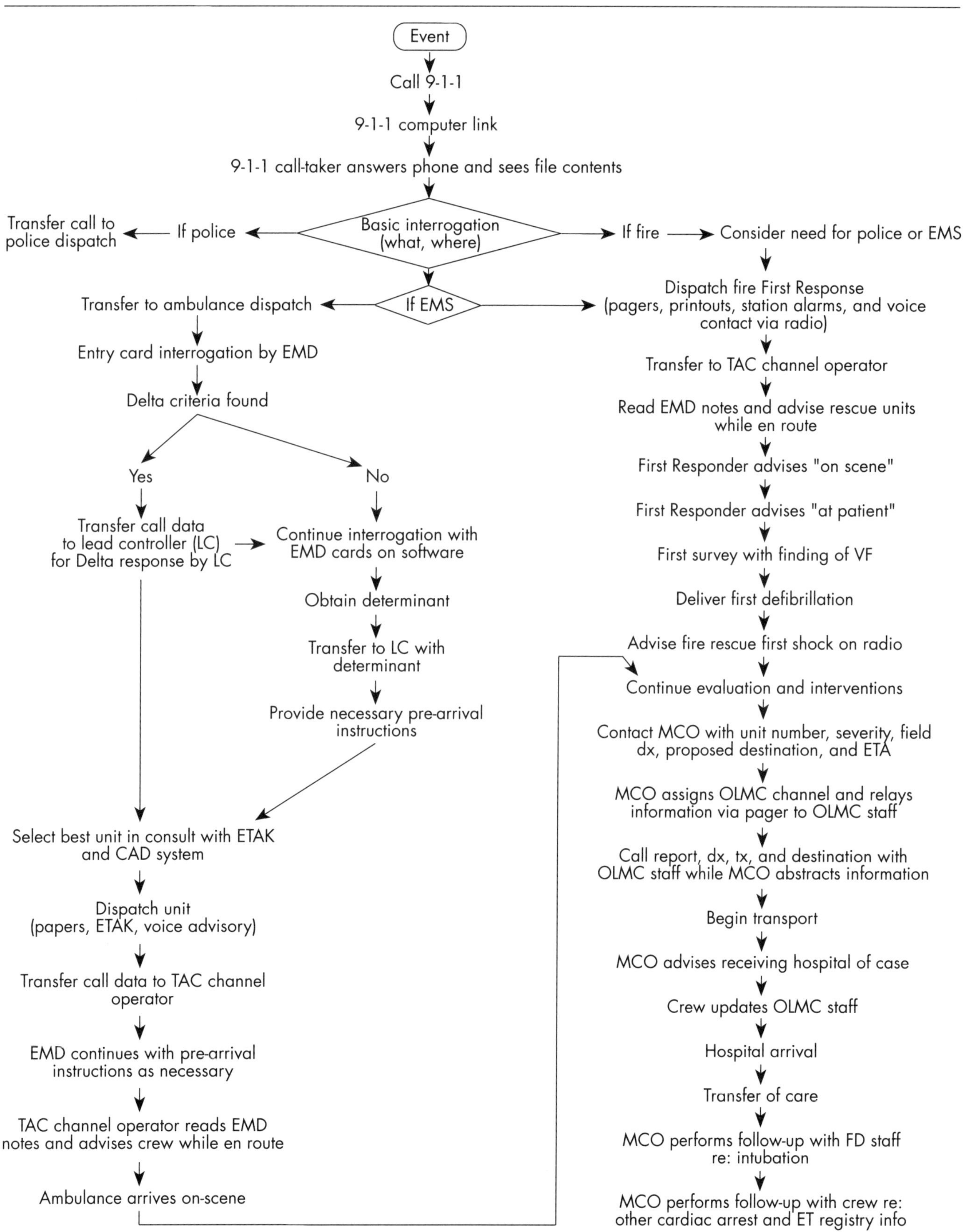

Figure 21-3. Process flow chart for an EMS system's response to sudden cardiac arrest. (Courtesy Pinellas County EMS, Largo, Fl.)

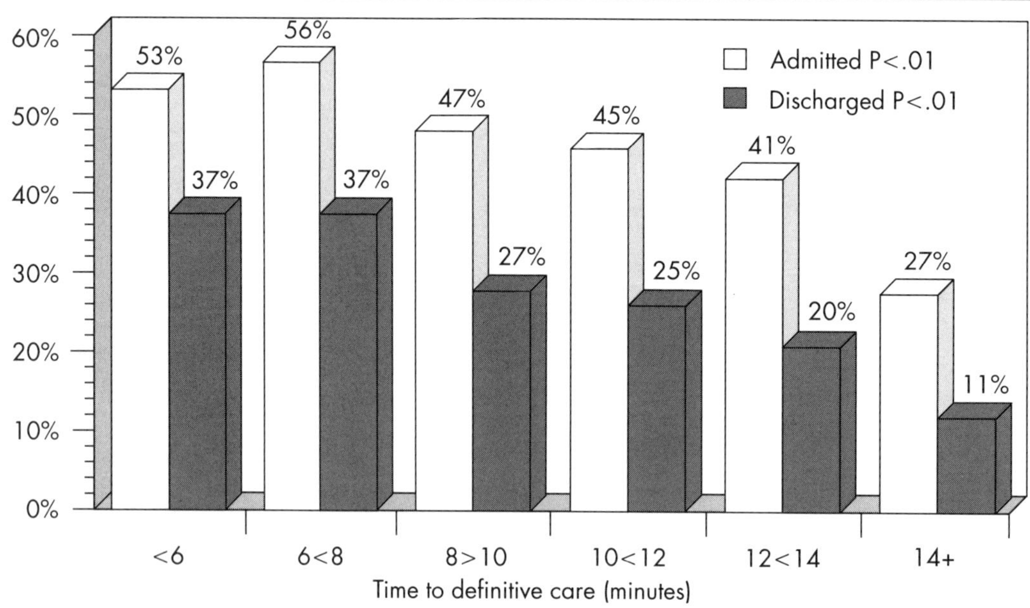

Figure 21-4. The window of survivability of sudden cardiac arrest in the community describes a fundamental design feature of an effective ALS system. (Modified from Eisenberg M et al: *Clinics Emergency Medicine* 2:13-25, 1983.)

all customers in an EMS service area should be the basic design feature of an EMS system. The needs of the customers are the standards of care for a system. The standards of care are the derivative of the needs of the customers of an EMS system.

The reorganization of emergency medical services in Kansas City, Missouri, from 1978 to 1979 is the best early example of the recognition and synthesis of these diverse customers' needs into the design of an EMS system.[24] As a result of public outcry following the tragic death of a police officer who exsanguinated after a 25-minute response by the EMS provider and a general perception by the public of unequal access to services among neighborhoods, the city government obtained consultation to reconfigure the system. The requirements of this new system (the customers' needs) were straightforward, yet profoundly impacted the delivery of care. All 9-1-1 customers were to be afforded equal access to care for life-threatening emergencies as prospectively defined by emergency medical dispatch.

Develop Product Features that Respond to Customer Needs

According to Juran, every product feature should meet a certain set of minimum criteria. The feature should first meet the needs of the customer. Those needs include stated needs, as well as perceived, real, and cultural needs. Second the product feature should meet our needs as a supplier including the needs of our internal customers. Next the product features should meet competition. Meeting the needs of external and internal customers does not ensure the customer will buy it—a competitor's product may be better or give better value. Meeting competition is an important criterion for developers. Last the product features should minimize the combined costs to both customers and suppliers. Each incurs costs involved with the product and seeks to keep their own at minimum. The optimum for society is when price reflects actual costs, and both are kept to a minimum.

The fundamental constructs of the reorganized EMS system in Kansas City were based on the standards of medical care defined by the consensus of community medical authority (the medical community-customer), the Emergency Physicians Advisory Board (EPAB). The citizens of the community (the patient-customer) were to be afforded equal access to timely and appropriate EMS that met their needs with 90% reliability at the 8-minute interval (the lower specification limit of the product). This response time requirement applied to all councilmanic districts of the city irrespective of call density or difficulties in coverage. *(Criterion #1—meet the customers' needs.)*

The city government, through the creation of a trust entity in the public's interest, would control all necessary aspects of delivery of service. *(Criterion #2—meet the needs of the supplier.)*

The Metropolitan Ambulance Services Trust (MAST), which is a type of public utility commission representing the government or civic customer, was created. It had several critical functions. It would (1) contract for the cost-effective provision of services by competitive bid for the entire market (making it economically feasible by directly controlling costs), (2) award, through performance contract with a single provider, exclusive market rights to the community (like an electric or water company), (3) monitor performance requirements, through its own activities and those of the EPAB, using objective criteria, (4) exercise contractual recourse for failure to perform including firing the contractor for breach if necessary. *(Criterion #3—meet competition and Criterion #4—minimize combined costs.)*

Develop Processes that are Able to Produce the Features

In QM terms a process is a "systematic series of actions directed to the achievement of a goal." Process development refers to process design and evaluation, process selection, provision of facilities, provision of methods and procedures for operation, and control and maintenance of the process.

SSM was developed out of necessity to provide the levels of coverage and response time reliability that meet the needs of system customers at an affordable cost. Consider the problem—most EMS systems seek to keep response times low and often it may seem they are doing so, as average response times are within acceptable ranges. This concept is critically flawed, however, from the customer's perspective. All systems have a heterogeneous pattern of call density. By responding to those needs with ambulance placement, it is possible to drive average response times down by providing short responses to high call density areas, sacrificing the lives of those in low call density areas (Figure 21-5).

However, using the principles of demand pattern analysis and peak-load staffing, equal access to care for patient-customers is provided. These SSM systems are driven by a fractile response time requirement (for example, an 8-minute response to life-threatening emergencies provided with 90% reliability over all subunits of a service area). This is known in QM as a lower control limit (LCL) or specification limit for a process and is a contractual requirement in many systems. The shift to this strategy in the Kansas City system resulted in a 35% increase in efficiency and afforded the system equal access to care (Figures 21-6 A-C, 21-9, 21-10, 21-11, and 21-14).[24]

Transfer the Resulting Plans to the Operating Forces

The transfer of processes from the planners to the operating forces is necessary to confirm that theoretical process capability can be accomplished on the production line. This commonly occurs through testing the process. These tests may be dry-runs, pilot tests, or

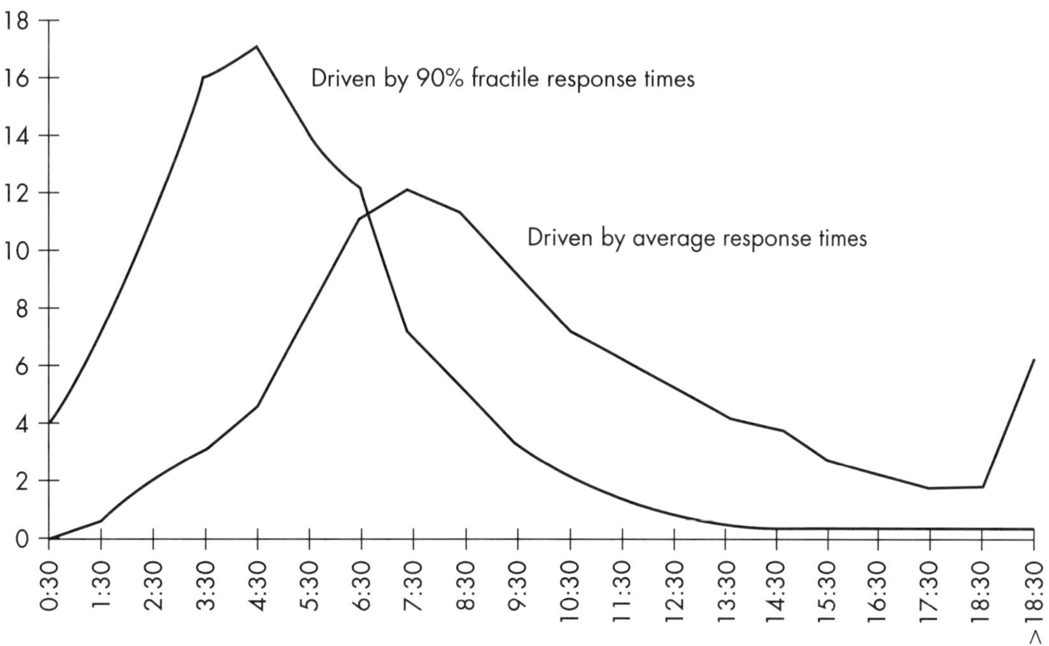

Figure 21-5. The differences in emergency response time performance between these two communities is striking. The system driven by fractile response time performance clusters 90% of emergency response with the 8-minute interval. The system driven by average response time performance has a much longer "tail." This design flaw severely limits the potential for survival from sudden cardiac death. (Courtesy Fourth Party Inc., West River, Md.)

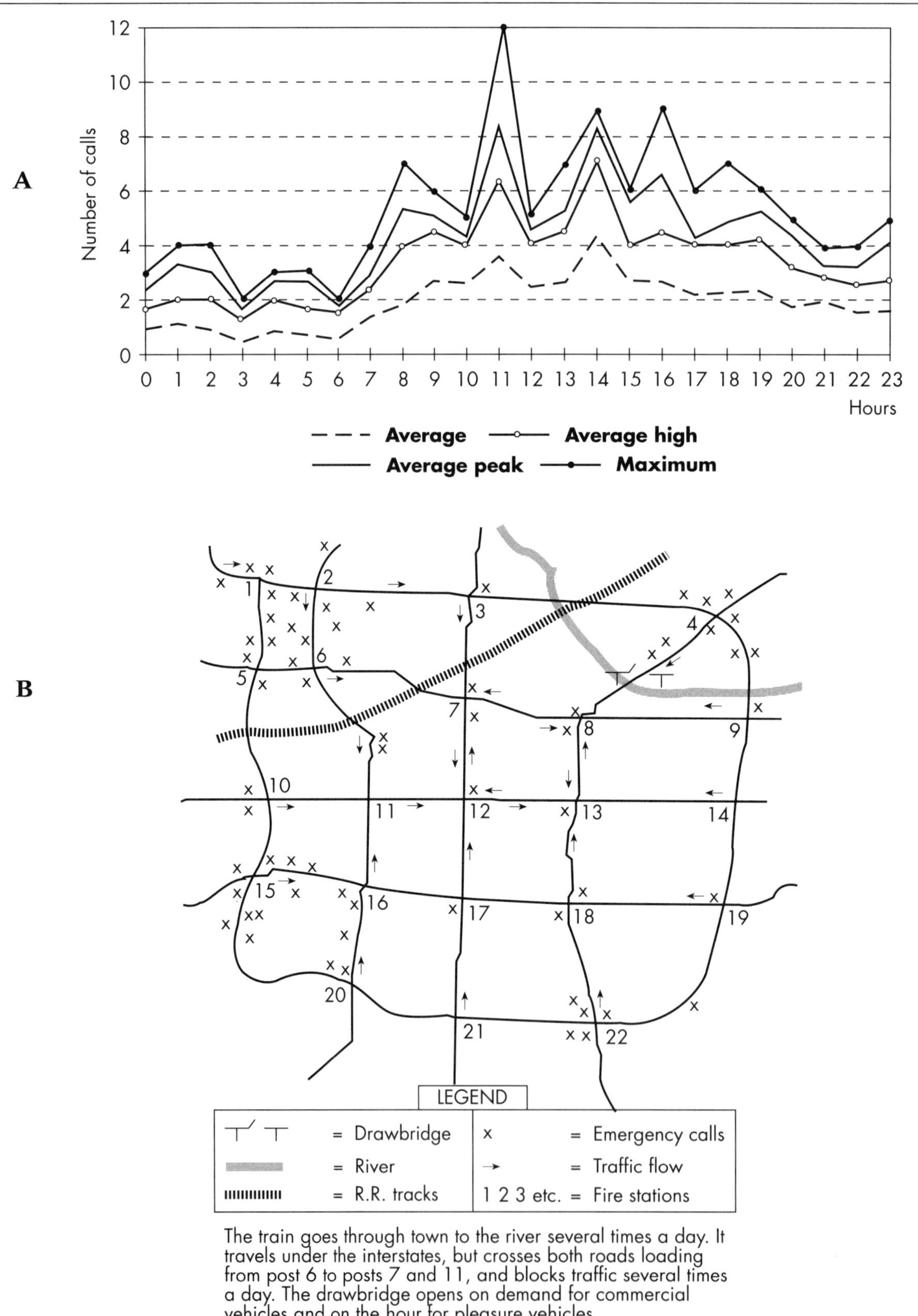

Figure 21-6. Temporal and geographic demand patterns are shown. By peak load staffing, the demand patterns for service are covered. **A,** Temporal demand pattern for service, Tuesday. **B,** Demand map for Monday, Hour 8. **C,** New schedule for Friday. (Courtesy Fourth Party Inc., West River, Md.)

C

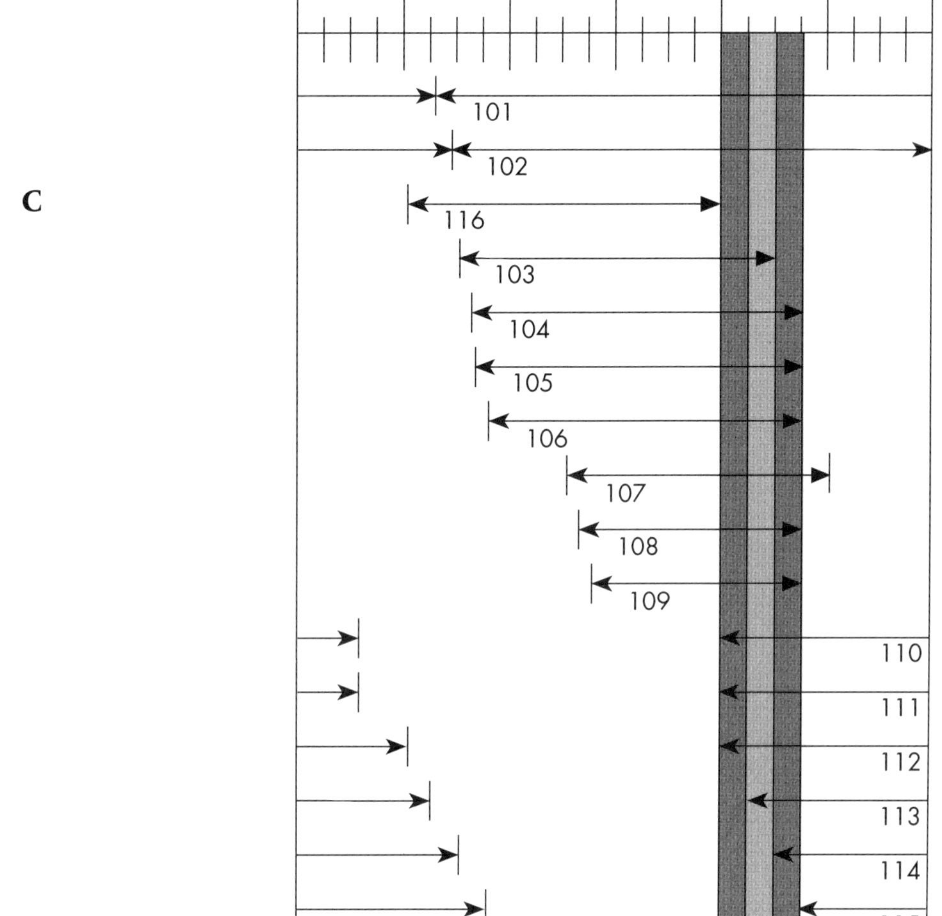

simulations. It is important that these approximate as closely as possible the real world events that they seek to reproduce. Often these are cooperative projects of the quality planning team and selected line personnel. The interaction of these groups is extremely valuable in refining process capability.

Process and Quality Control

Donabedian defines process as the characteristics of provider behavior in the management of health and illness.[8] Process deals with a set of activities between practitioners and patients. The observation of process is best done directly or secondarily by the study of documents of care.

Juran considers process from an operational viewpoint.[20] "The concept of control is one of holding the status quo"—keeping a planned process in its planned state so that it remains able to meet the operating goals. A process that is designed to be able to meet operating goals does not stay that way. All sorts of events can intervene to damage the ability of the process to meet goals. The main purpose of control is to minimize this damage, either by prompt action to restore the status quo or better yet by preventing the damage from happening in the first place.

The Controllability of Processes

If consistency and reliability are quality attributes of the processes of an EMS system, then they require strategies to assess and improve these features of care. There are obviously profound differences in machining ball bearings in a factory and delivering emergency care in the diverse and uncontrolled environment of the street. These are not conceptual differences, however, and should not cause us to reject the appropriateness of applying industrial process models to EMS. Rather, many emergency care processes can be controlled and are highly consistent and reliable in their production of quality care.

The Control Pyramid

Control of processes exists at all levels. Nearly all effective control of EMS care is exercised by the workers. The controllability of processes is largely a function of self-control by individual EMS providers. Overlying this is a layer of managerial control provided directly by the communications center and indirectly by the administrative supervisors. This pyramid differs significantly from those described by Juran for industrial processes. The level of automated controls in EMS is relatively small compared with the level of control by the workforce. Process control by management, communications, and field supervisors, usually at a distance, is also less (Figure 21-7).

The Concept of Statistical Process Control

Central to QM concepts of quality planning is the standardization of processes to increase their reliability and productivity. These standards are inherently quantitative, measurable, and suitable for statistical analysis. All measured processes exhibit elements of variation. The understanding of the distribution and patterns of variation in processes is a key feature of the industrial approach to quality control.

Variation in systems is attributable to the inherent randomness of the system (common causes) or to some specific event (special causes). The evaluation of any process first determines whether the process is stable.[6]

> A stable process, one with no indication of a special cause of variation, is said to be, following Shewhart, in statistical control, or stable. It is a random process. Its behavior in the near future is predictable. . . . A system that is in statistical control has a definable identity and capability. . . . In the state of statistical control, all special causes so far detected have been removed.

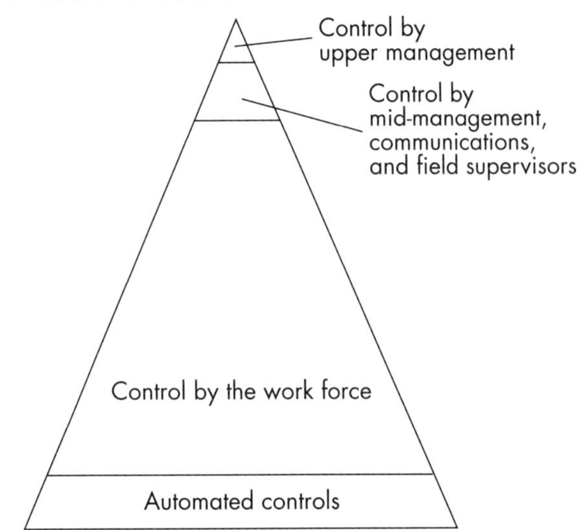

Figure 21-7. The pyramid of control of EMS process. (Modified from Juran, 1993, OMD)

Statistical process control as developed by Shewhart around 1924 refers to the application of analyses of the means, ranges, and standard deviations of a process quantifying its variability and randomness. These analyses are often represented and monitored by control charts that graphically illustrate the stability of processes and the common and special causes of variation (Figure 21-8).

Are the processes by which we provide medical care consistent (that is, in statistical control or stable); are their behaviors in the near future predictable?

No, with a few exceptions they are probably not stable. One need only review medical literature to recognize that these concerns are almost never acknowledged or addressed in published research. Most typically, clinical trials in which the process was flawed are simply discarded from the sample, labeled incomplete, or eliminated from statistical analysis. Infrequently reported ranges and standard deviations for study groups indicate that these concepts are not widely recognized in scientific medicine.

Do we have examples of processes in EMS that are in statistical control as defined by QM?

Yes, there are a number of tracked system processes that appear to be in statistical control. The following examples are predominantly found in so-called high-performance (HP) EMS systems: (1) reliability of preventative maintenance programs in production of critical failure-free miles for ambulances, (2) 90%; + reliability of 8-minute response time performance to life-threatening emergencies, (3) 98%; + reliability for non-emergency response times, (4) 100% reliability for 9-1-1 complaint answering in PSAPs, (5) 94% reliability for correct dispatch determinant selection by EMDs in Los Angeles.[23]

Juran's benchmarks for quality control are shown in the box below

Quality Control

- Evaluate actual product performance
- Compare actual performance to product goals
- Act on the difference

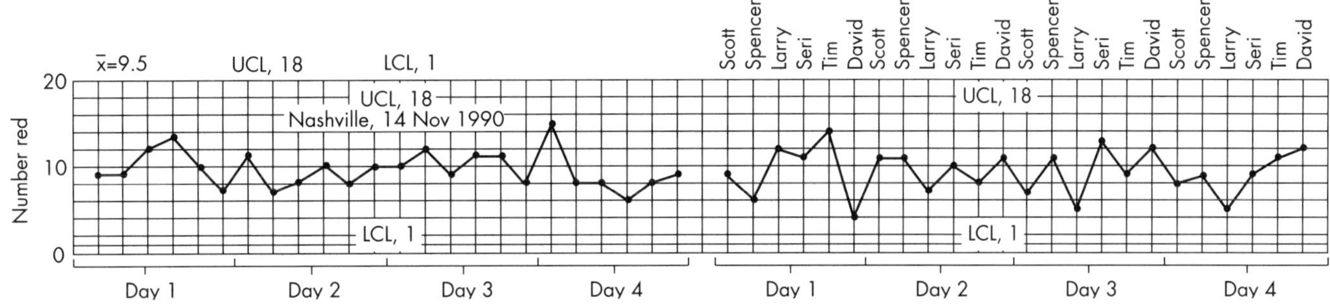

Figure 21-8. A statistical process control chart for the Red Beads Experiment. It illustrates the sequence of production runs for each of the willing workers over a 4-day period. The upper and lower control limits (UCL and LCL) are three standard deviations from the mean. (From Deming WE: *The new economics,* 1993, MTI.)

Evaluate Actual Product Performance

Eisenberg called the system audit of cardiac arrest the "best outcome evaluation of an EMS system's performance."[11] The characteristics are (1) the event is important, (2) the event has a clear case definition, (3) the outcome is measurable, (4) the intervention is straightforward, (5) the intervention has an effect, and (6) it occurs frequently. Cardiac arrest is the ultimate personal emergency and serves as a benchmark of system performance.

The measures and tools for evaluation of EMS processes are problematic but improving.[32] It is nearly impossible to directly observe the process of care in a systematic way. Rather, we depend on indirect observations (for example, real-time through radio communications or documents produced by the chain of internal processes). Significant progress has been made in the standardization of measurement and the exploration of new tools and technologies to refine field data collection.[25] Improvement in EMS systems fundamentally depends on the definition of essential data for field performance and reliable methods for its retrieval. These methods are only successful when field providers recognize their critical roles as clinician-investigators. Such efforts have to date been ambivalent at best.

SSM was implemented first in Kansas City, Missouri, as a result of that EMS system's reorganization. The performance of the system was measured on an ongoing basis through a number of statistical tools and was continually refined to equalize access to care and improve overall response times. Figures 21-9 through 21-11 illustrate actual measurements of performance improvement from 1979 to 1982.

The indirect but real-time observation of care has been used reliably in a number of systems. The

Month	1979 Pre-SSM (mean minutes/month)	1982 Post-SSM (mean minutes/month)	Change (%)
Jan	9.2	5.0	-46
Feb	8.2	5.3	-35
Mar	7.2	5.0	-31
Apr	6.4	4.9	-23
May	5.9	4.8	-19
Jun	6.4	5.0	-22
Jul	6.7	4.9	-27
Aug	6.1	4.6	-25
Sep	6.3	4.4	-30
Oct	6.2	4.4	-29
Nov	5.9	4.6	-22
Dec	7.3	4.6	-37

Figure 21-9. Comparison of monthly average emergency response time performance pre- and post-implementation of system status management, Kansas City, Missouri. (Courtesy Metropolitan Ambulance Services Trust 1984.)

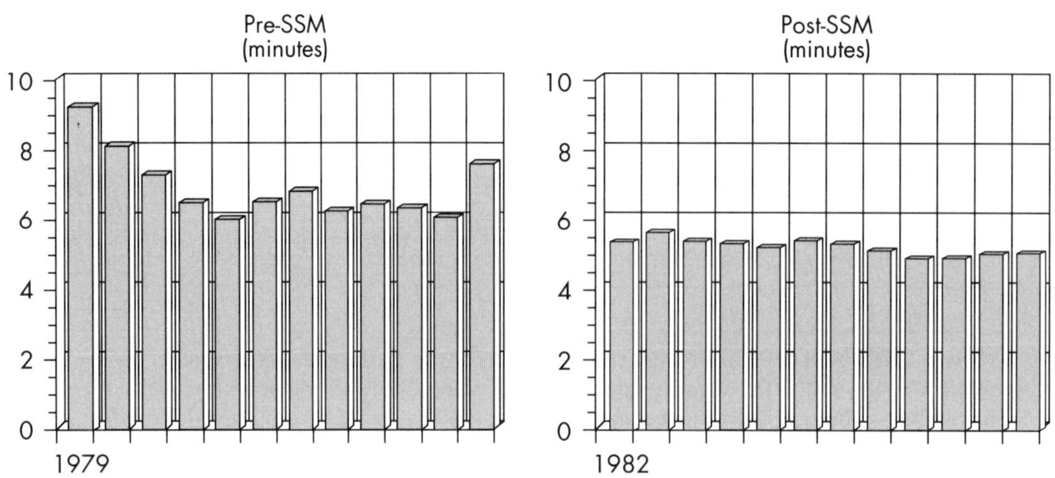

Figure 21-10. Measurement of performance improvement from 1979 to 1982. (Courtesy Metropolitan Ambulance Services Trust, 1984.)

unique vantage point of the EMS communications center provides the best practical "look" at overall system performance. This nerve center is equipped with a large number of "sensors" that can be used in quality control. An increasing number of computerized ambulance dispatching systems (CADs) are incorporating clinical features.[3] The medical communications officer (MCO) collects a number of ongoing registries of clinical information and actuates the feedback loops for quality control. The Pinellas Cardiac Arrest Registry data set is shown in Figure 21-12.

Compare Actual Performance with Product Goals

The process of quality control from an industrial perspective requires the application of a concept familiar to us from physiology—the feedback loop (Figure 21-13).

The implementation of SSM was accomplished initially by hand and then computerized to run on a 48K Apple II computer. The MICAD program informed dispatchers of historical demand patterns for service (system status plans). As calls were received and dispatched, their locations and time intervals were measured and recorded. Ongoing evaluation of this data produced subsequent refinement in system status planning. Although steady and significant improvements occurred in response time performance and efficiency, the 90% fractile performance goal was not achieved until 1982 (Figures 21-9, 21-10, 21-14, and 21-15).

Act on the Difference

How system leaders and managers act on the differences between system goals and performance will ultimately determine the success or failure of CQI in EMS. Davidson points out that there are two management styles.[5] First, to continue with the "bad apples" approach and close the loop through a cycle of fear or second, to enter a pathway toward a model of participatory management that focuses attention on the system of work and not individuals. Workers work smarter and not harder, having increased pride in their work and higher productivity, quality, and effectiveness.

Outcome and Quality Improvement

The third element of classical medical quality assessment theory is the analysis of outcome. Outcome as defined by Donabedian relates to changes in health status as a result of structure and process. Outcome is the most significant of the three elements; however, it is also the most elusive.[8] Particularly, in EMS the direct association of the process of care and its relation to outcome is often difficult to ascertain.

Juran's benchmarks for QI are described in the box below.

Quality Improvement

- Establish the infrastructure
- Identify the improvement projects
- Establish project teams
- Provide the teams with resources, training, and motivation to:
  1. Diagnose the causes
  2. Stimulate remedies
  3. Establish controls to hold the gains

Text continued on p. 234.

A

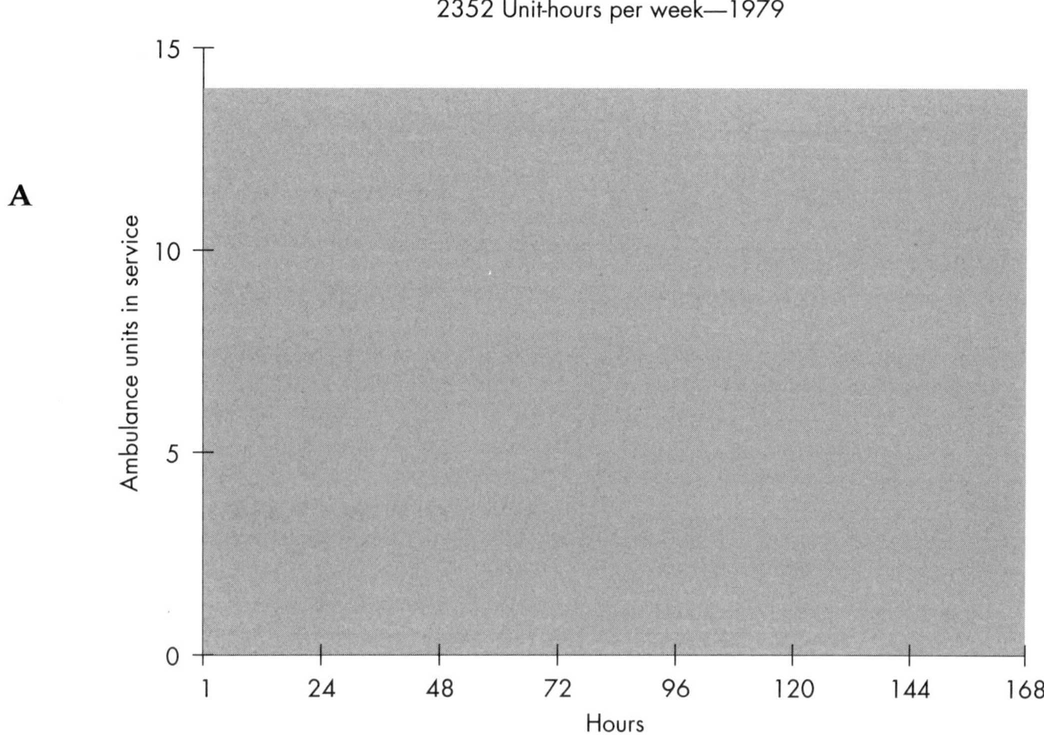

B

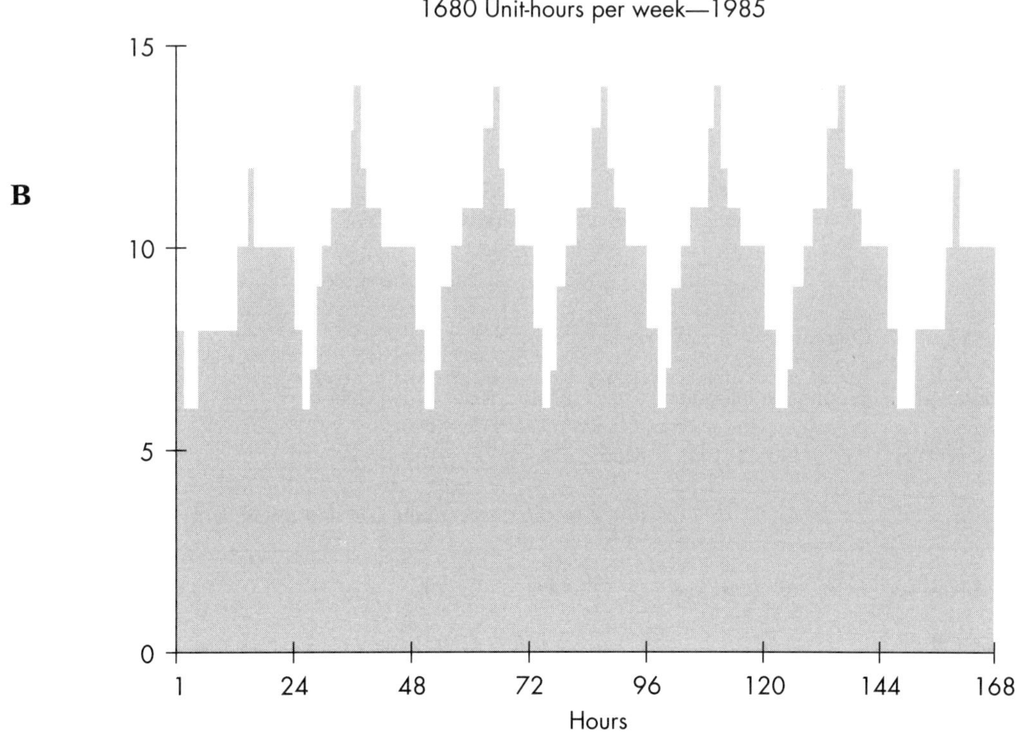

Figure 21-11 The effect of peak load staffing on unit-hour deployment in Kansas City, Mo. **A**, 1979; **B**, 1985.(Courtesy Metropolitan Ambulance Services Trust, 1985.)

CARDIAC ARREST AND INTUBATION REGISTRY/FIELD DATA FORM

Get the following information (from the 9-1-1 CAD only) before calling the ED:

Date: ________ Co. Inc. # ______________ SS Inc. # ______________ MOD/MD:________ Grid: ________

First arriving ALS unit: Agency:__________ Shift: __________ FD unit # ______________ SS unit # ____________

Dispatched: ____________ On-scene: _____________ Transp. time: _____________ Hosp. arrival time: ____________

Was "At-Patient" notification given in 9-1-1 notes? (circle one) Yes = 1 No = 2 At-Patient Time: ____ OLMC Time:______

Ask call-taker who was given pre-arrival: None = 0 EMS = 1 Bystander = 2 PD = 3 Nursing staff = 4 Family = 5 Other = 6

Call the ED and ask for the nurse in charge of patient care:

Who am I speaking with? ______________________ Can you confirm tube placement: (check one) ○ Yes ○ No
(nurses name)

If yes, who confirmed tube placement? (read list to nurse) (check one) ○ MD ○ X-ray ○ RT ○ RN

Ask to speak to paramedic in charge of patient care:

Patient Type: ○ Adult ○ Pediatric (0-17 yrs) Run Type: ○ Medical ○ Trauma

Intubation time: ______________________ Tube size:______________________

\# of attempts: (check one) ○ 1 ○ 2 ○ 3 ○ >3

Intubation method: (circle one) Orotracheal Nasotracheal Digital TTJV

Major difficulty: (circle one) None Anatomy Secretions/Vomitus Trauma Equipment failure Foreign body Environment Patient position Available light Other__________

Equipment/Manuevers used: (circle all that apply) None End tidal CO_2 Stylet Cricoid pressure Magill forceps Transillumination Other__________________

Other airways used: (circle all that apply) EOA EGTA OPA Nasopharyngeal Other _______________

Intubation performed: (circle one) On-scene En route ED

Reintubation because: (circle one) Esophagus intubated Dislodged Other _______________________

Intubation successful: ○ Yes ○ No Medic ID# ________________________________

If first medic unsuccessful, second medic ID#: ______________

Was intubation performed with cardiac arrest? (check one) ○ Yes ○ No

If NO, complete box below: ▼▼▼ If YES, go to other side. ➡ ➡ ➡ ➡ ➡ ➡ ➡

Name of MCO filling out form: ____________________________ Reviewed by: (circle one) D. Shepherd / M. Wallace
(REQUIRED)

CARDIAC ARREST AND INTUBATION REGISTRY/FIELD DATA FORM

(continued)

Historical data:

Lead medic in charge of patient care: ______________________ ID # ______________

Patient name: ______________________ (last) ______________________ (first)

DOB: ______________ Age: ________ (if <1 yr use 1) Sex: (circle one) M = 1 F = 2

Arrest witnessed by whom: (circle one) No Witness = 0 EMS = 1 Bystander = 2 PD = 3 Nurse = 4 Family = 5 Other = 6

Time CPR initiated: __________ By whom: (circle one) EMS = 1 Bystander = 2 PD = 3 Nursing Staff = 4 Family = 5 Other = 6

Initial presenting rhythm:

What was the initial presenting rhythm with no pulse: V-Fib = 1 V-Tach = 2 Asystole = 3 Idiovent = 4 Other = 5 ___

If initial rhythm was VF/VT, was "First Shock" notification given in 9-1-1 CAD notes? (circle one) Yes = 1 No = 2 Time:___

If no, ask medic the time of the first defibrillation/cardiovertion: ______________________

During the code, was there ROSC? (circle one) Yes = 1 No = 2 Time: ____________ *and/or*
was there ROSV? (circle one) Yes = 1 No = 2 Time: ____________

Circle the ROSC rhythm: N/A = 0 SR = 1 A-Fib = 2 1°HB = 3 2°HB-I = 4 2°HB-II = 5 3°HB = 6 Idiovent = 7 Other = 8

Blood pressure: __________ Pulse: __________ Resp: __________ IV access time: __________

Pt. Hx: (circle one) None = 0 Cardiac = 1 COPD = 2 HTN = 3 Seizure = 4 Diabetes = 5 CVA = 6

Patient outcome:

Ask the paramedic: Before arrest, was the patient experiencing CHF, cardiogenic shock, or chest pain or was the arrest of unknown etiology? If yes, circle Cardiac = 1

OR

Before arrest, was the patient in cardiac arrest due to etiology of trauma, COPD, CVA, or other condition? If yes, circle Non-Cardiac = 2

Hospital dest. #: H ______________ Patient outcome: (circle one) Died in ED = 1 Admitted = 2

Name of MCO filling out form: ______________ (REQUIRED) Reviewed by: (circle one) D. Shepherd / M. Wallace

Figure 21-12. EMS Cardiac Arrest Registry Data Entry Forms. These forms are used by communications center personnel to gather real-time information regarding cardiac arrests. The time and effort involved in tracking this important data is minimized by immediate follow-up. (Courtesy OMD, Office of the Medical Director, Pinellas County EMS, Largo, Fl.)

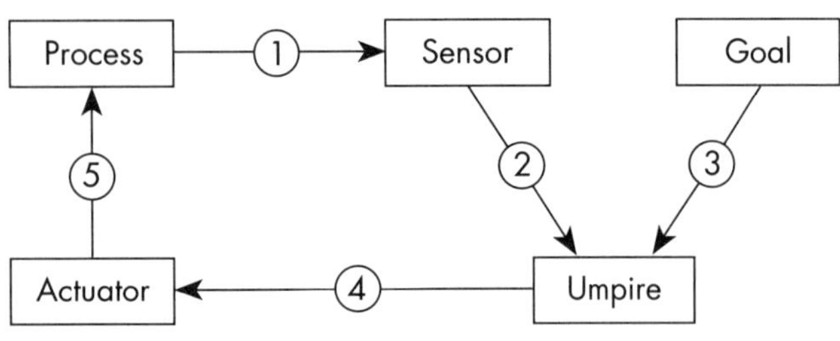

Figure 21-13. Industrial quality control feedback loop. 1) Each process is equipped with various sensors that quantify actual performance. 2) Those sensors are evaluated by an umpire who also receives information regarding the goals or standards for the process. 3) The umpire compares actual performance with the goals or standards and initiates an actuator if the process is out of range. 4) The actuator makes changes in the process to bring performance in line with goals. (From Juran Institute, Wilton, Conn.)

	1979 Pre-SSM	1982 Post-SSM	Change (%)
Emergency responses (yr)	14,600*	16,126	+10
Average responses (wk)	281	310	+10
Unit-hours (wk)	2352	1680	-29
Unit-hour utilization ratio	.12	.18	+35

*Average daily number of responses

Figure 21-14. Comparison of selected response parameters, Kansas City, Mo. EMS System (see Figure 21-15).

Although conceptually the QM process begins with quality planning, the mandate for change is often more difficult. Just as most medical directors do not design the system in which they function, most systems are not quality-oriented organizations at that point either. Most of the QM authorities recommend beginning the transition with a QI project that will catalyze the change.

Establish the Infrastructure

In *Kaizen, the Key to Japan's Competative Success,* Imai contrasts improvement in industrial organizations east and west.[16] Western management, he notes, "worships at the altar of innovation." The solution to most problems lies in quantum leaps in the wake of technological breakthroughs. In Japan, alternatively,

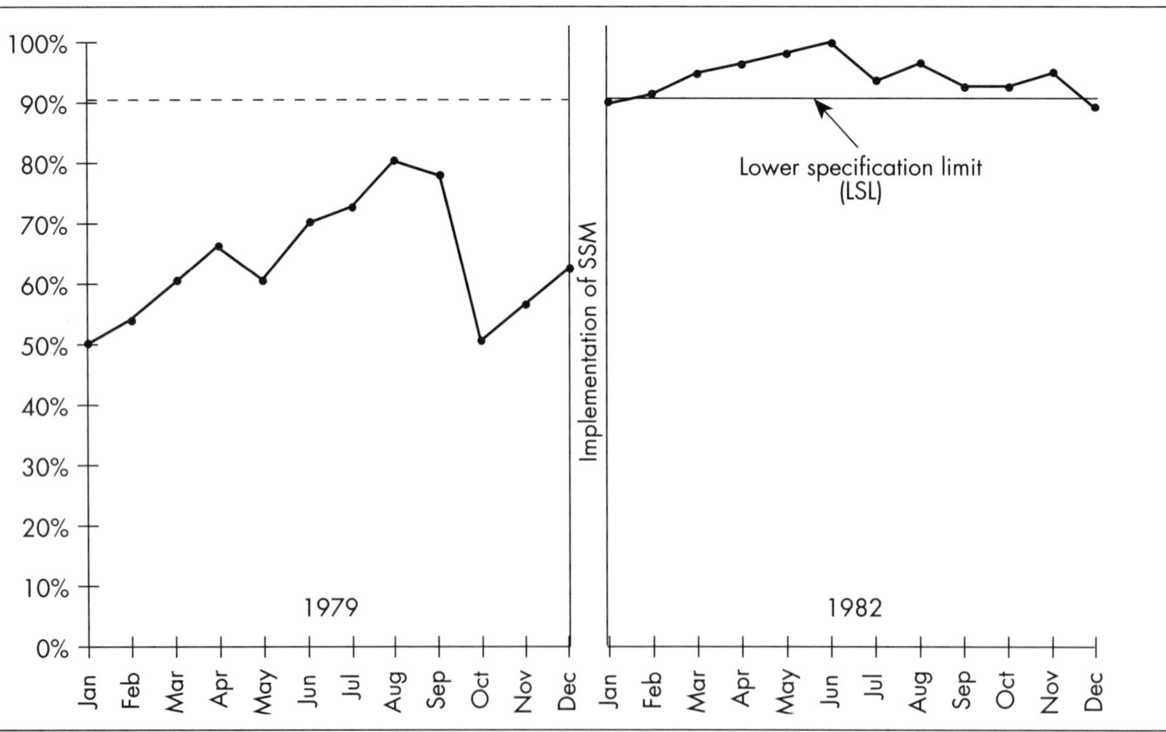

Figure 21-15. System efficiency and cost as shown by improvements in unit-hour utilization were large over the period of implementation of system status management. However, the goal of 90% fractile response time performance reliability was not achieved until 1982. (Courtesy Metropolitan Ambulance Services Trust, 1984.)

QI is subtle and gradual but pervasive in the organizational culture. *Kaizen,* which means improvement, is an ongoing process involving everyone in the organization from managers to workers. The kaizen philosophy is not confined only to the workplace but influences social and family life as well.

QI in EMS will most likely fail (as it has in many U.S. companies) if it is viewed as a quick fix. Witness the advent of automatic defibrillators (a technological breakthrough) and their ambivalent success in improving outcome from cardiac arrest.

Transforming organizations to this new way of doing business must be done carefully. Some organizations (such as the Public Utility Model systems) are equipped with design elements that facilitate these concepts (Figure 21-16). For most, however, these elements are less clear. Identifying a project and selecting and organizing a quality team are the key steps.

Physicians have suffered from the illusion that medical oversight was the necessary and effective reins of system performance. Evidence suggests that direct medical control is inconsistent, overexercised, and of little practical value.[13,41] Medical directors function best as leaders, role models, clinical experts, political champions, and consensus builders. The key to QM in EMS is for the medical directors to let go. Only when the worker (who has nearly all the ability to control the processes of care) is given the appropriate knowledge to choose, the responsibility for the results of their actions, and shares the authority to change the system will EMS be a quality-driven practice of medicine.

Identify the Improvement Projects and Establish Project Teams

These two steps are typically interrelated. At a strategic level, management identifies its agenda for improvement based on consensus and often with the special expertise of a quality engineer or external consultant. At an operational level, similar consensus building establishes common ground for the initial improvement project. The choice is critical. QM experts recommend a process that is significant to both management and the workers; one that has a relatively straightforward solution and will be a quick success to provide momentum for QI within the organization. The selection of the quality team reflects the cross section of management and workers necessary for the solution and interested in making a commitment to learn the process. Most EMS organizations cannot afford external consultants to facilitate the process. A useful and well-written guide to team building and working through projects is *The Team Handbook* by Scholtes.[27]

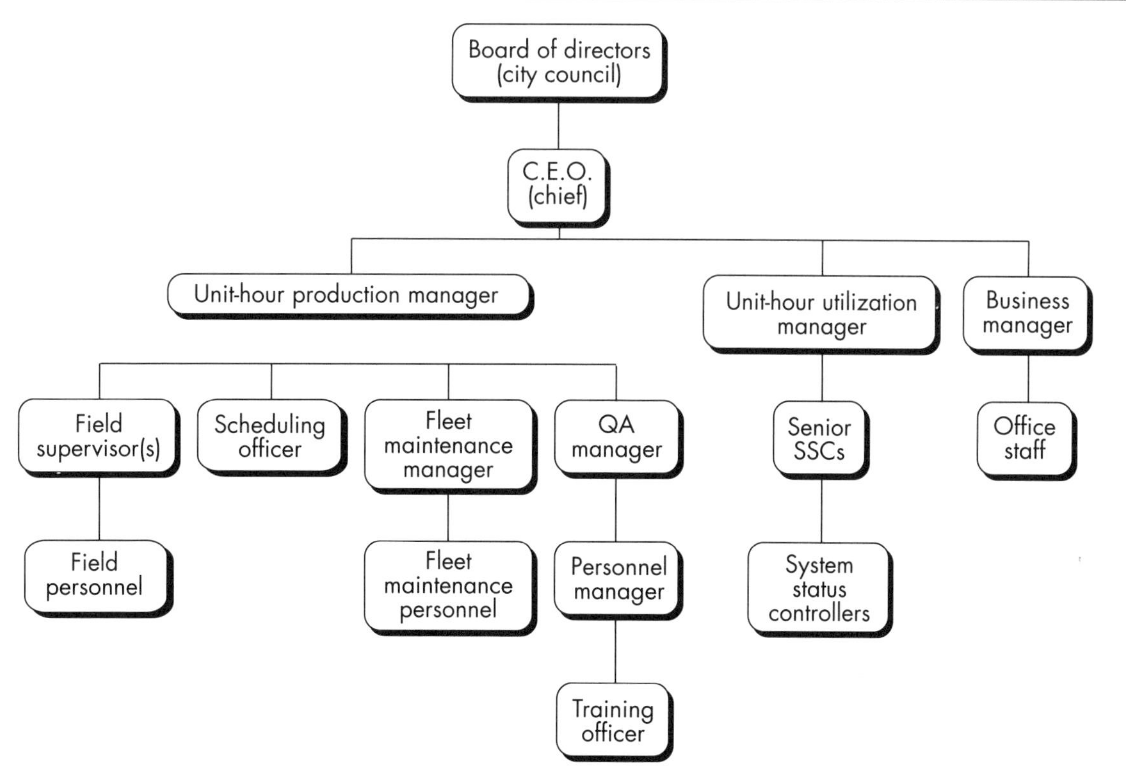

Figure 21-16. Effective organization in the SSM environment. (Courtesy Fourth Party, Inc., West River, Md.)

Provide the Teams with Resources, Training, and Motivation to Diagnose the Causes, Stimulate Remedies, and Establish Controls to Hold the Gains

Eastham has developed an excellent program for introducing the QI process to EMS organizations.[10] Provider-based quality assurance (PBQA) uses a form of nominal group process to define and prioritize QI issues. The program requires the support and commitment of leadership, and one individual must manage the program. By involving organizations from the ground up, the program increases the likelihood of early success and ongoing support. Eastham uses concepts of "just in time" training to enable team members to apply QM tools to practical problems in their organizations.

Seven Statistical Tools

QM uses seven statistical tools to evaluate the causes of poor quality. They are key to managing systems by fact and are in some cases familiar concepts to medical directors.

Process flow chart. As discussed in quality planning, the initial evaluation of processes through flow charts is revealing. A process flow diagram is a graphic representation of the sequential steps in a process. The actions of the team in constructing the chart often reveal hidden aspects of a process and hidden customers. By illustrating the interrelations of different elements, members of the team are afforded new perspectives of their areas effects on other parts of the flow (for example, the 9-1-1 complaint-taker and the emergency medical dispatcher). Flow diagrams illustrate critical steps, locate process flaws, and graphically elucidate the sources of inefficiency and rework. Figure 21-3 illustrates the complex sequence of steps necessary to provide definitive care in cardiac arrest.

Ishikawa or cause-and-effect diagrams. Cause-and-effect or "fishbone" diagrams (named for Kaoru Ishikawa) categorize and display in groups theories about how and why processes fail.[4] They serve, as do flow diagrams, to build the team's understanding of each member's elements and how individual perceptions of problems are often incomplete. They illustrate how the causes of problems are often interrelated. Ishikawa diagrams also point out the need for data points regarding elements of a process to quantify problems.

The fishbones relate associated elements using a number of conceptual threads. Often these are the "5 Ms" in manufacuring processes: man, machines, materials, methods, and measurements. In service industries the "5 Ps" are often used: patrons (external customers), people (internal customers), provisions (supplies), places (the work environment), and procedures (policies and protocols for work).

An Ishikawa diagram of causes of late responses and definitive care is illustrated (Figure 21-17).

Check sheets. In the evaluation of any process the quantification of quality or defects is based on data. Check sheets organize necessary data elements efficiently to allow for collection. In a sense the EMS prehospital care report (PCR) is a check sheet. More often these are matrices that allow the check-off of types of observations, allowing quantification of the frequency of defects by type.

The Pinellas County PCR was developed over a 3-year period by a team of field clinicians and medical control staff; it is an example of our evolution to a structured computer-oriented field record for care (Figure 21-18). Computer software based on this data set enables the provider to create an electronic record using clipboard computers at the patient's side or in the destination hospital.

A monthly check sheet illustrates PCR documentation accuracy by paramedics (Figure 21-19). The goal is 100% accuracy by all personnel. The ambulance contractor is required by contract (a performance specification) to sample 30% of records using an explicit criterion review technique. The check sheet (a Microsoft Excel spreadsheet) is entered by field training officers instructed in the process. Summary data are published for review by all personnel.

Histograms. A histogram is a frequency distribution chart of a process. The chart is a special form of line or bar graph that illustrates the variation of continuous data such as time, weight, size, or temperature. The histogram also illustrates the distribution of continuous data. Important concepts in the significance of these distributions is illustrated in the comparison of histograms of response times between an average response and a fractile response time-driven system (see Figure 21-5).

Run or trend chart. These graphic tools illustrate changes in a process over time. In industry they are frequently used with quality control samples to track the changing performance of an operation on the assembly line. They show the wear and loss of precision tolerances of a machine tool, for example. There are many processes that are observable in EMS by use of trend charts (see Figure 21-15).

Text continued on p. 241.

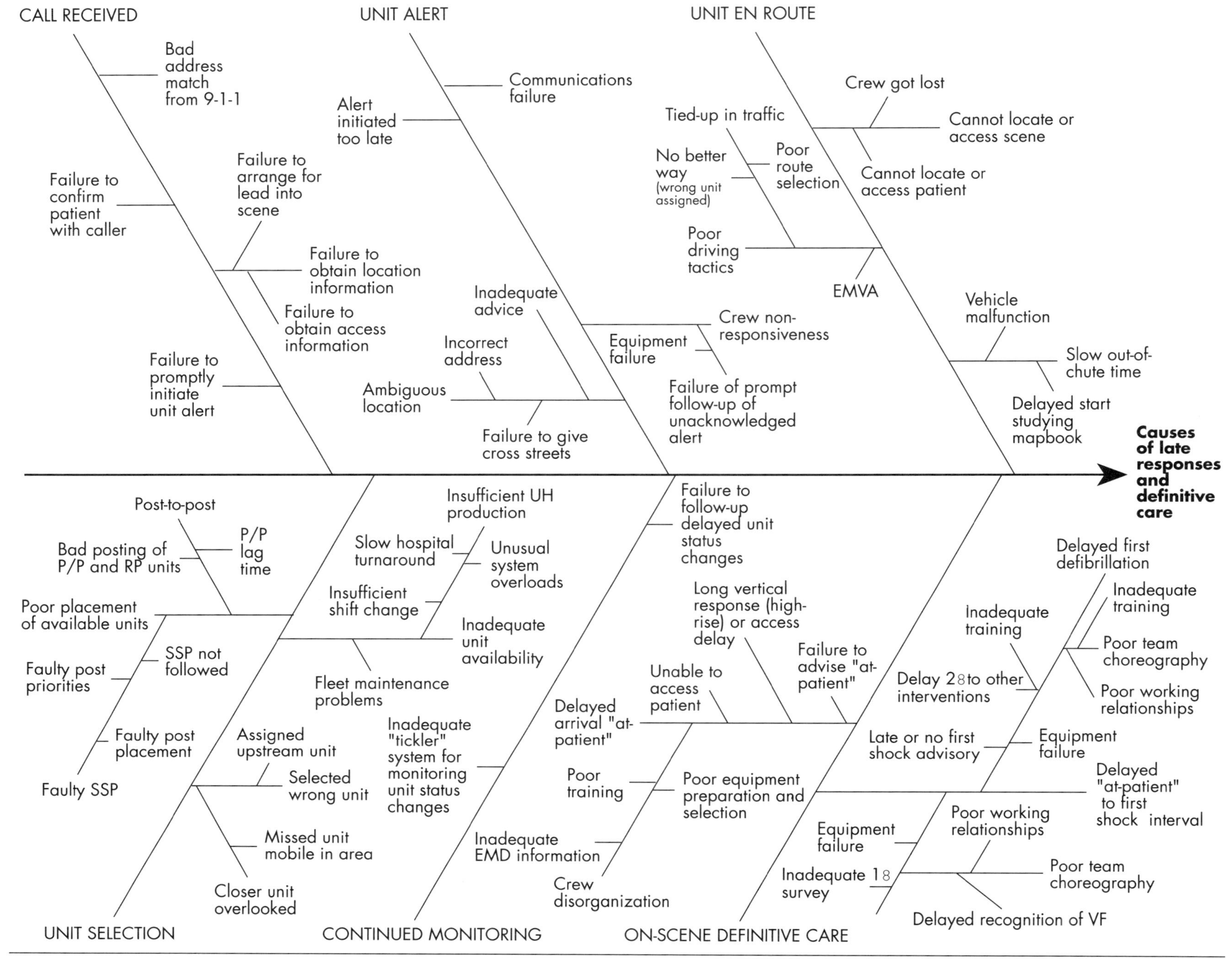

Figure 21-17. A cause-and-effect diagram of causes of late response and definitive care. (Modified from the SSM Workshops; courtesy Fourth Party, Inc., West River, Md.)

PINELLAS COUNTY EMS REPORT

CALL DATA

Date: | FD: Run #: | SS: Run #:

Call Location: | City:

Unit: F T | FD D Crew: | AMB D Crew: | Patients: FD AMB | Staged: FD ☐ AMB ☐

FD Medic: S☐ D☐ T☐ | Transport Medic: S☐ D☐ T☐

SITUATION

How/Where Found: | Action Taken: | Situation Found:

Patient Severity: R Y G B | CPR: Prior to Arrv. Y N | FA: Adequate? Y N | Time: | By: EMS ☐ PD ☐ Bystander ☐ Family ☐ Other ☐ Staff ☐ | Witness By: EMS ☐ PD ☐ Bystander ☐ Family ☐ Other ☐ Staff ☐

Patient Name: | Unk ☐ | Age: D M Y | Race: W H NA B A | Sex M F | DOB: | Wt. - KG.

Chief Complaint: Site, Duration, Severity (1-10)

Sec. Complaint: Site, Duration, Severity (1-10)

MECHANISM OF INJURY

Mechanism or Cause:

☐ Steering Wheel Deform
☐ Windshield Spider
☐ Dash
☐ Side Post
☐ Ejection
☐ DOA Same Vehicle
☐ Rollover
☐ Space Invasion >1 ft.

Fall (ft.)

Extrication Time (min.)

VEHICLE: FRONT 1; 8 7 6; 1 2 3 / 4 5 6 / 7 8 9 / 10; 2 3 4; 5

Air Bag: Y N NA | Seat Belt: Y N U | Helmet: Y N U

RESPONSE TIMES

Dispatch FD:
Dispatch AMB:
Respond FD:
Respond AMB:
Arrival BLS:
Arrival FD-ALS:
Arrival AMB:
At Patient:
Trauma Alert:
Time of Trans:
Arrival at Dest:
FD in Serv:
AMB in Serv:
Grid:

PATIENT SURVEY

Primary

	Pass	Fail	Intervention
Airway			
Breathing			
Circulation			
Disability			

GLASGOW COMA SCORE

EYES		VERBAL		MOTOR		
Spontaneous	4	Oriented	5	Obeys Commands	6	Total GCS Score
To Voice	3	Confused	4	Localizes to Pain	5	
To Pain	2	Inappropriate Sounds	3	Withdraws (Pain)	4	
None	1	Incomprehensible Sounds	2	Flexion (Pain)	3	
		None	1	Extension (Pain)	2	
				None	1	

Trauma Score — Adult

RESPIRATORY RATE:	RESP. EXPANSION:	SYSTOLIC BP:	CAP. REFILL:	GCS POINTS:	Total Adult Score
10 - 24 = 4; 25 - 35 = 3; >35 = 2; 1 - 9 = 1; None = 0	Normal = 1; Retroactive = 0	=/> 90 = 4; 70 - 89 = 3; 50 - 69 = 2; 1 - 49 = 1; None = 0	Normal = 2; Delayed = 1; None = 0	14 - 15 = 5; 11 - 13 = 4; 8 - 10 = 3; 5 - 7 = 2; 3 - 4 = 1	

Trauma Score — Pediatric

WEIGHT:	AIRWAY:	SYSTOLIC BP:	CNS:	OPEN WOUNDS:	SKELETAL:	Total Pediatric Score
>= 20 kg. = +2; 10 - 19 kg. = +1; <10 kg. = −1	Normal = +2; Maintainable = +1; Unmaintainable = −1	> = 90 = +2; 50 - 89 = +1; <50 = −1	Awake = +2; Obtunded/LOC = +1; Coma/Decerebrate = −1	None = +2; Minor = +1; Major/Penetrating = −1	None = +2; Closed Fx. = +1; Open/Multi. Fx. = −1	±

History of Present Illness:

Source:

Past History

Allergies: Codeine ☐ Caine Drugs ☐ Penicillin ☐ Morphine ☐ Sulfa ☐ Valium ☐ None ☐ Unknown ☐ Other:

Medications: ☐ ☐ ☐ ☐ ☐ ☐ ☐ ☐

Vitals: Time: | BP: | Pulse: | Resp.: | ID: | Patient's Physician: | Admits To:

Secondary

	SKIN	HEENT/NECK	CHEST	HEART	ABDOMEN	PELVIS/GEN/RECT	UP EXT.	LW EXT.	BACK
Normal									
INSPECT	F C P J	JVD TDR TDL Stoma	Accessory Muscles Flail: Rt Lt U L		Distention NE	Crowning Priapism Perineal Tear NE	DROM: R L NE	DROM: R L NE	
PALPATE	H C D	SQE NE	SQE	Pulse Deficit _____ NE	R G SQE Pulsating Mass NE	PIC PPC S U SQE NE	NBP: R L	NBP: R L	SQE NE
AUSCULTATE		Stridor NE	WH: Rt Lt U L I E Rales: Rt Lt U L	Heart: Y N Sounds: M NE	Bowel Sounds: Y N NE FHT _____/Min.				

NEURO — PUPILS: L: N C D NR Irr Cat | FINDINGS: ☐ Normal ☐ Combative ☐ Confused ☐ Dysphasia ☐ Hallucination ☐ Obtunded ☐ Post Ictal ☐ Seizures ☐ Tremor | DEFICIT: Hemiplegia R L; Cord Lesion A L

Physical Findings

Site:	Injury/Finding:	Comments:	Site:	Injury/Finding:	Comments:

Final Field Impression 1: | 2: | 3:

PRIMARY COPY

04/13/92

Figure 21-18: Data-oriented, structured prehospital call reports. Note that nearly every field is designed to be drawn from forced-choice look-up tables.

Treatment Protocol:	1st.	2nd.	3rd.	4th.	PINELLAS COUNTY EMS REPORT	V/S	BP	Pulse	Resp.	Skin	GCS	TS
						Meds	Dose	Route	Result	Change		
						ECG	Rhythm	Rate	Ectopy	Rate	Lead	

TREATMENT FLOW CHART

Time	Action		Performed By	Parameters						
		1 2 MC								
		1 2 MC								
		1 2 MC								
		1 2 MC								
		1 2 MC								
		1 2 MC								
		1 2 MC								
		1 2 MC								
		1 2 MC								
		1 2 MC								
		1 2 MC								
		1 2 MC								
		1 2 MC								
		1 2 MC								
		1 2 MC								
		1 2 MC								
		1 2 MC								
		1 2 MC								
		1 2 MC								
		1 2 MC								
		1 2 MC								
		1 2 MC								
		1 2 MC								
		1 2 MC								

REMARKS

MISC.

A.	B.	C.	D.	E.

Medical Control: MD MOD | Supplemental Sheets: | Abuse Registry ☐ Trauma Registry ☐ | Blood Consent ☐ Telemedic ☐ | Chapter ☐ 401 | Refusal on Back: ☐ Additional Sheets: | No. of Refusals: FD AMB

TRANSPORT DATA

FD Ride In: Y N | Trans To: | Destination Address: *City* *State* *Zip* | Odometer Start: Stop:

Hospital Selection: Patient Choice ☐ Nearest Facility ☐ Special Needs ☐ Diversion ☐ | Response Code: BLS ☐ ALS ☐ Standby ☐ Out of Town ☐ Cancelled ☐ | Wait Time: | Trans By: *Unit #* | Admitted: Y N

Moved to Ambulance: Walked ☐ Carried ☐ Chair ☐ Stretcher ☐ | Transport Position: Prone ☐ Supine ☐ Shock ☐ Sitting ☐ Left Lat. ☐ Recum. ☐ | Oxygen Supplied: Y N

BILLING

Patient *Address:* *City* *State* *County* *Zip* Unk. ☐ | Patient Phone:

Patient SS # : | Medicare # : | Medicaid # : | Ambulance Member #

Guarantor Name: *Last, First* | Guarantor Phone # :

Guarantor Address: *City* *State* *County* *Zip* | Worker's Comp.: Y N | Hospice: Y N

Employer Company Name: | Employer Phone # :

Employer Company Address: *City* *State* *County* *Zip*

Reviewed By: *FIRE*	Reviewed By: *TRANSPORT*	Reviewed By: *MEDICAL CONTROL*

PRIMARY COPY 04/13/92

Figure 21-18—cont'd: Only "history of present illness" and a section for remarks are free text. This design enables EMS data to be highly computerized and retrievable. (Courtesy Pinellas County EMS, Largo, Fla.)

RUN REPORT DOCUMENTATION ACCURACY PROFILES

PARAMEDIC	PR#	FTO	Reports Complete (%)	Reports Complete (#)	Reports Incomplete (#)	Audit TOTAL	BREAKDOWN OF MISSING OR INCOMPLETE ITEMS: Run #	Name/ date	Call lctn.	Actn. takn.	Sit. fnd.	Crew ID	Pt. C/O	Meds	Allrg.	Past hist.	Phys. exm.	Trma. score	Final assmt.	Prtcol. used	VS	Tx. flow chart	Trans. to	Mi	Guar. name	Addr. and zip	Pt's DOB	Soc. Sec. #	Insur. info.	Not legible	Rept. missing	Tr. reg.	Arrst. Reqst.
Paramedic 01	2194	VG	100%	9		9																											
Paramedic 02	2141	AB	100%	7		7																											
Paramedic 03	574	AB	100%	41		41																											
Paramedic 04	2043	VG	100%	7		7																											
Paramedic 05	943	AB	96%	49	2	51																		1		5							
Paramedic 06	2082	VG	96%	44	2	46															1					1							
Paramedic 07	888	VG	94%	46	3	49															1			1								1	
Paramedic 08	2027	NP	94%	45	3	48													2		2												
Paramedic 09	2123	LP	89%	41	5	46	1	1																3									
Paramedic 10	2143	AB	83%	40	8	48	2									1					3					3		1					
Paramedic 11	496	AB	82%	41	9	50					1									7												1	
Paramedic 12	1083	VG	81%	42	10	52	1														3			5		1							1
Paramedic 13	864	NP	79%	34	9	43					1	1	2			2	1				2			1		3						1	
Paramedic 14	2084	AB	78%	25	7	32																		2		3		1				1	
Paramedic 15	2128	NP	76%	29	9	38					1					1					1			4		3		1					
Paramedic 16	2171	VG	74%	26	9	35				1							1			1	1			2		5							
Paramedic 17	835	LP	67%	33	16	49	6													1	2			2		7		3					
Paramedic 18	2148	LP	67%	32	16	48	2		1				2		1				1	4	2			4		4						1	
Paramedic 19	2156	AB	67%	28	14	42									1					1	6					3						3	
Paramedic 20	754	NP	63%	30	18	48				1						1	1			9	3			2		4	1	3					
Paramedic 21	354	LP	58%	25	18	43	6	1					1	1	1					4	7			1		4							
Paramedic 22	2151	LP	57%	8	6	14								1	1	2			1							2		1					
Paramedic 23	512	NP	54%	22	19	41	1				1					1			1	7	2			3		7							
Paramedic 24	456	LP	50%	9	9	18								2	1						2			4		2		1					
Paramedic 25	2152	NP	48%	19	21	40	2			1	1	2								2				3		12						1	
Paramedic 26	500	AB	46%	19	22	41	1				1								2	3	3			1		2		9				2	
Paramedic 27	2144	NP	42%	22	31	53	3					1	3			21	2		1		24					3		1					
Paramedic 28	513	NP	41%	16	23	39	2					2							1	7	3			7		7		5					
Paramedic 29	2183	LP	34%	10	19	29	3				1	2							1	1	4		1	2		13				1		1	
Paramedic 30	764	AB	30%	3	7	10		1		1		1		1	1	2		2		2	1					1						1	
COMPANY AVERAGE			78.67%	2699	758	3457														118	# #	1	10	133	3	248	4	40	4	2	0	43	
Previous scores as of:																																	
10/31/91			47.60%																														
12/05/91			62.00%																														
12/17/91			64.00%																														
12/31/91			68.69%																														
02/01/92			77.39%																														
02/15/92			76.42%																														
03/01/92			77.58%																														
03/16/92			77.91%																														

Figure 21-19. A checksheet of causes of incomplete EMS run reports documentation. The use of a computerized checksheet (spreadsheet) enables the data to be analyzed and reports generated efficiently. (Courtesy Wayne Ruppert, National Director of Quality Improvement, LifeFleet, Inc., 1992.)

Pareto charts. Juran identified the "Pareto Principle" to separate causes of poor quality between the "vital few" and the "useful many."[19] By graphing the frequency of occurrence of defects by type from greatest to least, it is obvious where efforts should be prioritized to decrease defects. We used this concept to improve PCR documentation in cooperation with our ambulance contractor. This tool can be applied to a broad group of issues as a method of prioritization. The Pareto chart in Figure 21-20 illustrates prioritization of causes of incomplete PCRs.

Statistical process control chart. A special application of the run or trend chart is the statistical process control chart or "control chart" (Figure 21-8 and 21-21). The concept of statistical control is discussed earlier in this chapter. The control chart illustrates the trends in control of processes and graphically identifies some common and special causes of variation. There are a number of specific types of control charts, and each are applicable to different data types. Typically a basic chart shows the variability of sample or population data around its mean, and a companion chart quantifies the variation in the

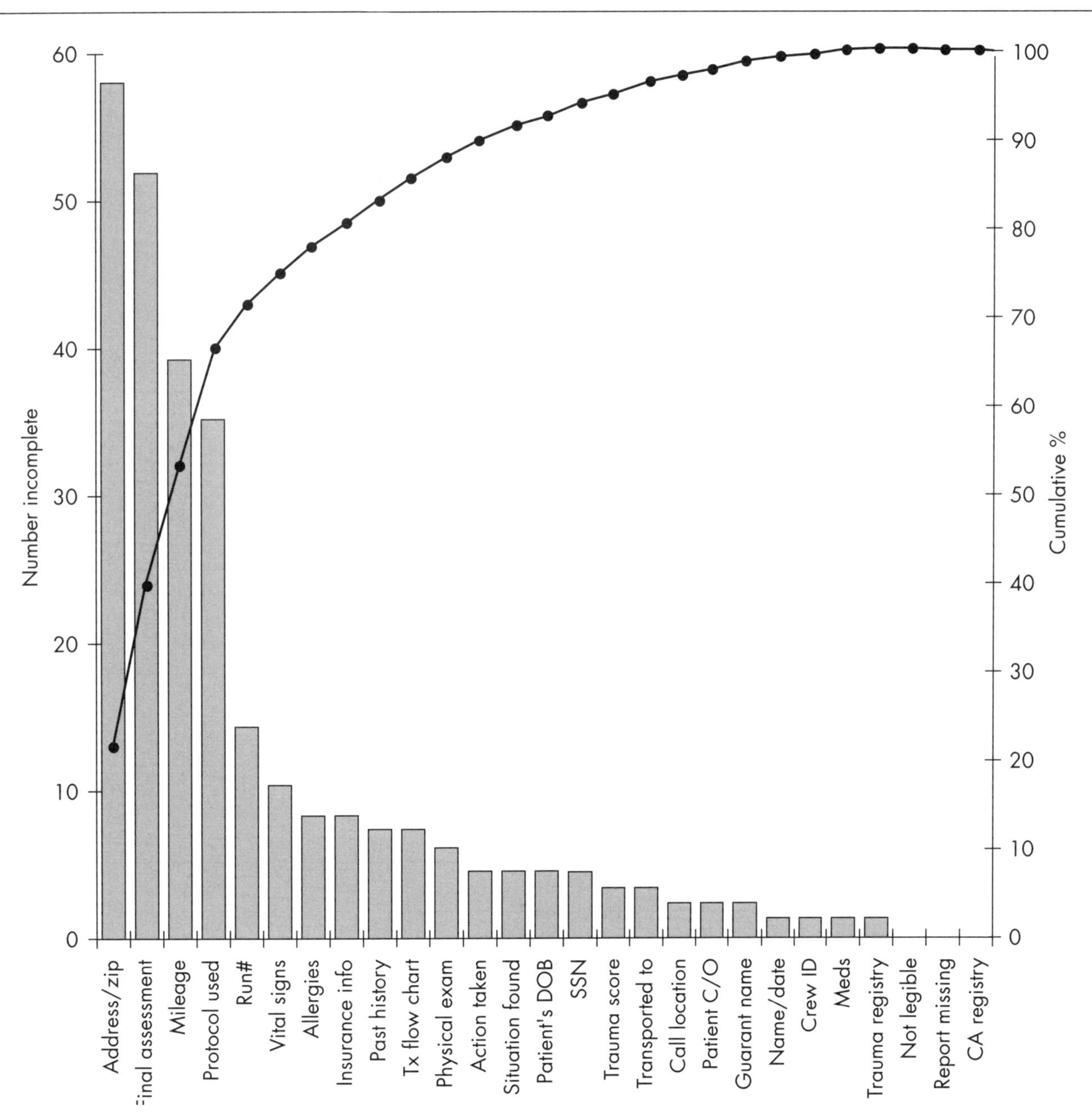

Figure 21-20. Causes of incomplete run report documentation in the first quarter of 1992. (Courtesy Pinellas County EMS, Largo, Fla.)

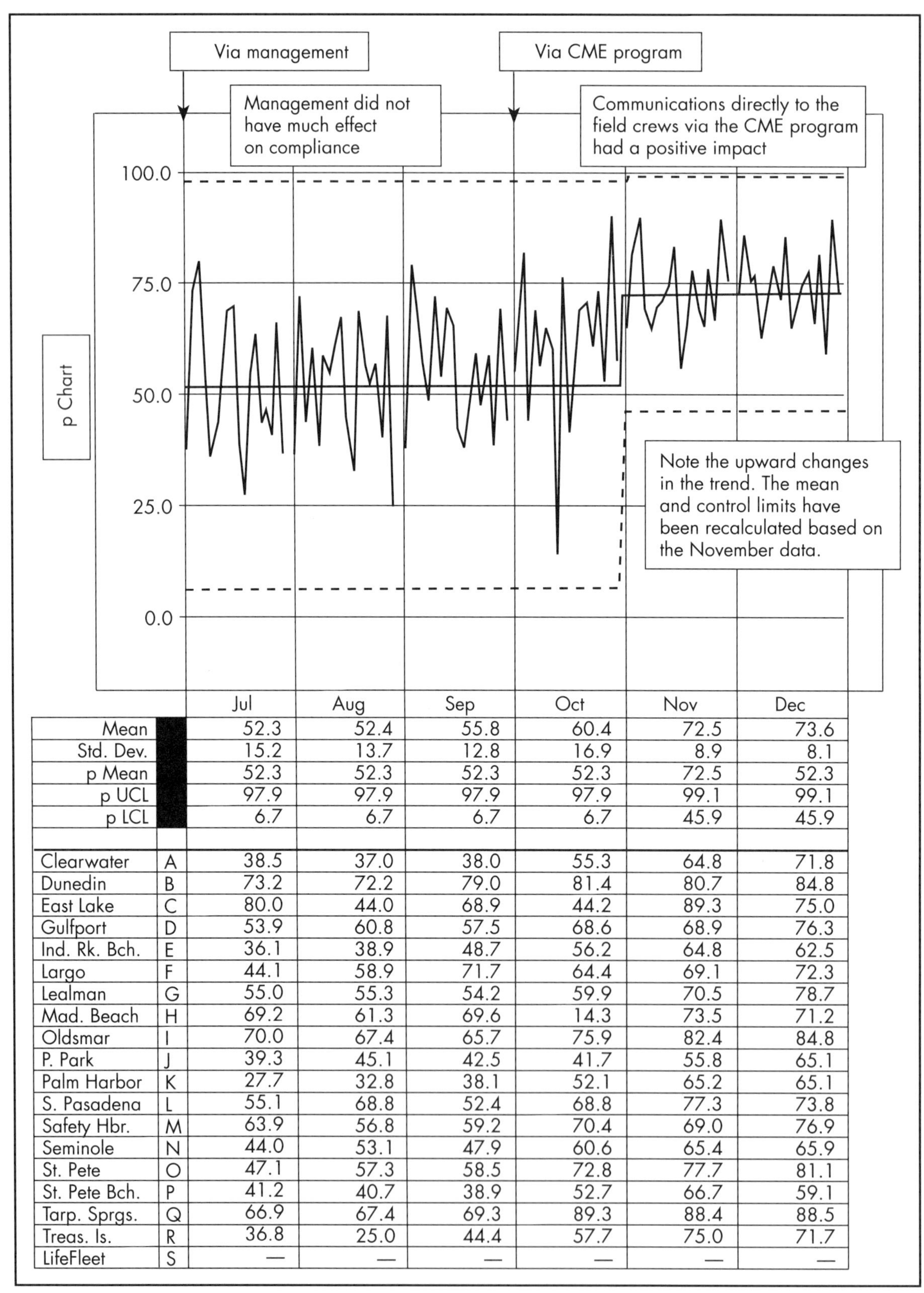

		Jul	Aug	Sep	Oct	Nov	Dec
Mean		52.3	52.4	55.8	60.4	72.5	73.6
Std. Dev.		15.2	13.7	12.8	16.9	8.9	8.1
p Mean		52.3	52.3	52.3	52.3	72.5	52.3
p UCL		97.9	97.9	97.9	97.9	99.1	99.1
p LCL		6.7	6.7	6.7	6.7	45.9	45.9
Clearwater	A	38.5	37.0	38.0	55.3	64.8	71.8
Dunedin	B	73.2	72.2	79.0	81.4	80.7	84.8
East Lake	C	80.0	44.0	68.9	44.2	89.3	75.0
Gulfport	D	53.9	60.8	57.5	68.6	68.9	76.3
Ind. Rk. Bch.	E	36.1	38.9	48.7	56.2	64.8	62.5
Largo	F	44.1	58.9	71.7	64.4	69.1	72.3
Lealman	G	55.0	55.3	54.2	59.9	70.5	78.7
Mad. Beach	H	69.2	61.3	69.6	14.3	73.5	71.2
Oldsmar	I	70.0	67.4	65.7	75.9	82.4	84.8
P. Park	J	39.3	45.1	42.5	41.7	55.8	65.1
Palm Harbor	K	27.7	32.8	38.1	52.1	65.2	65.1
S. Pasadena	L	55.1	68.8	52.4	68.8	77.3	73.8
Safety Hbr.	M	63.9	56.8	59.2	70.4	69.0	76.9
Seminole	N	44.0	53.1	47.9	60.6	65.4	65.9
St. Pete	O	47.1	57.3	58.5	72.8	77.7	81.1
St. Pete Bch.	P	41.2	40.7	38.9	52.7	66.7	59.1
Tarp. Sprgs.	Q	66.9	67.4	69.3	89.3	88.4	88.5
Treas. Is.	R	36.8	25.0	44.4	57.7	75.0	71.7
LifeFleet	S	—	—	—	—	—	—

Figure 21-21 Statistical process control chart (p chart) for EMS agency compliance with reporting of "at-patient" times. (Courtesy Office of the Medical Director (OMD) Pinellas County EMS, Largo, Fla.)

range of the values. The control limits of a process represent standard deviations from the mean.

The control chart is by far the most powerful of the statistical tools because it describes not only the causes of variation but also points us in the direction of solutions. A detailed discussion of the use of this tool is noted.[30,31] Last the control chart provides a method to hold the gains. By sampling processes that are in control on an intermittant basis, evidence can be found for the slipping of processes that may be readdressed by quality teams.

Results

The influence of CQI implemented in systems of prehospital care can be profound. Yet breakthroughs in quality are only the result of a diligent and relentless pursuit of optimization of the system. Experience with cardiac arrest survival illustrates these points.

Optimization of system design exists throughout the Pinellas EMS system. Established in 1986 as a public utility model system, it provides all prehospital care services to 1 million residents of Tampa Bay, Florida. The system responds to over 150,000 calls per year with fire service ALS First Responders and a single private ALS transport provider. An emergency response time interval (call received to unit on-scene) of 6.5 minutes is provided with 90% reliability through the use of SSM. A powerful SSM computer-aided dispatching system provides access to a wide variety of nonclinical performance data. MCOs monitor and track in real-time a broad group of clinical quality indicators from the EMS Communications Center.

Resuscitation is provided to more than 1200 field cardiac arrests annually. A paramedic-level emergency medical dispatch system and an aggressive communitywide CPR training campaign increased the frequency of bystander CPR from 11% to more than 50% in 2 years. The system anecdotally perceived itself as producing high quality care and a high survival rate from cardiac arrest.

Early in 1992 a cardiac arrest quality team was formed by the Office of the Medical Director (OMD) to implement an Utstein-style cardiac arrest registry. The team worked for several months constructing data collection and verification processes. Arrests were analyzed on a monthly basis, and reports were generated and refined (Figure 21-22). By June, reliable data showed the system had a survival rate for cardiac arrests of cardiac etiology of only 1.9%!

This realization was both shocking and confounding.

The group began dissecting the problem. The process was described using a flow chart to identify the parallel and sequential elements, as well as internal and external customers (see Figure 21-3). The elements of event reporting and data collection were recognized as integral to the process and included in the flow diagram.

The causes of late responses and definitive care were listed and grouped into an Ishikawa Diagram, showing major process categories to focus the team's attention (see Figure 21-17). The branch "on-scene/ definitive care" was added in recognition of the unmeasured interval between the customary "response time," that is, call received to unit on-scene, and the clinically important event, delivery of the defibrillatory shock.

The crossfunctional team developed and instituted a process to capture and integrate the measurement of "at patient" (the time of first physical contact with the patient) and "first shock" times (the delivery of the first defibrillatory shock). The process was piloted by a single high-volume rescue unit and then instituted systemwide.

The integration of this new process into the management of cardiac arrests was initially slow and problematic. Causes of unreported and incomplete data were reviewed by the team. Process analyses or refinements and positive competitive reinforcement of performance was widely distributed to field personnel. Graphic representations of current performance and process goals, as well as improvements in cardiac arrest survival were distributed and discussed at monthly CME seminars attended by all personnel (see Figures 21-21 and 21-22).

In February of 1993 the system achieved a survival rate of 14% for *cardiac arrests of cardiac etiology,* a seven fold increase in survival (see Figure 21-22). This improvement is remarkable in that process goals for "at patient-first shock" intervals had not yet been achieved, that is, 90% reliability at the 1-minute interval and 100% reliability at the 2-minute interval.

Becoming a Learning Organization

Deming's final admonition is to "take action to accomplish the transformation." He views this as a never ending quest to optimize the system that he called the "Shewhart Cycle" but has generally become known as the PDCA (plan-do-check-act) or Deming Cycle (Figure 21-23).

The ultimate goal of this transformation is a fundamental change in the organizational culture. In *The Fifth Discipline,* Senge describes this as a *metanoia* or trancendence of mind, "becoming' . . learning organizations, organizations' where people continually expand their capacity to create the results they truly desire, where new and expansive patterns of thinking are nurtured, where collective aspiration is set free, and where people are continually learning how to learn together."

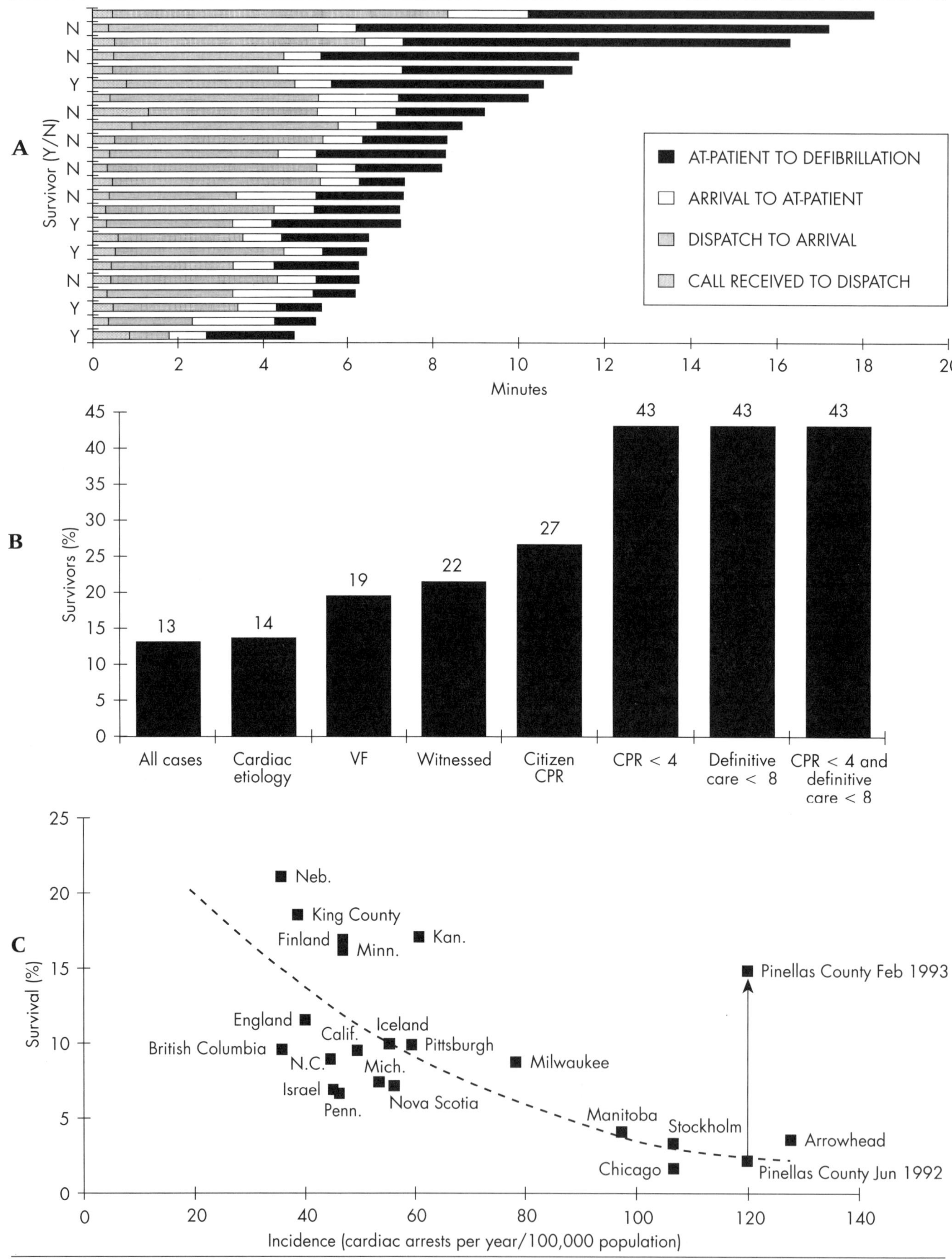

Figure 21-22. **A,** Cardiac arrest response time intervals from call received to defibrillation (n-97). **B,** Cardiac arrest survival to discharge, Pinellas County EMS, Feb 1993. **C,** Relationship of incidence and survival. (Modified from Becker L: Incidence of cardiac arrest: a neglected factor in evaluating survival skills, *Ann Emerg Med* 22:1, Jan 1993.)

1. **Plan**—What would be the most important accomplishments of this team? What changes might be desirable? What data are available? Are new observations needed? If yes, plan a change or test. Decide how to use the observations.
2. **Do**—Carry out the change or test decided on, preferably on a small scale.
3. **Check/study**—Observe the effects of the change or test.
4. **Act**—Study the results. What did we learn? What can we predict?
5. Repeat step 1 with knowledge accumulated.
6. Repeat step 2 and onward.

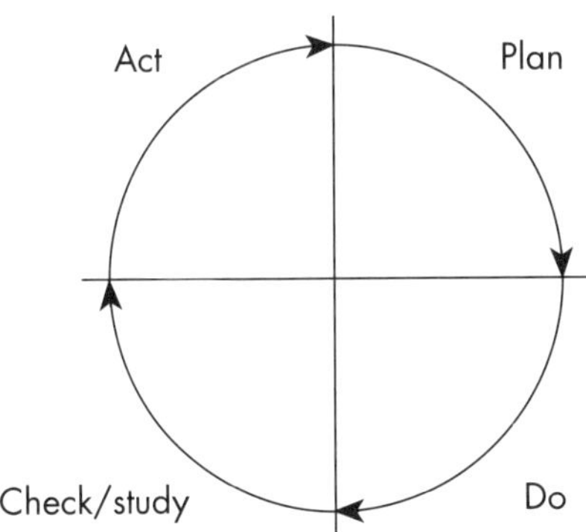

Figure 21-23. The Shewhart Cycle. (From Deming WE: *Out of crisis,* Cambridge, Mass. 1986, MIT Center for Advanced Engineering Study.)

He notes that what will ultimately distinguish learning organizations from traditional authoritarian "controlling organizations" is the mastery of certain basic disciplines. Organizations that master these disciplines can produce robust quality in their processes of care (that is, processes that are not only able to demonstrate benefit in the clinical laboratory, but also reliable quality in the street). "Quality is a virtue of design. The 'robustness' of products is more a function of good design than of on-line control, however stringent, of manufacturing processes."[39] The disciplines of the learning organization are personal mastery, mental models, building shared vision, team learning, and systems thinking (the fifth discipline).[29] This is what EMS is challenged to become.

Summary

CQI has been recognized broadly in medicine as the future of QM. These concepts have been successfully applied in EMS systems for a number of years. Largely through the influence of Stout, there are a number of well-established examples of CQI already up and running. The challenge is to transform the organizations by letting go of the "bad apples" approach and replacing it with principles of participative management that support the dignity and contribution of the field providers.

If we can accept the basic validity of the approach of CQI to medicine, there is a singular conclusion; the medical care system focused on the treatment and mitigation of illness and injury rather than the preservation of health is fundamentally flawed in concept. For EMS the true horizon lies beyond the foothills of QI in the unexplored realm of ideas.

Finally, although the processes of health care resemble industrial processes and benefit from efforts to understand their order and control their variability, health ultimately may not. Mankind's homeostatic tether to existence resembles not so well nature's systems of order, but rather the dynamic systems of sensitive dependence on initial conditions—the systems of chaos.[15]

REFERENCES

1. Berwick DM: Continuous improvement as an ideal in health care, *N Engl J Med* 320:53-56, 1989.
2. Berwick DM et al: Curing health care: new strategies for quality improvement, 1991, Jossey-Bass Inc, Publishers.
3. Clawson J: Pro QA: *A computer-based emergency medical dispatching system,* Salt Lake City, Medical Priority Consultants.
4. Davidson SJ: *Authority and empowerment.* In: *The National EMS Medical Directors Course and Practicum,* 1989, EMSAC Foundation.
5. Davidson SJ: *Closing the loop: discard the bad apples or continuously improve EMS?* In: Swor RA: *Quality management in prehospital care,* St. Louis, 1993, The CV Mosby Co.
6. Deming WE: *Out of the crisis,* 1986, Massachusetts Institute of Technology.
7. Deming WE: *Principles for transformation.* In: *Out of the crisis,* 1986, Massachusetts Institute of Technology.
8. Donabedian A: Definitions of quality and approaches to its assessment, 1980, Health Administration Press.
9. Donabedian A: *Explorations in quality assessment and monitoring,* 3 vols, 1980-1985, Health Administration Press.
10. Eastham JN: Assuring quality from the ground up, *JEMS* 16(5):48-59, 1991.
11. Eisenberg M: Quality assurance: is it possible? San Francisco, Nov 1987, EMS Forum ACEP Scientific Assembly.
12. Eisenberg MS, Bergner L, and Hallstrom AP: *Sudden cardiac death in the community,* 1984, Praeger Publishers.

13. Erder MH, Davidson SJ, and Cheney RA: On-line medical command in theory and practice, *Ann Emerg Med* 18:258-261, 1989
14. Garvin D: A note on quality: the views of Deming, Juran, and Crosby, *Harvard Business Review* 9-687-001:1-13, 1986
15. Gleick J: *Chaos: making a new science,* 1987, Penguin Books.
16. Imai M: *Improvement east and west* In: *Kaizen: the key to Japan's competative success,* 1986, McGraw-Hill Inc.
17. Ishikawa K: *The essence of quality control.* In: What is total quality control? the japanese way, 1985, Prentice Hall.
18. Ishikawa K: *What is total quality control? the Japanese way,* 1985, Prentice Hall.
19. Juran JM: *Juran's quality control handbook,* ed 4, 1988, McGraw-Hill.
20. Juran JM: *Juran on leadership for quality,* 1989, Free Press.
21. Juran JM: *Planning for quality,* 1989, Free Press.
22. Juran JM: *Leadership for quality,* 1989, Free Press.
23. Lifefleet Southeast, Mercy Las Vegas, Hartson/Medtrans San Diego, and Medical Priority Consultants: Personal communications, 1992.
24. Overton J: Personal communication, 1982.
25. Proceedings of the methodology in cardiac arrest research symposium, *Ann Emerg Med* 22:1 1993.
26. Ryan JL and Overton J: *An anticipatory ambulance deployment strategy for a large urban EMS system,* University Association for Emergency Medicine, 1985, (abstract).
27. Scholtes PR: *The team handbook: how to use teams to improve quality,* 1988, Joiner Associates Inc.
28. Scholtes PR: *The team handbook,* 1988, Joiner Associates Inc.
29. Senge PM: *The fifth discipline: the art and practice of the learning organization,* 1990, Doubleday & Co.
30. Shewhart WA: *Statistical method from the viewpoint of quality control,* Reprinted 1986, Dover Publications, Inc. (originally published in 1939).
31. Small BB: *The statistical quality control handbook,* ed 2, 1958, AT&T Technologies.
32. Spaite DW et al: Prospective evaluation of prehospital patient assessment by direct in-field observation: failure of ALS personnel to measure vital signs, *Prehospital Disaster Medicine* 5(4):383-388, 1990.
33. Stout JL: Measuring your system, *JEMS* 8(1): 84-91, 1983.
34. Stout JL: System status management, *JEMS* 8(1): 22-23, 1983.
35. Stout JL: How much is too much? *JEMS* 9(2): 26-33, 1984.
36. Stout JL: Ambulance system designs, *JEMS* 11(1): 85-89, 1986.
37. Stout JL: Wrestling with the big three policy issues, *JEMS* 13(6): 79-81, 1989.
38. Stout JL: *System design.* In: *The national EMS medical directors course and practicum,* 1989, *EMSAC* Foundation.
39. Taguchi G and Clausing D: Robust quality, *Harvard Business Review* Jan-Feb 1990.
40. Walton M: *The Deming management method,* 1986, Perigee Books.
41. Wasserberger J et al: Base station prehospital care: judgment errors and deviations from protocol, *Ann Emerg Med* 19:867-871, 1987.

SUGGESTED READINGS

Couch JB, editor: *Health care quality management for the 21st century,* Tampa, Fla, 1991, American College of Physician Executives.

deBono E: *deBono's thinking course,* New York, 1982, Facts on File Inc.

deBono E: *The mechanism of mind,* New York, 1969, Penguin Books.

deBono E: Sur/Petition: *creating value monopolies when everyone else is merely competing,* New York, 1992, Harper Business.

Eastes L and Jacobsen J, editors: *Quality assurance in air medical transport,* Orem, Ut, 1990, WordPerfect Publishing Co.

Geisel TS (Dr. Seuss): *On beyond zebra!* New York, 1955, Random House Inc.

George S: *The Baldridge quality system,* New York, 1992, John Wiley & Sons Inc.

Ohmae K: *The mind of the strategist: the art of Japanese business,* New York, 1982, McGraw-Hill Inc.

Osborne D and Gaebler T: *Reinventing government: how the entrepreneurial spirit is transforming the public sector,* New York, 1992, Penguin Books.

Pirsig RM: *Zen and the art of motorcycle maintenance: an inquiry into values,* New York, 1974, Quill, William Morrow & Co Inc.

Polsky S, editor: *Continuous quality improvement in EMS,* Dallas, Tex, 1992, American College of Emergency Physicians.

Swor RA, editor: *Quality management in prehospital care,* St. Louis, 1993, The CV Mosby Co.

Tenner A and DeToro I: *Total quality management: three steps to continuous improvement,* Reading, Mass, 1992, Addison-Wesley Publishing Co Inc.

22

Risk Management

Michael P. Wainscott, M.D., FACEP,
David L. Morgan, M.D.

In the practice of prehospital medicine the goal is to provide the best possible patient care. Many factors impact EMS patient care including primary training, medical supervision, and continuing education. Quality management (QM) is used to evaluate and improve patient care provided in an EMS system.

Prehospital risk management also enhances patient care and at times overlaps with QM: The term *risk management* traditionally implies that an adverse event has occurred and that actions are needed to mitigate damages to the patient, personnel, or institution.[8] Risk management in most EMS systems is a loosely defined mechanism for resolving patient care incidents, but it is important for this traditional view to be altered. Risk management includes not only a defined mechanism for managing patient care incidents, but in a broader sense, addresses multiple areas that facilitate improved patient care.

Prehospital risk management is a comprehensive mechanism for the identification, resolution, and disposition of medically related EMS incidents (adverse patient occurrences) including reporting, documenting, prioritizing, investigating, resolving, and defining disposition of those reported occurrences. It also includes the proactive assessment of other factors that affect patient care including primary training, preemployment screening, medical supervision, continuing medical education, documentation, and patient expectations. These areas are the major focus of this chapter.

Components of Prehospital Risk Management

Many factors influence patient care. A comprehensive prehospital risk management program should take the following components into account.

Primary Training

Primary training of prehospital personnel has great impact on patient care. A solid foundation of knowledge, skills, and attitudes is necessary for EMS personnel to function effectively and provide consistent quality patient care.[3] An awareness of the quality of primary training institutions and courses used to educate EMS personnel is important. Factors such as curriculum, teaching techniques, methods of evaluation, and clinical training have important roles in the student's preparation for a role as prehospital care provider. This knowledge is the responsibility of the EMS medical director, but EMS administrators should also be aware of this background. If the course medical director and the EMS medical director are different people, then communication between them is essential. In some EMS systems, primary training is provided as part of the individual's employment, and this facilitates involvement of the system's medical director in the training process.

Preemployment Screening and Orientation

If a potential EMS field employee received primary training outside the EMS system, it is important for this individual to be assessed in terms of medical knowledge and patient care skills before being released to function independently in the field. As a prehiring assessment, many systems use a written examination that may include tests of basic knowledge such as reading and math. Other assessments that are used include EMS knowledge-based written and skills testing, physical ability testing, interviews, and psychological screening. Most systems have standard administrative procedures such as background checks.[3]

New EMS employees should receive a field orientation and evaluation before functioning as patient care providers. Orientation is provided in administration, operations, and medical areas including protocols and field performance standards.

Medical Supervision of Prehospital Care

Assurance of quality EMS health care is provided through the process of medical accountability.[6] The medical supervision of prehospital care is discussed extensively throughout this book. The vital role of the medical director in defining patient care standards, establishing protocols, approving the level of prehospital medical care that may be rendered by all individuals in the system, and impacting positively all the operational aspects that affect patient care cannot be overemphasized. In addition, the medical director should be directly involved in the risk management program.

Continuing Medical Education

Continuing medical education serves multiple purposes in an EMS system, including updating personnel on protocol changes, providing reviews, presenting medical information and technology, and evaluating knowledge and skills of field personnel. A number of studies have demonstrated deterioration of knowledge and skills in EMS providers. In 1980 Latman and Wooley demonstrated that Emergency Medical Technician-As (EMT-A) lost 50% of basic skills proficiency, and paramedics lost 61% of basic skills proficiency within 2 years of training.[7] In 1987 Skelton and McSwain reported a correlation between the amount of technical skill deterioration and increasing length of time from completion of the training program.[13] One role of continuing medical education is to evaluate and enhance knowledge and skills of field personnel.

Other roles of continuing education include updates on protocol changes, run reviews, and new medical information and technology. It also serves as a forum for EMS personnel to provide feedback regarding patient care. In 1990 Goldberg et al published a review of litigation in a large metropolitan EMS system and suggested that medicolegal continuing education could protect EMS systems and paramedics from future litigation.[4]

Documentation

The Joint Commission on Accreditation of Healthcare Organizations (JCAHO) requires that a medical record is established and maintained on every patient seeking emergency department care.[2] The JCAHO mandates certain elements be included in the record; other elements may be added to conform with state regulations and hospital requirements. In comparing this with the prehospital arena, it is apparant that documentation requirements for EMS patient records vary widely. Patient records are required for all transported patients, yet specific elements of the record are far from universal. A number of states have a standardized EMS patient record, but use of such a prehospital care report (PCR) may not be not required.

Many systems maintain limited or no patient documentation if a patient is not transported. In 1992 Zachariah et al reported serious even fatal outcomes in patients not transported by EMS. Situations in which EMS personnel either denied transport (or mutually agreed with the patient not to transport by ambulance) were twice as likely to result in hospitalization than cases in which the patients declined transportation against the advice of the EMS personnel. In 1990 Selden studied medicolegal documentation of prehospital triage and suggested that rather than an abbreviated form or small section of the usual PCR the release form (when a patient is not transported) must be at least as detailed as the usual incident report.[11]

In 1985 Solar et al reported on the 10-year malpractice experience of a large urban EMS system and stated that a properly completed PCR is the best defense against a malpractice allegation.[14]

Other important areas of documentation include the new employee's application, preemployment screening, and field orientation. Some systems document the new employee's knowledge of protocols. Written protocols governing prehospital care should be available to EMS personnel. Some states require the presence of protocols on ambulances. All aspects of patient care incident management should also be documented.

Quality Management

Quality management (QM) of the patient care rendered in an EMS system may identify actual or potential risks to patients and the system. This identification allows for the proactive management of such risks and takes the EMS system out of the reactive mode of dealing with problems in patient care. The QM loop forms a continuous action loop starting and ending with protocols and education. Documentation of variance from or compliance with protocols forms the basis for analysis of the quality of care delivered.[10] QM and risk management are closely linked.

Other Factors

Other incidents may occur in an EMS system that have potential impact on patients. If an ambulance is involved in an accident, the patient may receive injuries directly or have increased morbidity from a delay in transport. In 1992 Bowers reported on 182 cases of alleged negligence involving prehospital care providers; 40% of the cases involved ambulance accidents (although some of these cases involved several identified categories of negligence).[1] This is compared with 42% of the cases that were related to negligence involving treatment or care. A provider who is injured while extricating a patient may no longer be able to provide patient care at the scene, potentially affecting patient care. Equipment malfunctions such as defibrillator failure may have direct bearing on morbidity and mortality for a patient. Steps should be taken to identify and address potentially preventable occurrences such as special driver training programs and regular equipment checks.

Patient Expectations

The concept of patient expectations concludes the components of prehospital risk management. Locales, socioeconomic status, cultural influences, and many other factors play a role in a patient's expectations of the EMS system. It is important that patient expectations are taken into consideration. As a group, patients come to the healthcare system with basically realistic expectations. They expect that the healing professionals will treat them with dignity and regard their welfare as a principal concern.[5] When the expectation of the patient is different than that of the EMS crew, conflict may arise. Discussions with EMS personnel regarding potential patient expectations and responses to possible conflicts may have significant positive consequences for an EMS system.

In a study of 17,271 emergency department (ED) patients the number 1 and number 3 factors that patients perceive as reflecting quality care are physician courtesy and nurse courtesy. The other factors cited follow in order of importance: comfort of waiting area, satisfactory answers to patient questions, protection of privacy, acceptable waiting time for treatment, cleanliness of treatment area, and satisfaction with pain control.[9] Extrapolation of these findings to the prehospital area is logical.

In healthcare, patient satisfaction remains the major product. When expectations are not met, patients feel they are not getting their "money's worth." Anger can be expressed in many ways in this culture, and filing a lawsuit is one of them.[9]

Table 22-1 Major Categories of Alleged Negligence Involving Prehospital Care Services or Providers

Category*	No.	%†
Treatment and care	78	42.85
Ambulance accidents	73	40.10
Dispatch and transport	50	27.47
Training, staffing and administrative	41	22.52

From: Bowers MA: Negligence cases involving prehospital care providers and the implications for training, continuing education, and quality assurance, doctoral thesis, Ann Arbor, Mich, 1992, University Microfilm International.

*In some cases, more than one category was identified and used in this table.

†Percent based on entire 182 cases.

Patient Care Incident Management

As a clearly recognized component of the healthcare system, EMS personnel are affected by the trend of increasing litigation. Over the 12-year period of Goldberg's review (1976 to 1987), claims made against the Chicago Fire Department EMS increased three-fold.[13] Of the 60 lawsuits presented, 47% named a paramedic as a defendant and 3% named the medical director. As the medical control physician is increasingly recognized as a fundamental component of quality prehospital care, correlative potential liability will necessarily follow.[12] It is likely that EMS physicians will be named more often in lawsuits as time progresses.

In 1992 Bowers reported on the major categories of alleged negligence in 182 cases involving prehospital care services or providers (Table 22-1). The category of "treatment and care" represented about 43% of the cases.[1] Goldberg reported 77% of the cases in his study involved alleged improper medical treatment.[4] It is important that the physician responsible for medical oversight grasps the full import of this information and responds by using an effective risk management system.

Patient Care Incident

A patient care incident or occurrence is any situation where there is a concern or complaint regarding patient care. This concern or complaint may be related to the commission or omission of actions on the part of EMS personnel, bystanders, other prehospital personnel, physicians providing direct medical control, or others. These actions either affected or potentially affected patient care and outcome of the situation.

At times, extenuating circumstances such as prolonged scene time may impact patient care, but could not have been prevented. Equipment failures, scene injuries to crew members, or accidents involving ambulances may impact patient care. The documentation and consideration of such problems are part of patient care incident management.

Establishing a Comprehensive Mechanism

Establishing a comprehensive mechanism for managing patient care incidents is an important aspect of a risk management program. This mechanism includes incident identification, incident investigation, investigation findings, indicated actions, documentation, and system impact. It is important that all are oriented to this mechanism, including field employees, supervisors, and senior level management.

Incident Identification

Incident identification occurs when a patient or other source expresses a verbal or written concern regarding EMS patient care. It also may result from an identified equipment failure or a crew's assessment of a difficult patient encounter such as a prolonged extrication.

Quality management studies and reviews may show areas that need improvement such as success rate for initiation of IVs. The risk management program itself may identify trends in patient care incidents that indicate necessary systemwide intervention. It is important that a mechanism be in place to identify, document, receive information, and initiate the process for handling a patient care incident.

Serious or Critical Patient Care Incidents

Serious or critical patient care incidents are occurrences that involve significant injury to a patient or impact negatively on patient care, morbidity, or mortality; they should be reported immediately. Usually the EMS system has a chain of command for reporting incidents, and it is vital that this chain includes contacting the medical director.

Incident Investigation

Incident investigation is a uniformly applied, prearranged mechanism for investigating a patient care incident. It includes a chain of command that identifies roles for all the players in the system and provides a routing mechanism for information and documentation obtained in the investigation. An investigation worksheet is a useful tool for the personnel investigating a patient care incident. This worksheet contributes consistency to investigations and also serves as a reminder for necessary actions to be taken and items to be obtained. A list of critical checklist ingredients is shown in the box above.

The personnel responsible for carrying out the investigation should be educated in this aspect of their work. These investigators should respond in a timely manner to patients or other sources expressing negative comments or concerns about patient care. Many complaints may be resolved quickly with the education of the person who calls or writes about some aspect of prehospital medical care. For example, a physician may be concerned because his patient was not brought to the appropriate hospital. Yet, when the EMS supervisor explains that the patient became critical, and it is the policy of the EMS system to transport critical patients to the closest hospital, the physician gains a better understanding of the process, and the problem may be resolved. However, the supervisor should always document the incident.

Some EMS systems require receipt of a formal written complaint before initiating an investigation. This is short sighted, and it profoundly limits the scope of risk management. Some systems have less formal requirements for when an investigation may be initiated; however, immediate documentation of all complaints and discussions is important.

EMS crew members involved in an incident should have the opportunity to respond verbally and in writing to a concern that is being investigated. These written incident reports serve as information sources and are a routine part of the investigation. Other individuals may be asked to make oral or written statements regarding the events surrounding an incident. For example, the ED physician who finds an endotracheal tube placed in the esophagus and notifies the EMS system should be interviewed

Incident Investigation Checklist

- Discussions with involved EMS crew members
  - Name/date:
  - Name/date:
- Documentation of discussions with EMS crew members
- Discussions with other personnel (patient, physician, etc.)
  - Name/date:
  - Name/date:
  - Name/date:
- Documentation of discussion with other personnel
- Crew member incident reports
- Patient care record (delete name and assign number)
- Other appropriate documentation
  - Photographs
  - Tape transcripts
  - Medical control records
  - Other
- Equipment or products causal to the incident

by the investigator. Documentation of the interview is mandatory.

Any other information, tape transcripts, PCRs, and equipment pertinent to the investigation should be collected. These materials are then collated with the incident reports and other documentation to formulate the summary of the investigation. EMS administration and the medical director should evaluate this information through a formal process and make a disposition of the incident. Further discussions, interviews, or investigations may be necessary.

Patient privacy must be respected, and the PCR should be treated as a physician record. This is a logical extension of the premise that providers function under the delegated authority of the physician medical director. States such as Texas protect PCRs in the same fashion as hospital medical records. Any unnecessary written or verbal reference to an incident report or its contents lessens the confidentiality of the report, contributes to potential negative repercussions, and minimizes the resultant value of its completion.[16]

In most states the limits on discoverability of hospital incident reports are much better defined than for EMS incident reports. In general, prepare only a few copies of the report and define clearly who receives them. It may help to clearly mark on each incident report that it is being prepared for possible use by legal counsel. Because there may be multiple regulations and statutes involved such as those protecting peer-review material, it helps to design the incident report and the risk management program with consultation from all appropriate medical, administrative, and legal entities.

All aspects of the investigation should be fair and involve due process for the employee, including the employee's prospective understanding of how the risk management program functions and how investigations are conducted. Some systems have review panels that include field personnel. EMS medical directors are the key individuals in the resolution of a patient care incident; therefore they should be made aware of the initiation of an investigation for minor incidents and be actively involved for more serious or critical incidents. Medical directors must have final authority on the evaluation of the clinical aspects of the incident.

Investigation Findings

Investigation findings are the conclusions from the investigation of a patient care incident. Results of the investigation may show that the incident was related to safety factors, environmental influences, training, employee clinical performance, judgment error, equipment failure, product deficiency, vehicle operation, incomplete documentation, patient expectations, protocol problems, employee behavior, actions of other personnel, or medical control. These may be presented and indicated in a checklist (see box on p. 250). The medical director must play an active role in evaluating investigation findings to determine appropriateness and accuracy in confirming.

Potential Investigation Findings

Results of the investigation show the incident was related to:

- Environmental influences
- Safety factors
- Training
- Employee clinical performance
- Employee behavior
- Judgment error
- Equipment deficiency or failure
- Incomplete documentation
- Patient expectations
- Protocol or policy problems
- Actions of other personnel
- Medical control
- Other: ____________________

Indicated Actions

Indicated actions depend on a number of factors, including seriousness of the incident from an administrative, medical, or media standpoint, system response to previous similar incidents or similar types of incidents, and the employee's long-term performance and disciplinary history. Indicated actions are administrative or medical. There is overlap at times, and communication between the administration and the medical director is essential.

Administrative actions usually fall into the generic classification of employee personnel actions. Medical actions generally fall into the categories of no action, policy or protocol revisions, product changes, remedial education, and corrective measures such as decertification. Remedial education actions include classroom education, clinical hospital education, testing, and supervised field preceptorship. Actions of an educational nature may also include systemwide training or retraining through continuing medical education. Potential corrective measures include counseling, probation, and decertification. The physician charged with medical oversight by contract has final authority on medical actions in response to patient care incidents.

Generally, for an initial employee performance problem the employee receives some type of counseling and retraining that is specific to their needs.

This process should be viewed as education-based rather than discipline-based, unless there are circumstances for which disciplinary measures are truly indicated. Even in the latter case the educational aspects must still play a vital role and represent a positive system response to a problem.

Documentation

Documentation of the investigation and resolution of patient care incidents cannot be overemphasized; it facilitates a more complete and consistent understanding of the investigation and ensures fairness and due process. Decisions regarding documents to be used and to whom information may be disseminated should be defined by the risk management program.

Summary

One major goal for the risk management program is to provide effective patient care incident management so the incident becomes part of the overall QM program and so it does not simply become an isolated circumstance with no system impact. Trends and patterns must be observed and interventions taken as necessary.

The goals for an EMS risk management program extend far beyond reactive management of patient care incidents. A good program allows for the prospective management and evaluation of all the medical care provided in an EMS system; it considers factors and influences that may negatively impact patient care even before a patient care incident occurs. The program affects protocols, continuing education, training, preemployment screening, medical oversight, and administration.

Change is facilitated through the identification of problems reactively and proactively; all personnel involved in the EMS system become part of the solution. The ultimate benefactors are the patients in the EMS system; their medical care improves through the changes and growth that result from the program.

In 1989 Valenzuela et al reported that less than 65% of emergency medicine residency training programs provided formal instruction in EMS risk management.[15] Both present and future EMS medical directors must become active, knowledgeable participants in prehospital risk management.

REFERENCES

1. Bowers MA: *Negligence cases involving prehospital care providers and the implications for training, continuing education, and quality assurance,* doctoral thesis, Ann Arbor, Mich, 1992, University Microfilms International.
2. Bukata WR: *Emergency department medical record.* In: Henry GL, editor: *Emergency medicine risk management: a comprehensive review,* 1991, American College of Emergency Physicians.
3. Cason D and Wainscott MP: *Training and evaluation.* In: Polsky SS: *Continuous quality improvement in EMS,* 1992, American College of Emergency Physicians.
4. Goldberg RJ, Zautcke JL, and Koenigsberg MD: A review of prehospital care litigation in a large metropolitan EMS system, *Ann Emerg Med* 19:557-561, 1990.
5. Henry GL: *Patient expectations.* In: Henry GL, editor: *Emergency medicine risk management: a comprehensive review,* 1991, American College of Emergency Physicians.
6. Krentz MJ and Wainscott MP: Medical accountability, *Emerg Med Clin North Am* 8:17-31, 1990.
7. Latman NS and Wooley K: Knowledge and skill retention of emergency care attendants, EMT-As, and EMT-Ps, *Ann Emerg Med* 9:183-189, 1980.
8. Little N: The quality assurance-risk management interface, *Emerg Med Clin North Am* 10:573-581, 1992.
9. National Emergency Room Survey: *Quality of care monitor,* Park Ridge, Ill, 1991, Parkside Associates.
10. Polsky SS and Weigand JV: Quality assurance in emergency medical service systems, *Emerg Med Clin North Am* 8:75-84, 1990.
11. Selden BS: Medicolegal documentation of prehospital triage, *Ann Emerg Med* 19:547-551, 1990.
12. Shanaberger CJ: *Legal issues in medical control.* In: Kuehl A, editor: *EMS medical director's handbook,* St. Louis, 1989, The CV Mosby Co.
13. Skelton MB and McSwain NE: A study of cognitive and technical skill deterioration among trained paramedics, *JACEP* 6:436-438, 1977.
14. Solar JM et al: The 10-year malpractice experience of a large urban EMS system, *Ann Emerg Med* 14:982-985, 1985.
15. Valenzuela TD et al: Evaluation of EMS management training offered during emergency medicine residency training, *Ann Emerg Med* 18:812-814, 1989.
16. Zeller CL: *Occurrence (incident) reports.* In: Henry GL, editor: Emergency medicine risk management: a comprehensive review, 1991, American College of Emergency Physicians.

23

Education

Bruce John Walz, Ph.D.
Gustave Pappas, B.S., EMT-P

A major, often neglected role of the EMS medical director is that of educator. When sophisticated medical information was first directed toward prehospital providers in the early 1960s, medical directors could have created learning environments that rewarded instructional excellence; unfortunately, that was rarely the case. The main reason was that in the early 1970s EMS providers were growing toward a consensus composite from two distinct, polarized philosophical roots—technicians who were trained and clinicians who were educated (Figure 23-1).

In 1972 the consensus composite was formalized with the introduction of the basic emergency medical technician (EMT-A) that was defined by the 72-hour curriculum. Since then the provider levels between "first aider" and physician have expanded by adding many hours of instruction and numerous skills modules. Ultimately a multitude of intermediate and advanced levels evolved; some levels are actually physician extenders (for example, paramedic), and some are independent providers of increasingly sophisticated first aid (for example, emergency medical technician-defibrillator). The educational dichotomy that existed before the development of the EMT-A curriculum has reappeared. For the paramedic, education often took a back seat to training that stressed rote memorization and electronically transmitted concurrent medical orders. For the EMT-A the same rote memory was required often without concurrent medical orders, and only the most perfunctory attempts were made to provide a medical background for the prehospital activities. With the further clinical sophistication of prehospital medicine in the later 1970s and 1980s, the need to provide higher quality adult education for all prehospital providers should have become obvious; however, it did not. Today, no EMS program of substance can exist without concomitant high quality educational activities. Presently the confounding problem is that there is a growing dichotomy between programs that strive to educate prehospital providers and those seeking to limit providers to a minimum number of interventions, requiring as little educational background and as few classroom hours as possible.

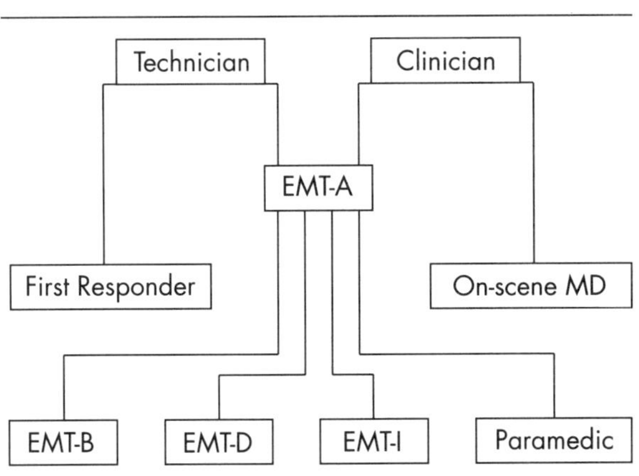

Figure 23-1. Consensus composite.

Roles of the EMS Medical Director

EMS medical directors must ensure that what is necessary for the adequate provision of prehospital care is both taught and learned, as well as ensure that education is provided efficiently and well. Medical directors need a working knowledge of the training curriculum completed by personnel under their direction. Such knowledge allows medical directors to provide guidance within the scope of practice of the providers and identify areas of needed training or change. In addition, medical directors will appreciate the level of expertise possessed by those working under their direction.

Medical directors must understand that in many jurisdictions the training curriculum and scope of practice of prehospital providers is set by regulation or law. The directors' role may be limited to that of a change agent, working with various constituent groups within a structured system. Depending on system design, the role of the EMS medical director may be that of educator, manager of education, or a combination of both.

Educator

Part of the directors' responsibilities may be the instruction of prehospital providers under their supervision. Such educational activities can include teaching a new procedure, introducing a new drug, teaching a section of the U.S. Department of Transportation (DOT) standard paramedic curriculum, or instructing an entire training course.

Most systems have established the position of non-physician instructor. This position may be regulated by law or regulation. Non-physician instructors are usually peer instructors who have demonstrated mastery of the curricular material and have completed formalized instructor training. Often nursing and allied health professionals serve in this role. Responsibility for course organization, administration, and student management is frequently handled by a non-physician instructor or program coordinator, thus freeing the medical director to concentrate on teaching-learning activities.

Medical directors possess medical expertise, but not all directors are teachers. Medical directors must realize their limitations in this area. The qualities of a good instructor discussed later in this chapter should serve as a guide for self-evaluation. Medical directors must also understand those they instruct. The volunteer EMT-A is not a first year medical student. The educational model used in most U.S. medical schools is not suitable for training prehospital providers, especially those with collateral responsibilities who cannot devote all their time to EMS-related training.

Education Manager

In addition to the opportunity to serve as an educator, medical directors may be required to fill the role of manager of education. This can be a complex and demanding task. Managing an educational program requires involvement across the spectrum of program planning, development, delivery, teaching, evaluation, testing, and overall administration. Unless specifically trained in educational administration, medical directors are wise to delegate this task to a non-physician administrator. Resources in even the smallest EMS systems usually include the hospital in-service coordinator, patient education coordinator, local community organizations, fire or police department training staff, and local school systems. A valuable resource in many locales is the community college. Affiliating with the college has many advantages, not the least of which is an established mechanism for delivery of educational programs. In addition, the community college adds the potential for providing college credit for EMS-related training, thus contributing to the professionalism of EMS.

Although medical directors may delegate administration of EMS education, they are nonetheless responsible for the quality of education being delivered. It is important to establish a quality assurance mechanism for training. Directors must recognize that determining quality of education and training is just as important and difficult as evaluating field care. Again, consultation with a trained educator may be helpful in establishing a quality assurance approach. However, medical directors must not be mislead by output statistics that may not reflect the outcome of the educational experience. Outputs are measures of how an education program is functioning. Measures such as number of students completing, student contact hours, and mean final grade reflect the output or final product of the educational program. Outcomes, however, are more nebulous and attempt to measure impact of the education on the EMS system. Changes in mortality and morbidity after conducting a training program for prehospital providers are examples of outcome measures. Outcome measures used to judge an educational program should be established before conducting the program and be of a measurable nature.

Education versus Training

Having discussed the role of the medical director in regards to education and training, the remainder of this chapter presents an overview of the educational process. It is important, however, to address a confusing aspect of any technical-based education program—the difference between education and training.

So far the terms training and education have been used synonymously in this chapter. This is the case in much of the popular education literature. However, there is a difference between the two terms. A common example of this difference is the cliche, "You train animals; you educate people." The connotation drawn from this is that training is something less desirable than education.

One of the simplest ways to discuss the difference between education and training is to look at the definitions of each term. *Education* is defined as[9]:

> The act of educating, teaching or training; the act or art of developing and cultivating the various physical, intellectual, aesthetic, and moral faculties; instruction and discipline; tuition; nurture; learning; erudition.

Training is defined as[9]:

> Teaching and forming by practice; the act of one who trains; the process of educating; education; drill; course of exercise and regimen.

From these definitions the difference between education and training may not appear cut-and-dried, especially given that both definitions refer to the other term. Perhaps there is no significant difference in the dichotomy as used today. However, the common perception of education and training is that education is directed toward the whole person; it is a holistic learning experience. Training, on the other hand, is perceived as a structured means to bring about a set change in knowledge and skill level. Another approach to this idea is that one educates the whole person, and one trains the individual for a given task.

Using field provider education as an example, a training program would focus on the student mastering the knowledge base necessary for functioning at the provider level. Drill and exercise would be used to develop mastery of the skills needed by a field provider. In contrast, using the idea of education as a holistic approach, the student would learn the knowledge and skills necessary to function as a provider and be exposed to the broader concepts and ideas of medicine. An educated field provider would have been required, for instance, to complete courses in anatomy and physiology, general chemistry, and psychology. The trained field provider may be equally qualified to perform the same skills as the educated provider but without a broad understanding of the underlying principles.

Training is not bad or less desirable than education. Many situations lend themselves well to the training approach, whereas others may allow for more extensive education. System constraints, budgets, personnel requirements and regulations, time, and instructional resources may all influence the degree to which EMS personnel are educated or trained. However, if the plan is to build lifetime career ladders for EMS professionals, then a lifetime of education makes the most sense.

Curriculum Development

To ensure a positive learning experience the instructor must be knowledgeable of the material presented and present the material in an ordered and logical way. Nothing is more frustrating for students than an instructor or speaker who obviously knows the material but loses the class because of a disorganized or inappropriate presentation. Hence the role of curriculum in the educational process.

Underlying the current development of curriculum in EMS education is the conflict of assessment versus diagnostic-based curriculum. Traditional medical education and by default prehospital education have been based on the idea that the student must arrive at a diagnosis to apply the appropriate treatment regime. Such an approach requires an extensive knowledge base and understanding of the underlying pathophysiology. Assessment-based education in contrast teaches the student how to react to specific signs and symptoms. For example, if presented with an overdose patient, diagnostic-trained EMT-As would conclude that they were dealing with an overdose and attempt to differentiate the type of overdose involved. The EMT-As would have been trained to recognize signs and symptoms associated with narcotic overdose, tricyclics, amphetamines, and alcohol. The assessment-based providers would understand that there are different types of overdoses, but they would react based primarily on how the patient presented. If the patient was unconscious, the providers would assure a patent airway. If hypotensive, they would treat for shock. It is important for medical directors to understand that these two methods of patient management exist and to recognize curriculum as belonging to one of the groups. Directors may be called on to select the appropriate approach for local training activities.

In EMS education medical directors have two options concerning curriculum. One is to use prepared curriculum developed either by national consensus groups or a commercial vendor. The other option is to develop a curriculum. The latter can be a lengthy, complicated, and arduous task.

Prepared Curriculum

To ensure uniformity in the instruction of national and regional training programs, such programs often provide a prepared instructor package along with student materials and standardized tests (see box at the top of the following page).

In addition to national consensus programs the various EMT-A and EMT-P textbook publishers provide instructor guides to accompany their textbooks, or they follow the national standard curriculum. Some of these commercial packages even include visual aids, student handouts, and tests. Most also include information similar to that presented in this chapter to assist the instructor who has had limited formal instructor training (see box at the bottom, left of the following page).

Examples of Nationally Available EMS Curricula

Basic Cardiac Life Support (CPR)—American Heart Association and American Red Cross, Complete student and instructor materials
Advanced Cardiac Life Support (ACLS)—American Heart Association, *Instructor's Manual for ACLS* and *Supplement to the Instructor's Manual for ACLS*
Advanced Trauma Life Support Program (ATLS)—American College of Surgeons, *Instructor Manual*
Basic Emergency Medical Technician National Standard Curriculum (EMT-A)—NHTSA, 1983, *Course Guide, Instructor's Lesson Plans,* and *Student Study Guide*
Emergency Medical Technician-Paramedic National Standard Curriculum (EMT-P)—NHTSA, 1985, *Course Guide* and *Lesson Plans*

Developed Curriculum

The development of instructional curriculum can be an involved process—entire books have been written on the subject. However, there are times when medical directors may need to prepare a training program, a series of lectures, or even an entire course for which no prepared curriculum is available or suitable.

Advantages and Disadvantages of Using Prepared Curricula

Advantages include

Standardization
Adherence to national standards
Lessons follow student texts
Reduced instructor preparation time, lesson can be delivered off-the-shelf less haphazardly
Supplemental material and visual aids often available
Prepared by professional educators

Disadvantages include

Lack of flexibility on part of instructor
May not adhere to local protocols
May not meet the needs of a particular student group or program parameters, instructor teaches "cookbook style"
May lead to poor instructor preparation due to off-the-shelf nature of material

The curriculum development process consists of the following five steps: needs assessment, objective formulation, course development, course delivery, and evaluation. An overview of the five basic steps is presented. Medical directors contemplating the development of a course of instruction would be well advised to seek the assistance of an educator.

Needs assessment. The needs assessment is designed to answer the fundamental question, "What do the students need to know?" Through needs assessment, assessors determine what the students know and compare this with what they should know. This difference or "gap" will be filled by the educational activity that is being developed. For instance, in developing a course to take providers from the intermediate level to the paramedic level, it is assumed that the students already know the material covered in the intermediate curriculum. The new course will focus on material needed to fill the gap to the paramedic level.

A needs assessment should not only focus on the learner's needs, but it should consider organizational and environmental needs as well. At the organizational level the question, "What level when?" must be answered. Environmental needs are those related to the environment that the prehospital provider will function in.

There are many different approaches to a needs assessment. Consideration should be given to using an outside consultant to prevent biased results (see box below).

Formulation of objectives. Once the needs have been established, they can be translated into behavioral objectives. First, though, the needs are screened against organizational goals and objectives, available resources, learner concerns, and environ-

Approaches to Performing an Educational Needs Assessment

Review of national standards
Comparison of training program with organizational goals and objectives
Surveys of providers, administrators, and consumers
Nominal group techniques
Review of EMS literature
Interviews with people involved in the system
Review of prehospital call reports
Reviews by advisory and technical committees
Formalized task analysis

mental considerations. For example, consider a hypothetical plan to train EMT-Bs to intubate. This plan requires that the student perform the skill successfully on five live patients. If clinical sites or approved preceptors are not available to handle the number of projected trainees, then this need is not feasible, and an alternative approach must be found. Similarly, plans to train paramedics to perform an advanced surgical skill such as peritoneal lavage would most likely be screened out by environmental parameters.

After the needs are screened, they are grouped. For instance, all those related to airway are in one group, fluid replacement in another, and fracture management in a third. The needs in each group are then prioritized considering such things as urgency, sequence, frequency, and course goal compatibility.

Objectives are prepared from the needs using a 3-step approach. First the specific behavior to be exhibited by the student is defined as an action statement. For example, "The student will be able to *list the bones of the upper extremity.*" Next, any conditions under which this behavior must occur are identified. These conditions should be as realistic as possible. Continuing with the example above, we would add, *"from memory and without assistance."* If this were a skill, conditions such as "while using universal precautions" or "while functioning as a team of two and given a simulated patient" would be added as well. The final step in developing an objective is to list the degree of acceptable performance. Again, adding to our example, *"to an accuracy of 70%."* The complete objective would read, "The student will be able to list the bones of the upper extremity from memory and without assistance to an accuracy of 70%." For a skill the objective might read, "The student will be able to demonstrate application of a traction splint while working as a member of a team, using universal precautions and given a simulated patient and traction splint, within 10 minutes and to the satisfaction of the instructor."

Objectives are the backbone of an educational activity. Not only do they define what the student must know and do, but they provide a means to measure performance. Objectives must be written to express a behavior on the part of the student that is measurable. For this reason, it is important to avoid terms such as "know" and "understand" when describing a behavior. Such words cannot be directly measured. What can be measured are terms such as list, identify, recite, order, describe, and state.

Course development. This intermediate step in the curriculum development process involves the actual formulation of the instructional events. To begin this process the developer arranges the behavioral objectives in logical groups. For example, objectives for an EMT-A course might be grouped into all objectives dealing with patient assessment, fracture management, burns, etc. These groups are the major topic areas or units of instruction; they are the chapters of a textbook.

Next the objectives in each group are prioritized. The needs assessment stage may have identified many needs, but not all of them can be met in one course or at one time. They are like a bulls-eye target; the bulls-eye is those objectives the student "must know." The next ring out is "should know," followed by "nice to know," and finally the outer ring is "related information." How far one is allowed to move off target is usually determined by the amount of time allotted for training.

Finally the objectives remaining in each group are arranged according to the teaching cycle. Objectives can be classified as belonging to one of the following three domains of learning: affective (attitudes), cognitive (knowledge), and psychomotor (skills). Affective information is presented first, followed by cognitive, and then any skill related to the knowledge. For example, to master application of a traction splint the student must first learn the importance of proper splinting (affective) and know the musculoskeletal system and the general concepts of splinting (cognitive) before practicing (psychomotor) the application. Once the objectives are prioritized and arranged, the instructional format for each unit can be determined.

Methods of instruction. Criteria for selection of the instructional method varies by the objective type, instructor preference, and resources. For instance, a verbal explanation of intraosseous infusion could be accompanied by slides and a demonstration using a training mannequin, or a cadaver. Each method is appropriate for a given time, class size, and resources. Many methods of instruction are available to the program developer and instructor. A useful typology developed by Knowles is presented in the box at the top of the next page.

After the methods of instruction are decided on, lesson plans for each unit are developed. This is essentially a process of "exploding" the objectives into teaching points and operations. The lesson plan is in essence an outline of the material to be presented during the course. It should not be too specific or it will become a textbook rather than a plan or guide. A common approach in education is "whole-part-whole." The instructor presents an overview of the entire subject or activity, then moves to the various parts of the material, concluding with putting the parts together again as a whole. Mager and Beach describe five techniques to use when arranging lesson material as follows[6]:

Methods of Instruction

Presentation techniques:

Lecture	Programmed instruction
Debate	Multimedia packages
Dialogue	Motion picture
Interview	Slides
Symposium	Dramatization
Panel	Recording, radio
Group interview	Exhibits
Demonstration	Trips
Colloquy	Reading
Audiocassette	Computer

Audience-participation techniques:

Question and answer period
Forum
Listening teams
Reaction panel
Buzz groups
Audience role playing
Expanding panel

Discussion techniques:

Guided	Problem-solving
Book-based	Case
Group-centered	Socratic

Simulation techniques:

Role-playing	Games
Critical-incident process	Section maze
Case method	Participative cases
In-basket exercise	Virtual reality

Other techniques:

T-group (sensitivity training)
Nonverbal exercises
Skill-practice exercises, drill, coaching

Modified from Knowles MS: *The modern practice of adult education: from pedagogy to andragogy,* (revised), Chicago, 1980, Follett Publishing.

1. General to specific
2. By area of interest (cover topics the student is most interested in first)
3. By logic (build upward from a foundation)
4. By skill
5. By frequency (cover the skills most often used or needed first)

Instructors should consider lesson plans a "personal thing." The program developer may write a lesson "guide," but it only becomes a lesson plan after it is personalized by the instructor. Individual instructors add notes, examples, illustrations, and stories as they prepare to present the material outlined in the guide.

The last task of the development process is the formulation of the student evaluation scheme. This stage, like those discussed previously, is based on the objectives. When each objective was written, a condition and degree was identified. This information is transformed into the student evaluation. For example, if an objective states that students will list something with an accuracy of 70%, then the appropriate evaluation is a written test question asking them to list the information. If the action word in an objective is discuss, then students are evaluated either through oral questioning or short answer or essay questions. For objectives requiring demonstration a skills test is appropriate, using the degree statement as the performance criteria (see the box below).

Program delivery. This step involves the planning for and the delivery of instruction. Program delivery activities include four items.

Scheduling—A workable schedule for delivery of the training must be set. Medical directors may

Common Types of Tests Used in EMS Education

Pretests are diagnostic tests useful in defining what material the students know initially. Posttests are summative and verify that learning has occurred by comparing pre and post results. Often the pretest and the posttest are the same.

Criterion referenced tests are designed to compare educational performance against a standard or behavioral objective. The main objective of criterion referenced testing is to evaluate mastery not to assign a grade or score.

Norm referenced tests discriminate performance levels among members of a class. Students are ranked competitively within the class.

Prescriptive tests are diagnostic and similar to pretests. They measure a students readiness to learn and knowledge base.

Progress tests are the typical quizzes, midterm, or unit test given to measure improvement in the students knowledge, skill, or attitude. Such tests not only provide an indication to students of how they are doing but also provide a check for the instructor.

Classification tests are similar to norm referenced tests. They are given not only to measure progress but to classify students, that is, to determine a grade. They should be based on the course objectives and passing criteria should be as specified in the degree section of the student performance objective.

have to consider restraints such as shift-work, restrictions on overtime compensation, volunteers, and their own work schedule. In addition, state or regional EMS system recertification and testing deadlines may influence the scheduling of training programs.

Facilities—Where training takes place is as important as the training itself. Concerns that seem extraneous such as student travel, travel cost, availability of alternative sites, and need for special facilities such as laboratories, anatomy labs, and field sites need attention.

The quality of the training site must be evaluated. Many institutions such as hospitals and fire departments have training facilities, but others do not. Will an ambulance have to be pulled out of the garage, folding chairs set-up, and a sheet taped to the wall as a screen before material can be presented? Distractions such as radio calls or on-call students who have to suddenly leave class need to be addressed. Parking availability and facility passes need to be arranged. All these things must be evaluated before the actual training session. The medical director should visit the proposed training site before a class begins to prevent any surprises.

Classroom arrangement—How students are arranged in the classroom can directly affect the learning experience. A group may require rearrangement for optimal teaching. If the class will be divided into small discussion groups, the seating arrangements must be changeable. Arrangements will also have to be made for skills practice space. Rearranging the classroom during a class takes time away from instructional activities.

All students must also be able to see and hear the instructor. When dealing with adults, visual and hearing changes can adversely affect the learning outcome. In addition, it is uncomfortable for adults to sit in desks designed for schoolchildren. If chairs are provided, students must be able to take notes or complete written exercises. The general environment including comfortable temperature, classroom accessibility, and rest rooms is also a concern.

Support materials—The development and selection of media to support a presentation could be the subject of its own book and is beyond the scope of this chapter. Nonetheless, it is an important consideration when planning and delivering a program. Instructors cannot assume that every training location has a selection of audio visual equipment; they should check in advance and be prepared to provide their own support. The rule to remember with visual aids is that they should support the message, not be the message.

Program Evaluation—Although listed as the last step, this is one of the first things the medical director and others involved in the program development process should address. The means and criteria for evaluating the educational experience should be decided early in the development process; thus the criteria will be established and evaluation continuous. Waiting until after the program is developed to design the evaluation criteria would be like conducting research and then writing the hypothesis.

Steele identified five program characteristics that should be considered when developing an evaluation of an educational exercise (see box below).

After deciding which characteristics to evaluate, the developer must decide with which criteria the learning experience will be compared. This is the "what should be" established during the needs assessment. Next, evidence to support the evaluation must be chosen. For instance, effectiveness of a program could be measured by how many students passed the state certification examination. Student evaluations using rating scales could be developed to measure the quality of instruction.

Evaluation can be a useful tool only if the results are used constructively. Feedback mechanisms to allow change and revision of the program need to be identified and available. The medical director and others must be willing to accept the results of the evaluation and use them to improve the learning experience.

Program Characteristics Requiring Evaluation

Quality—How good was it? What was the quality of the content, learning activities, media, and teacher's performance? How did people react to it?

Suitability—Did it meet the needs and expectations of the participants? Was it at the appropriate level of difficulty? Did it meet the expectations of the community? Was it within the mission of the programming unit?

Effectiveness—What did it accomplish? How well did it accomplish its objective?

Efficiency—Were the accomplishments sufficient for the amount of resources required from the agency and the participants? Was this the best use of resources?

Importance—How valuable was it to those who participated and to society? Was its importance sufficient to the resources that were involved?

From Steele S: Program evaluation: a broader definition, *Journal of Extension* (summer):13-14, 1970.

The Adult as a Learner

The course development process is important; however, it is just as important for the medical director to understand the recipient of all this activity—the learner. More specifically the adult as a learner.

Much of the current literature on adult learning centers around the work of Malcolm Knowles.[5] Knowles is best known for his idea of andragogy, which is the art and science of helping adults to learn. This concept contrasts the more traditional approach of pedagogy or child learning. Inherent in andragogy are four basic assumptions that are of use to instructors of adults.

1. The adult moves from childhood dependency towards self-autonomy. In terms of education, children depend on the teacher and the school system to determine what they must learn. Adults on the other hand are capable of self-directed learning. Additionally, learning changes from a full-time "occupation" to a part-time exercise.
2. The adult possesses an increasing reservoir of experience that can be used as a learning resource. This experience is often used by adults to define "who they are." Therefore, it is important that the learner's reservoir of experience be tapped in the learning experience.
3. The adult's readiness to learn is directed to current developmental tasks or social obligations. For example, you are reading this chapter because you are examining your role as a medical director. You have decided that you are now ready to learn more about being a medical director.
4. The adult's orientation to learning changes from delayed application to immediate application. Adults engage in learning activities that are usually related to their current life situation and needs. Thus they seek education that is problem- or performance-centered.

These four basic principles of adult learning can be applied directly to EMS education. In planning an educational activity the learners should be involved in the planning process as much as possible. This input allows the learners to feel empowered and in control of their own learning experiences. Giving the learner choices is another way to provide autonomy in learning. For example, a lesson on abdominal trauma could be offered in both lecture format and as a student-paced interactive computer learning program. Learners would be free to choose the activity with which they are most comfortable.

Asking students to share experiences or identify topics of interest based on their backgrounds provides an opportunity to use the students' reservoir of experience. Excessive "war stories" should be avoided, but such expressions allow students to integrate experience with the learning task. Methodologies such as role-playing and simulation exercises also make good use of learners' experiences.

Although a learner's reservoir of experience can be a useful learning adjunct, it can also be a barrier to learning. Adults pass all new material through a personal experiential filter. Thus it may be necessary early in the course or learning activity to break down such barriers, allowing the adult to be more objective and free of preconceptions. This is especially true of the adult who has had a negative experience with compulsory education. Such individuals may claim that they cannot learn. Providing opportunities for early success may help overcome this preconception.

Readiness to learn is exemplified by the new recruit or employee. One of the developmental tasks challenging young adults is getting started in an occupation.[4] Young persons selecting EMS as their occupation have an increased interest in learning about the profession. In contrast, they probably would show little interest in a course on planning for retirement.

The orientation of adults to early application of learning can be addressed by providing them with knowledge or skills that can be immediately applied. Many EMT-A courses provide time for the trainee to ride-along on actual calls after they have completed the initial part of the course. This provides an opportunity for the learner to see immediate application of material presented in class. In addition, it provides a problem-centered learning environment that is conducive to adult learning.

Beyond the four basic assumptions of adult learning already discussed, Knowles also identifies superior conditions of learning. The medical director should keep the following points in mind when planning learning experiences for adults[5]:

Conditions that influence learning by adults

- The learners feel a need to learn.
- The learning environment is characterized by physical comfort, mutual trust and respect, mutual helpfulness, freedom of expression, and acceptance of difference.
- The learners perceive the goals of a learning experience to be their goals.
- The learners accept a share of the responsibility for planning and operating a learning experience, and therefore they have a feeling of commitment toward it.

- The learners participate actively in the learning process.
- The learning process is related to and makes use of the experience of the learners.
- The learners have a sense of progress toward their goals.

Adult Motivation

The needs that bring the adult to an EMS educational program are as diverse as the individuals themselves. Ranging from the fire fighter who is being "made" to attend to the first year medical student who simply cannot get enough information fast enough, the mix and degree of students' motivations present the teacher with a complex and often insurmountable instructional challenge.

In an ideal institutional setting the teacher would be able to integrate the needs and goals of each student with the needs and goals of the content to be taught. Unfortunately, that idea presupposes that the teacher had the opportunity to assess the motivational needs of each student and has the skills, knowledge, and opportunity to tap into and reinforce students' needs throughout the course. Two fundamental realities of field provider education make this virtually impossible—large class size and the magnitude of student heterogeneity.

The ability to accurately assess a student's motivational needs requires individual interaction that is not easily performed in a class setting involving 20 or more individuals. While a teacher may assess the needs of a few students, because they are either patently obvious or through personal discussions, it is unlikely that the teacher can discover the individual needs of an entire class. Therefore, class size is a barrier to the effective teacher-initiated management of student motivation. The heterogeneity of most field provider classes exacerbates this barrier. In the usual absence of any screening or selection process for determining participation, most EMS provider classes are comprised of students with a diverse set of skills, background, competencies, and needs.

Because average class size is not going to shrink and standards for enrollment in EMS training are not forthcoming, the responsibility for motivated learning remains with the student and by default the instructor. The responsibility of the instructor is not only to be a content expert but also to be able to demonstrate a superior level of instructional effectiveness that supports the student's motivational framework. Therefore, the medical director must have a basic understanding of adult motivation.

No discussion of motivation is complete without mention of the work of A. H. Maslow. Maslow arranged human needs in a hierarchial order, beginning with basic physiological needs, followed by social needs, and finally what he termed *self-actualization*.[7] A graphical representation of Maslow's hierarchy of human needs is presented in Figure 23-2.

What Maslow's hierarchy means to the medical director-educator is that basic physiological needs such as room temperature, sound level, and setting need to be met before higher needs can be addressed. This is why the learning environment should be carefully considered. In addition, activities such as a friendly greeting for the learners, "ice breaking" exercises, and positive feedback help meet the psychological and social needs of the students.

The literature of adult education contains numerous theories of adult motivation; however, a few basic concepts are useful for the director involved in teaching adults. The following is a series of characteristics of adult health care professionals that affect motivation as it relates to continuing education in health care.[8]

- Most health professionals are motivated to continue their learning.
- Health professionals seek knowledge that has an immediate and pragmatic application in their current situation.
- Participation in continuing education is strongly influenced by an individual's past experiences.
- Efforts to improve the conditions of learning can influence the outcomes of continuing education.
- The realities of the practice world require that the health professionals know how to continue learning, stay abreast of new developments, and adapt to new environments.
- Continuing education should support health professionals' natural desire to learn.
- Health professionals should be encouraged to accept the personal responsibility of learning.

Pat Cross developed the chain-of-response (COR) model of adult participation in learning (Figure 23-3). The model shows that the decision to participate in a learning activity is influenced by a series of related positive and negative reinforcers. If the sum of factors is positive, the individual is likely to participate. If it is negative, participation is doubtful. In traditional adult education, getting the learner through the door is at least half the battle.

Meeting life cycle needs is a basic tenant of adult motivational theory. This sequential approach to adult development speaks of predictable crises or stages that confront the adult through life. Resolution of each stage is necessary before the next stage can be addressed. One of the methods used by adults to meet these challenges is education. The adult focuses on learning activities that will help him through each crisis or stage.

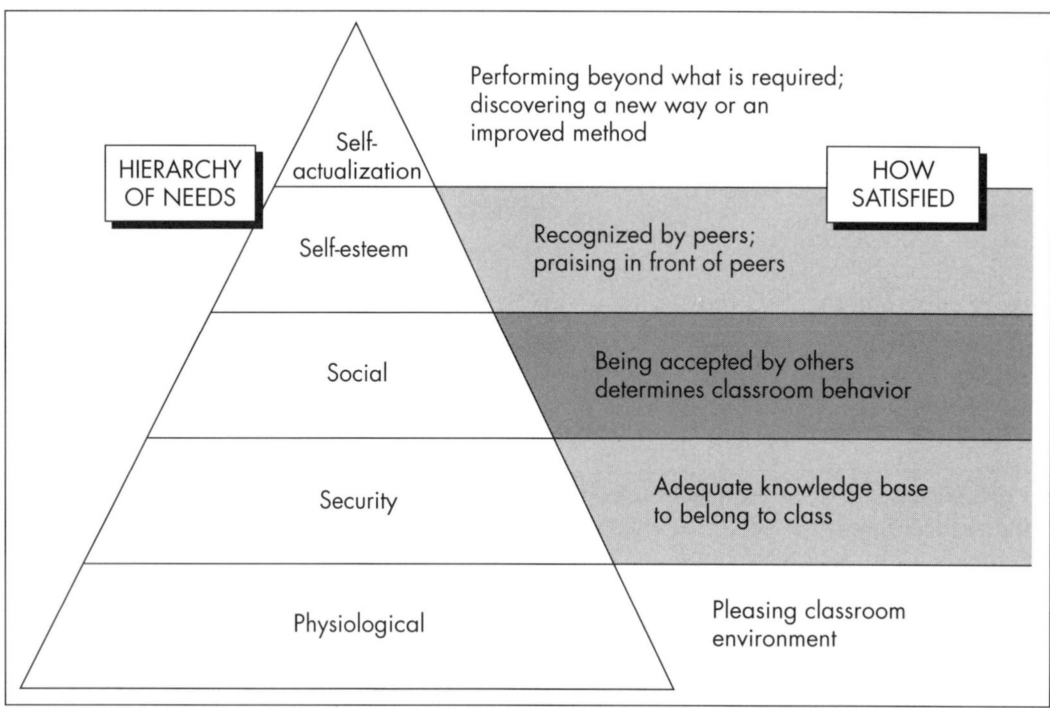

Figure 23-2. Abraham Maslow identified basic human needs and placed them in a sequential hierachy. (Modified from Knowles MS: *The modern practice of adult education: from pedagogy to andragogy,* Chicago, 1980, Follet Publishing.)

Although a useful approach, stage theory has come under increasing scrutiny in contemporary literature. Many of the studies were based on small samples of mostly middle class, married, white males.[2] Only recently has research focused on females or on the effects of cultural norms on development.[1] A prime question confronting stage theorists is whether movement between the stages is abrupt or fluid.[2] Regardless of the theoretical basis, adult development is nonetheless an integral part of the complex phenomenon of motivation.

A question often asked is what to do about the student who does not want to be in a provider class. Unless the student was physically bound and dragged into the classroom, a conscious decision has been made to attend the class. The motivation may not be that desired, but nonetheless there is some motivating factor. Take for instance, fire fighters who are told to take an EMT-B course. They may have no interest in EMS, having chosen the profession of fire fighting because of the excitement. However, if they do not complete the course, they will be terminated;

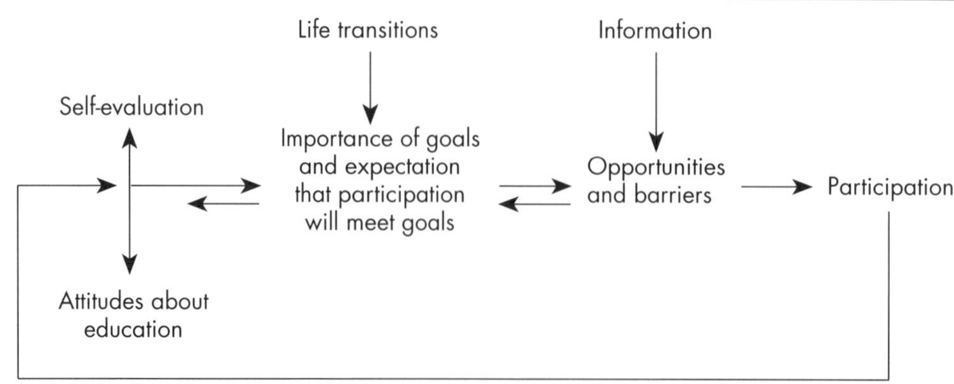

Figure 23-3. Chain-of-response (COR) model for understanding participation in adult learning activities. (Modified from Cross KP: *Adults as learners: increasing participation and facilitating learning,* San Francisco, 1983, Jossey-Bass.)

thus they will not meet their goal in life at that time. The challenge to the educator is to determine what motivates them and use that knowledge to accomplish the learning objectives. In the fire fighters' case the instructor could use an example such as talking about how they feel when responding to an alarm and relating their explanations to the affects of sympathetic stimulation. Everybody is motivated by something. Once that motivation is identified, it can be channeled into positive developmental change.

Disruptive Students

There may be adult learners who are unintentionally disruptive. These individuals often fit into one of the following stereotypes: (1) the sturdy battler who constantly challenges the leadership role of the teacher, (2) the friendly helper who attempts to have all the answers, and (3)the rigorous thinker who if left uncontrolled, can force the entire class to unnecessary depths of understanding.

By using the basic natural direction of the disruptive student's interest the experienced educator can move the student and the class in the appropriate direction. For example, by turning over a degree of authority and responsibility to the "sturdy battlers," they become invested in the success of the educational exercise. The friendly helpers, craving attention and approval, may be satisfied by being asked to present a later exercise. The rigorous thinkers must be carefully evaluated. If they truly know the required material, they may be allowed to "test out" and pursue an independent study in an advanced, related area. If the rigorous thinkers do not really understand the material, then that fact must be dealt with by the teacher, and a specific effort must be made to appropriately motivate the student by raising his awareness that behaviorally a change is beneficial.

Screening Students

Related to the problem student and the role of motivation in learning is the almost taboo subject of student screening. In many EMS systems, especially those staffed by volunteers, restricting entry or denying training to any interested student is met with great resistance. However, the medical director must decide whether to allow unqualified or educationally challenged individuals to occupy space that may be better used in times of economic restraint and public accountability. All too often "problem classes" are associated with instructor or testing problems when the real cause is the students. By not addressing the student population directly, the system is doing an injustice to both the instructor and the student. Marginal or below standard students take time and resources away from other, more capable students who have a higher potential to succeed and thus become an asset to the EMS system. Screening should be designed and used as a tool to assist the program director, instructor, and student. Job-specific and validated screening tests provide a baseline against which perspective students can judge their potential for success. In addition, testing provides a diagnostic profile of the class for the instructor. Testing should be job related and cover all critical domains of learning. Thus for most EMS training, psychomotor and cognitive testing should be used. Testing may also identify advanced or superior students who can be "fast-tracked" in an accelerated course.

Other Educator Roles

In addition to the education of personnel in the traditional classroom setting, medical directors may engage in a number of specialized educational activities.

Preceptor

One of the more rewarding and to some degree more challenging roles of the medical director is that of preceptor. In this role, directors have a unique opportunity to not only precept other health professionals, but to grow professionally themselves.

Preceptoring is the process of working one-on-one or with a small group in a clinical setting. The medical director's role becomes that of a coach or mentor, rather than that of a teacher in the more general sense. Most physicians engage in some form of mentoring on a regular basis such as explaining a procedure to a resident or showing paramedics a technique in the emergency department (ED) are all examples of informal mentoring. A preceptoring program can benefit the preceptor, as well as the student. It can also present many disadvantages (see the box on the following page).

Despite the disadvantages to preceptoring, if planned and executed properly, it can be a rewarding experience for both the preceptor and the student. To ensure success, it is important for the medical director to continually monitor the performance of the student and the preceptor. Students should not just be "dumped" into a unit or assigned to a prehospital provider, physician, or nurse without some prior interaction and a clear understanding of the preceptor's role.

The preceptor experience has the potential to be less controllable than a classroom or lab setting; it can also be less dependable. The case mix presented to the student usually cannot be prearranged, especially in the field setting or in an ED. Personnel

Advantages and Disadvantages of Precepting

From the preceptor's perspective

Advantages

Professional stimulation (Opportunity to watch others learn can be very rewarding.)
Improves knowledge and skills (Preparation for precepting may require the preceptor to review infrequently used knowledge and procedures.)
Allows the preceptor to demonstrate leadership and interpersonal skills
New information can be learned from students
May serve as an incentive for continuing education

Disadvantages

Time consuming both in preparation and during precepting
May interfere with scheduling
Requires preceptor to balance work responsibilities with needs of student (especially true if preceptor is functioning in normal work capacity)
Requires additional work outside the actual precepting time (for example, completing student evaluation forms)
May be stressful as preceptor is under constant observation by student (In addition, preceptor may find need to perform "by the book" interferes with job function.)
Preceptor may be called upon to deal with nonclinical situations

From the student's perspective

Advantages

Opportunity to practice role socialization in a controlled environment
Reduces reality shock by allowing the student to "practice" profession
Conflicts that may develop can be addressed directly and resolved with the help of the preceptor
Close supervision allows for direct feedback and immediate resolution of problems
Student's confidence is increased through skills practice and knowledge application
Student's confidence is increased by opportunity to practice in the "real world"
Allows tailoring the experience for the individual

Disadvantages

Takes more time than group instruction
Less flexibility in scheduling (especially a problem with shift workers)
Possibility for incongruence with preceptor
Can be stressful (Students may feel they are always "on stage.")
Student may get "dumped on" by preceptor (may be given menial tasks that preceptor does not want to do)
Student may learn bad habits, incorrect procedure, or poor attitude

changes such as sickness or work schedules may alter or change the preceptoring activity.

To ensure a quality experience, preceptors need to be committed and willing to participate. In addition, they should possess exemplary clinical skills and ability. A difficult aspect of preceptoring is dealing with the stressed or incompetent student in a crisis situation. A student who freezes in the middle of a cardiac arrest needs to be firmly but compassionately dealt with. Training in student counseling and evaluation techniques may also be required of the preceptor.

Clinical performance objectives should be established for the program. These not only add structure to the experience but also serve as the basis for student evaluation. A simple skills check-off sheet may be used until formal objectives are available.

Skills Instructor

The medical director may be called on not only to provide didactic instruction but skills instruction as well. Teaching a skill usually involves the demonstration method of instruction. The concept underlying the demonstration method of instruction is whole-part-whole. The instructor presents the whole of the procedure or skill, then the individual parts of the whole, followed by a review of the whole again. This approach allows the student to develop the proper set necessary to master the skill. In addition, repeating the whole serves as a summary to reinforce the steps and key points presented.

As during lecture, students are passive during the demonstration, but unlike the lecture, hearing is not the only sense stimulated. The students must be able to both hear the instructor's explanation and see his actions. Thus good visuals are an important part of the demonstration process. This can be achieved by good classroom set-up and design and proper class size. The use of "larger-than-life" equipment or cutaway models can also improve visibility.

Equipment used in the demonstration should be identical to that used in the field. Expended or outdated equipment may confuse the student. Asking the student to pretend or visualize something distracts from the psychomotor skill learning process.

The instructor should also check that equipment for the demonstration is working properly and all necessary ancillary supplies are on hand. Unfortunately, when Murphy's Law strikes in education, it is usually during the most critical point of a demonstration.

Although instructors may be presenting a skill that they have performed numerous times before, practice and rehearsal are still necessary. As the experienced providers become accustomed to performing a skill, they unconsciously alter and change the procedure in subtle ways. They may also become "sloppy" and not follow the procedure as outlined or required. It may help to review a skill or procedure manual in preparation for the demonstration. Also helpful is demonstrating the technique to a colleague, asking them to provide feedback from a student's point of view.

Not only should teachers present the skill correctly, but they need to be sensitive to the motor and sensory aspects of the procedure and how best to relate them to the learner. Take for example teaching the placement of an IV catheter. It is easy to describe the site preparation, angiocath preparation, and approaches to vein cannulation; however, what is difficult to "teach" is the feel of entering the vein and advancing the stylet a short distance before moving the cannula. For the teacher, this may be an almost automatic response that is overlooked in demonstrating the skill, but it is a critical action for the student to master.

Another aspect of skills instruction that teachers need to be cognizant of is coupling of activities. As they become more familiar with a skill or procedure, they may subconsciously link or combine small steps or stages of a skill or procedure together. When the skill is taught, it is important to separate these connections so the student is exposed to the intricate nuances necessary to master the skill. The use of a skill flow sheet or performance check sheet is helpful to ensure that critical steps are clearly presented and explained.

It is important for the skills instructor to appreciate that students will exhibit various levels of mastery as they attempt to learn a skill. Limits on skills practice preclude the student from leaving the instructional experience at much more than the demonstration stage of skills mastery. Following a demonstration, the student will be motivated to practice. Ample opportunity and facilities should be provided for student practice and review.

Skills Evaluator

Related to the teaching of skills is the role of evaluator of skills competence. This role is most often fulfilled during the practical examinations required for certifications such as paramedic. As with any evaluation process, it is important that the evaluation be intimately related to the objectives. The condition and degree statements provide the criteria for the evaluation. The steps and related knowledge that are determined in the occupational analysis form the skills check-off list and sequence.

As with skills instruction, it is important to realize that the student is not an experienced master but essentially an imitator. In addition to a limited ability to perform the skill the student may be intimidated by the teacher or evaluator. Nervousness and sudden forgetfulness are common. A simple smile or statement acknowledging the student's stress will not alter the evaluator's objectivity but will put the student at ease.

Instructor Evaluator

As a manager of education the medical director should evaluate instructors working in the local program. Therefore it is important to understand some of the characteristics of a good instructor.

The process of instruction is in essence a specialized form of communication. Therefore it is imperative that instructors effectively communicate with people and understand human behavior. A student-teacher relationship built on mutual understanding and respect is a tremendously positive aid to learning.

Enthusiasm and a sincere desire to teach are also necessary qualities of a good instructor. If an individual is forced to teach or does so without enthusiasm, the learning experience will be mediocre at best, resulting in a lost opportunity for the system. In some systems, residents are required to teach parts of prehospital provider training programs. If they are not skilled at teaching or just not interested, this needs to be addressed by the medical director. Regardless of the outcome, how instructors perceive their role transfers directly to students. Therefore enthusiasm on the part of the instructor has a good chance of stimulating enthusiasm in the students.

Loyalty to the instructional program and the overall field of prehospital care is as necessary as any other trait in a good instructor. To effectively teach, instructors must believe in what they are teaching and in their students. Mutual respect and support, just like enthusiasm, motivate the student; they also add credibility to the instructor.

Instructors need to be resourceful and creative. The great diversity of field provider levels and educational programs require instructors to be flexible and dynamic. Nothing can be more frustrating to EMT-B students than a physician giving a lecture from notes and visuals designed for third year medical residents. The ability to adjust the level of instruction to meet the needs of the students and the system is a valuable asset in an instructor.

Related to resourcefulness and creativity is the need to show empathy and sensitivity toward students. In volunteer systems a student who is late to class because he was held at his job needs support and assistance, not chastisement. The instructor's ability to see the world through the student's eyes can go a long way toward making the educational experience rewarding for both.

To ensure the quality of instruction the medical director must plan for not only instructor evaluation but also instructor selection and education. Either directly or through others the director must arrange for continual instructor evaluation during instruction, as well as a postcourse review and critique.

The Future

There is currently a nationwide epidemic of clinical, physical, and emotional burnout of experienced prehospital providers, most of whom will not be administrators, teachers, or dispatchers. An educational and operational continuum must be created in the near future. Soon *all* EMS education will be individual, interactive, and computer driven. There will be no more lectures; students will learn at their own speeds, and psychomotor skills will be learned through virtual reality.

Summary

EMS medical directors spend years learning a great deal of material; they have a responsibility to share that knowledge with field personnel. Too often the physician has either not learned to teach effectively or has not applied those lessons to the educational task at hand. Educating prehospital providers is a fulfilling and uplifting experience that has the potential to affect the lives and well-being of many people. By understanding and appreciating the many facets of education in their roles as both educator and manager of education, EMS physicians can better accomplish their ultimate goal to provide sound, professional medical oversight.

REFERENCES

1. Bardwick JM: *The seasons of a woman's life.* In: McGuigan D, edition: *Women's lives: new theory, research and policy,* Ann Arbor, 1980, University of Michigan Center for Continuing Education of Women.
2. Boucouvalas M and Krupp JA: *Adult development and learning.* In: Merriam SB and Cunningham PM, editions: *Handbook of adult and continuing education,* San Francisco, 1990, Josssey-Bass Inc, Publishers.
3. Cross KP: *Adults as learners: increasing participation and facilitating learning,* San Francisco, 1983, Jossey-Bass Inc, Publishers.
4. Gould R: *Transformations: growth and change in adult life,* New York, 1978, Simon & Schuster Inc.
5. Knowles MS: *The modern practice of adult education: from pedagogy to andragogy,* (revised), Chicago, 1980, Follett Publishing.
6. Kuehl AD: *Thoughts on the future of EMS education.* In: Bournss: The EMS medical advisor 3:2, 1993.
7. Mager RF and Beach KM Jr: *Developing vocational instruction,* Belmont, Calif, 1967, Fearon-Pitman Publishers.
8. Maslow AH: *The farther reaches of human nature,* New York, 1971, The Viking Press.
9. Pennington FC, Allan DME, and Green JS: *Learning theory, educational psychology, and principles of adult development,* In: Green JS, Groswald SJ, Suter E, and Walthall DB III, editors: Continuing education for the health professions. San Francisco, 1984, Jossey-Bass Inc, Publishers.
10. Thatcher VS, editor: *Educational book of essential knowledge: an edition of the Webster encyclopedic dictionary of the Eng-lish language,* 1966, Educational Book Club.

24

Authorization and Empowerment

Steven J. Davidson, M.D., M.B.A., FACEP

EMS medical directors gain a role in an EMS agency through the specific authority of law and contract. However, power derives only slightly from authority; more correctly an EMS medical director should recognize that properly structured and implemented authority provides the *opportunity* for the EMS physician to gain and exercise power.

Medical oversight in EMS is usually at the service of external forces. The forces that have the greatest relevance and impact on an EMS medical director include state statute, the statute's attendant regulations, case law subsequent to the adjudicative processes involving the statute, and applicable regulations.

On the local level, county or municipal ordinances and corresponding regulations may affect the EMS medical director. Lastly the realities of contract, budget, reporting structures, personnel policies, ego, and turf all inevitably come into play.

Although not all these issues can be resolved in the medical director's favor or entirely avoided, the framework in which they are addressed can substantially affect medical directors' fulfillment of their responsibilities and the pleasure or pain with which they are able to do so. This chapter discusses the issues surrounding authority that an EMS physician should address when accepting the responsibility of EMS medical director for an EMS agency and the structures including the written contract that can most directly influence the success and desirability of the medical director's position.

Authorization by Contract

The EMS medical director most specifically obtains authority by contract with the EMS agency. This contract is an agreement between the EMS agency and the physician medical director. When written in accordance with state law and "The Uniform Commercial Code," the contract is enforceable by civil law processes.

The EMS medical director's contract must address internal components of the system into which the medical director is to be incorporated. For example, personnel rules and the presence or absence of a union bargaining group with a concomitant contract between the provider organization and its unionized work force can substantially influence the way the medical director focuses energies to make medical control effective. Budgetary considerations including availability of funds in capital and operating budgets can force certain realities on the medical director.

Lastly of course, many softer points including turf issues, dealing with the other system managers, and in political models dealing with appointed agency leaders who obtain their positions through the political process all influence the effectiveness of the medical director. To avoid conflict, it is highly desirable to spell out in exquisite detail these aspects of the medical director's responsibilities, authorities, and compensation.

Contractual Responsibilities

In discussing the job description and activities that account for the responsibilities of the medical director, it is important to define exactly the medical director's title and rank within the organization. That is, is the medical director merely a consultant to the operating managers or is the medical director serving as the agent of the medical community? Accountability to and support from the medical community as a whole suggest that the medical director will be able to enforce a level of compliance with patient care requirements.

The nature of the organization and the independence of the medical director are contingent on the overall organizational structure. Restructuring a system is inevitably a political process, and while some have proposed and even implemented models in which the medical director serves as the agent of the medical community, in reality few systems begin this way; it is only with great effort that systems evolve to such an ideal. Therefore the putative medical directors should concern themselves with the nature of the position and how it will be organized in the EMS agency for which they assume responsibility.

Authority

Authority obtained through law, regulation, ordinance, contract, and chain of command leading to the medical director is all well and good, but how will that authority be operationalized? Are the responsibilities that come with this authority stated in terms of broad system responsibilities or merely articulated as functional responsibilities for which the medical director is specifically accountable to senior system managers? Is there an opportunity to truly influence policy, or will the medical director merely serve as management's agent in keeping the medical community "in line" by fulfilling the necessary tasks of quality activities, training, and meeting attendance?

If the activities of the medical director are described in simple terms of day-to-day tasks such as quality activities, training, medical advisory committee staffing, and direct medical control with no input into the policies that determine the structure and broader organizational roles of these tasks, then it is likely that the employing authority is not seeking the medical director's input in policy development but only in policy implementation.

In assessing whether the medical director's attention is focused solely at a component or functional level or extends to a system and policy level, it may help to consider specific examples. Does the contract permit or encourage the medical director to accept the full responsibility for overall quality of patient care? The difference between a contract requirement for routine quality assurance audits and a contract provision for implementation of a modern quality improvement program speaks volumes to the agency's interest in the medical director's role.

However, specific examples alone are not sufficient to determine whether the medical director will indeed have a role in policy. The tone of the proposed relationship should be explored. When all parties have known one another for a long time, this may be an easy task; otherwise, efforts should be made to get a broad range of opinion about what is really being sought by naming the medical director and why the EMS agency is choosing this time to do it.

Does the system offer the opportunity for participation in agency policy development including input in operations, capital and operating budgets, overall staffing, unit placement strategies, and dispatch management? Other chapters point out still other opportunities for medical director participation.

For example, in personnel issues (a *key* requirement for definition in your contract), do medical directors have the authority to determine whether a paramedic may provide field service to patients? Are they able to participate in hiring and firing decisions? Do they have input in a disciplinary process that specifically includes medical considerations? Medical directors should strive to assure that promotions incorporate medical input so that those promoted are not simply good managers but also exemplary providers.

Activity

In addition to the need for participation at a policy level, specific activities such as quality activities that begin in a setting where they influence the general tone of medical direction including the development of training and treatment policies represent a positive sign or at least the opportunity for influence.

Does the system or service conduct training internally? Many systems conduct their own continuing education, but few conduct full paramedic training or recertification training. If the system does train, what is the medical directors responsibility for that training? Are they to serve as the training institute medical director or simply accept the output of a community college program in which they have no input on the details of training and curricular coverage? Negotiating responsibility for agencywide continuing medical education may be a foot in the door.

Specific responsibility for development of treatment protocols and standing orders provides an opportunity to extend the medical director's reach to policy development. However, if these roles are not articulated in the contract, the opportunity will not develop.

The continuum of responsibility for quality activities can and should be defined in the medical director's contract. What is expected? Is it merely review of patient care through prehospital care report audit, review of communications, and conduct of morbidity and mortality conferences with providers and hospital personnel? Medical directors whose agencies permit the development of a modern, sophisticated quality management approach find themselves challenged yet more integrated into the overall functioning of the agency.

Meeting participation can be a significant issue because of the time that is required in larger systems. Many meetings with field providers, system managers, and higher levels of authority including state agencies may be required; substantial time may be consumed in meeting attendance. Support for the meeting time and travel if necessary should be specified in the contract.

What about field activities of direct medical control? Inevitably, medical directors stumble upon events requiring EMS. Indeed, they may participate by riding along with a paramedic unit to observe or through patrolling. What is the expectation, and whether it is fulfilled directly by the medical director in a smaller system or by a combination of the medical director and agents in larger systems should be defined in the contract.

What about special conditions such as disasters, mass casualties, or prolonged extrications? Is there a responsibility for the medical director to personally respond, or is the expectation greater still that a hospital will be chosen to provide additional medical resources? Offering to provide these services through a hospital or group practice to an agency that has not considered them positively influences both the negotiation process and the ultimate relationship. Indeed the commitment for a larger organization to respond under special conditions is valuable because it is often seen by the contracting agency as filling a vital need even though the occurrence is so unusual that the commitment has little impact on the day-to-day activities of the medical director, hospital, or group practice.

In some situations the medical director provides personal health services to system or ambulance provider employees. Are employee physical examinations, evaluation for disability, and return to work part of the responsibility? What about administration of hepatitis vaccine or regular tuberculosis skin testing? These personal health services may or may not be part of the expectations of a given agency. As with all the points discussed above, these issues and responsibilities should be defined in advance.

Insurance and Indirect Support

Another component of the contract should include the medical director's liability. This is not simply the medical director's liability for medical negligence but also liability for operational decisions. Certainly, issues regarding medical malpractice liability should be carefully reviewed. Do state laws and regulations cover the medical director's activities; is there any possibility that state Good Samaritan statutes will provide a degree of protection? If a medical director is compensated for providing medical oversight of an EMS agency, it is unlikely that Good Samaritan statues will afford any protection. However, the issues of medical oversight should be explored with medical malpractice carriers to determine any restrictions or endorsements on your coverage.

The downside of participating in broader policy development and implementation is the risk of suit for negligence in this role. This kind of insurance coverage is not usually included in medical malpractice insurance. Therefore the EMS agency or service should provide insurance coverage for administrative decisions made by medical directors so that they are appropriately protected (for example, a provider may choose to litigate an adverse personnel decision in which you participated).

Indirect support (support of the medical director's overhead) is equally important for the medical director to accomplish the tasks required. What support services will be available to the medical director? Are a secretary and other staff, telephones, fax machines, and computers all resources available? What about a vehicle? Provision of a vehicle if an emergency response is ever anticipated or support for some fraction of the medical director's own vehicle are all appropriate negotiating points. Specialized equipment and clothing including turnout gear may be appropriate as well.

Compensation

Compensation is of course a key issue. How are medical directors to be compensated for providing services as medical experts to the EMS agency? This is a thorny issue. An hourly rate of compensation is unlikely to match the loss of income from direct clinical practice, yet it is the only way for most medical directors who serve in a part-time capacity. Incorporated municipalities are generally familiar with appropriate compensation levels for professionals, because they commonly employ a city attorney and judge.

The fortunate few who, in association with larger systems and agencies, can serve half-time or more frequently negotiate a compensation package pegged to that fraction of their total compensation for which they are providing services to the system. For example, a half-time medical director and half-time emergency physician may arrange compensation from the agency back to the group practice or organization that employs them at a rate intended to maintain their preexisting income level.

Compensation for system or regional medical oversight can also be pegged to regional levels for emergency department physician directors. Because the EMS medical director is typically responsible for more patients than even the largest emergency department in the area, it is appropriate to peg the EMS medical director's compensation to the ninetieth percentile of all (public, academic and private) emergency department physician directors in the region.

Another approach for compensating system or regional medical directors is to set their salary demands at a level similar to that of the medical examiner for the congruent service area. This approach is a particularly apt comparison because both the EMS medical director and medical examiner positions are often created by statute and described by regulation. Furthermore, fully qualified individuals for each position are equally scarce.

Other support including pro rata support of benefit packages, membership dues, subscriptions, and continuing medical education may fall into the realm of direct support and compensation.

The relationship between the EMS agency and the medical director may provide for compensation through a variety of models. The simplest of course is one where the physician works directly for the EMS agency. Other examples include models in which the medical director is employed by or contracted to an organization that has general responsibility for the EMS services. This is common in public utility models in which a medical board is constituted as part of the organization; the medical director is employed by the organization and is accountable to that organization through a medical board. Alternatively, such medical boards, rather than contracting directly with an individual, may contract with a hospital or other organization such as an emergency physician group practice to provide anywhere from a fraction of a full-time equivalent to one or more full-time equivalents of medical expertise and medical oversight support.

A Brief Example

The medical director of the Philadelphia Fire Department and Philadelphia EMS region, I enjoy authority granted through the Emergency Medical Services Act and regulation Department of Health 28 Pennsylvania Code Chapters 1001-1013. Published in 1989 (4 years after enactment of the statute) because of the extensive input of organized groups including emergency physicians, this relatively progressive state EMS law when combined with regulations recognizes the necessity for medical control of the modern EMS system. No City of Philadelphia ordinances specifically address EMS, but executive order 88-7 identifies the fire department as the lead EMS agency in Philadelphia.

The regional EMS medical director is responsible for all paramedics in the region. This individual is authorized to recommend providers for recertification or deny them permission to sit for recertification examination if, for example, the field provider has not maintained sufficient skill at various invasive procedures. In addition, the medical director may "... temporarily suspend EMS prehospital personnel from medical care duties. . . ."

The contract between the City of Philadelphia and the medical director's employer, the Medical College of Pennsylvania, is constrained in part by the Philadelphia Home Rule Charter, which prohibits contractors from having authority over city employees. Thus the medical director has no direct authority over fire department paramedics or other field providers. However, the contract does acknowledge the medical director as the sole source of authority regarding medical oversight matters for the EMS system.

The present and previous fire commissioners routinely have consulted with the medical director in the development of medically relevant policies. This consultation has become more frequent and has begun occurring earlier in the planning process over the course of the last 5 years. The medical director participated in planning the introduction of First Responding engine and ladder companies and more recently the upgrading of these units with automated external defibrillators. Currently, policy and planning focus on staffing levels, numbers of units deployed, and the implementation of alternative training programs.

Summary

This chapter discusses the sources of authority for an EMS medical director including laws and regulations, which are a given, and the contract that the medical director negotiates. Power comes to medical directors through the careful exercise of authority and through the expertise that they bring to EMS through their ability to negotiate the interests of all while serving as a consultant to everybody, thereby enhancing everyone's ownership of issues and solutions. In this fashion rather than serving as a single voice on high whose opinion is delivered as if *ex cathedra*, the medical director serves at every opportunity in the role of physician expert, consultant, and educator, facilitating and bridging the multiplicity of political interests into consensus. Together, authority and power empower the medical director.

Suggested Readings

Brislin RW: The art of getting things done: a practical guide to the use of power, New York, 1991, Praeger Publishers.

Fisher R and Ury W: Getting to yes: negotiating agreement with out giving in, New York, 1983, Penguin Books.

Ury W: Getting past no: negotiating with difficult people, New York, 1991, Bantam Books.

Section Three

Interpersonal Elements

Whereas portions of both Sections One and Two were integral to the first edition, the following section is entirely new. It is placed here as a transition between the basic historical, structural, and medical oversight elements and the more complicated, multifaceted operational issues.

Just before the publication of the first edition, an inherent design weakness in the text caused by its overwhelming focus on the analysis of purely structural elements was identified. Consequently, the first edition Epilogue was added to serve as a philosophical counterbalance to the dense information in the remainder of the book. Ironically, many readers of the first edition remember best the lessons of the Epilogue. Therefore, Section Three has been created as the philosophical counterbalance of the second edition. The thought-provoking chapters on ethical and legal issues help the reader smoothly segue into the latter chapters that examine expanded roles for prehospital providers and demonstrate how members of the EMS team expect to participate. The four concluding chapters of the section describe due process, team building, critical incident stress management, and political survival in terms that are not medically oriented but are comprehensible to even the most inexperienced provider of medical oversight.

25

Ethical Issues

James G. Adams, M.D.

Ethics is often thought of as a philosophical discipline removed from the daily operational and medical challenges of emergency services. In reality, ethical dilemmas are common and often difficult. When a provider of prehospital medical care recalls the most difficult, challenging, and frustrating cases, ethical dilemmas were probably present. When a person in medical crisis refuses care, when the family refuses to allow resuscitation of a loved one, or when resources are stressed by non-emergency calls, ethical dilemmas are highlighted. In attempting to resolve these difficult situations, it is necessary to understand the fundamentals of ethical thought, recognize legal and social realities, and stay abreast of evolving trends.

This chapter introduces the ethical principles prominent in prehospital care. The discussion is not philosophical and remote, but rather directly applies to EMS. Ethical problems are raised, current philosophies reviewed, and possible resolutions proposed.

Fundamentals of Ethics

During the last two decades, an evolution has taken place regarding ethical analyses in health care delivery. The trend clearly disfavors paternalistic undertakings by the medical community. Instead, patient autonomy must be respected. EMS is not an enterprise that deals easily with patient autonomy; prehospital care providers are more comfortable providing care that the provider deems necessary. EMS often functions appropriately in a beneficent mode, acting in the perceived best interests of the patient. The providers must act according to the wishes of the patient. The guiding principle is respect for patient autonomy. This fundamental legal and ethical premise grants patients the right to decide what will be done with their own bodies, even if the decision is contrary to medical advice.

Once these principles are understood, dilemmas that are routinely faced can be recognized. A dilemma arises, for example, when a prehospital patient in medical crisis seems to be making an irrational decision by refusing care. Dilemmas also arise when providers lack mechanisms to honor patients' requests to limit interventions such as intubation or cardiopulmonary resuscitation (CPR), even when those requests are carefully thought out and painstakingly defined in anticipation of crisis.

Do Not Resuscitate Orders

Along with the increased recognition of patient autonomy came the recognition that patients could make known their wishes to refuse attempts at resuscitation. EMS, however, begins with another premise. When EMS is activated, the duty is to provide full medical and resuscitative interventions with the assumption that the patient wants such attempts. At the time of crisis, the provider must not make judgments about the likelihood of recovery or presumptions of what the patient would want. The duty is clear—preserve life and health. Even verbal requests by the family cannot be relied on as an ethically, medically, or legally appropriate directive to limit resuscitation. Furthermore, the provider cannot assume that unfamiliar written documents were constructed with the informed and competent consent of the patient.

An acceptable advance directive to limit resuscitation reflects the reasoned wishes of the patient and is verifiable to those expected to honor it. Because of

*The views expressed do not necessarily represent the position of the United States Air Force or the Department of Defense.

these difficulties, living wills and traditional do not resuscitate (DNR) orders were intended only for in-hospital use. Specifically, acceptable DNR orders were originally defined as those written by the physician in a hospital chart, and they were authorized only while that patient was hospitalized. Increasingly, orders to limit resuscitation of terminally ill patients are being recognized in the prehospital setting. The principles underlying these orders are the same. The patient's physician must ensure that the order reflects the informed wishes of the patient, that it is familiar and clear to those who will honor it, and that any concerns or questions can be resolved in advance. The prehospital setting, however, is relatively uncontrolled. There is rarely standard communication, authorization, or formulation for such orders, no ability to review such orders in advance of the crisis, and no prior knowledge of the patient's illness, wishes, prognosis, or personal values. All of these concerns figure prominently in the formulation of an appropriate advance directive. Providers must also decide how to respond when a family member wishes to overrule an advance directive. The prehospital environment presents great challenges to the implementation of an acceptable policy to withhold resuscitation. Ethical analysis clearly supports the limitation of resuscitation in the prehospital setting only when the instrument has been reviewed in advance, found to be medically and legally appropriate, and clearly and specifically reflects the patient's wishes.

Living wills in particular often present confusion. Fundamental aspects of a living will provide the following:

- The living will is executed while the person is competent and remains effective when the person becomes incompetent.
- The directive is to be implemented when the person suffers from a terminal or irreversible illness.
- Written instructions guide the use of artificial life support.
- Living wills have significant drawbacks; the specifications may not include circumstances unanticipated at the time it was written.

Statutes may restrict the conditions for which living wills can be used. Some states specify that a "terminal condition" must be present. The document may not apply to irreversible diseases that are not terminal (for example, severe Alzheimer's disease or persistent vegetative conditions).

Living wills do not necessarily imply the presence of a terminal illness. Living wills can express wishes in case of future illness. If providers are presented with such a directive, confusion regarding its applicability may result. Prehospital caregivers will be challenged to ensure both the applicability and validity of a living will, especially at the time of crisis. In general the living will is of limited utility in the prehospital setting. A specific, clear, legally and operationally defined DNR order is best.

Some systems attempt to standardize mechanisms that are recognizable to the field providers, so resuscitation can be withheld in certain terminally ill patients.[5,6] The private physician then bears the burden to address the issue of limitation of attempted resuscitation. This physician must advise the family when emergency personnel should and should not be called, as well as ensure that the DNR document is appropriately completed. What is meant by DNR must be defined. Is atropine given for bradycardia? Are intravenous fluids given to a dehydrated patient? In general a DNR order applies only at the time of cardiac arrest. Clear and careful definition must be provided to the prehospital providers. All care beyond the limits of the order must be offered.

In Hennepin County, Minnesota, the EMS Council adopted DNR guidelines for long-term care facilities and hospice agencies. The system reports success with this venture, noting considerable appreciation from the medical community. In general, their guidelines recommend the following[2]:

- A DNR order must be written in the medical record, signed by the physician, and dated within the past year.
- The order is defined as, "In the event of an acute cardiac or respiratory arrest, no cardiopulmonary resuscitation will be initiated."
- The patient is eligible for all services of the EMS except those specified in the order.
- Verbal orders are not acceptable unless the physician is on the scene to assume responsibility.

Additional protections such as validation stamps and standardized forms have been used in private homes.

The administrative, legal, and operational challenges to implementing a system of portable orders that limit resuscitation are obvious but not insurmountable. Currently, several states have mechanisms such as legal opinion, state EMS protocol, and statutory law that enable such orders in the prehospital setting. Ideally, there is immunity for the provider who honors an advance directive in good faith; such protection is provided by a Montana law.[8] Other states address the issue or will do so in the near future. Legislative, legal, administrative, and logistical considerations are the most common barriers to implementing a prehospital policy to withhold resuscitation attempts.[9]

The trend is toward developing appropriate mechanisms to honor a patient's wishes to limit resuscitation. Federal legislation mandates that hospitals and nursing homes have mechanisms to honor requests to withhold resuscitation.[4] If EMS systems are to provide for the best interests of their patients, they are obligated to find acceptable solutions. Whether the directives are signed documents, wallet cards, or names in a central registry, technical hurdles must be cleared and unwanted attempts at resuscitation prevented. Wrist bracelets that are identifiable to providers are becoming more widely used. Such a standardized and recognizable means of identification promotes portability from the home, nursing home, or hospice to the emergency department and the in-hospital setting.

Patient Consent: Informed, Implied, and the Emergency Rule

The concept of informed consent is central to the ethical and legal frameworks of all medical care. Although prehospital medicine frequently operates under exceptions and assumptions regarding patient consent, the importance of consent must not be overlooked. Instead of minimizing concerns for patient consent in this unique environment, EMS medical directors must hold great concern for the wishes and interests of the patient.

To maximize respect for the patient's participation in prehospital medical decision-making, prehospital personnel must understand the facts and fallacies of informed consent. The Presidential Commission on Bioethics defined general criteria for informed consent as follows[7]:

> The patient must demonstrate a clear understanding of the nature of the disease and the proposed treatment, must be able to think clearly, must recognize the risks of the proposed interventions, and must be willing to accept the balance of risks and benefits in the decision to proceed with medical care.

Informed consent is the ideal authorization to proceed with care, but such requirements are difficult to achieve in the prehospital setting. The providers should not have to discuss risks versus benefits of treatment and transport. Prehospital medical services are usually provided under the authority of implied consent. It is assumed that reasonable individuals wish to have all measures undertaken to preserve their life and health, especially if the interventions present little risk of serious complications. When patients cooperate with the prehospital care providers, this is accepted as implied consent.

Another important element in prehospital care is the emergency rule. When patients are unconscious or otherwise unable to express their preferences, it is assumed that they wish to have necessary interventions performed to preserve their health. The law grants this authorization on the basis of a universal obligation to provide for the health and well-being of the citizens. EMS shares this obligation. Some states have developed statutes that define this doctrine. For example, Washington law states that in life-threatening circumstances, if no proxy consent can be reasonably obtained and the health provider is acting in good faith,[3]

> no physician or hospital licensed in this state shall be subject to civil liability, based solely upon failure to obtain consent in rendering emergency medical, surgical, hospital or health services to any individual regardless of age where its patient is unable to give his consent for any reason.

Medical professionals must not provide interventions exceeding those necessary to allow sufficient recovery of the patient to discuss their wishes, and known wishes of the patient must not be violated.

Based on these premises, EMS generally operates comfortably. Discomfort arises when a patient in medical need will not consent to care.

Refusal of Care

When patients refuse care or revoke consent, they are exercising their right to terminate the relationship with the EMS system. This assumes that patients understand their illness, realize the potential harm of refusing care, and are able to interpret this information, coming to a reasoned decision to refuse care. If these assumptions are true, then the patient is expressing an autonomous decision that supersedes the system's obligation. If the providers disregard the patient's wishes, they are acting paternalistically and risk assault and battery charges. The EMS system does not allow a competent patient to refuse care, rather patients allow the EMS system to provide care.

When patients with a minimal illness are thinking clearly, are substantially healthy, and are acting rationally, there is generally no conflict when they refuse care. However, some patients who refuse care have significant, perhaps life-threatening, illnesses. Some controversy exists about the appropriate approach to these patients. If the patient is unconscious and cannot consent or refuse, there is no dilemma. The patient is treated as a reasonable person would wish to be treated; that is, care would be provided. If the patient is minimally responsive, the "reasonable person" standard would still apply. However, not all patients fit easily into one of these categories. There are patients with severe, perhaps life-threatening, medical crises who are awake, talking, and oriented to person, place, and time. When these patients impulsively refuse care, great caution and concern must be exercised. Refusal of care by these patients should not be routinely construed as informed.

Difficult questions arise. Should such patients ever be forcibly transported? How should transport of an uncooperative but seriously ill patient be carried out? Is assault and battery committed if the patient is restrained and transported? Is the patient "abandoned" if he is not transported? The answers to these questions rest on whether the patient is capable of making an autonomous, informed judgment regarding health care.

When the patient is unable to make an autonomous, informed judgment, the EMS system must respect its obligation of beneficence and provide care for the patient. When a patient with a life-threatening illness refuses care, there is a greater burden on that patient to demonstrate an understanding of the illness, an ability to reason, and the goals that will be achieved by the refusal. The decision to refuse care must be consistent with the patient's established values and previous judgments. If the patient is unable to demonstrate such capacity when a life-threatening illness is present, then transport to the emergency department should be carried out even if restraint is required. Police might be of assistance, but they are often reluctant to become involved. Judicial determinations of incompetence establish the legal authority to treat patients against their expressed wishes; however, such determinations take time.

Research

The prehospital setting is an important arena for research. Great strides will be made in resuscitation and the treatment of acute medical crises if appropriate clinical investigation is performed. However, operational and logistical factors make such studies daunting. One of the challenges of prehospital investigation is the requirement for informed consent. Obtaining a clear and acceptable informed consent is not easy in the prehospital setting; some would argue that medical and logistical factors make it impossible. There are ethically appropriate mechanisms for establishing consent for prehospital research that allow sufficient analysis and concern for the patient.

Before conducting a study in the prehospital setting, it should be recognized that the patients will never be fully informed of the details of the research. Time limitations and potential physical and psychologic impairments of the patients make this point fundamental. Still, research that is constructed appropriately can still find acceptable mechanisms for obtaining consent. Such alternatives must maximize the patient's information and provide an opportunity for the patient to either consent or refuse. Some general guidelines regarding patient consent for participation in prehospital research are listed in the box below.

These general principles for participation require that the research minimize risk to the patient, provide relevant information to the subject, ensure that participation is voluntary, and provide potential benefit to the patient.

Although the general guidelines may be appropriate for conscious patients, resuscitation research presents dilemmas when minutes are critical and there is no time for discussion. In such circumstances, deferred consent can be used if the need for intervention is immediate and the prognosis otherwise hopelessly grave.[1] There are specific conditions under which deferred consent is appropriate; the individual must be comatose, the experimental therapy must need to be initiated immediately, intervention must offer no meaningful additional risk, and the investigator cannot know based on current scientific knowledge whether standard or experimental therapy is better. In

Guidelines for Patient Consent for Participation in Prehospital Research

1. The patient or a legal surrogate must be informed of the study and must be aware of potential risks and benefits of the intervention.
2. The safety and efficacy of the proposed intervention must have been demonstrated if possible in other, more controlled clinical situations before assessment in the prehospital environment.
3. Adequate protection of the rights and welfare of the patient must be assured and the risks to the patient minimized.
4. There must be potential benefit to the patient that is at least comparable to that of standard therapy.
5. The information must be unobtainable by other means and must be beneficial and substantially important.
6. The study design and hypothesis must be scientifically sound and appropriately approved.
7. The patient or surrogate should have the opportunity to withdraw from the study at any time.

addition, no potentially beneficial therapies can be withheld. In other words the patient must have the full benefit of the current standard of care, and experimental therapy must not create a meaningful risk of harm. At the earliest time possible the patient's surrogate must be informed of the experimental interventions. The surrogate must then provide consent for continued participation in the project.

Before any prehospital investigation and especially before implementing a study using deferred consent, the protocol must be reviewed by an institutional review board (IRB). Such review assures that the study is ethically appropriate, scientifically sound, and of minimal risk to patients. Some IRBs are not familiar with the environment of prehospital care and may have to be educated. The challenges of research must be continually confronted in the prehospital setting. EMS has a large patient base, the potential to improve the care for thousands of patients, and an obligation to continue improving prehospital medical therapy; therefore a continued effort to carry out effective prehospital research is indicated.

Justice

Ethical issues may be understood in terms of specific challenges that arise between the provider and the patient; however, there are also ethical imperatives within the EMS structure. Most prominent is the principle of justice, which is highlighted by two very real concerns in EMS—allocation and rationing.

Allocation decisions concern the distribution of finite resources. Allocation requirements determine which drugs are carried, which equipment is purchased, and how personnel is distributed. Allocation decisions are common and necessary for medicine in general and EMS in particular. Ethical concerns simply dictate that allocation is fair and judgments are reasoned.

When there are insufficient resources to care for all people who request aid, rationing decisions must be made. Decisions regarding rationing are almost always preceded by allocation decisions. In busy systems, rationing decisions are made initially at the moment of the first call prioritization by dispatchers; later the field providers make rationing decisions if they refuse to transport patients with minimal complaints. Presumably, rationing decisions allow for more efficient care of patients in acute need. The ethical imperative of justice must be recognized. Clear guidelines are necessary for the providers told to make decisions that may delay treatment or deny transport; obviously, quality assurance mechanisms must be in place to review the allocation and rationing practices.

Confidentiality

Maintaining confidentiality of patient information must remain a foremost concern. The field provider may act as a physician surrogate and therefore assume many of the obligations of the physician. One prominent duty is to maintain confidentiality; this duty may also be required by legislative statute. Numerous potential threats to patient confidentiality exist in the prehospital setting. Radio communication, family, friends, bystanders, police, media, and curious others may threaten the confidentiality of the patient. Only communication that is directly necessary for the care of the patient should be carried out. Reports of intoxication, seizure, infectious disease, and even routine illness can profoundly affect the personal, social, and professional life of the patient. Neighbors, employers, and even family members should not be given diagnostic or prognostic information. Prehospital providers must always conduct themselves with the utmost concern for the patient's well-being, including respect for confidentiality.

Dilemmas may arise when police, media, or outside agencies desire information. Systems should have policies regarding such interaction or appoint a spokesperson for the case. If the individual provider is ever in doubt, nothing should be discussed; everything should be deferred to a supervisor. Potentially devastating personal consequences can result from the dissemination of information regarding drunken driving, HIV seropositivity, assault, rape, or any of a number of other situations that prehospital providers encounter daily. In general the less information shared with those assuming no direct care of the patient the better.

Summary

Ethical issues figure prominently in the routine of prehospital care. The EMS medical director must be aware of these issues and should be prepared to resolve dilemmas when they arise. In several areas, laws clarify obligations and promote the best interests of the patient. EMS medical directors should be familiar with applicable local laws. The law does not, however, define all of the moral obligations of EMS. Prehospital providers must be sensitive to the ethical elements of the care they provide. Ethics is not a static discipline; it continues to evolve. EMS medical directors must direct the evolution by working toward resolution of current problems and preparing to confront issues that are sure to arise. Furthermore, field personnel require guidance in how to respond to the dilemmas that they will face. Development of protocols and objective guidelines is crucial, but reason and judgment will always be necessary.

REFERENCES

1. Abramson NS and Safar P: Deferred consent: use in clinical resuscitation research, *Ann Emerg Med* 19:781-784, 1990.
2. Crimmins TJ: The need for a prehospital DNR system, *Prehospital and Disaster Medicine* 5:47-48, 1990.
3. First Extra Ordinary Session: Laws of 1971, Chapter 305, May 20, 1971.
4. Greco PJ et al: The patient self-determination act and the future of advance directives, *Ann Intern Med* 115:639-643, 1991.
5. Marshall L: Resuscitating the terminally ill, *JEMS* 24-8, 1985.
6. Miles SH and Crimmins TJ: Orders to limit emergency treatment for an ambulance service in a large metropolitan area, *JAMA* 254:525-527, 1985.
7. President's Commission for the Study of Ethical Problems in Medicine and Biomedical Research: *Making health care decisions,* vol 1, 1983, US Government Printing Office.
8. Rouse F: Case studies, *Hastings Center Report* 19, Nov-Dec 1989.
9. Sachs GA, Miles SH, and Levin RA: Limiting resuscitation: emerging policy in the emergency medical service, *Ann Intern Med* 114:151-154, 1991.

26

Legal Issues

Carol J. Shanaberger, EMT-P

Medical oversight in prehospital care is distinctly different than any other physician supervisory professional activity. Although it is acknowledged as an integral element of an EMS system, medical oversight as a function of medical directors has been a bit of a mystery to the law, the public, and the medical community. Despite the immense responsibilities in providing medical oversight, medical directors were rarely defendants in litigation during the first 20 years of EMS.

There have been obvious improvements in the sophistication of EMS systems since the early days of "invalid coaches" staffed by "ambulance drivers." However, prehospital medical care is often misunderstood, and consequently the role of the medical director is often not understood by lawyers, citizens, and even some physicians. As recently as 1989 an appellate court judge referred to an ambulance as a "medical taxicab" rather than a mobile intensive care unit.[15]

Ignorance and misperceptions affect medical directors. They face confusion, misconceptions, and uncertainty in the day-to-day events of medical direction and in the legal crises that may erupt. The medical profession has had decades to develop standards and predictability in legal rulings. However, only recently has a patchwork of legal decisions involving EMS activities solidified sufficiently to provide some predictability. In a few states, trends about liability issues that help define responsibilities of EMS systems or prehospital providers and interpret immunity statutes governing prehospital care are evolving. Medical directors may benefit from the few legal precedents established by other participants in this unique and developing body of medical care. However, any medical director, whether a novice or an expert, must keep in mind that there are many unresolved issues surrounding EMS medical direction.

In most states the birth of EMS, with its "call to arms" by countless physicians, paraprofessionals, and citizens, preceded the enactment of enabling legislation authorizing this unique delivery of medical care.[23] When federal grant funds were offered, every state eventually enacted EMS legislation to qualify; however, intense physician supervision was not necessarily mandated in these statutes, many of which remain in effect more than two decades later.[10]

During the development of EMS systems, immunity from liability for the rescuer gradually became a focus of many state legislatures. It was assumed that immunity was a prerequisite for volunteer (uncompensated) provider involvement in emergency response, although there was no evidence to substantiate this proposition.[21] In a 1978 appellate court ruling absolving from liability rescuers that failed to oxygenate a patient in cardiac arrest, the court reasoned that immunity laws were essential because of the difficulty in obtaining insurance and because unlimited liability could "be enough to drive many providers of ambulance service out of business and greatly discourage others from entering."[17] Immunity for the prehospital provider became common and remains rooted in EMS law. Eventually laws were passed to protect the trained rescuer and professional paid responder, as well as the "Good Samaritan." Governmental immunity also became a strong shield from liability for the public agencies. Immunity for the Good Samaritan physician became commonplace, and immunity for the supervising physician was seen as early as 1976.*

It is important that the medical director realize that medical oversight as a component of an EMS system has not been recognized with uniform enthu-

*As of 1979, 82% of the Good Samaritan statutes pertained to physicians, 55% pertained to paramedics, and 36% pertained to EMTs, according to Norris.

siasm in EMS legislation. Although physician participation (often side by side with paramedic personnel) existed in the early mobile cardiac care units, legislative mandates for physician involvement varied tremendously from state to state. Physician involvement commenced only at the hospital door for the majority of volunteer basic life support (BLS) units that covered the expanse of highways and hillsides across the country. Even as EMS passes into the 1990s, medical directors still are not required to supervise the medical care of many non-paramedic services, particularly in rural, nontransporting EMS services.* However, the delivery of medical care in the prehospital setting has matured largely to the credit of many physicians willing to divide their medical practices between patient care in emergency departments or private practices and the care of patients miles from the hospital.

Despite the years of muted development of medical control, the silence of the courts regarding the role of the prehospital medical director has begun to change. Medical direction will become increasingly recognized in the legal arena as a fundamental component of quality prehospital care, especially as medical directors become more active and more informed. Potential liability is the inevitable corollary that shadows the development of responsibilities in medical control.

Sources of Accountability

The role of the medical director involves multiple and diverse responsibilities. Aspects of administration, medical care, personnel management, and education all occupy the medical director's daily activities in the oversight of an EMS system. Consequently, liability concerns are also multifaceted. As with any form of medical practice the physician's conduct must conform to accepted standards of care. Sources that may provide some definition of standards are discussed here.

State Statutes and Regulations

Responsibilities and qualifications. Although the role of the medical director is complex, the statutory provisions that directly affect the role are often brief. Each state statute has supplemental regulations concerning the responsibilities of medical directors to the EMS personnel they supervise or the EMS system in which they function. There are different regulatory structures and varying degrees of specificity. For example, some state laws provide little more than a short definition of the medical director as a licensed physician responsible for the supervision and training of EMS personnel. Some regulations only generally state the responsibilities of the medical director, and it is assumed that the medical director will engage in certain supervisory activities. In other states the regulations identify the responsibilities of the medical director in detail. Florida statute requires, for example, that the medical director "establish a quality assurance committee to provide for quality assurance review of all emergency medical technicians (EMTs) and paramedics under his supervision."[8] Medical directors are required to ride with the ambulance services in Oregon.[3] In Washington, rules expressly provide that the "medical program director" is certified by the EMS regulatory authority and can be terminated for failure to perform the duties of the position.[34] Clearly, trends are emerging in the regulatory arena to abolish the "paper doc" and mandate quality supervision.

Increasingly, states are attaching qualifications to the role of medical director beyond mere state licensure to practice medicine. In Oregon the Board of Medical Examiners must review and approve an application for the position of prehospital medical director.[1] Certification in emergency medicine or family practice and advanced cardiac life support are required in Missouri.[20]

State regulations also cover the scope of practice, licensure or certification, and training of the prehospital personnel. The medical director must ensure that protocols delegate medical functions consistent with each prehospital care provider's certification and training. On more than one occasion an unwary medical director has conceded to an EMT's request to perform a medical act not legally authorized by statute or covered in the EMT's training. Some skills are subject to extra reporting requirements. For example, EMT-Defibrillation (EMT-D) programs involve considerable reporting to the state agency and documentation of skills proficiency. In addition, specific testing or training requirements may exist for registered nurses who function in the prehospital setting; the medical director should keep abreast of these regulatory provisions.

Another common regulatory provision is the prerequisite that the medical director provide written authorization for a provider to qualify for certification. Quite often the medical director signs a form making a statement such as ". . . I understand that I am legally and professionally responsible for the directed medical actions of this EMT-Paramedic." This language is quite explicit and certainly im-

*Colorado requires all levels of EMTs have a physician advisor as of April 1, 1992. Colorado Rules Pertaining to Emergency Medical Services Physician Advisors bring all levels of EMTs under the supervision of a physician.

poses significant legal responsibilities on the medical director. The medical director who makes a commitment on paper must ensure that the prehospital provider is capable and can practice with reasonable skill and safety. Available evaluation or risk management tools should be used. At the very least, documentation of proficiency or capability from reliable sources such as training institutions or employers should be provided.

Medical directors must be aware of these regulatory constraints that define and affect their role. They should not rely on an apparent lack of enforcement by the state regulatory authority to justify ignoring legally imposed responsibilities. A shortage of prehospital providers in a community should never be justification for authorizing a person with serious deficiencies in skills or poor judgment. New medical directors are wise to contact state and local EMS offices early in their tenure to be sure that they are in compliance in these matters. Veteran directors will hopefully have maintained communication channels that enable them to use regulatory agencies as a reliable resource.

Immunity laws. Some states have statutes that provide immunity from liability for acts performed by medical directors as long as they act in good faith or in a non-reckless manner.[45] Immunity statutes for EMS providers have successfully shielded EMS providers from liability for negligent conduct, but providers remain accountable for grossly negligent or reckless conduct. The medical directors' immunity laws may therefore give a medical director a sense of comfort that the courts will forgive some misjudgments in medical control activities. These statutes have not yet been the subject of review at the appellate court level. However, the responsibilities of the medical director remain unchanged, and only the payment of damages is avoided. In addition, the physician remains accountable to the state licensing board for his medical control functions.

Local ordinances. The medical director will encounter additional layers of codifications in county and municipal government. City ordinances and county resolutions often address activities not addressed by state regulations. Such provisions can be very stringent and sometimes quite outdated. Although the sanctions imposed on ambulance services for violations are sometimes insignificant fines, misconduct may lead to revocation of an ambulance service's permit to operate in the jurisdiction. These provisions may require proof of protocols, insurance, and proper staffing and may restrict the response activities of the ambulance service. Medical directors who give orders that conflict with local laws set their service up for trouble with the "city fathers." Local government politics can be a major source of consternation, and seemingly minor infractions can seriously complicate community relationships.

County attorneys and plaintiff lawyers scrutinize the "black letter law" of these various codifications and hold the physician accountable to the "letter of the law" and the "spirit of the law" as circumstances warrant. The medical director must know and operate within these legal statutes, regulations, and codes. Sound legal advice should be sought if there is a question of interpretation or application, preferably before a legal conflict has materialized. Competent private counsel, city and county attorneys, and state regulatory boards can provide valuable guidance in the medical director's decision-making.

Court Decisions

Case law is a source of law in which a written decision by a judge or panel of judges interprets statutes or the applicability of legal principles to a case. Often referred to as "judge-made law" or common law, these rulings can determine the merit of a plaintiff's negligence claim or interpret a statute. For example, in recent years, interpretations of the working of immunity statutes and what conduct constitutes "gross negligence" have abounded. However, because of varying facts from case to case, varying interpretations from state to state, and because years often transpire between the date of the incident and the court's ruling, case law is sometimes an ineffective educator.

State court decisions are not binding on any other state; however, the discussions and issues in state case law reveal the success or failure of legal theories proposed by plaintiffs, thereby highlighting the kinds of conduct that attract the attention of judges and juries. An awareness of the legal arguments by plaintiffs seeking recovery from EMS agencies and prehospital providers can guide the medical director in areas where acceptable protocols and negligent conduct have not been well-defined. Specific areas of EMS case law important to the medical director are discussed further.

Remarkably, few legal decisions have discussed medical oversight or implicated the medical director in allegations of EMS providers' misconduct. One of the few negligence actions that addressed the role of the medical director resulted in a ruling adverse to the medical director. In Florida an appellate court upheld a jury verdict against a medical center, because the EMS medical director failed to properly supervise, train, and instruct the paramedics.[45] A 5-

year-old female patient was assessed at her home by paramedics who decided no emergency medical care was needed; the young patient died hours later of congestive heart failure. The EMS medical director admitted that there was no written protocol for "how to take a history or how to distinguish between an emergency and non-emergency situation," or for taking a pediatric patient's vital signs. Instead the medical director depended on the paramedics' prior schooling and experience to provide the necessary guidance. The jury concurred with the plaintiff's contention that the medical director was responsible for developing procedures "and deviated from the standard of care by not having established such written procedures."[47]

Constitutional law. Federal case law involving prehospital providers has revealed some warnings in the application of the Fourteenth Amendment of the United States Constitution that states, "No person shall be deprived of life, liberty and the pursuit of happiness, without due process of law." A federal statute, 42 U.S.C. Section 1983, provides a remedy for an individual to seek redress for deprivation of constitutional rights. This claim is significant because state immunity statutes do not affect the ability of the plaintiff to sue and seek damages. A few examples demonstrate why these "1983 actions" can be significant in prehospital care.

The decision of *Doe v. Borough of Barrington* was rendered in 1990.[49] It ruled that a city violated a citizen's rights because the city failed to train police officers about acquired immune deficiency syndrome (AIDS) and the need to keep confidential the identity of a person infected with human immunodeficiency virus (HIV). Reasonably extrapolated to EMS agencies, failure to train public employee prehospital providers about the transmission of AIDS and patient and confidentiality may result in liability if medical treatment and confidentiality are not correctly managed because of the ignorance on the part of the prehospital providers.

An obstetric patient argued that she had a constitutional right to direct a county ambulance to the hospital of her choice in *Wideman v. Shallowford Community Hospital, Inc.* The patient contended that when an ambulance transported her to a county hospital that was the ambulance service's direct medical control facility, she was deprived of her "constitutional right to essential medical treatment."[51] However, the appellate court held that there was no constitutional right to prehospital treatment and transport to the facility of the patient's choice.*

*The *Wideman* ruling is some indication that the courts may not consider EMS an essential public service, as fire and police are often viewed.

Medical directors face constitutional issues when a prehospital provider contests termination from employment based on due process. Grievance procedures involve matters of notice, efforts in remediation, and qualifications of personnel that may involve the medical director's participation. Understanding due process may prevent unnecessary review proceedings. For example, in *Baxter v. Fulton-DeKalb Hospital Authority,* a federal court ruled on the due process claim of a paramedic who had been cleared of misconduct in a hospital investigation of field performance.[50] The medical director, who was employed by the hospital and supervised the paramedic who was employed by a public hospital, refused to reinstate the paramedic, even though the paramedic had been cleared of misconduct. The court ruled that the paramedic's claim against the hospital should not be dismissed because the hospital deprived the paramedic of due process by acquiescing to the medical director's decision.

Areas of Liability

Absent any judicial interpretation of medical oversight, the legal claims against medical directors that will prove successful for the plaintiff's attorney can only be surmised. The relationship of the medical director to the prehospital provider is unique, although there are similarities to the relationships between nurse and physician or physician assistant and physician. Extrapolating from these medical-professional relationships and from general medicolegal principles, a few theories are worth noting. These legal theories are the pathways by which a medical director can be linked to liability.

Direct Liability

Failure to perform responsibilities. A clear source of liability is negligence or malpractice committed by the medical director. Through statute and regulation, medical directors are obligated to perform certain tasks such as providing direct medical control, establishing protocols, and auditing the performance of field personnel. In addition, expert testimony by medical directors gives substance and shape to the professional duties of colleagues when litigation arises. Despite many variations among EMS systems and state laws, standards of conduct in medical control for the medical director have taken shape. Therefore a malpractice action against a medical director could be a valid cause of action if the plaintiff can establish the requisite elements of malpractice including standard of care, breach, proximate cause, and damages. This was successfully argued in the case of *Tallahassee,* discussed previously.

Negligent supervision. A claim of negligent supervision requires proof of the duty to supervise and breach of that duty that proximately causes harm to another person. Negligent supervision might be argued if the medical director failed to take action to correct deficiencies such as (1) the medical director observes a paramedic's poor intubation technique, (2) a supervisor of an ambulance service reports a series of patient care incidents involving a paramedic who verbally abused patients, or (3) the medical director fails to establish medication protocols consistent with current standards of medical practice, thereby letting the paramedic exercise unfettered discretion in the field. If a physician fails to act on knowledge, whether acquired from direct observation, field audits, patient complaints, or other sources, that a paramedic is lacking in skills or is practicing in a dangerous manner, the physician is duty-bound to remove, restrict, or otherwise prevent the prehospital provider from continuing to render substandard care. This responsibility would likely be shared (although not necessarily equally) with the paramedic's direct employer. This duty to supervise arises from the statutory role of medical directors, as well as by virtue of the medical directors' delegation of medical practice. A jury would likely view medical directors, with their superior training and their authority to have taken corrective action, to be culpable because of failure to exercise their lawful authority. Although errors in judgment regarding the capabilities of a particular prehospital provider can still occur, negligence claims against medical directors are less likely to materialize if they are active, informed, and involved.

Medical directors usually do not have complete control over the employment or membership of a prehospital provider in an EMS agency. However, active involvement in the personnel aspects of an EMS service is important because the skills and judgment of prehospital care providers directly affect the quality of patient care. The authority of medical directors to determine who may practice under their license was the focus of a ruling from the state of Minnesota, *County of Hennepin v. Hennepin County Association of Paramedics and Emergency Medical Technicians.*[42] A county paramedic who was a member of a union had been terminated by the county because of patient care related conduct. After a hearing for reinstatement, an arbitrator ruled that the paramedic should be reinstated. The case was appealed and the testimony of the medical director was important because he had stated that he could neither trust the paramedic nor be certain that the paramedic would perform safely and appropriately even if on probation. The appellate court ruled that the medical director could not be forced to authorize the paramedic to work under his medical license. The unique relationship of medical directors extending their license to the paramedic could "impose potential tort and disciplinary liability on the medical director for actions of unfit paramedics." Therefore the medical director may exercise "medical judgment" to decide who should or should not work as a paramedic, according to the *Hennepin County* decision. It was noted that the paramedic could have been assigned to a position not involving direct patient contact.

If an employer such as a fire department fails or refuses to impose restrictions, the medical director's ability to invoke conditions on a prehospital practitioner's scope of practice may seem complicated. Medical directors are not forced to continue extending their license to a prehospital provider employed by an uncooperative agency, whether in a paid or volunteer service, if the prehospital provider has demonstrated incompetence in patient care. The employer hopefully would be persuaded to follow the medical director's recommendations for remediation. Such scenarios can be quite divisive and are best averted by being addressed before they occur such as at the time of contract negotiation.

Indirect Liability

A second type of liability that the medical director should be aware of is indirect liability, often referred to more specifically as vicarious liability. This legal doctrine provides that the negligent conduct of one person is imputed to another person because of the relationship between the two persons. The common phrase "Let the master answer" exemplifies vicarious liability. The "master" (employer) is accountable for the actions of the employee even if the employer's conduct is faultless, as long as the employee was acting within the scope of his employment and presumably benefiting the employer. This form of liability is not new to the medical profession. It has been the source of liability for physicians in situations in which the physician was considered "the captain of the ship." This doctrine evolved when hospitals generally were immune from liability as charitable or governmental institutions; the negligence of the nurses was not imputed to the institution but rather was imputed to the surgeon.[11] It was reasoned that because the nurse functioned under the direct control and supervision of the surgeon, the injured patient could seek compensation from the surgeon even if the surgeon committed no act of carelessness.[32] This legal theory eroded over the years in response to the increased independent professional responsibility assumed by professional nurses and increased liability imposed by the courts.

The theory of indirect liability has not surfaced in EMS case law; it may have very limited applicability in the prehospital scenario. Of course, it is to the medical director's benefit that this principle not apply. Although the term "direct medical control" may seem to create a claim of vicarious liability, actual over-the-shoulder supervision is not typically involved in the relationship between the prehospital provider and the medical director. The element of control is diminished in the context of contact through radio and protocols. The factor of control is pivotal in cases involving nurses acting on physicians' orders. The principle necessitates scrutiny of the extent of control the physician exercises over the particular action of the prehospital provider, the authority of the medical director to exercise control over the prehospital provider at the particular time, and the prehospital provider's skill and training in the specific medical act. Just as the nurse usually has independent professional and dependent medical functions when acting on a physician's orders, it is likely that the courts would examine the prehospital provider's medical functions.

The administrative medical director or indirect medical control physician can clarify responsibilities and authority through frank discussion and written agreements.

System Concerns

By definition, EMS is a network of resources and therefore medical directors must construe their role and responsibilities jointly and cooperatively with the other components and players of the EMS system. Modern EMS is often tainted with antiquated principles that define structure by political boundaries rather than patient needs. Medical directors rarely have an opportunity to implement the EMS system of their choice. More likely, they are saddled with a machine that is in terrible need of repair, functioning suboptimally, and probably not up to code. Nonetheless, medical directors' responsibilities cannot be shirked; certainly they are no less accountable, and perhaps over time even more so, if they acquiesce to the unabated continuation of the problems in the system.

System problems such as regionalization, patient destination, and use of paramedics or aeromedical transport can cause a damaging ripple effect in an EMS system. Competing EMS agencies can compromise patient care if coordination and cooperation are not promoted by the medical director. These politicolegal battles in EMS are among the most vociferous and most costly. Often, problems are the result of parochialism, competition for patients, or simply ignorance. Medical directors often can be instrumental in correcting the errant habits and customs of an EMS system, although it may take years of patience, debate, and befriending. However, if they do not make the effort, both they and the system are destined to fail.

Entire EMS systems, not just individual EMS providers, are increasingly under legal scrutiny. Although medical directors usually are not identified as the negligent defendant in these cases, medical directors are not an unwitting appendage to an EMS system. They should be the quarterback of all EMS resources. The following system concerns can become less daunting when addressed with protocols and policies founded on and driven by the principle of optimal patient care.

Response

How a fire department staffs rescue units or uses medical personnel to respond to a medical emergency is as much a medical decision as is the choice of intravenous solutions. Optimal patient care is sacrificed by the poor placement of ambulances, the lack of coordination of tiered responses, and many other political, emotional, and business factors. Medical directors must objectively study the components and agencies within their EMS system; the goal of quality patient care must dictate system management decisions.

An example of a failed system is *Brooks v. Herndon Ambulance Service, Inc.* The care of a patient was compromised when an EMT-A unit responded to a call. The patient, a student in a gym class, began seizing and then arrested.[44] The ambulance that received the call had difficulty finding the address, then equipment malfunctioned on-scene, and finally the ambulance broke down en route to the hospital with the patient. Ten minutes from the school was a fire department with a paramedic unit that was never notified. Modern EMS will not tolerate such provincialism and uncooperative practices.

Volunteer systems are not immune to attack. Many communities depend on the willingness of individual, uncompensated volunteers to respond on emergencies. However, such EMS services still must meet minimum standards. The volunteer spirit and contribution must not compromise patient care. A promise to provide EMS through the formation of a fire department or fire protection district supported by public funds creates obligations, irrespective of the uncompensated status of the responders or the absence of charges to the patient. The duty for these providers to act reasonably is not altered by the gratuitous services. For example, a volunteer fire department with so few EMTs that there are no adequately staffed ambulances to respond to a call may invite liability if the delay in response was avoidable. This issue was raised in a Virginia case where a volunteer rescue service repeatedly had a shortage of personnel during early morning hours. The dispatcher was not notified of this problem and as a result did not request the assistance of a neighboring agency until the local rescue service failed to acknowledge the requests.[22] Unless medical directors are actively involved in these aspects of an agency, the care rendered in the field may be less than optimal thus inviting legal complications. Medical directors must show prehospital personnel how such operations endanger or compromise patient care. They can encourage other options to be considered by the service and perhaps lead efforts for systemwide improvement that had not yet been recognized as necessary by the community. Mutual aid arrangements and insistence that only qualified personnel accept patient care responsibilities are examples of the input the medical director may offer to minimize legal risk.

The issue of several appellate court decisions has been the use of personnel and equipment, but liability has been defeated because of the protections of immunity laws. For example, in *Malcolm v. City of East Detroit* fire fighters trained only in first aid were dispatched to care for a man complaining of chest pain, while available EMT-A fire fighters stayed at the station.[40] The patient arrested and the firefighters attempted to ventilate with a bag-valve mask, although the patient was aspirating. The jury decided the city's action was willful and wanton, and therefore immunity protections did not apply. However, the judgment of $500,000 was vacated by the state Supreme Court, which gave an expansive interpretation to the governmental immunity statute.[5] The message is that the law may excuse substandard care, but scrutiny and evaluation of EMS resources must still be pursued by the medical director of the system.

Destination

The wrath of the courts has surfaced in decisions addressing the destination policies of EMS systems. When transport of a patient is not dictated by medical concerns and the patient's best interests or is hindered due to nonmedical reasons, juries have been harsh in their verdicts. In *Hospital Authority of Gwinnett County v. Jones,* the plaintiff convinced a jury that the transport of a patient who had sustained serious burn injuries was dictated by economic gains for the receiving hospital. The jury awarded punitive damages against the hospital in the amount of $1.3 million and $5000 against the ambulance service. A burn facility was approximately 15 to 20 minutes away by helicopter, and the defendant hospital was closer by ground. Rather than transporting the patient directly to the burn facility by a helicopter already en route to the scene, the patient was brought to the defendant hospital by the ambulance, thereby necessitating another transfer of the patient to the burn facility. Arrangements for this second transport caused further delay. When lifting off from the hospital en route to the burn facility, the helicopter crashed, killing the pilot and crew but sparing the patient. The helicopter landing area had been used for years but was not approved by the Federal Aviation Administration. The jury returned its verdict with an additional powerful message, "We the jury find that there should be more stringent regulations of the ground and air ambulance services in the state of Georgia".[13]

The case of *Moreno v. South Hills Health System* involved the limited paramedic resources of the city of Pittsburgh. One issue of the case was whether paramedics were negligent in not accepting an interhospital transfer of a gunshot victim. The paramedics had responded and transported the patient to the nearest hospital. The patient then required transport to another facility where a trauma surgeon awaited. At that time the City of Pittsburgh had only four paramedic ambulances for First Response calls and emergency transports; private ambulances handled non-emergent interhospital transports. A nurse asked the paramedics to handle the transfer, but she did not explain that the transfer was an emergency, which the unit was authorized to accept. Consequently the paramedics declined the transfer, according to their protocols; the surgical treatment had to be delayed until the transfer was ultimately completed. "Due to this shortage of vehicles it was the policy of the service to not make interhospital transfers," the court noted. The court deferred to the policy and held that the duty of the emergency ambulance service was completed upon transporting the patient to the nearest facility; absent knowledge that the transfer was of an emergent nature, there was no basis for negligence in the paramedics' refusal to accept the transfer. Ambulances in an EMS system should not be used or viewed as an unlimited resource, and sound policies are defensible.

The authority of the patient to direct the ambulance to a specific hospital poses troubling issues. A state court found no liability against a direct medical control physician who advised EMT-As to comply with a patient's preference to be transported to a Level II hospital.[30] The providers had assessed the patient's injuries and felt that transport to a Level I facility was more appropriate. However, the patient's stated preference was honored, which was consistent with a protocol approved by the regional EMS authority. The patient died from a ruptured aneurysm while awaiting treatment at the Level II facility. The father's claims against the physician and hospital providing medical control were dismissed because the father failed to produce evidence that the patient would have survived the injury at the Level I facility. This state court ruling emphasizes the need for protocols that reflect sound medical principles, even when the patient's outcome may not be optimal.

Failure to Transport

Emergency responses in which the patient is not transported can seem like wasted effort. In some systems, these ambulance encounters consume time and resources, yet they constitute a significant patient population the medical director never sees.[27] These EMS calls are a medicolegal quagmire involving issues of patient autonomy, consent, medical assessment, and ill-defined legal duties. Patients denied transport or convinced by field personnel to forego ambulance transport have been a source of numerous claims and case law.*

When field personnel are called to a scene and do not transport a patient because they discovered no medical reason for the patient to be taken by ambulance to the hospital, questions of liability are easily raised if the patient suffers deterioration or demise. If the patient refuses the transport despite apparent medical need, the questions focus on whether the patient's refusal was an informed refusal of ambulance transport. Claims of liability in either case depend on the following two factors: (1) the thoroughness or accuracy of the prehospital provider's field assessment and (2) the adequacy of the prehospital provider's communication with the patient about the findings of the assessment and the need for medical treatment.

The principle of consent is well-known to the practicing physician. It is established that adults of sound mind have the right to refuse medical treatment, even if the refusal of treatment may result in death.[26] The medical profession also requires that refusal of treatment be informed refusal.[4] However, there are indications in EMS that there is no constitutional right for a patient to be transported to the hospital by a governmental EMS agency.[25] In addition, there is some indication that the patient may insist on transport to a hospital less qualified to provide necessary emergency care.[30]

Several issues make "no transport calls" troublesome. To minimize the risk in these calls, short of transporting every patient the medical director must understand the legal pitfalls inherent in the protocols or absence of protocols for these calls. First, although it is repeatedly impressed on EMS providers that they cannot "diagnose" illness, they are often directed by protocol to determine whether a patient is mentally "competent," which is a diagnosis and arguably a legal conclusion.[14] Second, prehospital providers have only basic training in assessing mental capacity or lucidity to evaluate a patient's ability to refuse treatment. Typically, they are instructed to ask only simplistic, routine questions about orientation such as "awake, alert, and oriented times three." This training is insufficient for evaluating mental status and providing information to patients for purposes of informed refusals. Third, there is no clear standard of the validity of mental status evaluations made outside the clinic or hospital environment.[36] These cases are further complicated by the lack of established legal standards regarding what constitutes informed refusal in the prehospital environment, to what extent consent is warranted for transport, and to what extent the duty to establish consent or refusal can be delegated by the medical director.

Another important issue is the scope of informed consent in the prehospital environment. Decades of case law in medical malpractice regarding the principle of consent involve patients seen in doctor's offices and hospitals, but the field environment is different. It may therefore be unrealistic to assume that the physician's duty to obtain informed consent or informed refusal applies to the prehospital provider, particularly given the dearth of training in EMS for this task.

Similarly, there have been no judicial interpretations of the relationship between a patient contacted in the field and a prehospital provider or the medical director. Arguably a physician-patient relationship is created in both cases. Similarly, there is no judicial statement that the prehospital provider must contact the base station to terminate the patient relationship in a no transport situation. However, sound medical oversight dictates that the medical director consider direct medical control essential or that very clear and precise protocols be in place if the patient-prehospital provider relationship is terminated without such supervision.

Factually, legal cases involving nontransport often involve glaring deficiencies in the assessment performed by the EMS provider; often, they reflect lack of discipline by the providers in adherence to protocols.[12,28] Liability can befall prehospital providers who leave the patient in the field without thorough and adequate assessment; medical direc-

*From Handler H: Vice President, The American Agency, 1988.

tors may be responsible if they fail to provide sufficient protocols that detail the circumstances under which patients can be left in the field.

Denial of ambulance transport. *Wright v. City of Los Angeles* expounded on the paramedic's duty to assess in a costly incident of failure to transport.[38] Police summoned EMS personnel for a man found lying on the sidewalk. He appeared to have been involved in an altercation. The paramedic did only a cursory assessment and decided ambulance transport was not necessary; he advised the police officers that the patient could be checked by a physician before booking. In fact, the patient was in sickle-cell crisis. The court held that if the paramedic had conducted an examination consistent with the standard of care, he should have been able to determine that the patient was in need of immediate treatment. There was no contact with the direct medical control for approval of the nontransport; the paramedic testified that he "saw no symptoms indicating such a call was necessary."[38] Minutes after the paramedic left the scene the patient arrested and died. The paramedic thought that the patient was simply intoxicated. The court found that the paramedic's failure to provide "even a scant amount of care" was an "extreme departure from the standard of care for a paramedic in such a situation." Therefore governmental immunity did not shield the defendant from liability in this state court ruling because the conduct was deemed grossly negligent. Although the medical director was not implicated in liability in *Wright,* the case exemplifies how direct medical control contact might have averted a death and a costly lawsuit.

The medical director should evaluate the substance of the prehospital provider's radio report when request is made for a nontransport disposition. Although the prehospital provider has the best direct view of the patient's situation, the medical director or direct medical control physician may have the medical expertise to evaluate the complications or implications of the patient's signs and symptoms; therefore the need for consultation and careful supervision is certainly warranted. The medical director should also carefully monitor radio contacts and ensure that all physicians providing direct medical control know the protocols for nontransport situations.

An example is provided in *Green v. City of Dallas,* which involved paramedics who failed to transport a 35-year-old male patient complaining of chest pain. Because of the patient's age, the fact that he was on no medications, and the observation that he was exhausted from playing basketball, the paramedics reasoned that the pain was not cardiac in nature. Five minutes after the crew departed the man arrested; the ambulance was sent back to the scene, but the man could not be resuscitated. The City successfully avoided liability through governmental immunity.

The decision in *Hialeah v. Weatherford* demonstrates that the time between the EMS contact with the patient and the patient's demise need not be brief to establish proximate cause.[43] In this case the patient died 24 hours after the ambulance crew left. The patient's wife had called for assistance; the prehospital providers observed her husband lying naked and stuporous when the ambulance arrived. The ambulance crew refused to transport the man, despite his wife's requests. The patient was transported 24 hours later when his wife again called for an ambulance; he died shortly afterward. The court held that there was sufficient evidence of proximate cause between the failure of the first crew to transport and the man's death more than 24 hours later, notwithstanding the wife's delay in requesting an ambulance the second time.

Nontransport situations also occur when the patient refuses to be transported to the hospital, despite the EMS crew's request and advice. Often a relative has summoned the ambulance and wants the patient transported. Liability claims may still be argued against the EMS agency. In *St. George v. City of Deerfield Beach* an ambulance was summoned by a visitor of a man found bleeding extensively from tooth extraction.[35] The paramedics failed to transport the man who was "obviously drunk and bleeding, but he absolutely and continually refused examination or treatment." The visitor called 9-1-1 a second time about 20 minutes later, but the dispatcher refused to send an ambulance. The appellate court rejected the defendant's motion to dismiss and ruled that sovereign immunity did not apply.

Patient Refusal

Sometimes a patient adamantly refuses transport, although the EMS crew feels transport is necessary. These cases are troubling for the prehospital providers who feel that it is in the patient's best interest to receive medical care. In addition, some prehospital providers have been instructed by medical directors who would rather take the risk of forced transport than leave an injured patient. Therefore transport is accomplished so the physician can evaluate the patient and establish informed refusal in a controlled setting. It can be argued that transport is warranted because the patient is unable to give informed refusal, if circumstances or the injuries appear to impair the patient's ability to comprehend the risks and consequences of refusal. On the other hand, in the absence of a life-threatening injury an adult of "sound mind" is allowed to refuse medical treatment; patients have the right to make medical treatment decisions that may result in deterioration and even death.[16]

Transport against the patient's express desires, particularly if restraints are used may constitute false imprisonment. The pivotal issue is whether the detention of the patient is justified under the circumstances.[35] There is some legal authority for a physician to forcibly restrain a person in need of treatment by virtue of a qualified privilege.[2] In any event, deprivation of a citizen's liberty is a serious and risky matter.

A few states have statutes that provide legal authority for peace officers to direct EMS personnel to take a person to a hospital, if it reasonably appears that medical treatment is needed. Such statutes usually require the peace officer or transporting personnel to act in "good faith" to gain the protections of immunity.[9] These statutes provide both authority and legal protection in the unwilling transport dilemma; however, medical control oversight is no less important and may be evidence of "good faith." The medical director must understand the circumstances under which such laws may be used. Consultation with local law enforcement may be vital for the effective application of protective custody efforts.

Many EMS agencies and medical directors require that the provider contact direct medical control in every patient refusal encounter. This is useful only if the quality of the contact is not superficial. The EMS provider must be thorough, accurate, and honest in the report to the physician. The physician must be diligent in listening, questioning, and evaluating the soundness of the information. The medical director must tailor the protocol for patient refusals according to the EMS system and the prehospital providers' skill and experience. Quality supervision by a medical director thereby diminishes claims of negligent failure to transport or patient abandonment.

Documentation of the refusal. Careful patient assessment and instructions or advice regarding refusal of treatment must be documented. The documentation on the prehospital care report (PCR) should unequivocally demonstrate an assessment adequate for an informed decision regarding the need for transport. Liability might arise for the medical director who fails to retrospectively review cases of nontransport or patient refusal to identify deficiencies in assessments or information provided to patients.

The use of releases, waivers, or other such documents that the patient signs in the field has limited legal merit for several reasons. First, courts frown on documents that attempt to deprive a person of recourse to the courts through such language as "release of liability." Therefore as a matter of public policy, these documents are construed against the party placing them in use. Some state court rulings have rejected the medical professional's efforts to contract away potential liability for negligent medical treatment.[31] Release from liability for negligent care has been rejected when the patient has little choice in where these services may be obtained.[33] Many of these forms are written in nearly incomprehensible legalese, which further invalidates their use. Therefore documents purporting to relieve the prehospital provider from liability might be invalid. Second, "promise not to sue" language in these documents does not preclude the necessity of obtaining an "informed refusal" of treatment and transport from the patient.

Obtaining a patient's signature may be beneficial for simply demonstrating the patient's physical and cognitive abilities. Such a document may be appropriate if used as a statement of acknowledgment by patients of their voluntary refusal of treatment. It may serve as a testimonial of the efforts made to educate and persuade the patient to be transported. However, such forms should be supplemented with appropriate documentation of the patient's physical and mental condition as assessed by the prehospital provider. The document should reflect attempts to warn the patient of the risks of delaying treatment and alert the patient that the prehospital provider may not be aware of the full extent of the injuries.[29] The medical director should not permit a release form to be used until it has been evaluated by legal counsel.

In summary the medical director should consider the following in the management of nontransport calls:

1. The medical director should have an accurate understanding of local and state laws regarding patient rights and the circumstances if any under which the physician may authorize or direct treatment and transport without the consent of the patient.
2. The medical director must ensure adequate training is provided to prehospital providers on specific techniques for evaluating mental status in the field.
3. Protocols must be appropriate for the prehospital providers' respective skill and experience levels. A review by competent legal counsel of the protocols and release form is recommended.
4. Contact with direct medical control if not required should be encouraged in all cases in

which a patient is not transported. Moreover, medical control contact should not be a mere formality; it should be a consultation.

5. Ongoing review and audit of radio reports, prehospital care reports (PCRs), and follow-up patient contact to evaluate the quality of field releases and patient refusals is imperative.
6. All use of restraints should be reviewed by the medical director.
7. The protocol for field releases and patient refusals should be reviewed periodically by the medical director and altered as needed.
8. If the release form used by the EMS agency is of questionable legal merit, then the medical director should prohibit use of the form.

Transfers

Interhospital transfers have evolved as one of the more lucrative profit centers for ambulance services. Transfers generally mean non-emergent use of ambulances and thus for many prehospital providers these patient contacts seem less exciting and less deserving of their medical skills. For example, these calls could include the "routine transfer" of a debilitated nursing home patient to and from a clinic appointment. It could also be a neonate in an incubator or the cardiac patient with multiple intravenous lines infusing medications. Obviously, transfers can be as diverse and critical as 9-1-1 calls.

A variety of problems can arise in the management of transfers. For example, the "transfer car" may be staffed with less experienced personnel, which can create risk in these sometimes medically complex calls. In addition, research shows that physicians may fail to use the appropriate level of skill for the patient's medical condition and, more important fail to stabilize patients adequately before transport.[19] Transfers are often initiated by persons unfamiliar with EMS systems and ambulance service management. This is evidenced by the requesting party directing the non-emergent response of the ambulance; it is also evident in the reimbursement problems that arise when the transport destination is based on physician convenience. Transfers can also be a source of liability for physicians and hospitals if a patient is unnecessarily put at risk because of the transfer.

With the enactment of federal legislation that regulates interhospital transfer of patients in the Consolidated Omnibus Budget Reconciliation Act (COBRA) of 1985, planning and preparation of transfers became serious business.[37] The law may actually protect prehospital providers from being "dumped on," as well as create more paperwork for emergency departments. The COBRA law only pertains to the transfer of "unstable" patients and mandates that transfer be "effected through qualified personnel and required transportation equipment."[7] The law may also affect destination policies because the patient must be transported to a qualified facility. The law can impose significant burdens on small ambulance services, which the medical director should attempt to limit. For example, in rural EMS systems the need to transport an unstable patient to a higher level of care may be valid. However, the service may have only BLS personnel available and a limited number of ambulances. Nonetheless, qualified personnel and equipment must accompany the patient. It becomes imperative that the medical director educate hospital staff of the transport capabilities of the ambulance service for transfers. The medical director should also be careful that "convenience transfers" do not misuse ambulance resources, exposing the rest of the EMS system to risk. Additionally, political and economic decisions should not dictate the movement of patients. One court considered it egregious to refuse ambulance service to a patient because of political interests. A hospital that refused to allow use of its ambulance unless the patient was brought to its facility (where the patient's attending physician did not have privileges) supported a verdict for outrageous conduct in *DeCicco v. Trinidad Area Health Association*.[48]

The medical director must vigilantly ensure that an ambulance service accept transfers only if adequately trained crews are available. This may entail careful examination of individual skills and prospective identification of specific medications that the prehospital provider may monitor. In addition, there may be need for cooperative arrangements between the hospital nursing staff who accompany the patient in the ambulance and the ambulance personnel. The respective responsibilities of nursing personnel and the EMS crew should be clarified *before* transports are initiated. There should be no question of "turf" or responsibilities in the back of a moving ambulance with a critical patient utterly dependent on the attendant caregivers assigned to the transfer.

Documentation

Paperwork has been the bane of existence for many medical professionals otherwise skilled in the provision of patient care. Training in this critical area has been largely overlooked and improvement has been dependent on retrospective audits. Poor documentation has persisted, and prehospital providers tend to believe that the trip reports are insignificant in a patient's medical record or ignored by the hospital health care providers. Lack of immediate feedback and tolerance of poor report writing by emergency department staff and medical directors undermine documentation efforts.

The PCR is a measure of accountability for the EMS provider, just as the medical record substantiates the hospital health care providers' patient care. The ambulance run report should reflect the quality of patient care and assessment. Adherence to protocols should be evident in the PCR report. Although the medical director may audit every paramedic's PCR to monitor their emergency care performance, EMT-A providers have less training and are often less experienced both in patient care and documentation. Therefore their PCRs warrant greater efforts for improvement of report writing skills. Many medical directors supervise providers who run just a few calls each month; thus each PCR should be reviewed and used as an opportunity for quality improvement.

Patience and persistence by the medical director can lead to improved PCR preparation and patient care. The medical director should develop useful PCR forms and writing formats and discourage formats and forms that impede quality documentation. Every PCR should address unique aspects such as scene factors or observations, patient positioning when first encountered, the apparent mechanism of injury, scene interventions, and extrication difficulties. Documentation of responses to interventions, justifications for interventions or for failures to treat, and the condition of a patient upon arrival at the emergency department are also important on the PCR. The medical director should take a proactive role in the quality management efforts of documentation.

Finally, legibility remains a critical factor in the usefulness of documentation. The medical director should insist on legible PCRs; only if the information in the PCR is legible can it be useful to subsequent health care providers, quality improvement efforts, and possible legal proceedings.

Equipment

To some degree the skills and capabilities of EMS providers have been confounded by equipment or more precisely the compulsion to employ equipment in the "technical imperative."[24] From the insistence to dispatch a helicopter when rational assessment would obviate the expense and expedite patient care to the forceful plunge of a 14-gauge angiocath when an 18-gauge would suffice, the use and abuse of medical equipment have been implicating factors in many claims and lawsuits. Aided by the use of poorly drafted treatment protocols, the "technical imperative" has caused endotracheal tubes to be forcefully pushed into airways rather than deferring to oropharyngeal airway and bag-valve mask ventilation; it contributes to misuse of precious time consumed on-scene where rapid transport of a trauma patients is warranted. Medical directors should be the source of authority for the use of equipment, procedures, and protocols because they will be responsible for the consequences attributable to misuse of equipment.

At least one court has ruled that the equipment that is carried on an ambulance and used in patient care is a matter of "medical judgment."[18] The medical director should impress on EMS providers that new equipment must have a demonstrated capability to improve patient care to be implemented. Medical directors should consider the legal protective measures listed in the box below for equipment usage by the EMS personnel under their supervision.

Control Through Contracts

The role of the medical director is complex and demanding. The physician newly recruited as a medical director can benefit from predecessors. One of the lessons to be learned is that accepting a position of responsibility for an EMS system and all patient care rendered within that system should be preceded by a frank and detailed discussion of roles and responsibilities. The job is more manageable if medical directors have clear and unequivocal authority to accomplish the tasks with which they are charged. A contract in which the medical director's responsibilities and authority are delineated and agreed on is not an unreasonable formality; it is simple sound business practice.

Medical directors must acknowledge the fact that they are accountable regardless of how much time

Equipment Usage Protective Measures

1. Exercise authority in the selection and implementation of equipment such as defibrillators, drugs, and restraints.
2. Require skills check-off with new equipment through direct observation of each EMS provider to ensure proper use.
3. Implement clear, concise protocols that facilitate appropriate use of the equipment, and review the protocols periodically.
4. Remove hazardous or ineffective equipment from use or disallow its use if problems are not corrected.

they devote to medical oversight and regardless of the number of field personnel practicing under their license. Medical directors must also realize the risks, the means, and the goals of this position and not hesitate to address these factors before accepting the position. Moreover, accepting the responsibility without the authority is an invitation for frustration, as well as risk. It is important to also recognize limitations that exist in the EMS system and negotiate the means and resources necessary to meet the goals of the job. For example, medical directors may insist that the fire department assume certain responsibilities in training and documentation and that practice restrictions invoked by the medical director be honored. They might insist that a coordinator position be established or equipment upgrades be made. If a private ambulance service has a contract with a city and has promised certain response times, potential medical directors must evaluate whether they can accept the constraints of that performance contract before they become the medical director for the ambulance service.

The medical director who cannot engage a written contract may accomplish some goals by using written protocols or establishing a quality improvement program with performance standards. However, it is likely that the medical director has implied authority to impose certain restrictions and standards despite the absence of a formal written contract. In most states, medical directors extend their medical license to EMS providers as physician extenders, at least at the paramedic level. Inherent in that extension is the authority to exercise medical judgment in matters including who can function under their license. This was recognized in *County of Hennepin v. Hennepin County Association of Paramedics and Emergency Medical Technicians.* A state court ruled it a matter of medical judgment for medical directors to determine who can function under their license; the employer or the paramedic union could not force the medical director to accept a paramedic the medical director felt was incapable of practicing with reasonable skill and safety.[6]

There is no standard contract, but there are certain minimum issues any contractual arrangement should address (see box at right). Prospective medical directors should carefully scrutinize the EMS agencies' strengths and weaknesses, the political tone and community support for EMS, and other factors that may impact their goals. The detail and complexity of the contract will differ if it is an understanding between the medical director and each EMS provider rather than between the medical director and the county commissioners or a municipality.

The substance of the contract may differ, depending on the agencies, the patient populations, the training and staffing of the prehospital providers, and the different needs for immediate and long-range goals for quality improvement measures. The medical director's role must be formalized because many systems consist of multiple management heads with decision-making authority spread amongst fire chiefs, company owners, city managers, and medical directors. Medical directors must identify the correct party or parties with whom they must negotiate. A contract with the city health department may be meaningless if the city fire department chief has unbridled discretion regarding who is hired whether paramedics, EMT-As, or First Responders are dispatched to certain medical emergencies, and whether attendance at continuing education sessions is mandatory.

Minimum Provisions of Contractual Arrangement

1. Responsibilities of both parties must be clearly delineated. For example, the medical director likely will be responsible for creating protocols, and the service agency is responsible for distribution of protocols to all prehospital providers.
2. The authority to fulfill the responsibilities must be provided. For example, the medical director should be allowed to impose education requirements and practice restrictions on any paramedic who demonstrates inadequate performance.
3. The medical director should have a clear understanding of the person or entity to whom he is responsible. At the same time, it must be understood that the medical director is at all times a patient advocate.
4. The terms of payment, duration of the contractual arrangement, and the recourse for nonperformance by either party should be delineated.
5. The medical director must have the authority to participate in all aspects of the EMS system that affect patient care including dispatching, information about all patient complaints, equipment selection, and review of all contracts that may impact the medical director's responsibilities.

Summary

The role of a physician in medical oversight is complex and time consuming; it is a mixture of medicine, administration, public relations, and engineering. Careful delegation of tasks to field coordinators and hospital staff alleviates the burden quantitatively but does not lessen the physician's responsibility qualitatively. The benefit of interactions with field personnel is not merely for risk management. Medical directors who exercise and practice meaningful medical oversight gain by knowing their system, understanding its operations, and participating in its improvement. Passivity or acts of omission such as failure to provide protocols, failure to discipline, or failure to implement quality management audits place medical directors at great legal risk and deprive the prehospital providers and the community of the expertise and leadership that good indirect medical control should provide. Medical oversight is seldom hazardous unless the medical director serves only by signature. The days of passive, uninformed medical oversight are hopefully shortening. Risks arise when the EMS physician fails to keep informed of accepted standards of prehospital medical practice, confuses politics or economics with good patient care, and acquiesces to inappropriate or inept actions by EMS providers. Through development of systemwide protocols, quality management systems, and personnel policies, the medical director should be secure.

Legal hazards and pitfalls are nothing new to the emergency physician who is constantly presented with the unexpected, vagaries of caring for strangers, community pressures, and unrecognized sacrifices. The delivery of prehospital medicine is as complex and uncertain as emergency medicine, perhaps more so. Despite the medically and legally uncharted territory in prehospital care, the apparent variations and questions of duty in all aspects of medical oversight rely on the basic principles of medical practice—paramount concern for patient care and professionalism in the delivery of health care. The EMS medical director has a unique opportunity to serve innumerable patients, prehospital providers, and EMS systems in a challenging arena.

REFERENCES

1. Ambulances and Emergency Medical Personnel, 847-35-020(2).
2. *Blackman v Rifkin,* 759 P 2d 54, 1988.
3. Board of Medical Examiners: Oregon administrative rule 847-35-020.
4. *Canterbury v Spence,* 464 F 2d 772, certification denied, 409 US 1064, 1972.
5. *City of East Detroit v Malcom,* 468 2d 479, 1991.
6. *County of Hennepin v Hennepin County Association of Paramedics and Emergency Medical Technicians,* 464 2d 578, 1990.
7. The Emergency Medical Treatment and Active Labor Act, 42 USCA 1395dd(c)(2).
8. Florida Public Health Law 401.265.
9. Florida statutes, Section 396.072(1), 1979.
10. Highway Safety Program Standard Number 11: Emergency Medical Services, 23 CFR 1204.4, Nov 14, 1968.
11. Holder AR: *Medical malpractice law,* ed 2, New York, 1978, John Wiley & Sons.
12. Holroyd B et al: Prehospital patients refusing care, *Ann Emerg Med* 17:957-963, Sep 1988.
13. *Hospital Authority of Gwinnett County and Gwinnett Ambulance Services Inc v Jones,* Case 46956, Supreme Court of the State of Georgia, Brief of Appellee.
14. Kaplan K et al: The clinician's role on competency evaluations, *Gen Hosp Psychiatry* 11:397-403, 1989.
15. *Kowalski v Gratopp,* 177 A 448, 442 2d 682, 1989.
16. *Lane v Candura,* 376 2d 1232, 1978.
17. *Little v Davenport,* 251 2d 250, 242 Ga. 751, 1978.
18. *Lyons by Lyons v Hasbro Industries and Arrow Medical Services,* 509 2d 702, 1987.
19. Martin G et al: Prospective analysis of rural interhospital transfer of injured patients to a referral trauma center, *J Trauma,* 30(8):1014-1019, Aug 1990.
20. Missouri Rule, 19 CSR 50-40.160, *Missouri Register* 15:4, Feb 15, 1990.
21. Norris JA: Current status and utility of emergency medical care liability law, *Forum* 15:377-405, 1980.
22. *Overman v Occoquan, Woodbridge, Lorton Volunteer Fire Department,* District Court, 90-42A, 1990.
23. Page J: *The paramedics,* Morristown, Penn, 1979, Backdraft Publications.
24. Rosen P et al: The technical imperative: its definition and an application to prehospital care, *Topics Emerg Med* 79-85, Jul 1981.
25. *Salazar v City of Chicago,* 840 F 2d 233, 1991.
26. *Schloendorff v Society of New York,* 105 2d 92, 1914.
27. Selden BS et al: The "no-patient" run: 2,698 patients evaluated but not transported by paramedics, *Prehosp Disaster Medicine,* 6(2):135-142, 1991.
28. Selden BS et al: Medicolegal documentation of prehospital triage, *Ann Emerg Med,* 19:547-551, 1990.
29. Shanaberger C: Why releases don't work, *JEMS* 13:47-49, Feb 1988.
30. *Smith v East Medical Center,* 585 2d 1325, 1991.
31. *Threadgill v Peabody Coal Co.,* 526 P 2d 676, 1974.
32. *Tonsic v Wagner,* 329 A 2d 497, 1974.
33. *Vasquez v Board of Regents, State of Florida,* 548 2d 251, 1989.
34. Washington statute WAC 248-15, revised 1987.
35. *Wideman v DeKalb County,* 409 A 2d 537, 1991.
36. Zun L: A survey of the form of the mental status examination administered by emergency physicians, *Ann Emerg Med* 15:916-922, Aug 1986.
37. 42 USC 1395dd.
38. 268 A 2d 309, 1990.
39. 386 2d 120, 259 Ga. 236, 1989, 111 S C 1298, 1990.
40. 447 A 2d 860, 1989.
41. 462 A 2d 680, 1983.
42. 464 A 2d 578, 1990.
43. 466 2d 1127, 1985.
44. 475 A 2d 1319, 1985.
45. 543 A 2d 770, 1989.
46. 545 A 2d 284, 1986.
47. 560 A 2d 778, 1991.
48. 573 P 2d 559, 1977.
49. 729 F S 376, 1990.
50. 764 F S 1510, 1991.
51. 826 F 2d 1030, 1987.

27

Prehospital Providers in the Emergency Department

Michael P. Wainscott, M.D., FACEP
James M. Atkins, M.D.

The unique role of EMS personnel in the prehospital environment is understood by most emergency and medical personnel. However, the function of EMS personnel inside the emergency department (ED) is more obscure, leading to potential misunderstandings and conflicts. Through a clear understanding of the various roles and interactions of prehospital providers in the ED, EMS medical directors may serve as facilitators for the ED medical director, nurse director, and providers.

There are three major areas of interaction between ED and prehospital personnel. The first interaction occurs during training. The second interaction happens when the provider transports a patient to the ED. The third interaction is when the provider is actually employed in a patient care role in the ED. Each of these areas of interaction requires definition of both responsibilities and performance guidelines.

In the sections that follow, potential roles and functions of the traditional prehospital provider are presented to assist in the development of guidelines for the ED experience.

Students in the Emergency Department

The importance of quality initial education for EMS personnel is undisputed. A solid foundation of knowledge, skills, and attitudes is necessary for EMS personnel to function effectively and provide consistent quality patient care.[3]

The roles and responsibilities of students in the ED must be well-defined. It is important to recognize the goals of training students in the ED. Prehospital providers perform a different function than physicians, nurses, or any other hospital personnel; their training should reflect this difference.

Clinical Supervision

Clinical supervision of the student in the ED is a vital consideration. The course director, course instructors, and course medical director must establish clearly defined goals and objectives, lists of procedures to be performed, and performance evaluations for clinical training. Involvement of the ED nurse manager and ED medical director in the development of the clinical curriculum is also valuable.

During clinical training in the ED, students are typically supervised by ED nurses. It is important to orient those nurses to the educational needs, limitations, and performance parameters of the student. This orientation becomes especially important when there are multiple levels of field providers being trained. Preceptors from the training programs should also be present and are an excellent way of coordinating and enhancing the training experience.

Focus on Role and Function

In the prehospital environment the provider becomes a *substitute* set of eyes, ears, and hands for the physician. In the hospital, nurses and technicians are an *additional* set of eyes, ears, and hands, but they are not usually a complete substitute. A nurse assesses the patient before, during, and after the physician's management and collaborates with the physician to diagnose and treat the patient. A nurse maintains both parallel and complementary patient care roles with the physician. Nurses generally triage, assess, initiate and provide treatment, reassess, and ultimately discharge the patient. This integral role of the ED nurse in coordinating patient care delivery reflects the extent of education of the nurse, as well as the broadly defined role of the ED nurse on the ED team. On the other hand, a field provider functions as the sole caregiver without the direct involvement of the physician is the only source of information for the physician and has a more narrow and well-defined role in patient care.

Because field personnel are trained for different functions than most other health care providers, the educational goals are also different. These differences in goals impact the depth and breadth of training. Even paramedics are not trained as deeply in pathophysiology as nurses. Extensive training in pathophysiology allows the nurse to make independent and parallel judgments with the physician. Because the prehospital provider is acting in the absence of a physician, there is usually no parallel judgment. The provider makes some independent judgments within the parameters of protocols but is taught to function in the absence of physicians.

The field provider performs patient care using focused protocols. These protocols are important in gathering and transmitting patient care information and in determining the treatment of the patient. The provider responds in a relatively rigid and reactive manner. On the other hand, nurses have a broad base of education and generally do not function in a rigid protocol-driven fashion. The use of protocols by ED nurses is present in some EDs to establish triage criteria and facilitate early initiation of treatment. Clinical ED training of prehospital students must reflect these differences in ultimate function and goals.

Prehospital students need to learn the progression and outcome of various medical conditions. In the field, they evaluate and treat patients for a relatively brief time. It is important for the educational goals to include an understanding of how to recognize patients that may deteriorate. Visualizing and discussing progression of illness, response to therapy, and patient outcome are valuable aspects of clinical ED training. This interaction also enhances the students' awareness of their role on the emergency care team.

The curriculum should also include patient assessment and management specific to the types of medical care usually rendered by prehospital personnel. However, adequate amounts of such focused clinical training may be difficult to obtain. Factors that interfere with the role of the preceptor include a lack of understanding of the educational objectives, disagreement over the perceived clinical freedom enjoyed by field providers, a lack of trust in the relatively untrained individuals, and a fear of medicolegal consequences of actions taken by the students. Hospital personnel may also feel uncomfortable or even threatened by the expertise of paramedics in skills such as intubation or electrocardiogram (ECG) rhythm strip recognition. In considering the role and function of prehospital students, such potential problems or conflicts need to be addressed and appropriate intervention taken as necessary.

Often, exposure to prehospital care facilitates understanding by the ED staff. It is extremely beneficial for the ED nurses and physicians to occasionally ride with EMS units. This brings into focus the role of the prehospital care provider as a member of the emergency care team. ED physicians and nurses have an obligation to integrate prehospital care into the overall care of the patient, much like they integrate respiratory therapy. Only by comprehending the role of the prehospital provider will the ED staff become effective educators.

Goals

The ED can provide the student with an extremely valuable learning experience. Goals for this experience can be divided into the following three areas: patient assessment, skills performance, and the integration of both. These objectives must be clear to the student and the preceptor.

Patient Assessment. Prehospital providers receive much of their patient assessment training in the ED; thus a good learning experience is essential. Prehospital assessment is similar yet quite different from assessment by nurses and physicians. Limited numbers of personnel at the scene and austere environmental working conditions (such as inadequate lighting, scene hazards, no radiographs, and no laboratories) portray the limited resources of providers working in the prehospital arena. They must make judgments from history and physical findings, using only limited diagnostic adjuncts such as rhythm strips, ECGs, glucose sticks, and pulse oximeters.

Comprehensive histories and physicals are usually inappropriate in the field. Yet it is essential that the prehospital trainee develop strong history and physical evaluation skills, first in the classroom and then during clinical training. Physical evaluation skills include scene survey, primary survey, status decision, measurement of vital signs, and secondary survey. As assessment skills are developed, students must be taught to focus and then to prioritize the information needed to make rapid field interventions. Full understanding of these concepts impacts both scene time and patient care.

During training, much attention is addressed to the primary survey. The student is taught to make critical interventions in response to problems found during the primary survey such as airway difficulties. The amount of detail in the assessment and management depends on the provider's perceived urgency of the situation. The goal of assessment in the field is to rapidly define the need for specialized prehospital care such as airway, defibrillation, intravenous (IV) fluids, cervical collars, and backboards. Critical interventions are initiated as indicated.

The skills employed in the field vary from system to system, and clinical training should reflect appropriate assessment and skills performance necessary for a given system's patient care needs. Special emphasis should be placed on specific types of assessment done in the field. For example, if a medical director wishes a paramedic to perform pleural decompression for tension pneumothorax, then the paramedic must be taught more detailed anatomy and to recognize the signs and symptoms of a tension pneumothorax.

Skills performance. Adequate performance of psychomotor skills is another key area for prehospital students learning in the ED. In the classroom the students learn skills using artificial training adjuncts such as IV, cardiopulmonary resuscitation (CPR), and intubation mannequins. Many training programs allow IV practice on other students. All skills should be appropriately mastered before entering the clinical phase of training. Although practice sessions in the classroom are useful, direct supervised participation in ED patient care is essential. For example, cardiac monitoring, electrical cardioversion, endotracheal intubation, IV cannulation, CPR, and ventilation are skills to be performed with nurse or physician supervision in the ED during prehospital clinical training.

Increasingly, prehospital educators stress a symptom or assessment-based approach to patient evaluation and care. This process begins in the classroom and must continue in the clinical training setting. The goal is not to have the provider determine the diagnosis, but rather to initiate treatment based on the presentation and evaluation of the patient. As a result of the problem-oriented approach, overuse of some procedures such as cervical spine immobilization, IV cannulation, and medication requests from direct medical control personnel may occur. ED personnel must realize that overtreatment may be appropriate.

A number of studies have demonstrated deterioration of knowledge and skills in EMS providers, although the significance of this deterioration remains unclear.[3] In 1980 Latman and Wooley demonstrated that emergency medical technicians-ambulance (EMT-As) lost 50% of basic skills proficiency, and paramedics lost 61% of basic skills proficiency within 2 years of training.[5] In 1987 Skelton and McSwain reported a correlation between the amount of technical skill deterioration and increasing length of time since completion of the training program. They also concluded that basic skills even when used frequently deteriorate with time.[6] These studies confirm the need for adequate continuing education and retraining of EMS providers, perhaps eventually using the ED. The studies also emphasize the need for adequate initial education of EMS providers and the instillation of a practice ethic.

Patient management knowledge integration. Prehospital students must integrate their assessment and psychomotor skills into an overall patient management concept in order to make appropriate patient care decisions in the field. It is essential that the student recognize when to use certain skills based on assessment of the patient's problem and presentation. Active physician, nurse, and other preceptor involvement in this learning process cannot be overstated.

Effective Behavior Patterns

Interpersonal skills and behavior patterns of prehospital providers concerning patients and other health care professionals may be improved in the ED. Mutual respect among prehospital providers, nurses, and physicians can be fostered by developing rapport during clinical training in the ED. Frequently the ED is the first significant contact with physician and nursing personnel for the students. The students see the physicians and nurses as role models for patient care encounters. This role model concept should not be taken lightly; it should be viewed as a vehicle to teach and reinforce appropriate behaviors.

Thus the emergency physician and emergency nurse play extremely important roles in training prehospital providers. These roles can neither be ignored nor delegated. The care given to patients in the field is a reflection of the provider's clinical training. Often, that training depends on the ability of the ED nurse and physician to teach and effectively interact with the student. Preceptors of clinical training should be oriented to the prehospital environment and the specific needs, limitations, and performance parameters of prehospital training.

Clinical Interface: The Emergency Department

The ED is the interface between the prehospital environment and the hospital. Prehospital providers render care until the patient can be turned over to an equal or higher level of care. Most frequently, this transfer of patient responsibility occurs in the ED. All pertinent information must be efficiently and briefly relayed to ED personnel so appropriate triage can be performed. ED and EMS policies must carefully and precisely describe this interface of the prehospital and ED personnel.

Prehospital care personnel sometimes assist in the ED until adequate personnel are present to care for the patient. This role is important for critical patients who need immediate resuscitation. For example, when an ambulance crew transports a cardiac arrest patient to the ED and only one nurse and one physician are present, the crew may perform CPR until other hospital personnel arrive, allowing the nurse and physician to administer advanced life support.

Emergency departments vary dramatically in size, patient volume, and number of physicians, nurses, and other personnel. In some EDs it is customary for the triage nurse to initiate assessment of all ambulance patients. In other EDs the physician or the nurse and physician accept the patient. A smooth transition must occur to effectively transfer patient care responsibility from the EMS crew to ED personnel.

Information regarding mechanism of injury, patient presentation, treatment en route, and change in the patient's condition during transport is helpful in the management of the patient, often directly impacting initial patient care. This information should be obtained in a professional, structured, and courteous manner, recognizing that prehospital care is an important part of the overall medical care of the patient.

Feedback about prehospital care can be given directly by the emergency nurses and physicians. Logically, this is done out of hearing range of patients and the ED staff. Such immediate feedback enhances prehospital patient care and functions as a quality improvement mechanism.

The providers should understand the role of personnel at a given ED in the medical oversight system. If the EMS staff do not know the role of the specific nurse or physician in the provision of formal indirect and direct medical control, there can be embarrassment and confusion.

Traditional Prehospital Providers Working in the Emergency Department

A health care crisis in the United States has occurred as a result of patient acuity, increased admissions, and insufficient resources to optimally meet demand. This has led hospitals to seek alternative staffing options such as the use of caregivers other than registered nurses to provide patient care needs.[3] In addition to licensed vocational nurses, licensed practical nurses, and physician assistants, many EDs now employ emergency medical technicians-Basic (EMT-Bs) and paramedics in various clinical capacities. Job titles for these individuals include emergency department technicians, EMTs, orderlies, and nursing assistants.

In December 1991, a survey of emergency physicians conducted by the American College of Emergency Physicians (ACEP) showed that 43% of respondents use prehospital providers in the ED for patient care.[2] This was an increase from 1985, when Allerman et al published a study indicating that about 27% of responding hospitals were using or planned to use prehospital personnel in their EDs.[1] The ACEP survey also showed that 59% of the respondents began employing prehospital within the previous 2 years.[2]

The role for prehospital providers in the ED depends on the needs of the particular ED and should be defined accordingly. It is helpful for the ED physician, nurse, and administrative staff to develop a scenario of "ideal" patient care in their ED. From this ideal the types and numbers of personnel needed to render care are extrapolated including duties and functions. These needs must then be matched with the qualifications of the personnel. This can also be reinforced for the ED that already has prehospital personnel and is considering expanding service or personnel.

The decision to employ field providers in some EDs is initiated by nurses. Nursing may identify areas where patient care is slowed due to inadequate numbers of ED staff. If aspects of these areas such as phlebotomy, IV cannulation, taking vital signs, splint application, and gait training with crutches may be performed by prehospital personnel, then consideration may be given to formalizing a new role in the ED.

As the potential roles and duties are considered, it is essential to review state laws and regulations regarding EMS personnel functions. Rules may be so specific in some states that they preclude the use of EMS personnel in the ED. In other states broader definitions may be interpreted as allowing paramedics to provide more ED care. Malpractice coverage is also an important consideration. Written legal opinions should be obtained from the hospital's attorneys and from the state, regarding this matter.

The physician must carefully define the role of the prehospital provider in the ED. There may be a specific role or job title established in the hospital, and qualifications for the role may include, for example, EMT-B training. However, the actual title of EMT-B or paramedic may not exist in the hospital. Once roles and responsibilities are defined, individuals are hired and orientation is provided. Some EDs require further training and supervised performance for the prehospital providers before they assume their new role in the ED.

EMT-Bs function in a limited and mostly technical capacity in the ED. Their responsibilities might include taking and charting vital signs, performing CPR, applying sterile dressings, applying bandages, administering oxygen, applying physical restraints, assessing pupillary reaction, immobilizing suspected extremity fractures, performing oral suctioning, ventilating with the bag-valve mask, cleaning equipment or rooms, setting up equipment, transporting patients and supplies, stocking rooms, teaching patients crutch walking, and assisting within the defined limits of the role. In most states it is difficult to philosophically explain how the EMT-B or paramedic logically functions as a nurse "extender."

Paramedics may be allowed to perform skills additional to those already mentioned for the EMT-B. These include placing a patient on a cardiac monitor, IV initiation, blood drawing, performing a spun hematocrit or urine pregnancy test, and checking fetal heart tones. If laboratory tests such as spun hematocrits, pregnancy tests, or urine dip tests are performed by prehospital personnel, the provider must be trained and supervised according to the federal Clinical Laboratory Improvement Act of 1988 (CLIA). In some EDs, the paramedic provides triage functions. These skills require much nursing time in a typical, busy ED, and by transferring some of these tasks to paramedics, the ED nurses are able to spend more time performing other tasks such as patient management, administrative matters, and patient education. It is unusual but not unknown for a paramedic to intubate, defibrillate, and administer medications in the ED. Medications are to be given only in accordance with state laws. Paramedics have training in the administration of a very few drugs. It is clear that a paramedic in the ED is not a substitute for an emergency nurse; yet the paramedic can provide a valuable service. A paramedic in the ED technically acts as a physician extender under most circumstances, although they assist and are often supervised by ED nurses.

The relationships among the paramedic, nurse, and physician staff must be delineated. The paramedic ED role must be planned with care. All personnel in the ED must be oriented. Supervision for the paramedic must be clearly defined. The 1991 ACEP survey showed that in 65% of EDs the nurse supervised prehospital providers, and in 33% of EDs the physician supervises.[2] In some EDs where the physician is ultimately responsible the nurse actually supervises, because the nurse coordinates the patient care. As mentioned before, this may not be a technically legal relationship.

In 1989 Sklar et al reported on a 15-year experience using ED technicians; they described a program of training and graded responsibility for ED technicians, focusing on laceration and wound care, splinting, IV catheter placement, and other procedures for critically ill or injured patients. These technicians had been either military medics or civilian paramedics before entering the program to become ED technicians. They then received extensive additional training. Nurses supervised the activity level of the technicians, and attending physicians supervised specific procedures and were ultimately responsible for them.[7] The program described was much more complex than simply bringing the prehospital personnel into the ED. The care provided by prehospital providers in the ED should be reviewed as a part of the quality improvement program for the ED. As problem areas are identified, specific solutions can be developed. In addition, periodic evaluation of the roles and responsibilities of prehospital personnel ensures appropriate use to meet the needs of the ED.

Summary

Field providers interface with the ED in a number of roles, as students, prehospital patient caregivers, and employees. The ED nurses and physicians must take an active role in the clinical training of students including understanding the curriculum, teaching, and serving as role models. The proper transfer of care from prehospital personnel to ED personnel requires both good communication and recognition of the field provider as a member of the emergency care team. Fostering open communication among emergency physicians and the physician responsible for medical oversight is crucial to facilitating the interface of field personnel and ED personnel.

Field personnel may be actively involved in ED patient care. Responsibilities should be outlined, and supervision should be defined. In addition, because of the variation in state regulations and individual hospital policies, it is crucial to evaluate the medicolegal and operational aspects of EMS personnel employment for patient care in the ED setting. This is especially true if they are responsible to non-physicians.

REFERENCES

1. Allerman G, McKay JI, and Novotny-Dinsdale V: Use of prehospital care providers in emergency departments: a national survey, *Journal of Emergency Nursing* 11:33-39, 1985.
2. American College of Emergency Physicians: *1991 leaders survey: use of EMT's/Paramedics in the ED,* Dec 1991, The College.
3. Cason D & Wainscott MP: *Training and evaluation:* In: Polsky SS, editor: *Continuous quality improvement in EMS,* 1992, American College of Emergency Physicians.

4. Emergency Nurses Association: *Position statement: the use of non-registered nurse caregivers in emergency departments,* Jun 1990, The Association.
5. Latman NS & Wooley K: Knowledge and skill retention of emergency care attendants, EMT-A's, and EMT-P's, *Ann Emerg Med* 9:183-189, 1980.
6. Skelton MB & McSwain NE: A study of cognitive and technical skill deterioration among trained paramedics, *JACEP* 6:436-438, 1977.
7. Sklar DP et al: Emergency department technicians in a university-county hospital: a 15-year experience, 18:401-404, 1989.

28

Prehospital Providers

Brenda M. Bruns, M.D., M.S.M.
Michael Osur, EMT-P

Previous chapters in this text describe the background, rationale, and format of a prehospital medical care system. EMS medical directors must clearly understand these conceptual components to successfully design and manage an EMS system. Additionally, they must create an atmosphere of cooperation and enthusiasm for the processes required to develop and maintain high quality prehospital medical care. To attain these goals, medical directors must establish functional relationships not only with those who help manage the system (the direct medical control and administrative personnel) but also with those affected by that management (the prehospital providers). The "management-labor" aspects of these relationships are well-delineated in the section on medical oversight (see Chapter 18). This chapter outlines alternative modes of interaction between the EMS physician and prehospital care providers and demonstrates how selective extension of the provider role beyond its traditional boundaries enhances system relationships and hence quality.

Currently the major role of prehospital providers is the frontline delivery of prehospital care. Under the authority of EMS agencies or state law they serve as the extension of physicians into the community. They do hold management positions, but for the most part these are with the employer or volunteer corps (for example, ambulance company, fire department, or public agency) and involve strictly operational responsibilities such as scheduling, supply distribution, and enforcement of company policies. Prehospital providers are less commonly found in systemwide positions of authority or as members of committees that develop protocols and policies.

This exclusion may be counterproductive to the goal of quality medical care. Important to the efficacy of any system is acceptance of its policies by the persons who must use them. One method of facilitating such acceptance is to enlist the assistance of those members during the system development process. Applying this management tactic to EMS suggests that one of the best ways to make prehospital policies, protocols, and plans effective is to encourage participation of field practitioners in the management activities of the EMS system. Field providers frequently express concern regarding the relevance and applicability of EMS policies. They feel that the EMS agency is distant from the field and has insufficient comprehension of its reality. Enlisting providers in the authority camp not only increases acceptance of EMS processes but also deemphasizes the "we-they" atmosphere. In addition, experienced providers offer a wealth of field expertise; integrating this with the medical expertise of physicians makes EMS plans more effective.

If this process is to be successful, it must be well-defined and carefully supervised by the EMS medical director. Otherwise, overextension of the providers' roles, antagonism among providers involved and those not involved in activities, and infringements on personal and system confidentially ensue. Careful analysis of the relevant concerns of both medical control and prehospital personnel should occur before implementing such participation to optimally benefit the EMS system as a whole.

This chapter describes areas of EMS system management in which prehospital provider participation might occur. Examples of potential and existing mechanisms for such participation are provided. Although an extensive literature review and an informal survey of other EMS systems were conducted, the majority of the examples are garnered from the San Francisco Bay area counties in California. California's EMS system is proscribed by state legislation (Division 2.5 of the Health and

Safely code) and organized through county (or regional, in less populated areas) EMS agencies. The state EMS Authority provides guidance and direction for the local EMS agencies, but the responsibility for the overall planning, coordination, and monitoring of prehospital emergency care is delegated to county governments.

Each county establishes an EMS agency and appoints an EMS medical director. The duties performed by the local EMS agencies include the following[1]:

1. Organization and planning for EMS system maintenance and improvement,
2. Certification or authorization of prehospital personnel (including nurses or physicians who provide direct medical control),
3. Approval of prehospital training programs and continuing education,
4. Designation of trauma centers, base hospitals (direct medical control), and other specialty care centers,
5. Administration of contracts with provider agencies and hospitals,
6. Provision for direct and indirect medical control,
7. Developments and promulgation of policies and procedures, and
8. Distribution of EMS funds (acquired either through direct EMS tax assessments or from the general county or city tax funds.

Despite the specificity of state legislation for EMS systems in California, there is no delineation or guidance for incorporating prehospital providers into the EMS decision-making authority. Hence the issues described and exemplified below may apply to any EMS system currently lacking such roles for prehospital providers, even if the structure of the EMS system is different than that of California.

Formation of Policies and Protocols

The development and revision of prehospital policies, procedures, and protocols is one of the major tasks of an EMS agency. The discipline of prehospital care is rapidly evolving both medically and technically; it encompasses a wide spectrum of medical problems, focusing on provision of care in the first moments of acute injury or illness. Because of this complexity, the EMS agency should receive ongoing input from experts in all aspects of field care.

Medical Advisory Committee

The forum for medical and technical input in most systems is a medical advisory committee (MAC). The EMS system medical director usually serves as chairman of the committee. Members may include the base hospital medical directors, base hospital coordinators, medical directors of provider agencies, other physicians with specific areas of expertise, EMS educators, and representatives from the EMS agency.

In addition, the EMS medical director should consider including field practitioners as members of the MAC. Prehospital providers have extensive knowledge of field operations such as the emergency vehicle and its equipment, extrication methods and times, traffic problems, prehospital conditions, and capabilities and availability of fire and other public safety personnel. They can determine the feasibility of performing specific procedures or using specific equipment during extrication, scene care, or transport of patients. Although it behooves the EMS staff and physicians to experience and understand field care, the presence of field personnel on the MAC allows on-the-spot "field testing" of protocols and policies. Open exchange of information is educational not only for medical control personnel but also for the providers. Field and medical advisory personnel are often unaware of the financial implications of their recommended changes in field practices. Although medical care should not be totally governed by monetary considerations, cost-benefit analyses are involved in governmental decisions. Similarly, administrative and field personnel are not always cognizant of the most recent medical developments. Presentation, explanation, and discussion of operational, financial, and medical issues at the MAC clarifies for the field personnel the rationale behind the ultimate design of policies and protocols, which they in turn can relay to fellow practitioners.

The exact format of provider representation should be well-delineated in the description or bylaws of the MAC. Decisions to be made include the number of provider members, whether all provider agencies and all levels of providers should be represented, whether members should be practicing field personnel or supervisory personnel, whether there should be representatives from both union and nonunion providers, and whether providers should be voting or nonvoting members. The answers to and the relative significance of these decisions depend on the structure of the specific EMS system. Because one of the goals is to share information with, impart knowledge to, and promote a sense of involvement among the field providers, designating committee positions to them should be a high priority.

Several of the San Francisco Bay area EMS systems include providers in their MACs. Field and supervisory personnel are represented. Contributions from these members have included consensus reports from the paramedic associations, presentations of EMS literature reviews, and membership on subcommittees that develop protocols. For instance, a subcommittee of the Alameda County MAC, which includes two paramedics, recently suggested revisions of all the prehospital treatment protocols in accordance with the current American Heart Association standards and recent prehospital research. The paramedics' operational expertise and field experience enhanced the practicality of the protocols. The often lively interchange among physicians, nurses, and paramedics promoted understanding and acceptance of the final product.

Special EMS Advisory Committees

Frequently, *ad hoc* committees are created by the EMS medical director to address specific issues or design new programs. Developing relevant protocols and policies is the goal of such committees. An example of provider participation in this process is the San Francisco Emergency Medical Dispatch Committee. This committee was established to totally revise and update the dispatch system, develop a curriculum for a new dispatch training course, and design and enact an effective dispatch quality management (QM) program. The committee members included the EMS and prehospital provider agency medical director, a representative from the EMS agency, the supervisor of the dispatch division, and two field paramedics—one with extensive computer expertise and one with extensive dispatch experience (in San Francisco, dispatchers are paramedics). The committee developed a dispatch survey and sent it to 15 cities with similar population and ambulance response structures. Additionally, information from current dispatchers regarding job satisfaction, suggestions for changes in dispatch, and the actual dispatch method they used was obtained. Simultaneously the medical director for the paramedics reviewed problem dispatches and conducted an informal study of random calls that were initially dispatched at Code 2 (moderate mode) yet were ultimately transferred to hospitals as Code 3 (lights-and-siren mode).

After obtaining the data, the committee chose an appropriate dispatch protocol structure and developed specific dispatch guidelines and protocols. Although there was resistance to the new system, the presence of paramedics on the dispatch committee not only made the protocols more "field worthy" but also increased the acceptance of the protocols by dispatchers, because they respected the paramedic members of the committee and listened to their explanation of the rationale and necessity for change. Again the direct interaction between paramedics and physicians has fine-tuned the final product and made the authoritative flavor of the changes more palatable.

To prevent delays in the advancement of an EMS system, the EMS physician must carefully select the prehospital providers who participate on advisory committees. This is exemplified by the experience many systems had with the implementation of EMT defibrillation and fire department First Responders.

For example, in the early 1980s an EMS systems planning group was developed in New York City to determine the optimal EMS structure and to logically integrate the fire department, volunteers, and private providers into the system. Implementation of a proposed fire department First Responder program met with heavy resistance by the EMS providers because of concerns regarding infringement on the future of their practice. EMS providers recommended significantly decreasing ambulance response times rather than adding First Responders, even though other members of the committee, the EMS literature, and the financial considerations supported the concept of fire department First Responders. During the selection of prehospital provider representatives, consideration should be given to ensuring that the chosen representatives place medical concerns above personal and political agendas, that they are up-to-date on the current literature in their area of expertise, and that their recommendations or votes express a consensus opinion of the group or union they represent. Although these criteria are appropriate for all committee members, the EMS medical director must be particularly conscious of them when appointing prehospital providers because this is a relatively new and experimental practice in most parts of the country.

Supervision and Administration

As EMS systems become increasingly complex, the ability of the EMS medical director and EMS agency to make expeditious and informed decisions may be enhanced by direct and ongoing input from prehospital providers. In many EMS systems such input is provided solely by nurses, physicians, and administrators employed by the EMS agency, the hospitals, or the ambulance providers. Placing specially trained prehospital providers in a role directly reporting to the decision-making individual or body provides an additional and valuable perspective. Examples of these specific roles are described.

Paramedic Prehospital Care Coordinator

In California, EMS agencies are usually staffed by prehospital care coordinators (PCCs). Paramedics have been hired as PCCs; they add an additional dimension to the role of prehospital providers. PCCs can be a valuable resource to the EMS medical director because of their field experience and understanding of what it is really like to work in the EMS system at the street level. With such a PCC on the staff, medical directors can more objectively receive input from provider agencies and other field practitioners regarding system development and change.

The transition from field practitioner to EMS agency PCC can be a difficult one; not all prehospital providers have the special skills and educational background to fill such positions. These persons must have the confidence of their fellow practitioners, the skill to communicate effectively with all EMS system members, and preferably formal management training.

In addition, the role of the PCC in EMS QM cannot be overlooked. In Alameda County, California, the paramedic PCC is the "triage officer" for all the written unusual occurrence reports (that is, problem calls or incident reports) received by the EMS agency. The paramedic PCC's ability to understand the issues and determine which merit further investigation is key to retrospective review of the hundreds of such reports received by the EMS agency annually.

Field Evaluator

Field evaluators (FEs) are prehospital personnel recognized for their clinical and interpersonal skills. They perform concurrent evaluation of field personnel to provide requested specific performance information to the EMS medical director or other system medical directors.

Examples of several successful FEs exist. In the Seattle Fire Department paramedic program, senior paramedics ride-along with junior paramedics on a regular basis to evaluate field performance. Pons et al described a field instructor program to evaluate and guide newly hired personnel and provide refresher instruction to long-term employees requesting or displaying need for an updated performance evaluation.[7]

In Alameda County, California, FEs ride with newly certified paramedics during their first 6 months in the EMS system. Using established criteria, they evaluate new paramedics on all aspects of prehospital care. In addition, the FEs clarify policy questions and emphasize the "system" way of treating patients, conducting radio calls and completing prehospital care reports (PCRs). FEs may also ride-along with paramedics who are undergoing remediation programs. For the EMS agency the FE can function as a representative of the medical director. For the prehospital provider agency the FE can provide an unbiased viewpoint regarding the ability of the paramedic in question.

These positions may be filled by paramedics employed by the EMS agency or ambulance provider; there are advantages and disadvantages to both options. If FEs are employed by the EMS agency, they are more likely to be objective in the evaluation of the field practitioner. On the other hand, FEs employed by the ambulance provider have a vested interest in ensuring that the employee performs at a level sufficient for the ambulance provider to maintain quality performance. Clearly the FE must be a field provider with exceptional skills and knowledge of EMS policies and protocols. FEs can also train other individuals in new procedures and policies and participate in pilot studies or research projects.

Clinical Field Supervisor

In contrast to the FEs who may not perform clinical duties during the performance of their role, clinical field supervisors (CFSs) provide hands-on medical supervision and education, as well as performance evaluation at the scene. San Francisco's Department of Health Paramedic Division recently developed a formalized clinical field supervisor program that enables specially trained and experienced paramedics to provide on-scene clinical guidance and assessment of all paramedic providers on a regular basis and to perform advanced or complicated procedures. Alameda County's private paramedic provider service is beginning a clinical "mentor" program for similar purposes. Common to these programs is the selection of senior paramedics who have been recognized for both their outstanding clinical and interpersonal skills.

Quality Management

The successful functioning of an EMS system depends on the effectiveness of its QM program. A QM system consists of the following four basic components: (1) structure—protocols, policies, standards of care, and scope of practice, (2) process—monitoring of actual care delivered, (3) outcome—measurement of the efficacy of care delivered, and (4) feedback—alterations in structure based on analysis of outcome.

Essentially a QM system evaluates the performance of the system's structure and personnel. This is accomplished by prospective, concurrent, and retrospective audits. Results of these audits are analyzed and produce revision of structure. This revision can take many forms including changes in policies or protocols, development of new programs (for example, EMT defibrillation), revision of system design, and provision of educational programs that increase adherence to or understanding of protocols and policies.

Currently, participation in QM by physicians, mobile intensive care nurses (MICNs), and administrators is common. EMS agencies monitor overall system performance, set standards for prehospital personnel certification, develop system policies and protocols, and coordinate the investigation of unusual occurrences. Direct medical control and provider agency medical directors audit radio calls and PCRs and participate in ride-alongs. Base physicians and MICNs provide direct medical control. Outcome data from these sources is collated and analyzed by the EMS agency. It is then the responsibility of the EMS medical director to determine the necessity for and character of system revisions. In many EMS systems a QM committee (either a separate entity or part of the MAC or trauma audit committees) advises the medical director regarding QM issues. Prehospital providers are often not members of such committees nor do they participate in many of the previously cited QM activities.

Field personnel are interested in participating in QM because it significantly affects the quality and security of their vocation. This is a reasonable concern, especially if field practitioners view their chosen employment as a profession. Members of a profession determine and guide the evolutionary process, scope, standards of practice, and qualifications of members of the profession. An additional characteristic of professionals is a high level of commitment to performance excellence. Emergency medical technicians-ambulance (EMT-As) have traditionally been viewed and are referred to as technicians. Yet many prehospital providers participate in associations and unions that focus not only on job quality and benefits but also on enhancing quality of patient care. The future viability of field practitioners as professionals depends on their ability to participate in meaningful activities. Because "professionalization" of field personnel will ultimately lead to increased provider interest in the delivery of high quality care, EMS physicians should promote this trend.

Including field personnel in EMS QM activities may increase their satisfaction and cooperation with the QM process and provide a more balanced QM perspective to all system members. Field providers often relate that the QM system exists solely to monitor and critique their performance. Their dissatisfaction with QM processes stem from seeming inconsistencies of disciplinary actions and the lack of concurrence between their assessments of individual performance and the results of QM analyses. Because the system appears personally assaultive, field personnel respond defensively to QM activities. Additionally, many providers feel that they are more capable of identifying suboptimal colleagues than are medical control personnel. Hence they engage in QM not only to protect themselves from inaccurate or unfair QM assessment but also to improve policing of their profession.

Although some of these perceptions are valid, this is a narrow view. Focusing on the "witch hunt" QM mentality can ultimately be destructive to the system. Unrestrained incident investigations, audits, and interviews threaten both practitioner and patient confidentiality and promote antagonism among field providers and other system participants. It is important to clarify for all members of the system that the goal of a comprehensive QM program is to evaluate the system in its entirety and provide a format for overall system improvement. This occurs by monitoring each part of the system, as well as assessing how the parts interrelate and how the prehospital medical care system interfaces with other portions of the patient care process. Of course, if analysis indicates that an individual practitioner's performance is repeatedly associated with poor patient outcome, specific retraining and if that fails discipline or dismissal may be necessary. Clearly, emphasizing to the providers that the QM system is an educational tool and a mechanism for attaining systemwide excellence enhances its efficacy and acceptance. Encouraging participation in the QM process by representatives of all system members promotes this goal. Additionally the QM process should be well-described, formal, confidential, and provide positive and negative feedback so it is not perceived as arbitrary and punitive.

Activities

Once the concept of field practitioner participation in QM is accepted, an appropriate forum must be selected. Formal involvement with well-delineated roles allows opportunity for provider participation yet maintains sufficient medical control.

For better or worse, retrospective review of prehospital care is the focus of most EMS QM activity. Retrospective activities consist of audits of prehospital provider records and base hospital written reports and tapes, investigation of unusual occurrences, statistical review of system data, and trend analysis. Until recently, few EMS systems allowed field provider participation in these processes. In California, physicians and nurses for the EMS agency, base hospital, and ambulance provider are not only responsible for supervising such activities but also for performing them. Support for involving field personnel is growing. Field personnel are increasingly represented in the prehospital literature and specifically are participating as data abstractors and evaluators. In a descriptive study by Swor et al, paramedics performed reviews of prehospital records and assisted in the development of performance criteria for the review.[11]

Many provider agencies are adding field personnel to their QM departments because such expertise is valuable for on-scene evaluation and MAC's or special advisory committees. Retrospective review has many limitations including reliance on the completeness and accuracy of documentation. Prehospital providers are often more attuned than medical control personnel to the significance and validity of information documented on PCRs and tapes. They may be better able to "read between the lines" and determine if a particular procedure, scene time, or extrication time was reasonable and whether the field provider understood the clinical situation and used protocols appropriately. Investigation of unusual occurrences requires review of relevant PCRs, tapes, and interviews with the involved field personnel. The first step in many investigations is development by the EMS service of an incident report based on these sources. Field personnel assigned to QM or risk management departments may provide assistance ascertaining the actual chain of events by providing a "reality check" and decreasing the defensiveness of the involved field personnel. Their practical experience and understanding of field conditions are respected by other prehospital providers; hence the efficacy of interviews and counseling if indicated is enhanced.

Advisory Committees

Membership on formal EMS QM advisory committees offers additional opportunities for prehospital providers to participate in QM activities. As mentioned earlier, field personnel are often not included on such committees. This trend is changing. In the Bay area, EMS committees that focus on QM include paramedic peer review committee (PPRC), trauma audit committee (TAC), and the quality management committee (QMC). The issues pertaining to the appointment of field providers to these committees and the delineation of the provider role on these committees are discussed in the following sections.

Quality management committee. In many EMS systems, this committee serves as an advisory committee to the medical director on general issues concerning quality of prehospital care. The committee assists with the development of a systemwide program for monitoring prehospital care, identifying and investigating system problems and assigning responsibility for problem-solving. The focus of the committee is trend analysis of performance and formulation of appropriate system revisions rather than inspection and discussion of individual performance. Occasionally, specific cases provide the impetus for further analysis. Hence the QMC membership is restricted, and members must sign a statement of confidentiality. Field providers are interested in participating on this committee to relay their consensus opinions, have input into the development of the QM insight into the activities and goals of the QMC. The need for confidentiality regarding committee discussions and decisions could interfere with the latter goal. To enhance mutual trust among physicians, medical directors, and providers, these issues must be discussed openly and clarified.

Trauma audit committee. Many EMS systems have developed or are developing committees specifically designed to perform trauma system QM. San Diego and Alameda County, California, have well-delineated committee processes. In Alameda County, paramedics participate on subcommittees of the main TAC that perform the initial review of trauma care given individual patients. Field providers specifically examine field care reports for extended scene or transport times. Their input is invaluable in analyzing quality of care from moment of injury to definitive treatment.

Peer review. Development of peer review in the Bay area has been more difficult because of controversy over the format, function, and scope of the process. Prehospital providers envision the peer review structure as a liaison between indirect medical control and the individual field practitioner. Many are less interested in engaging in QM activities that identify performance trends (chart and tape audits, and ride-alongs) than in performing career-development activities that would increase their experience with assessment and review of prehospital care, giving them an opportunity to advise and counsel other field practitioners. This latter activity is pivotal to the prehospital provider's concept of peer review—involvement with the investigation of unusual occurrences. For example, if paramedics have a seemingly unfair report filed against them, counsel from the peer review group could be obtained. The group would investigate the incident, develop a consensus opinion, and submit its conclusions and recommendations to the EMS medical director before the institution of any official action. From the perspective of medical directors in states where the paramedic is a physician extender or literally uses the physician's license, this suggestion may sound too democratic.

The medical director and other indirect medical control personnel consider peer review to be too limited; it focuses exclusively on the punitive aspects of QM rather than on a systemwide approach to quality care and risk management. Indeed, it is useful to obtain field practitioner input when controversial incidents involving individual providers occur; however, conducting an investigation that could ultimately threaten a provider's occupational future exposes the investigators, the EMS agency, and the medical director to legal risks. Therefore in most systems a formal review board is the forum for such considerations. Positions for providers exist on such boards; placing field practitioners in these positions (perhaps as representatives from a peer review committee) would be a useful compromise.

The key to establishing a successful peer review committee is direct interaction and integration with the overall system QM program. An idealized EMS peer review system is described as follows. Prehospital providers participate in all aspects of the QM process. They conduct chart and tape audits and perform ride-along peer evaluations. Projects are initiated at the recommendation of the EMS medical director with input from the members of the peer review committee. Members assist with data collection and research. Although some of these activities result in the identification of problem paramedics, they also address the more constructive QM goals of delineation of performance trends, improvements in policies and procedures, and identification of educational and training needs.

Prehospital provider involvement should occur at all levels of the QM process and should be closely supervised by a medical control physician. Results of these activities should proceed through normal channels. Confidentiality of all material must be maintained to protect the legal and personal rights of reviewed field practitioners and their patients. The goal of field practitioner involvement is to provide significant and acknowledged input so dissatisfaction with and perceived deficiencies of the system are identified and remedied before problems develop.

Summary

Prehospital provider participation in EMS system management is feasible and desirable, especially in the areas of policy and protocol development and QM. This chapter describes the processes that a system must implement to integrate field personnel into the authority structure. The issues are universal and often controversial, particularly in large urban areas where providers are typically unionized, vocal, and more experienced. If the structure is carefully planned, the outcome is rewarding. The quality of the system and the atmosphere of interactions in the system will improve. Hence the common goal of delivery of high quality medical care becomes more attainable.

REFERENCES

1. *Alameda County EMS Policy Manual,* 1991, Alameda County Health Care Services Agency.
2. Holroyd BR, Knopp R, and Kallsen G: Medical control: quality assurance in prehospital care, *JAMA* Aug 22-29 1986.
3. Kresky B, and Henry MC: Responsibilities for quality assurance in prehospital care, *QRB* 231-235, Jul 1986.
4. Luterman A et al: Evaluation of prehospital emergency medical service (EMS): defining areas for improvement, *J Trauma* 702-707, 1983.
5. Maio RF and Burney RE: Improving reliability of abstracted prehospital care data: use of decision rules, *Prehospital and Disaster Medicine* 15-20, Jan-Mar 1991.
6. Pointer JE: The advanced life support base hospital audit for medical control in an emergency medical services system, *Ann Emerg Med* 557-560, May 1987.
7. Pons PT et al: The field instructor program: quality control of prehospital care, the first step, *J Emerg* 421-427, 1985.
8. Stewart RD et al: A computer-assisted quality assurance system for an emergency medical service, *Ann Emerg Med* 25-29, Jan 1985.
9. Stout J: Organizing quality control in EMS, *JEMS* 67-74, Mar 1988.
10. Swor RA and Hoelzer MH: A computer-assisted quality assurance audit in a multi-provider EMS system, *Ann Emerg Med* 19:286-290, 1990.
11. Swor RA, Bocka JJ, and Maio RF: A paramedic peer-review quality assurance audit, *Prehospital and Disaster Medicine* 321-326, Jul-Sep 1991.

29

Nurses

Beth Lothrop Adams, M.A., R.N., EMT-P
Major Peggy Trimble, M.A., B.S.N.

History

Every history of prehospital care credits Pantridge with the mobilization of coronary care.[10] Perhaps he should also be credited with moving nurses into some EMS services initially staffed by interns and nurses. Soon after mobile coronary care began, came the National Academy of Sciences and National Research Council report on trauma deaths. The military experience in Vietnam provided trained trauma experts in the form of recently discharged military medical personnel.[10] When the newly developed Department of Transportation (DOT) training standards for paramedics blended coronary and trauma care, nurses bridged the gap for these experienced trauma care technicians by assisting the EMS physician with the necessary training. Since that time, nurses have been instrumental in the initial and ongoing education of prehospital providers.

The administrative demands of system development and implementation often exceeded any one person's abilities. Soon, nurses with their broad-based education and team leadership skills were augmenting the EMS physician in this area as well. In those early days, there was no abundance of educated, experienced field personnel to assist the burdened medical director with program and system development. Boyd in Illinois and Cowley in Maryland relied heavily on nurses to build their state EMS systems.[2] Trauma nurse coordinates and nurses in EMS system administration were implemented in these states. These nurses participated in designing systems, developing applications, formulating designation criteria for trauma centers, and educating other providers.

Overview

Today, in many parts of the country, nurses work closely with physicians, government agencies, and field personnel to establish and maintain EMS systems. As EMS continues to evolve and mature, it is appropriate to develop EMS systems that maximally use the capabilities of all team members. As members of the team, nurses contribute skills such as (1) communicating with and coordinating the efforts of many disciplines to address patient or system issues, (2) applying organizational skills for the management of multiple endeavors at a variety of levels (for example, patient or family, interdepartmental, interagency, interhospital), and (3) focusing on the well-being of the patient or family as the goal of EMS. These skills are foremost goals of professional nurses' education and experience bases.

The maturing EMS system should examine potential contributions from nurses for three reasons. First, an EMS system includes responsibilities ranging from prevention through rehabilitation. When seen as a system that includes multiple high-risk populations (trauma, burns, cardiac, high-risk maternal and neonatal, behavioral, and poisoning), the value of a professional nurse as a member becomes clear.[3] Much of the work of EMS is well-matched to the skills of the nurse. Professional education and guided experiences acquired during many nurses' careers have even developed some EMS areas of concentration into specialties. For example, patient and family teaching principles readily adapt to community efforts in prevention, fund-raising, system access and awareness, legislation, lobbying, and staff work for special projects.

In addition to the skill match of professional nurses to EMS needs, nurses are often the largest provider group in an EMS system. Professional nursing organizations such as the American Association of Critical Care Nurses (AACN), the Emergency Nursing Association (ENA), and the Society of Trauma Nurses (STN) can be valuable allies when EMS efforts are underway locally or nationally (see box below). Often, nurses access many networks by collaborating with professional organizations and interacting in the patient care delivery system of many health care agencies. This enhances the value of nurses as members of the EMS management structure because these networks and organizations are natural vehicles for communication. They provide a process for EMS systems to address such work as the collection of data, special projects, quality management, protocol and policy dissemination, and problem-solving. A nurse-to-nurse process often works best here. Even when the process calls for a non-nurse lead, the partnership with nursing adds a dimension in patient and professional sensitivity possibly not present otherwise.

As a third consideration of nurse leaders in EMS, the phase of the EMS system beginning when the patient reaches the hospital and phases that follow need to be included and addressed by the EMS system. To date, the in-hospital phase has lagged behind the prehospital phase in system development and formalization. Overcrowding, reimbursement, and societal issues continue to challenge systems in their efforts to ensure not only that the high-risk patient *gets* to the right place at the right time but that the hospital and staff there will be *able* to care for the patient in spite of other competing and confounding demands. The in-hospital and post-acute care settings are familiar territory for nurses. Additional progress in *system* management could occur when nurses address issues of resource allocation, organization of care environment, and critical communication linkages.

Nursing Associations with Interest in EMS

American Association of Critical Care Nurses
American College of Nurse Midwives
American Practitioners for Infection Control
Association of Rehabilitation Nurses
Association of Operating Room Nurses
Emergency Nurses Association
Organization of Nurse Executives
Nurses Association of the American College of Obstetrics and Gynecology
Society of Post Anesthesia Nurses
Society of Trauma Nurses
National Association of Orthopedic Nurses

In an EMS system, however, the role of nurses depends on several variables including (1) state or local laws, (2) the EMS director, (3) the type of EMS agency or system, and (4) economics, especially supply and demand.[4] To address legal aspects first, existing state and local laws govern the scope of practice for registered nurses (RNs) in all states. To date, no states have laws that allow the independent licensure of field personnel. In contrast, RNs are independently licensed and legally must function according to the Nurse Practice Law in their states. As one example of legally integrating the traditional nurse-physician relationship into prehospital EMS, some system medical directors have delegated the responsibility for direct (online) medical control to nurses within a framework of indirect medical control protocols.[5] This is not a great departure from the advanced role coronary care nurses have accepted in managing Advanced Care Life Support (ACLS) situations using medical protocols in an in-hospital setting. In some systems, failure to implement this nursing role would significantly limit the availability and delivery of prehospital care.

The second variable influencing the role of the nurse in EMS is the EMS director; the director establishes and promotes the vision for a system. Whether this vision includes an interdependent, multidisciplinary team directly determines the inclusion or exclusion of the nurse in a recognized, legitimized role. Often the experience of the director influences the selection of vision and paradigms supported. Some directors have experienced collaborative practice with professional nurses and value the enhanced delivery of care because of such first-hand knowledge. For others, this model represents a departure from strongly held beliefs, an element of risk-taking, and perceived loss of control. The inclusion of this chapter in this book is for visionary risk-takers who recognize the potential for system enhancements that professional nurses offer.

The successful EMS medical director must be intimately and actively involved in all aspects of the system from administration and education to standard setting, quality assurance, and research. Yet no one person can or should provide all that a system may need. Collaborative, collegial relationships with EMS nurses have strengthened systems by enabling directors to maximize time and efforts. For example, verifying that education requirements for entry and recertification as EMS care providers are met can be a Herculean task and as such may necessitate delegation to a non-physician training coordinator if the EMS medical director is to fulfill any other obligations and responsibilities.

As a third variable, the type of EMS agency or system affects the extent of nurses' participation and involvement. Systems with medevac often use nurses in partnership with other patient care experts as caregivers on the flight team. Although it seems that a hospital-based prehospital service is more likely to employ nurses in a variety of roles, Houston and Seattle (both fire-based systems) use nurses in prehospital response. The Houston system created the role of prehospital nurse clinician, which serves as a model for other systems.[5]

Lastly, although it might be a matter of medical preference to use physicians and experienced paramedics to fill all roles and functions within an EMS system, economic pressures, availability of qualified practitioners, and especially standards of care in many parts of the country necessitate sharing the responsibility with nurses or other non-physicians. As examples, the burden of delivering prehospital emergency care in rural America often cannot be born by a limited number of available physicians and field personnel.

Education and Training

As a means of assessing the extent of involvement of nurses in EMS, a survey was sent to nurse participants at the NAEMSP Annual Conference (Houston, June 1990), graduates of the Pediatric EMS Training Program (Children's Hospital National Medical Center, Washington, D.C., 1986-1987), nurse participants at the Emergency Cardiac Care Conference (Albuquerque, April 1990), the nurses who attended the Critical Incident Stress Conference (Brainerd, Minnesota, June 1990). For the purpose of the survey, EMS involvement was broadly categorized into the following five areas: education-training, quality assurance, administration, clinical, and support staff. A total of 150 surveys were distributed nationwide. Forty surveys were completed and returned (27%), representing 25 states and including 32 nurses (80%). Twenty-one of the nurse respondents are currently certified EMS providers (66%); 11 are certified paramedics (34%).[1] The extent of EMS involvement by these nurses is displayed in Figure 29-1.

Ninety-one percent of the respondents are involved in the education and training of First Responders, emergency medical technicians (EMT-As), and paramedics. These activities include initial course work, in-service and refresher programs, and continuing education and specialized training (for example, ACLS, Basic Trauma Life Support (BTLS), Pediatric Advanced Life Support (PALS), or extrication and rescue).[1]

When prehospital certification is not required, many nurses and others find that such training and certification facilitates their acceptance and ability to relate to others in prehospital care. Taking into account state or local statutes, the required EMS training should depend on the role to be filled and the EMS director's preference. Certainly, if the individual is to function as a prehospital provider of emergency medical care, competence must be equivalent to that of peers.

Broad-based nursing education provides a sound framework of knowledge that along with the appropriate clinical experience and certain personal attributes equips the nurse for a role in EMS education throughout the continuum. In addition to required nursing process and skill courses, nurses complete course work in anatomy and physiology, cardiology, medicolegal aspects, microbiology,

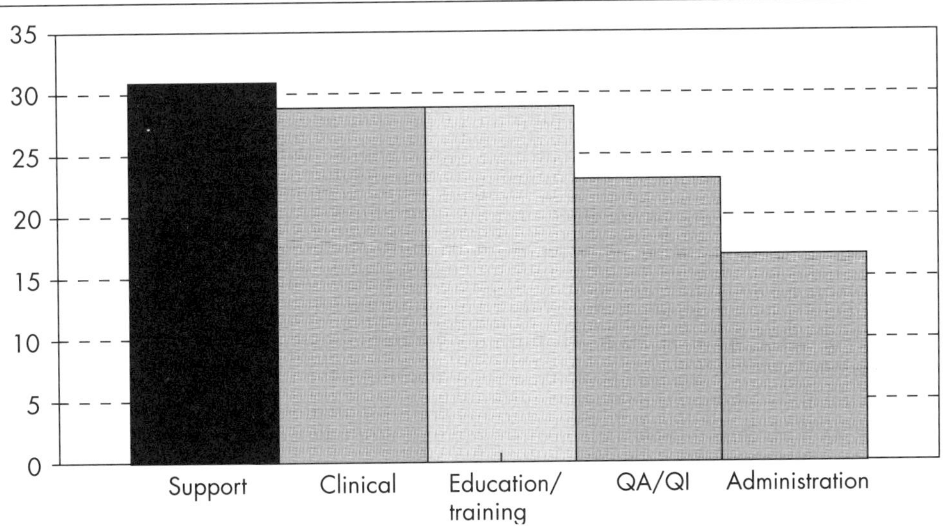

Figure 29-1. EMS roles of nurses, 1990 survey results.

obstetrics, pathophysiology, pediatrics, pharmacology, and psychology. Although all of this course work may not translate directly to the delivery of prehospital care, the depth of knowledge such a background provides is very beneficial in training.

It is not sufficient to merely know as much about a given topic as one's student. To teach successfully, one needs a broader depth of knowledge, as well as the ability to convey complex medical concepts in an easily understood manner. For nurses this capability often results from formal training and experience in providing education to patients and families in a clinical environment. Hence the experienced nurse is often an experienced educator upon entering EMS. These teaching skills can be applied at many points along the continuum. Prevention initiatives in the community, fund-raising addresses to contributors, interagency continuing education, and multidisciplinary training programs are only a few examples.

In the prehospital arena the global patient perspective, which is the essence of nursing, is a valuable adjunct for the education of prehospital personnel. Physician educators often focus on history, diagnostics, and disease; paramedics tend to be more task-oriented. This can limit one's ability to adapt when patient complaints or physical findings fall outside defined parameters. Patient management problems often have psychosocial aspects or fall under the "interpersonal relationship" category. Again, these processes responses are extensively addressed by nurses who impart their skills to other EMS providers. Nurses are well-prepared to blend the two perspectives—the priorities of the "golden hour" and the patient's overall status and chief complaints that extend beyond it.

As the spectrum of technical skills required of prehospital personnel continues to expand, initiation of therapeutic modalities in the field necessitates a working knowledge of infusion pumps, oximeters, and other monitoring devices, as well as the ability to calculate dosages and prepare drugs for infusion. Experienced nurses are a valuable resource for training others in the set-up, maintenance, and troubleshooting of such equipment, and they can relate the patient responses to the technology in training programs. This allows for application rather than the "cookbook" approach.

Clinical experience is an essential component in the training of all levels of prehospital personnel. For instance, the DOT curriculum standards require a minimum of 10 hours of in-hospital patient care experience for EMT-As and a minimum of 232 hours for paramedics.[11,12] It is advantageous to have a nurse who is familiar with EMS facilitate, coordinate, and ideally supervise student clinical experience. Often, nurses design clinical training activities that maximize student experiences most likely to result in skill mastery needed for care in the field. Nurses easily interact with the various departments and facilitate student adjustment in the hospital environment, having worked within that milieu themselves. Acceptance by hospital staff is most frequently negotiated on a nurse-to-nurse basis as is the approval and implementation of the clinical programs.

For EMS patient populations that do not originate at the roadside or in similar prehospital environments but rather enter EMS at the interhospital level, the interhospital link is paramount. Nurses are often key policy or protocol supporters, educating and coaching staff. Packaging the patient for transport and transmitting vital information usually is performed by the community hospital nurse. An EMS system that attends to the education outreach for these nurses will see an impact on care and transfer compliance.

Nurses in many systems have become experts at specific clinical aspects of EMS. Trauma registries, high-risk neonatal transport, infectious disease management, and patient support groups are examples. These nurses are the best educators for sharing their expertise regardless of the learner population. As EMS challenges continue and systems evolve, resources should be identified and applied appropriately. Enlisting the educational support of nurses from organizations such as the Association of Practitioners for Infection Control (APIC) to educate prehospital providers about principles of self and patient infectious disease protection, cleaning of equipment, and regulation compliance are examples of nurse partnership in EMS that reduce cost, improve patient care, and increase provider competency through education and training.

Quality Management

In the questionnaire mentioned previously, 75% of the respondents are involved in quality assurance activities such as developing standards of care and concurrent and retrospective monitoring to ensure compliance with system standards.[1] Realizing that quality management (QM) is the *sine qua non* of the present and future of any EMS system, it is imperative that the EMS medical director have a pivotal role in all aspects of QM. In most systems, almost all prehospital care is rendered under the medical director's license. Even for aspects of the system that are not delegated medical tasks, QM remains the framework for assessing areas for improvement and ensuring that the system is attaining the goals that the public entrusted it to meet. Once standards are established, it seems unrealistic and imprudent use of physician resources for the medical director to perform the routine, day-to-day monitoring activities. This is particularly true in large systems in which such an undertaking would be a great burden or those in which the EMS medical director role is an additional duty for a practitioner. The logical conclusion is to delegate such monitoring to nurses or other non-physicians. Collectively, nurses are known for their attention to detail and as such are well-suited for QM monitoring activities if they are knowledgeable of the existing EMS standards. Because the scope of nursing practice differs from that of prehospital care, it is beneficial if not essential that the nurse have EMS training and ideally field experience, if they are to be perceived as credible auditors of prehospital care by field personnel.

Many EMS systems have capitalized on the willingness of nurses to cross agency and geographic barriers to address patient care issues. If a nurse is at the EMS system QM level, the identification and facilitation of these opportunities for improvement are more readily evident. Conceptually and in implementation, the QM aspect of system EMS is rudimentary at most. It is an excellent match of work to nurse talents. Including nurses may add significant momentum to further develop this important but difficult aspect of EMS.

Administration

The role of management is to enable the workers to do their job. Although this demands that an administrator know and respect the job to be done, it does not require that they have done the job. The qualities that enable nurses to be successful contributing members of the EMS community as educators or QM coordinators also stand them in good stead as administrators. Communication and organizational skills, the nurse's work experience in a professional environment, and the resultant understanding of legal issues and regulatory agencies are valuable assets for any administrator.

Again referring to the survey conducted, 55% of the respondents (Fig. 29-1) fill administrative positions. The majority of these are managers or supervisors. Other positions include training division coordinators, regional or state EMS coordinators, and assistant or advisor to the medical director. Only 10% serve as field supervisors.[1] Although the domain of the EMS agency may limit the potential for nurses to move into administrative positions (particularly in a fire-based system), other systems have vast potential for including nurses in administration.[5]

In Maryland, for example, nurse administrators manage the high-risk neonatal and high-risk maternal programs. They are responsible for budget, protocols, and QM. In many states, nurses administer EMS-related grants. Most EMS trauma systems include trauma nurse coordinators in the management staff. The box on p. 312 provides an inventory of trauma nurse coordinators' responsibilities. Research projects are another example of nurse management skills put to good use because this concept is another part of the profession's fundamental education.

Patient Care

Currently, controversy exists regarding the legal and professional practice requirements for nurses delivering care in the prehospital environment. The National Association of Emergency Medical Technicians (NAEMT) position maintains that nurses practicing in the prehospital setting are certified as EMTs only after completing the appropriate DOT standard curriculum.[6] The ENA is developing a modified curriculum that combines the emergency nursing focus with the DOT paramedic curriculum. The modified curriculum intends to establish a core curriculum for prehospital nursing practice.[8] Various state boards of nursing are researching the issue also.

Nursing education makes it possible to readily grasp the scope and content of paramedic course work, but it does not prepare students for all the necessary technical skills or the reality of delivering patient care outside of a controlled hospital environment. On the other hand, requiring nurses to duplicate components of their education creates barriers to entry in areas where additional advanced life support personnel in prehospital care are needed. Additionally the regulation of nursing practice by entities other than state boards of nursing violates the regulations of some states.

The prehospital patient care environment of an ideal EMS system incorporates the physician-extender role of the paramedic and acknowledges that high quality patient care depends on a collaborative, interdependent effort and mutual respect among caregivers. This model does not dilute the medical director's authority; it supports it. Prehospital care personnel interact daily with physicians; they also interact with nurses on a daily basis in extended care facilities, clinics, and emergency departments. In a mature EMS system, these prehospital caregivers benefit from exposure to the comprehensive patient perspective of nurses, the scientific perspective of physicians, and the technical expertise that experienced EMT-As and paramedics provide. In this model a team concept is the essential basis for effective patient care.

Trauma Nurse Coordinator Role Functions

Research	Clinical Practice	Education	Consultation	Administration
Data collection	Clinical rounds	Inservice New equipment New protocols Orientation to team roles	Develops protocols	Implementation of protocols and standards
Trauma registry	Patient care follow-up	Continuing education Trauma nursing course ATLS ACLS	Liaison with community EMS council	Change agent
Identifies and monitors specific investigations with the trauma population	Applies primary and secondary assessment and interventions based on ATLS guidelines for trauma resuscitation	Outreach Prehospital Nursing Public	Liaison with prehospital care providers	Preparation of trauma program reports
Initiates nursing research for trauma	Formulation or supervision of written care plans for trauma patients	Role model for other trauma nurses through demonstration	Participation in planning and ongoing management of multidisciplinary programs	Preparation and management of trauma or trauma program budget
Interprets and communicates recent nursing innovations and research findings	Integration of team approach to trauma	Trauma patient care conferences	Consults with discharge planners Rehabilitation programs Special support services Home care Medical staff	Staff for trauma management committee
Translates relevant scientific knowledge into trauma nursing practice	Monitors nursing care of patient through the trauma care continuum			Monitors effectiveness of trauma program through QM activities
Experiments with new patient care modalities and practice models	Patient advocate within trauma system			Initiates corrective action measures for problems identified in trauma programs
	Gives feedback to nursing staff of referring hospitals			Marketing trauma programs
				Legislative activities

From Beachley M, Snow S, and Trimble P: Developing trauma care systems: the trauma nurse coordinator *J Nurs Adm* 18(7,8):34, 1988.

In the clinical section of the survey, 91% of the respondents had clinical responsibilities for prehospital EMS including mobile intensive care nurses (MICNs), flight nurses, field or emergency department preceptors, and ride-alongs (with or without patient care responsibilities).[1] Probably the most evolved nursing clinical role in EMS systems is that of trauma nurse coordinator. Beachley et al discussed this role, which began in some states as long ago as 1971.[2] Although the position is used in many systems today, variations in organizational structure and job descriptions exist (see box below).

Sample Job Description for a Trauma Nurse Coordinator

I. Major Functions—Works closely with the hospital's medical staff, administrators, department heads, and nursing personnel to coordinate all aspects of trauma care; Provides in-service education for the trauma team; Supervises and evaluates overall trauma team performance

II. Duties and Responsibilities
- A. Trauma Program Management and Clinical Responsibilities
  1. Participates in planning, developing, implementing, and evaluating the trauma program
  2. Demonstrates individual accountability for clinical practice and serves as a clinical resource by participating in providing trauma care
  3. Coordinates nursing care aspects of the trauma program with appropriate nurse managers
  4. Establishes, in collaboration with the trauma director, resuscitation protocols setting priorities for care
  5. Reviews plan of care for each trauma patient to ensure that trauma protocols are initiated and followed
  6. Assists staff in problem-solving related to care of trauma patients
- B. Education Responsibilities
  1. Maintains current knowledge of trauma care via literature review, trauma rounds, and trauma conferences
  2. Updates trauma skills performance for all trauma team members
  3. Supervises orientation for all new trauma team members
  4. Participates in hospitalwide trauma education for support ancillary services
  5. Co-chairs the trauma management committee with medical director
  6. Participates with communitywide trauma education programs for both prehospital care providers and general public
- C. Quality Management Responsibilities
  1. Daily review of emergency department log to determine problems with triage
  2. Conducts daily rounds on all trauma patients for concurrent review of care
  3. When feasible, conducts immediate posttrauma resuscitation critiques
  4. Provides follow-up on problems identified during trauma care critiques and documents action taken
  5. Coordinates trauma care rounds or care conferences
  6. Maintains trauma registry, supervises the data collection, analyzes data, prepares reports, and distributes reports to appropriate team members
  7. Conducts nursing audits
  8. Analyzes the trauma care system for efficiency, safety, and effectiveness of standards and protocols established
  9. Participates in multidisciplinary case review
- D. Liaison and Consultant Responsibilities
  1. Develops collaborative relationships with staff in all departments to facilitate cooperation and support for the trauma program
  2. Coordinates ancillary services to ensure a comprehensive multidisciplinary approach to trauma care
  3. Fosters good public relations for the hospital trauma program
  4. Acts as liaison for hospital with community and regional EMS providers

III. Qualifications
- A. Registered nurse with current license in state
- B. Minimum 5 years' experience in nursing program caring for trauma patients
- C. Advanced skills in critical care nursing
- D. Good communication, interpersonal, and analytical skills
- E. Self-directed
- F. Masters in nursing preferred
- G. Flexibility in working hours

From Beachley M, Snow S, and Trimble P: Developing trauma care systems: the trauma nurse coordinator, *J Nurs Adm* 18(7,8):34, 1988.

Unlike the care given by physicians who move throughout the hospital environment with the patient, nursing care is delivered based on unit assignment. These specialty units (for example, operating, recovery, and critical care) should be considered part of the EMS system. The nurse providers in the units need to be adequately connected to the system and prepared to provide the appropriate care for the specialty populations—adults, children, or neonates—in the acute care hospital. The trauma nurse coordinator is the logical choice as the organizational connection for these specialty areas for trauma patients. Other nurse specialists would be logical for nontrauma population.

In at least one setting at the University of California-Davis Medical Center, the trauma nurse practitioner position is being explored in an effort to provide service where workload exceeds available trauma physician staff. This model has been used successfully for many years in the postoperative through rehabilitative phases of care for neurotrauma patients in the Maryland system. Likewise the National Children's Hospital in Washington and The Johns Hopkins Hospital Children's Trauma Center in Baltimore have used nurse specialists to coordinate care from the acute hospital, to rehabilitation, and to home.[9]

The public criticism that EMS and trauma systems save lives but provide inadequate follow-up must be addressed. Existing home health care and rehabilitation services can be recruited into the EMS system continuum just as acute care hospitals and rescue squads were recruited in the earlier days of system development. Where gaps exist, efforts can be focused on filling them with plans developed as part of a system that best serves the patient. For example, specialty follow-up clinics may need to be created. Again, nurses are predominant caregivers and administrators in home health services and rehabilitation agencies. A nurse coordinator or administrator who facilitates communication and bridges patient connections across agencies at the "back door" of the system can improve not only continuity but also outcome of patient care.

For a number of patients and their families, community support groups serve an important role during recovery in re-establishing healthy behaviors. Nurses have been instrumental in establishing these groups for trauma, burn, and cardiac patients and in conducting the programs. Although not the motivating factor for organizing, such groups often take on the role of system supporters. Examples of this are lobbying for services, backing prevention legislation, and educating their own communities.

Support Staff

Ninety-seven percent of the respondents in the 1990 survey fill support staff functions, primarily as staff assistants and designated resource persons. Other support functions include infection control, peer counseling, critical incident stress debriefing (CISD), research and public relations, and participation in advisory groups and disaster planning.[1]

The experienced nurse with a good understanding of the prehospital environment and the EMS system is a valuable resource. Although their specific roles may vary from system to system, depending on the availability of other resources and the agency needs, nurses are often comfortable with an ombudsmanlike role. They are trained to deal with the psychological needs of caregivers and patients, as well as the integration of research and clinical practice. The wide array of support roles filled by nurses attests to the flexibility their education and training give them to address patient care via many different EMS avenues. Their ability as professionals to move throughout agencies and across disciplines is unmatched.

Summary

How should nurses be used in EMS? Responses range from the traditional to the innovative. Certainly, some aspects of EMS are better suited for nursing involvement. Although controversy exists regarding preparation for roles, consensus exists in many areas. Licensure as an RN alone is not sufficient for successful integration of the nurse into EMS just as licensure itself is not qualification for a physician to serve as an EMS medical director. Although the role of nurses in EMS may not be as clearly defined as that of the field provider or medical director, nurses contribute to the delivery of EMS care throughout our country on a daily basis.

If one accepts the premise that "critical care begins in the streets," then it is reasonable that nurses continue to be part of that team along with EMS physicians and other providers.[7] Each member brings a unique perspective and expertise to the delivery of patient care. If EMS systems accept the mission to serve the critically ill and injured based on a continuum of care, nurses will continue to be valuable assets in areas where specialized nursing care is required (for example, critical care transport), where interagency interface is important (for example, development of protocols and policies), or when skilled educators are required (for example, interosseous infusion and community prevention efforts).

One of the challenges that has always faced EMS pioneers is how to progress in spite of constrained resources. The nurse talent in EMS is to a great extent untapped. EMS systems have made major strides. Perhaps the 1990s will be the decade in which EMS recognizes the potential for growth through collaboration with nursing. Models already exist but others must be developed.

EMS has a history of attracting the innovative practitioner. Opportunities for expanding and improving systems abound. Nurses have responded to EMS in small numbers considering the population available. The ability of the EMS director to mobilize nursing support is directly proportional to the ability to include nurse leaders in the organization and practice collaboratively.

REFERENCES

1. Adams BL: Unpublished data, 1990.
2. Beachley M, Snow S, and Trimble P: Developing trauma care systems: the trauma nurse coordinator, *J Nurs Adm* 18(7,8):34-42, 1988.
3. Boyd D: The conceptual development of EMS systems in the United States. II. *Emergency Medical Services* 11(2):26-35, 1982.
4. Lyle NA: Prehospital nurse clinician: job description and evaluation tool, *Journal Emergency Nurse* 15(6):365-369, 1989.
5. Moore HS: MICNs: who can help? *Journal Emergency Nurse* 13(6):325-327, 1987.
6. National Association of Emergency Medical Technicians: *Role of the registered nurse in the prehospital environment,* Official position statement, Mar 1990, The Association.
7. Ramsey Emergency Medical Services: *Motto,* St. Paul, Minn.
8. Robinson K: Development of ENA national standard guidelines for prehospital nursing curriculum, *Journal Emergency Nurse* 18(1):48-53, 1992.
9. Spisso J et al: Improved quality of care and reduction of house staff workload using trauma nurse practitioners, *J Trauma* 30(6):660-665, 1990.
10. Stewart R: *Historical perspective.* In: Rousch W, editor: *Principles of EMS Systems,* Dallas, 1989, American College of Emergency Physicians.
11. US Department of Transportation, National Highway Traffic Safety Administration: *Emergency medical technician-ambulance national standard curriculum,* 1984.
12. US Department of Transportation, National Highway Traffic Safety Administration, *Emergency medical technician-paramedic national standard curriculum course guide,* Washington, DC, 1985.

30

Volunteers

Joseph J. Fitch, Ph.D.

Volunteerism is a tradition that dates to colonial times. As the United States transformed from an agrarian to an industrial society, the concept of "neighbors helping neighbors" continued to flourish. However, as the nation became a more mobile, motorized society, cities and suburbs replaced family farms and villages. Volunteering for the local ambulance corps or rescue squad became a socially accepted way for individuals to continue the volunteerism tradition. As society moves toward the twenty-first century and into an advanced information-based environment, however, EMS volunteers are becoming an increasingly endangered species. In this chapter the strengths and weaknesses of volunteer organizations are reviewed, the special sensitivities needed for working with volunteers outlined, and the benefits of the continued involvement and development of volunteer squads emphasized.

A Changing Environment

Volunteer rescue squads make a significant contribution to health care in America. The heaviest concentration of independent volunteer ambulance corps (often referred to as rescue squads) is in the Northeast region of the country. However, EMS volunteers are found as part of volunteer fire departments in most parts of rural America. According to a study published by *Firehouse* magazine, 65% of the nation's EMS providers are volunteers, supplying EMS service to more than 30% of the population.[3] Outside the Northeast, volunteers most frequently provide care to lower population density areas. These areas would otherwise be underserved; because of low call volumes, it would not be cost-effective to operate a career service. In recent years, many volunteer squads have been negatively impacted by changes in rural society. As rural areas became more suburbanized with access to cable television and other "advancements," the lack of discretionary free time has drained the pool of available volunteers. The Congressional Office of Technical Assistance (OTA) in a comprehensive study of rural health care called the volunteer drain "one of the most salient problems confronting rural EMS systems."[1] According to the OTA report, many rural EMS programs lack specialized providers and resources, operate with inadequate transportation and communications equipment, and are not part of a regional EMS system.

The volunteer drain is not limited to the rural area. Urban and suburban areas have been hit especially hard. For example, in a 1990 study of America's largest cities, only three of the largest 200 cities reported EMS service being provided by volunteers.[2] The state of Pennsylvania, which has long been an area in which EMS volunteerism flourished, reports major declines in recent years. Pennsylvania statistics indicate that 5 years ago volunteers represented 90% of those involved in EMS, but only 40% are involved today.[5] Squads are closing, using paid personnel, or being absorbed by either public or private ambulance services.

There are a number of reasons for that phenomenon. Volunteer agencies typically relied heavily on young, single members. That group is getting smaller. According to the U.S. Department of Labor's Bureau of Statistics there is a declining pool of 18-24 year olds. Members of that age group are moving into the entry level job market, and many must work two jobs. Many cannot afford to live in the communities in which they grew up. The cultural norms of the "twentysomething" generation also impact volunteer agencies. Popular literature has characterized that group as members of the "me generation." Fewer individuals see the value of volunteering. Similarly, potential volunteers who are "thirtysomething" are often deeply enmeshed in careers. Many married volunteers are part of two career households. Children, the pressures of balancing two careers, and the availability of leisure activities reduce the time available for volunteering.

There are a number of additional reasons for declining EMS volunteerism. They include commuter lifestyles, concerns about Acquired Immune Deficiency Syndrome (AIDS), and training requirements. Several decades ago most workers lived in the community in which they worked. Employers permitted individuals to leave work, enabling an occasional ambulance call to be answered as part of the employer's civic responsibility. In our commuter society, this practice declined because often neither the employer nor employees have strong community ties. The fear of AIDS and other infectious diseases make some individuals reluctant to enter the health profession, and most likely this fear also negatively influences those who consider volunteering.

Increased training and continuing education requirements are the reasons most often cited as barriers to volunteerism in EMS, in recent studies conducted by Fitch & Associates. Being a volunteer has changed from a "club" atmosphere to one requiring a continuing commitment to competence. Twenty-five years ago, anyone could stop by the station and become a volunteer with an evening or two of training. Today, it requires at least 110 hours to become an Emergency Medical Technician-Ambulance (EMT-A) and depending on local requirements, 500 to 1000 hours of training to become a paramedic. With the evolution of paramedics as the minimum standard of care for urban and suburban areas, increasing training requirements have compounded the problem for volunteers.[4] Not only is it harder to find volunteers, but they now must obtain and maintain a higher standard of training than was required in the past. The standard should not be lowered or exceptions granted for volunteers because competence is required: increased training opportunities and flexible scheduling are better options to reduce the perceived barriers.

Volunteer organizations throughout America are in transition. They must either meet expanding care expectations with fewer resources or categorically resist change, ultimately resulting in their organizational demise. Communities desiring to maintain volunteerism can work with squads to include them in progressive EMS systems without denigrating care. It takes time, energy and patience; however, the rewards for both the volunteers and the community can be great.

The city of Richmond, Virginia, is a good example of such an approach. Richmond embraced those local squads willing to make the commitments to provide predictable, sophisticated prehospital care and to become an integral part of the system. Parts of Richmond had been served by volunteer rescue squads for more than 30 years; when the City undertook a complete redesign of its fragmented EMS system in 1989, special attention was paid to providing opportunities for volunteer participation. The city required that participating squads meet all citywide requirements established by the medical control board, including providing advanced medical service and responding to life-threatening emergencies within 8 minutes 90% of the time. Richmond is the only public utility model EMS system that has an active volunteer component.

The squads initially resisted change and exerted considerable political pressure to continue a tiered system. Once the medical community made it clear that level of care was not a negotiable item, the squads were given an ultimatum to comply with the standards or cease operations. To facilitate compliance, the city provided new medical equipment, advanced training, and daytime staffing during the transition period to facilitate the training process. The system has been functional since 1990.

Positive Factors

There are a number of common positive descriptors that can be associated with excellent volunteer ambulance services. They include a variety of attributes, some of which are discussed here.

Tenacity, Desire, and Confidence

Many volunteer services survive because of the sheer will and perseverance of key members. In any group there are those who are halfheartedly involved, those who are committed, and a few who are passionately committed. It is this latter core of individuals that have a true love for EMS. Their passion comes from a deep desire to serve. In the best volunteer agencies the passion and commitment are patient-centered rather than internally focused on the squad. Confidence is another common descriptor of successful squads.

Flexibility and Willingness to Experiment

The limited size of most volunteer services often makes them more flexible than either business or government. By their very nature, volunteer squads can often be more responsive than business or government in meeting the needs of a specific neighborhood or community. Volunteer organizations understand that there are many ways to attack a problem, some of which may not be practical for other entities. The best volunteer services are on the cutting edge of care and technology issues and are always willing to experiment with equipment or procedures that may better serve patients. For example, Cypress Creek (volunteer) EMS in Houston was among the early groups to use monitor-defibrillator-external pacemaker systems and a computer-aided dispatch system. Forest View Volunteer Rescue Squad in Richmond, Virginia, was part of a multisite epinephrine study. Numerous volunteer squads have been at the forefront of advancing prehospital care.

Access to Private Funds and Volunteer Labor

Volunteer ambulance services are positioned to receive funds from practically every philanthropic source, ranging from the largest institutional donor to individual neighbors. Local corporations and individuals like giving to volunteer rescue squads because they see the results at work in the community and they may need service at some point in the future. Volunteer labor, when effectively harnessed to meet the clinical, operational, and administrative needs of the squad, provides unique advantages because volunteers provide EMS service at a fraction of the cost of private and government operations.

Community Spirit

The very act of beginning a volunteer EMS group has the potential to develop a valuable community force not just for emergency health care but across the breadth of society. The Bedford-Stuyvesant Volunteer Ambulance Corps, located in an area of Brooklyn heavily populated by minorities, was recognized by President Bush in 1991 as part of the Points of Light program. The organization serves as a community educational and organizational focus, in addition to its EMS role. Another volunteer squad to receive the Points of Light award was Sun City Center (Florida) Emergency Squad number 1, which has no member younger than 57 years old and answers 6,000 calls each year. It provides van transfers for those who do not require an ambulance and a wheelchair exchange for the retirement community that it serves.

Challenges

There are also several common challenges faced by volunteer ambulance services. These challenges include the following and others.

Lack of Clarity About Goals and Purpose

Many volunteer ambulance services cannot articulate the reason they exist. Other than stock phrases such as "providing care to our community," when asked hard questions about local needs, program delivery, and community response, many squads reveal glaring holes in their organizational methodologies. Like many voluntary organizations, rescue squads often believe that their survival no matter how difficult or necessary is their purpose. The worst believe that it is their right to preserve their "club" no matter what the consequences for the patient or the community. Volunteer organizations may resist improvements in the local EMS system simply because it is not to their organizational benefit. In sum, squads must adequately meet patient needs before attempting to meet the needs of the rescuers.

Ineffective Leadership

Many volunteer services lack leaders with strong management skills. Some squad leaders shun the notion that they must be strong leaders by saying, "we're just volunteers." Leaders are elected. In many cases elections are based on popularity rather than competence. Management shortcomings in volunteer squads are often masked by sacrifice, avoidance, or ignorance of the problem. Many organizations appear to be in better shape than they actually are. Most members join a volunteer rescue squad to provide care not to get bogged down in administrative matters. Leading and managing a volunteer organization requires additional skills; and it is often difficult to attract and promote individuals prepared to provide the nurturing leadership necessary for long-term success.

Insufficient and Undependable Financial Support

The fiscal life of volunteer ambulance services has been increasingly difficult in recent years. While the fund-raising techniques have become more sophisticated, the competition for donations has also increased. Squads often rely heavily on individual donors, and they are expending more effort raising funds than in the past. Most members do not enjoy asking for money. A common refrain is, "That's not the reason I joined; I want to save lives." As fiscal pressures increase, a number of squads have had to delay both equipment replacement and facility repairs; some have simply folded. The billing of consumers and insurance carriers remains a foreign concept for many squads. It is often equated with becoming a private ambulance service rather than recovering the costs necessary for the squad's survival.

Public Invisibility

Most members of the public are oblivious to EMS, until they need help. The needs of the local volunteer rescue squad are not usually a high priority of the average citizen. Squads often fail to adequately state their needs for fiscal support, leadership resources, and line personnel. Even those who have been provided service by a volunteer ambulance squad quickly forget among the cacophony of other societal activities. In many areas, EMS is regarded as a jurisdictional responsibility; users may not recognize the degree of volunteerism involved in the specific area.

Working With Volunteers

Encouraging a volunteer agency to maximize its strengths and minimize its weaknesses to benefit its patients and its members is not an easy task. One organization that is working to accomplish those goals is Cypress Creek EMS. Cypress Creek uses both career and volunteer staff and operates five advanced level units in a 250-square-mile area that borders Houston. The following 10 ideas for working with volunteers were offered by Cypress Creek's former executive director, David Almaguer.

Focus on Need and Pride as Motivators

Volunteers are motivated by need and pride. The more the need to provide a service, the greater the desire from the volunteer. A person must be needed to perform work for free. The less the perceived need for the volunteer, the more incentive programs are necessary to keep up the membership. Although some organizations are looking at pension plans and merit systems for regularly riding members, the primary reason volunteers perform is pride in their job. Perks are good, but they are also an indication that volunteers are not getting satisfaction from their work and need more reinforcement. Need brings in the volunteers; pride and job satisfaction keep them.

Recognize the Time Required for Training

It is increasingly difficult for a volunteer to commit the time necessary for learning and practicing the level of medical expertise required. Most EMS organizations, especially those providing sophisticated prehospital care, require more training, certifications, and continuing education than ever before. The more the medical capability expands, the more time commitments are necessary from the volunteer provider to obtain training and demonstrate proficiency.

Hold Volunteers to the Same Standards as Paid Personnel

Volunteers must be held to the same standards as paid personnel or the volunteer feels less professional. There cannot be two standards of care. Although it may be more difficult and require more time for a volunteer to maintain higher levels of training, by achieving those standards the volunteer feels as professional as any paid provider.

Limit Turnover

The reason a volunteer leaves an organization is usually a change in personal priorities such as children or a new job. Volunteers and paid personnel do not "burnout" in the same way. Paid individuals usually show stress and burnout symptoms that can be dealt with, whereas a volunteer may have no signs of burnout or problems before leaving the organization. Internal organizational politics, clashes of personalities, or loss of need and pride in the organization are other reasons volunteers leave. Internal strife is usually tied to either a lack of direction or weak leadership in the organization. People working together for a common goal are usually too busy attaining the goal to worry about power struggles.

Avoid Comparing Volunteers with Paid Personnel

Volunteers are very sensitive about being compared to paid professionals. They want to be treated and perform at the same or a higher level than paid personnel. Always using paid personnel as positive examples or using phrases such as "You're just a volunteer," should be avoided. Never refer to only the paid providers as "professionals."

Focus Competitive Energy on Personalized Service

The attitudes and approaches of volunteers to patients are often excellent. This is one area where competition between paid and volunteer personnel may be healthy. Paid personnel should be challenged to provide the same high levels of personalized service as the volunteers. The medical director should direct energy toward improving the level of personalized service given by both the volunteer and paid staff.

Educate Rather than Test for Competency

Volunteers have a natural desire to do their best. Instead of testing their abilities, as is common for paid personnel, educate! The volunteer needs support in attaining the goals that are set. If the goal is for volunteers to be proficient in Cardiac Pulmonary Resuscitation, train them on the procedures and allow them the opportunity to reach that goal. Make sure that the volunteers also accept it as their goal. If the volunteers buy into the goal, they will be working to accomplish their goal, not someone else's. Spend incentive dollars on education not perks like coffee cups, license plate holders, and beer blasts.

Facilitate Information Dissemination

Because volunteers do not work with the organization every day, they must have a clear and direct avenue to receive information and direct their concerns and questions. Clear-cut operations procedures are essential. The chain of command is very important; everyone must know who is responsible for correcting problems and effecting change. This clarity of authority also decreases the problem of getting the run-around about a problem. One person must have the responsibility and authority of leadership.

Provide Specific Goals

Volunteer organizations require a better mission statement than "to provide emergency medical care." They need direction toward obtainable goals. Once a major goal such as a new building or an award has been achieved the group may stagnate. Certification in a higher level of care is an example of a short-term goal for a member. There also needs to be clear and consistent long-term goals for the organization. This is particularly important since many volunteers are not exposed to the organization on a daily basis, and the leadership in many volunteer agencies can change with the popular vote of the membership. The organization should establish long-term goals that do not change with the whims of the new administration.

Put the Right Person in the Right Job

Good field providers are not necessarily good fundraisers. However, volunteers have the advantage of being experts in other fields of work that can be useful to the organization. Tap members for both medical and operational expertise. Volunteers are eager to help in areas they understand but shun areas that are unfamiliar such as asking for funds or discounts. It may be helpful to designate a group or an individual specifically for that difficult or unusual task.

Summary

Volunteerism in America is changing. To continue to be an effective force in EMS, volunteers need to embrace rather than resist enhanced levels of care and other advances in providing service. Special care must be taken by medical directors to recognize the strengths and limitations of volunteer squads. In many suburban and rural areas, volunteers are strategically located to work with the EMS system and the medical director to bridge geographic or organizational service gaps.

REFERENCES

1. Congress of the United States, Office of Technology Assessment: Rural emergency medical services, Special report, OTA-H-445, 1985.
2. Keller RA: EMS in the United States, *JEMS* 15:79, 1990.
3. McNally VP: A history of the volunteers, *Firehouse* 11:49, 1986.
4. Ornato J: The need for ALS in urban and suburban EMS systems, *Ann Emerg Med* 19:151, 1990.

SUGGESTED READINGS

Division of Medical Science, National Academy of Science-National Research Council: *Accidental death and disability: the neglected disease of modern society,* 1966, Washington, DC, The Council.

Allison EJ et al: Specific occupational satisfaction and stresses that differentiate paid and volunteer EMTs, *Ann Emerg Med* 16:676-679, Jun 1987.

Bachman JW: The good neighbor rescue program: utilizing volunteers to perform cardiopulmonary resuscitation in a rural community, *J Fam Pract* 16:561-566, Mar 1983.

Carter HR: Is the volunteer fireman an endangered species? *Rekindle* 14:12, 1985.

Congress of the United States, Office of Technology Assessment: *Rural emergency medical services,* Special report, OTA-H-445, 1985.

Daily RC: Understanding organizational commitment for volunteers: empirical and managerial implications, *Journal of Voluntary Action Research* 15:19-31, 1986.

Drucker PF: *Managing the nonprofit organization,* New York, 1990, Harper-Collins.

Gilbertson M: The volunteer crisis, *JEMS* 6-7, Jun 1988.

Gora JG and Nemerowicz GM: *Emergency squad volunteers: professionalism in unpaid work,* New York, 1985, Praeger Publishers.

Hudgins E: Volunteer incentives, *JEMS* 58-61, Jun 1988.

Karter MJ Jr: Taking the measure of the fire service, *Fire Command* 52:17, 1985.

Keller RA: EMS in the United States, *JEMS* 79, Jan 1990.

McNally VP: A history of volunteers, *Firehouse* 49, Mar 1986.

Miller A: The new volunteerism, *Newsweek* 111:42-43, Feb 8, 1988.

Ornato J et al.: The need for ALS in urban and suburban EMS systems, *Ann Emerg Med Serv* 151, Dec 1990.

Perkins KB and Metz CW: Note on commitment and community among volunteer firefighters, *Sociological Inquiry,* 57:117-121, Mar 1987.

Perkins KB: Volunteer fire departments: community integration, autonomy, and survival, *Human Organization* 46(4), 1987.

Smith DH: Altruism, volunteers, and volunteerism, *Journal of Voluntary Action Research* 10:21-36, 1981.

Swan TH: Keeping volunteers in service, *JEMS* 13:50-54, Jun 1988.

Swan TH: Recruiting EMS volunteers, *JEMS* 50-54, June 1986.

31

Discipline with Due Process

James O. Page, J.D.

The definitions of discipline portray the topic in very different ways. For example, "training that develops self-control, character, or orderliness and efficiency." In other words, a positive, nonpunitive effort to create desired attitudes and behaviors through training. From the same source, however, are the following definitions of discipline: "strict control to enforce obedience" and "treatment that corrects or punishes."

It should be apparent that the first of these definitions ("training that develops self-control, character, or orderliness and efficiency") is the preferable approach to discipline. But when that approach fails, it may be deemed necessary to employ the negative, punitive approach to discipline.

In the EMS field, there have been fairly recent requirements for quality management (QM) programs, presumably to assure that the quality of emergency medical care consistently meets minimum standards. While there have been elaborate designs developed for QM programs, almost all seem to avoid a critical issue: how to correct behavior and performance of an individual when the QM process reveals behavior or performance deficits. Most QM proposals simply advise that when errors are detected, the employer or regulator should "take appropriate corrective action."

What is "appropriate corrective action"? Is it a concentrated period of training that attempts to improve the self-control, character, orderliness or efficiency of the individual? Is it strict control to enforce obedience? Is it treatment that corrects or punishes (such as suspension of employment or certification, or revocation of certification and/or discharge from employment)?

Whenever the punitive approach is selected, the stage is set for a collision between the authority of the employer and/or the regulatory agency and the constitutional rights of the individual who is to be disciplined. In most states, regulations have been developed to guide and control the process. Often, they are poorly written and/or confusing. Furthermore, EMS agencies, medical control hospitals and medical directors tend to apply those regulations inconsistently, sometimes without apparent regard for the certificate holder's right to due process.

The purpose of this practice guide is to provide useful information and guidance to all parties—regulators, employers, EMS personnel, and their representatives. All parties have an undeniable responsibility to assure and protect the high quality of emergency medical care. To the extent that discipline plays a part in that process, this document is intended to help define and traverse the narrow line between the rights of the public to quality care, and the rights of certified EMS personnel to due process.

Discipline with due process is possible. It requires time, thought and extra effort. It is complex and sometimes frustrating. But it is a necessary balance of power in a free society.

Generally, people don't appreciate the importance of due process until their rights to property or their employment or their professional reputation are at risk.

Due Process

The Fourteenth Amendment prohibits any state of local government from depriving any person of life, liberty or property without due process of law (US Constitution, Amendment XIV).

According to the Random House Dictionary of the English Language, due process of law is, "A limitation in the U.S. and State constitutions that restrains the actions of the instrumentalities of government within limits of fairness."

*With permission of James O. Page, 1991.

Black's Law Dictionary, sixth edition (1990), offers the following definition:

> Due process of law implies the right of the person affected thereby to be present before the tribunal which pronounces judgment upon the question of life, liberty, or property, in its most comprehensive sense; to be heard, by testimony or otherwise, and to have the right of controverting, by proof, every material fact which bears on the question of right in the matter involved. If any question of fact or liability be conclusively presumed against him, this is not due process of law.

Perhaps the case of *Vaughan v. State* (456 S.W.2d 879, 883) best captures the spirit and intent of due process: "Aside from all else, 'due process' means fundamental fairness and substantial justice."

It is the "property" and "liberty" elements of due process which affect EMS employers and regulators with regard to disciplinary action. The "liberty" interests will be discussed later.

An individual's employment is considered "property" in many cases and thus state or local governments (or individuals or entities operating under the authority of state or local government) may not deprive the individual of that "property" (their employment or required certification) without due process. The actual steps (or mechanics) of due process will be described later. But first, let's explore the broader aspects of this constitutional protection.

Who is entitled to due process protection?

The courts have held that it exists if under state or local law, contract or administrative regulation, standards for retention are specified. *Board of Regents of State Colleges v. Roth*, 408 U.S. 564, (1972); *Perry v. Sindermann*, 408 U.S. 593, 609, (1972); *Bishop v. Wood*, 426 U.S. U.S. 341 (1976).

What does that mean?

It means that if there are any statutory, administrative or contractual standards for retaining employment (or certification), then the individual has a "property" interest in his/her employment (or certification), and that the employment (or certification) cannot be taken away from the individual without due process.

But doesn't that apply only to public agencies?

Prior to about 1980, private employers and their employees were deemed to be outside the requirements and protections of due process with regard to employment. Employees of private companies were deemed to be employed "at-will" (at the will of the employer) and had no constitutionally protected employment rights.

Since 1980, there have been several California cases which have held that there was an implied contract between the private employer and his/her employees. For example, *Cleary v. American Airlines*, 111 Cal.App.3d 443, 168 Cal. Rptr. 722 (1980); *Pugh v. Sees Candies*, 116 Cal.App.3d 311, 171 Cal. Rptr. 917 (1981). Also see *Walker v. Northern San Diego County Hospital District*, 135 Cal.App.3d 896, 185 Cal. Rptr. 617 (1982) for an example using the same theory of implied contract to erode the at-will doctrine. Note: Even though these cases apply only in California, it does tend to be a bellwether state in terms of legal developments.

But the 14th Amendment specifically applies to state and local governments. How can it apply to private ambulance companies?

Prior to 1980, most private ambulance services in the U.S. operated in an unregulated environment. Their relations with their employees was very much at-will. Now, however, private ambulance companies in many locations are functioning as legal and operational adjuncts of local governments, either through regulated monopoly franchises, protected zone arrangements, subsidy agreements or shared services. They are strongly regulated by EMS agencies, including quasi-governmental management entities, and many companies have entered into contractual agreements with employees ranging from labor-management agreements to individual employment contracts.

Consider the following material from the current Policy and Operations Manual of one unnamed private ambulance service:

> The employee, by virtue of accepting employment, assumes the responsibility to:
>
> Conform to all applicable governmental laws, regulations, ordinances, policies, procedures and protocols governing emergency medical services personnel, EMT's and paramedics, including all state, local and Company continuing education and in-service requirements.

In essence, the above provisions create a contract between employer and employee. Does that meet the standard of the Roth case? Probably so. The Roth case requires that standards of retention be specified under state or local law, contract or administrative regulation. This company's Policy and Operations Manual creates a contract with the employee and then adopts all applicable governmental laws, regulations, ordinances, etc., as the standards to be met if the employee is to retain his/her job.

Furthermore, the private company has an exclusive franchise in the community it serves, and the city also subsidizes the company. Though there have been no reported cases dealing with the question of a private ambulance employee's "property" or "liberty" interest in their employment, it could be argued persuasively that many private ambulance companies have become quasi-governmental.

The same company has entered into an agreement with its employees' union. That agreement includes a requirement for "progressive discipline." The progressive discipline system is defined and requires that employees are to receive advance notice, whenever possible, or problems regarding their conduct or performance in order to provide them with guidance and an opportunity to correct any problems. The labor agreement also details the progressive discipline procedure, which includes most of the elements of due process.

Even without the contractual links between employer and employee (discussed above), the structure and intent of current EMS law and regulation in many states seems to treat the private ambulance provider as a quasi-public agency. With such status there is a concomittant relationship between employer and employee.

How does the "property" interest apply to medical control hospitals and medical directors?

Although the authority delegated to medical control hospitals and EMS medical directors may vary from state to state, generally it includes the suspension or revocation of medical command or direction to an individual certificate holder (such as an intermediate EMT or paramedic). In many cases, this is tantamount to suspending or revoking the certificate itself.

To the extent that suspension or revocation of the individual's certification adversely affects their "property" interest in their employment, this infringement may be subject to due process protections. In other words, if the medical director has the power to take away an individual's certificate (or the necessary medical command or direction), thus depriving the individual of the opportunity to continue working at the same status or level of compensation, their "property" interest in their employment is adversely affected.

To date, there are no reported appellate court decisions involving due process violations by a medical director or medical control hospital. However, given the extensive powers conferred upon medical directors, and the potential for harm to the "property" interests of certificate holders, it is highly probable that the courts would formally impose upon medical directors certain requirements. Most likely, these would include pre-action procedural due process similar to that spelled out in *Skelly v. State Personnel Board,* 15 Cal.3d 194, 124 Cal.Rptr. 14, 28 (1975) and post-action evidentiary administrative hearings as defined in *Arnett v. Kennedy,* 416 U.S. 134 (1974).

Are due process requirements necessary when placing an employee or certificate holder on probation? Probably not. The Skelly pre-action procedure generally is required only in cases of significant punitive action, such as discharges, demotions or lengthy suspensions. Disciplinary actions such as warnings, reprimands, and 'improvement needed' performance evaluations, or suspensions of less than five days are not considered significant enough to warrant the pre-action procedure.

Even where a pre-action procedural due process hearing or a post-action evidentiary administrative hearing is described in state law or regulations, and is made available in cases of certificate suspension or revocation, or where renewal of a certificate is denied, such hearings may not be required in cases of lesser discipline, such as probation, or written or verbal reprimand. Careful study of applicable state law or regulations may be necessary to clarify this issue.

On the other hand, it could be argued that imposing probation on an individual's employment or certification may have adverse economic consequences (loss of opportunities to work overtime, suspension of transfer and time-off privileges, denial of promotional opportunities, ineligibility for step pay increases). If an otherwise benign imposition of punishment carries with it secondary economic consequences for the individual, it may be prudent to conduct the pre-action or post-action hearings, even though they may not be formally required.

What if the public needs immediate protection?

On occasion, it may become apparent that a certificate holder represents an immediate threat to the public. If the medical director or the certifying agency, based on a review of credible evidence, finds that such an individual represents an "imminent threat to the public health and safety," he or she may feel obligated to suspend the individual's certificate immediately.

The key to such action lies in the word "imminent." The immediacy implied by that word justifies taking action without the pre-action due process procedures. However, it is imperative that the medical director act only on credible evidence (which generally means detailed written information, rather than gossip or undocumented verbal reports).

Even where the medical director deems that immediate suspension is necessary to protect the public health and safety, the individual's employer should place him/her on paid leave until the facts can be presented in a post-action evidentiary hearing. By keeping the individual on paid leave during the process, his/her "property" interests are less likely to be injured.

If the evidentiary review is conducted properly, and if it confirms that the suspension (and possibly a subsequent revocation) were warranted by the facts, due process requirements will have been met and the individual can be removed from the payroll. If the evidentiary review determines that the suspension was not warranted, no injury will have been suffered by the certificated individual (since s/he remained on the payroll during the process).

The U.S. Supreme Court has addressed this issue as follows: "Before a person is deprived of a protected interest, he must be afforded opportunity for some kind of hearing, "except for extraordinary situations where some valid governmental interest is at stake that justifies postponing the hearing until after the event." *Boddie v. Connecticut,* 401 U.S. 371, 379 (1971)

Why should an employer pay an employee whose certification is suspended and who can't work?

Technically, the employer might get away with not paying the employee whose certification has been suspended. Indeed, some labor-management agreements in the EMS field specify that the employee must have a current certificate in order to be entitled to compensation. This is a short-sighted view, however, and is likely to cost the employer more in legal fees, administrative time and general disruption in the workforce.

The experience of law enforcement can be instructional. Whenever a police officer is charged with misconduct, the officer almost always will be placed on paid leave until the allegations can be examined, the officer (usually represented by legal counsel) is given an opportunity to make a written or verbal statement, witnesses can be examined and cross-examined, evidence can be evaluated, and a decision reached by an unbiased administrative panel.

If the administrative panel conducts a proper hearing and concludes that the officer was not at fault, his/her "property" (employment) rights have not been breached. If the panel concludes that the allegations are correct, due process will have been afforded and disciplinary measures can be implemented.

What is the "liberty" interest?

As indicated above, the Fourteenth Amendment prohibits any state or local government from depriving any person of life, liberty or property without due process of law. In California, the courts have consistently held that where the discipline involves charges that stigmatize the employee's reputation, the substantive right to liberty may be implicated to provide the employee with due process rights, even if the employee is found to have no property right in his/her job (as in the case of a temporary or probationary employee). *Board of Regents of State Colleges v. Roth,* 408 U.S. 564 (1972); *Lubey v. City and County of San Francisco,* 98 Cal.App.3d 340, 159 Cal.Rptr.440 (1979); *Wilkerson v. City of Placentia,* 118 Cal.App.3d 435, 173 Cal.Rptr. 294 (1981); *Jablon v. Trustees of the Cal. State Colleges,* 482 F.2d 997 (9th Cir. 1973); cert. denied, 414 U.S. 1163 (1974).

The liberty interest cases involve only terminations. Also, in those cases, the liberty interest is not an issue where the employee is charged only with incompetence or inadequate performance. However, where there are charges of immoral or dishonest conduct, the employee has a right to a hearing that affords him/her an opportunity to clear his/her name. *Williams v. Department of Water and Power,* 130 Cal.App.3d 677, 181 Cal.Rptr. 868 (1982); *Shimoyama v. Board of Education,* 120 Cal.App.3d 517, 174 Cal.Rptr. 748 (1981).

In order for the information (which stigmatizes the employee's reputation) to be damaging—and thus involve the liberty interest—it must be dispersed to others. If that information is considered and discussed in a closed meeting, and not broadcast, reported or shared with the public or the community, it does not impinge on the constitutionally protected liberty interest. *Burris v. Willis Ind. School District,* 537 F. Supp. 801 (1982); affirmed in relevant part, 713 F.2d 1087 (1983).

In a fairly recent case, a temporary deputy sheriff's liberty interests were implicated where his discharge was based on charges of misconduct, as well as incompetence. However, the court ruled that the employee had been afforded an adequate opportunity to clear his name without a full evidentiary hearing, where the employee was notified of the charges, allowed to explain his conduct to the officers making the termination decision and file a written response, and allowed to appeal to a higher-ranking officer before the termination was effective. *Murden v. County of Sacramento,* 206 Cal.Rptr. 699 (1984) (petition for hearing before California Supreme Court pending).

Can the "liberty" interest be implicated in the discharge of employees of a private company, or members of a volunteer organization?

Thus far, the courts have limited its application to employees of public agencies.

The Mechanics of Due Process

In California, the landmark Skelly case spells out certain minimal due process procedures to be taken by public agencies (and possibly private companies operating in a quasi-governmental capacity) before taking serious disciplinary action against "tenured" employees.

In the Skelly case, the California Supreme Court ruled that as a minimum, (the) pre-removal safeguards must include the following:

1. The employee (or certificate holder) is to receive a preliminary written notice of the proposed action stating the date it is intended to become effective and the specific grounds and particular facts upon which the action will be taken.
2. The employee (or certificate holder) is to be provided with any known written materials, reports or documents upon which the action is based.
3. The employee (or certificate holder) is to be accorded the right to respond either orally, in writing, or both to the proposed charges.

What is meant by "tenured" employees?

The Skelly case involved a physician who was employed by the State Board of Education. He was considered a permanent employee and, by the agency's own rules, permanent employees could not be dismissed or disciplined except for good cause. For purposes of the Skelly safeguards, "permanent" and "tenured" status is the same.

Ordinarily, in cases of discharge, due process requirements apply only to such "permanent" employees. Probationary and "exempt" ("at will") employees, who may under the employing agency's rules be terminated for any or no cause, are not legally entitled to such pre-action due process procedures (nor to a subsequent post- action evidentiary hearing).

There are some important exceptions in cases where a probationary or exempt employee's reputation may be stigmatized by the disciplinary action, cases involving arbitrary, long-term at-will private sector employees, and cases involving peace officers. Those cases and the exceptions are beyond the scope of this document.

How does that apply to EMS training institutions and certifying agencies?

While there have not yet been any reported cases specifically on point, reasonable analogies may be drawn. For example, an EMS trainee, or applicant for an EMS certificate, probably has no due process rights (to a diploma or certification). If a trainee is dismissed from the course, or if the applicant is denied a certificate, they probably have no right to a pre-action Skelly-type process, or a post-action evidentiary hearing.

On the other hand, once the individual is certified, their property interest in their certified status probably solidifies. Especially where the certificate is essential to gaining and keeping EMS employment, the property interest in the certificate would seem to be as tangible as the property interest in employment itself. Therefore, it can be reasoned that certificate holders are as much entitled to due process protections as are permanent employees.

Do due process requirements apply to all disciplinary actions?

No. According to one of the best sources on the topic, the disciplinary action must be "significant punitive action." Actions such as warnings, reprimands, improvement needed performance evaluations, and suspensions of five days or less may be administered without according the Skelly-type pre-action process. On the other hand, the employing agency is free to establish its own procedures for such minor disciplinary action, and it may provide for either pre-action processes or post-action reviews. Usually, these occur through a grievance process.

When punitive discipline is absolutely necessary a fair and consistent procedure for imposing it is essential. The next section of this chapter offers an algorithmic approach. The algorithm is an adaptation from a practice guide that was based on California's EMS Personnel Certification Review Process Guidelines. For this national version, all references to California regulations and procedures have been removed, and the algorithm has been reconstructed for possible use in all states.

Although the discipline algorithm attempts to provide a generic process, some portions of it may conflict with local statutes and regulations. It should be used—if at all—in connection with local statutes and regulations and, where local statutes and regulations differ or conflict with the algorithm, the local statutes and regulations must prevail.

NOTE: In locales where disciplinary procedures and regulations are being developed, or existing procedures and regulations are in need of revision, the discipline algorithm can be used as a guideline. Before adoption, however, it should be reviewed by competent legal counsel.

Summary

Generally, people do not appreciate the importance of due process until their own rights are at risk. Nonetheless, due process rights are among the most fragile and precious of freedoms enjoyed by Americans. Balancing those rights against the need to assure quality in health care present the EMS medical director with a complex dilemma. Although complex, time-consuming and sometimes very frustrating, due process is possible while guarding patients and the public against imminent risks. As with most technical processes, discipline can be divided into a series of questions, decisions and action steps. To guide EMS personnel, their employers, their regulators and their representatives, a recommended process is organized and illustrated in the following algorithm.

A Proposed Discipline Algorithm

Information is received, which, if true, would be evidence of a threat to public health and safety

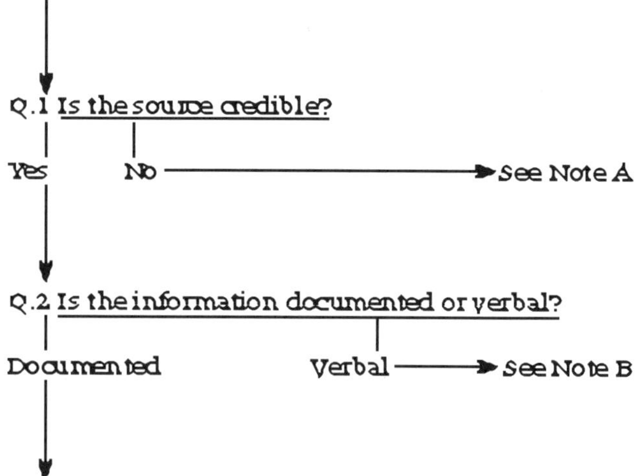

ACTION STEP 1: Evaluate the information relative to the potential threat to the public health and safety and determine if disciplinary action appears to be warranted. Proceed to Q.3

Q.3 Does this information refer to an individual who is NOT presently certified but has applied for certification?
No
Yes
Proceed to Q.12

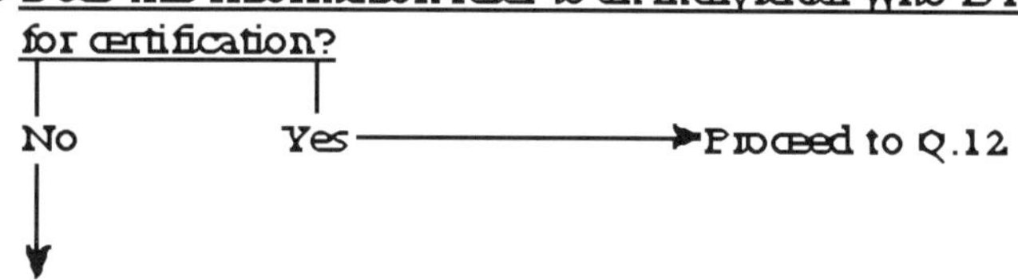

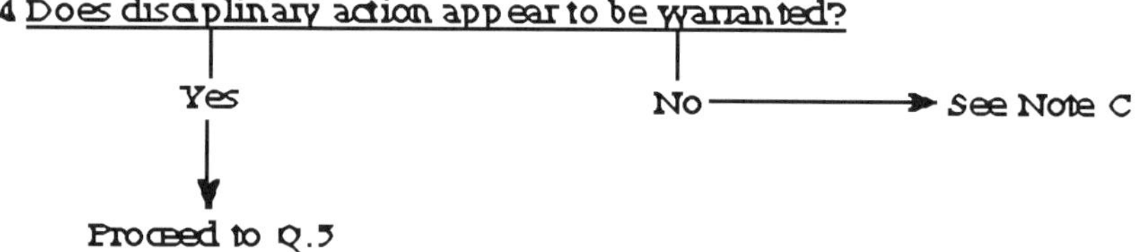

Q.5 Is an immediate suspension necessary to ensure the public health and safety?

Yes
No
Proceed to Q.6

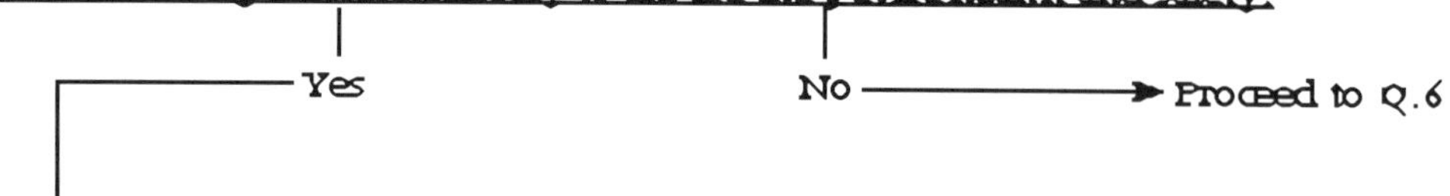

ACTION STEP 2: Certificate holder and his employer(s) shall be notified prior to or concurrent with initiation of the suspension. The notification should:

- Be by certified mail;
- Specify allegations and/or circumstances which caused the medical director or certifying agency to immediately suspend the certificate;
- State that the certificate is suspended immediately, and also specify the duration of the suspension;
- Identify the certificate(s) the action applies to in cases of multiple certificate holders;
- Inform certificate holder that he has the right to request a hearing to review the facts which necessitate the immediate suspension;
- Include a statement that the certificate holder must report the suspension if he applies for employment, certification or authorization from another employer or agency during the period of the suspension.

Proceed to Q.6

Q.6.................................. Is further inquiry into the situation necessary?

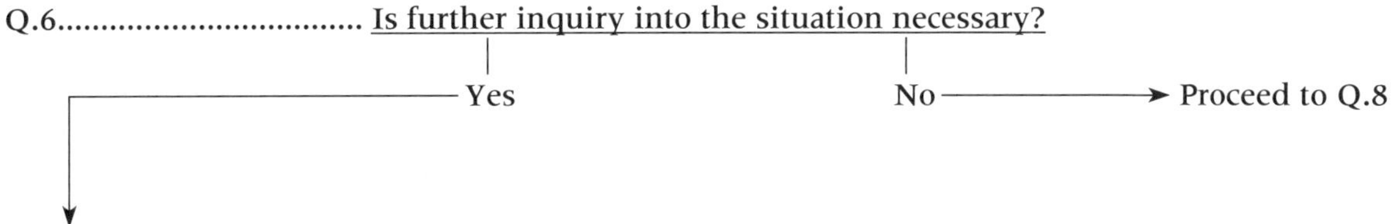

ACTION STEP 3: Begin formal investigation. Proceed to ACTION STEP 4

ACTION STEP 4: At a point in time when a formal investigation is begun, the certificate holder or applicant and his/her employer shall be notified of the investigation, and the notification shall:

- Be by certified mail;
- Notify certificate holder or applicant of a formal investigation;
- Include a statement of allegations against the certificate holder or applicant;
- Include a statement that the allegations, if found to be true, constitute a threat to the public health and safety and are cause for the medical director or certifying agency to take action;
- Include an explanation of the possible actions which may be taken if the allegations are found to be true;
- Include an opportunity for the certificate holder or applicant to present a written response to the allegations;
- Include an opportunity for the certificate holder or applicant to submit in writing any information which s/he feels is pertinent to the investigation, including statements from other individuals, etc.;
- Inform the certificate holder or applicant of the date by which information must be submitted;
- Include an explanation of the hearing process if suspension, revocation, denial or denial of renewal of a certificate may occur.

Proceed to Q.7

Q.7 Does the certificate holder request a hearing? (applicable only in cases of immediate suspension)

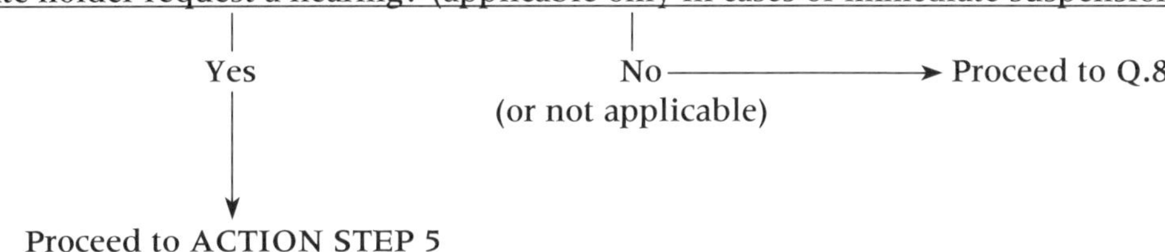

Q.8 Does the medical director or certifying agency conclude that the infraction or performance deficiency requires suspension, revocation, or denial of renewal of the certificate?

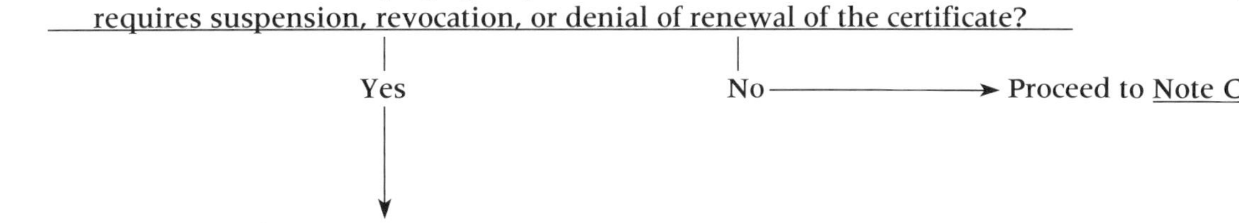

Q.9 Does the medical director decide to convene a hearing to assist in establishing the facts of the matter?

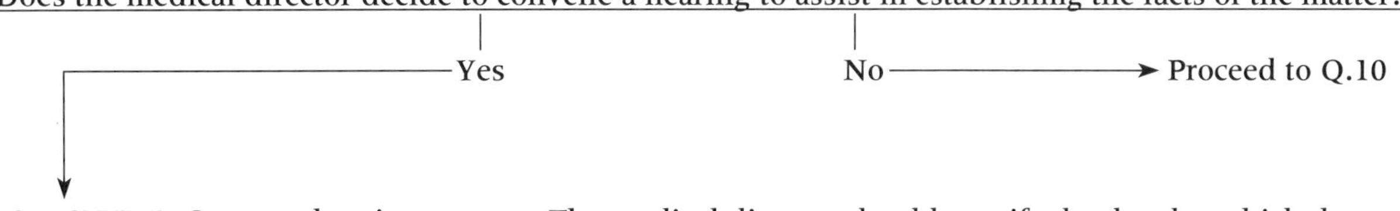

ACTION STEP 5: Convene hearing process. The medical director should specify the date by which the arbiter or panel shall make its report. The arbiter or panel shall make a written report to the medical director or certifying agency within the time limit. Proceed to Q.10

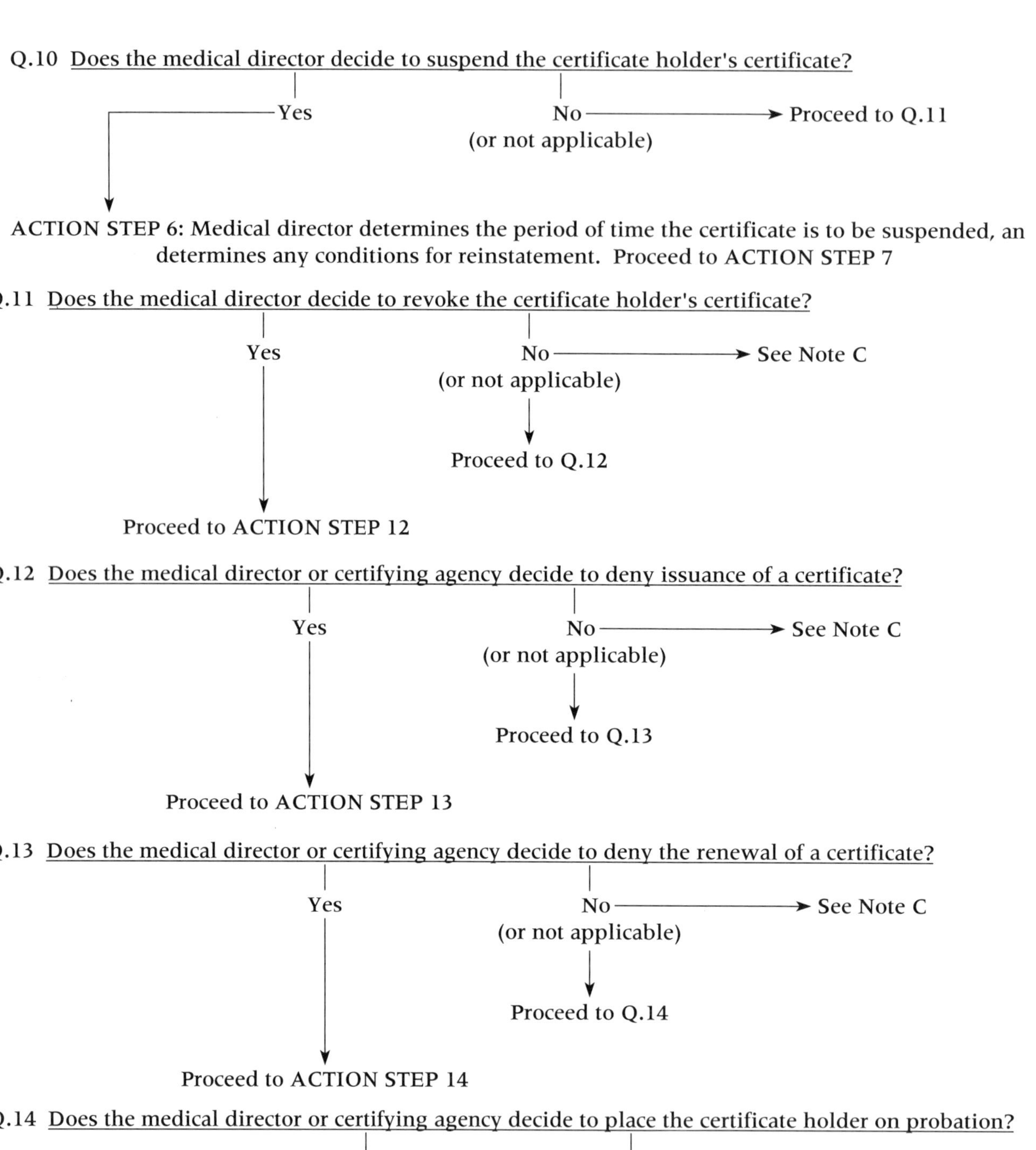
Q.10 Does the medical director decide to suspend the certificate holder's certificate?
Yes
No
(or not applicable)
Proceed to Q.11
ACTION STEP 6: Medical director determines the period of time the certificate is to be suspended, an determines any conditions for reinstatement. Proceed to ACTION STEP 7
Q.11 Does the medical director decide to revoke the certificate holder's certificate?
Yes
No
(or not applicable)
See Note C
Proceed to Q.12
Proceed to ACTION STEP 12
Q.12 Does the medical director or certifying agency decide to deny issuance of a certificate?
Yes
No
(or not applicable)
See Note C
Proceed to Q.13
Proceed to ACTION STEP 13
Q.13 Does the medical director or certifying agency decide to deny the renewal of a certificate?
Yes
No
(or not applicable)
See Note C
Proceed to Q.14
Proceed to ACTION STEP 14
Q.14 Does the medical director or certifying agency decide to place the certificate holder on probation?
Yes
No
Proceed to Note C
Proceed to ACTION STEP 15

ACTION STEP 7: The certificate holder and his/her employer(s) shall be notified within (a specified number of) days after the medical director or certifying agency determines the period of time the certificate is to be suspended, and any conditions for reinstatement. The notification shall:

- Be by certified mail;
- Specify allegations and/or circumstances which caused the medical director or certifying agency to suspend the certificate;
- State that the certificate is suspended, and also specify the duration of the suspension;
- Specify any conditions that must be met in order for reinstatement of the certificate to occur at the conclusion of the suspension period;
- Identify the certificate(s) the action applies to in cases of multiple certificate holders;
- Include a statement that the certificate holder must report the suspension if he applies for employment, certification or authorization from another employer or agency during the period of the suspension;
- Include an explanation of how to request a post-action hearing.

Proceed to Q.15

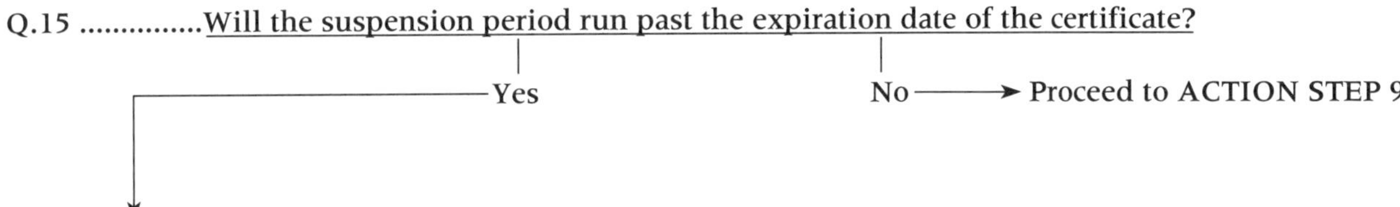

ACTION STEP 8: Calendar the expiration date of the certificate. On or before that date, the medical director may: (a) allow the certificate holder to renew the certificate by the usual process, or (b) require him to demonstrate that he sufficiently retains the necessary knowledge and skills. Proceed to Q.16

ACTION STEP 9: At the conclusion of the suspension period, determine whether the conditions for reinstatement have been satisfied. If they have been satisfied, notify the certificate holder that the suspension is rescinded and the certificate is reinstated. If the conditions have not been satisfied, notify the certificate holder that the suspension will remain in effect until the conditions are satisfied, or until the certificate expires, whichever occurs first. See NOTE E regarding the addition of conditions or extension of the suspension.

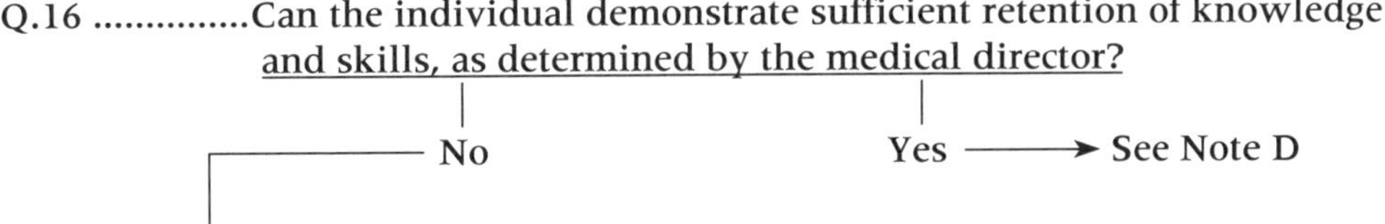

ACTION STEP 10: The medical director may require the individual either to complete specific retraining requirements or reapply for his certificate as if he were a new applicant. Proceed to NOTE E

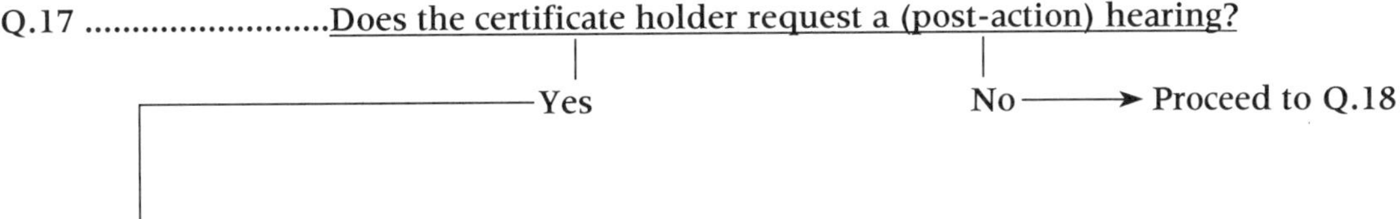

ACTION STEP 11: Determine whether the certificate holder is entitled to a (post-action) hearing? See NOTE F

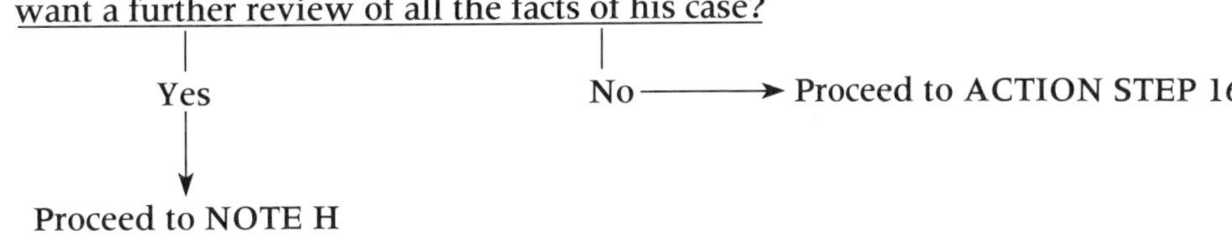

Q.19 Is the request for a (post-action) hearing made within (a specified number of) days of the date that written notice of action taken is received by the certificate holder?

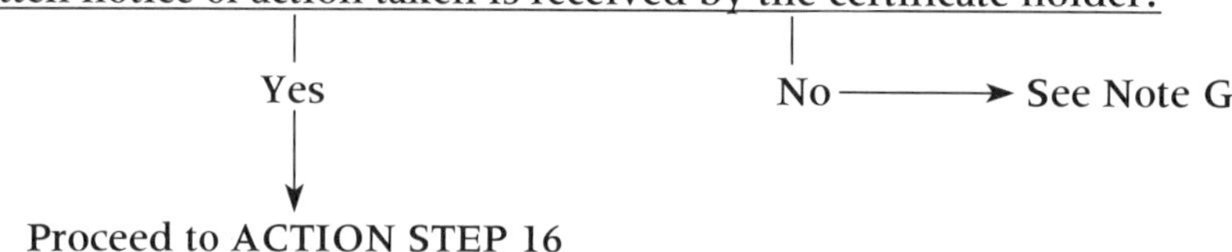

Q.20 .... Even if the regulations do not provide for a (post-action) hearing for certification applicants or where probation is imposed on certificate holders, or even if a certificate holder's request for a (post-action) hearing is not made within time limits, does the medical director decide to convene a hearing in this case?

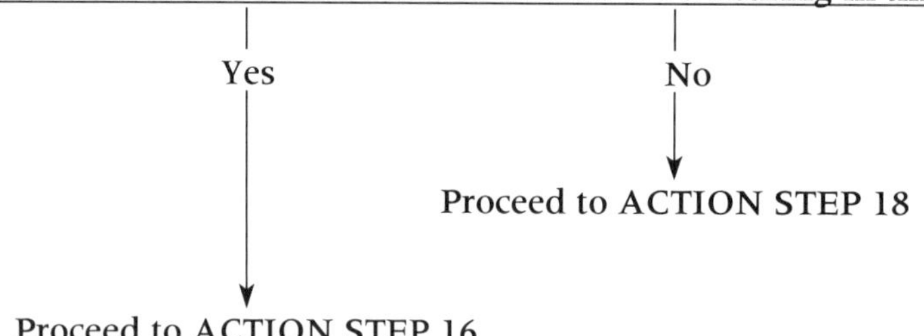

ACTION STEP 12: The medical director shall complete and place in the record a signed and dated statement certifying his decision. The certificate holder and his/her employer(s) shall be notified (a specified number of) days after the medical director makes a final determination to revoke the certificate holder's certificate. The notification shall:

- Be by certified mail;
- Specify allegations and/or circumstances which caused the medical director or certifying agency to revoke the certificate;
- Summarize the findings of the investigation (if an investigation occurred), including the findings of the hearing, if one was convened;
- Inform the certificate holder that his certificate(s) are revoked;
- Identify the certificate(s) the action applies to in cases of multiple certificate holders;
- If no hearing was convened, an explanation of the individual's right to request a post-action evidentiary review of the revocation;
- Include a statement that the individual must report the revocation if he applies for employment, certification or authorization from another employer or agency, and that his application may not be accepted or processed unless he presents documentation which, in the opinion of the medical director or the certifying agency demonstrates that the threat to the public health and safety which necessitated the revocation is no longer applicable.

Return to Q.17

ACTION STEP 13: The medical director shall complete and place in the record a signed and dated statement certifying his/her decision. The applicant shall be notified within (a specified number of) days after the medical director makes a final determination to deny the issuance of a certificate. The notification shall:

- Be by certified mail;
- Specify allegations and/or circumstances which caused the medical director to deny the issuance of a certificate;
- Summarize the findings of the investigation (if an investigation occurred), including the findings of the pre-action hearing, if one was convened;
- Inform the applicant that issuance or renewal of a certificate is being denied;
- Inform the applicant that he must report the denial of issuance of a certificate, or the denial of renewal of a certificate, if he applies for any certificate to provide prehospital emergency medical care (during a specified period of time).

ACTION STEP 14: The medical director shall complete and place in the record a signed and dated statement certifying his/her decision. The certificate holder and his/her employer(s) shall be notified within (a specified number of) days after the medical director or certifying agency makes a final determination to deny the renewal of the certificate holder's certificate. The notification shall:

- Be by certified mail;
- Specify allegations and/or circumstances which caused the medical director to deny the renewal of the certificate;
- Summarize the findings of the investigation (if an investigation occurred), including the findings of the (pre-action) hearing, if one was convened;
- Inform the certificate holder that his/her certificate(s) will not be renewed;
- Identify the certificate(s) the action applies to in cases of multiple certificate holders;
- If no (pre-action) hearing was convened, an explanation of the individual's right to request a (post-action) evidentiary review of the decision to deny renewal of the certificate(s);
- Include a statement that the individual must report the denial of renewal if he or she applies for employment, certification or authorization from another employer or agency, and that his/her application may not be accepted or processed unless he or she presents documentation which, in the opinion of the medical director or the certifying agency demonstrates that the threat to the public health and safety which necessitated the denial of renewal is no longer applicable. Return to Q.18

ACTION STEP 15: The medical director may place the certificate holder on probation (any time an infraction or performance deficiency occurs which, in the opinion of the medical director or certifying agency, indicates a need to monitor the individual's conduct in the EMS system in order to protect the public health and safety). The medical director may also set the term of the probation and any conditions, including the requirement that the certificate holder's performance shall be reviewed periodically during the probationary period, in accordance with the certifying agency's policies and procedures. Return to Q.17

ACTION STEP 16: Convene (post-action) hearing process. The medical director specifies the date by which the arbiter or panel shall make its report. The arbiter or panel shall make a written report to the medical director within the time limit. Proceed to ACTION STEP 17

ACTION STEP 17: The certificate holder shall be notified of the medical director's or the certifying agency's final decision, if notification has not already occurred. If a hearing was convened, this notification shall occur within (a specified number of) days of receipt of the request for the hearing. The notification also shall include the arbiter or hearing panel's recommendation.

ACTION STEP 18: Notify the applicant or certificate holder that the applicable statutes and regulations do not provide for a (post-action) hearing in cases where non-certified applicants are denied certification, where certificate holders are placed on probation, or where the request for a hearing is not made in a timely manner.

NOTES

Note A

Concluding whether a source of information is credible (believable) can be very subjective. Among the factors to be considered is the relative status and position of the informant. For example, is the information coming from a disgruntled former employee or partner? Or, is it coming from an EMS physician?

The requirement that information be from a "credible source" places a burden on the employer or medical director. That is, he must guard against activating the disciplinary process on the basis of representations by an informant who may be unreliable, dishonest and/or motivated by malice, revenge or ego.

If there is any question, the credibility of the source should be evaluated or challenged before evaluating the information itself. Once the test of credibility is met, return to Q.2.

Note B

Whether or not required by regulations, it is advisable that the employer or medical director insist that such information be presented in writing by the source or informant. The disciplinary process is very powerful and has the potential for depriving certificate holders of some of their constitutional rights. It is prudent to subject the reported information to this simple test before exercising the power of the disciplinary process.

Quite often, the circumstances that generate questions or concerns (about a certificate holder being a potential threat to the public health and safety) are emotionally charged. Those emotions tend to color descriptions of what happened. The process of reducing the information to writing invariably tempers emotions and subjects the information to an initial test of context and credibility.

Where the information is from a first-line supervisor and concerns the actions or performances of his/her subordinates, it is recommended that the information first be reviewed within the provider organization, one or two levels above the certificate holder's immediate supervisor. This follows the advice of legal experts regarding implementation of the "Skelly" standard.

This subjects the information to still another detached and unemotional review. It prevents a first-line supervisor from inappropriately unleashing a powerful disciplinary process against a subordinate. It also gives employers an opportunity to protect themselves against civil liability which could result from first-level supervisors taking untruthful or exaggerated information directly to the medical director or certifying agency.

If information is taken directly to the medical director or certifying agency by a first-line supervisor (especially verbal information), and if that information proves to be insufficient to substantiate the supervisor's allegations or the disciplinary action that results, the certificate holder may have a cause of action against the certifying agency, its medical director, the first-line supervisor, and the employer. After documented information has been acquired from a credible source, return to ACTION STEP 1.

Note C

If the medical director or certifying agency decides to take no action against the certificate holder or applicant, discontinue the evaluation of information, or the inquiry or investigation. If the original information was received from a source outside the certifying agency (e.g. employer, public safety agency, base hospital, patient, etc.), that source should be informed in writing that the information has been evaluated (or investigated) and that the medical director has concluded that no further action is warranted (or that the applicant should not be denied a certificate).

Special note: The evaluation of information of this nature, or an inquiry or investigation by a medical director or certifying agency, has the potential of stigmatizing a certificate holder, thus adversely affecting his 14th Amendment "liberty" interests. It is important for the medical director or certifying agency to make reasonable efforts to prevent and/or eliminate any stigma if and when it is determined that disciplinary action is not warranted (or that the applicant should not be denied a certificate).

Note D

Notify the certificate holder in writing that the suspension is rescinded. The notification process should be as prompt as possible. Suspension of certification adversely affects a certificate holder's ability to seek and obtain gainful employment, and that right is one of the "property" rights protected by the 14th Amendment. If a certifying agency fails to promptly notify a certificate holder that his suspension has been rescinded, that agency is, in effect, depriving the individual of a protected right without due process.

Note E

In requiring the certificate holder to complete specific retraining requirements or to reapply for his/her certificate as if he or she were a new applicant, the certifying agency or medical director should avoid imposing conditions which would (a) extend the period of suspension or (b) expand on the conditions for reinstatement which were specified in the notification of suspension (ACTION STEP 8). To add conditions or extend the period of suspension without an additional hearing could be viewed as a denial of due process. Also, such open-ended discipline has the effect of placing the certificate holder in a state of continual jeopardy. Proceed to Q.17

Note F

There are only two situations where a certificate holder may NOT be entitled to a (post-action) hearing. One is where probation has been imposed as the only form of discipline. The other is where the medical director denies certification to an individual who is NOT already certified. As a matter of practice, some certifying agencies provide for a (post-action) hearing process in cases of probation even though technically the certificate holder may not be entitled to it.

If the individual IS a certificate holder and is entitled to a (post-action) hearing, proceed to Q.19 at page 8.
If the individual is an UNcertified applicant for certification, or a certificate holder being placed on probation, proceed to Q.20.

Note G

Although technically the burden may be on the certificate holder to request a (post-action) hearing within (a specified number of) days of the date that he or she receives written notice from the medical director or certifying agency, it is probably not wise to deny the request if it is received late (within a reasonable period after the deadline). When confronted by disciplinary action that threatens one's livelihood and professional identity, many people become emotionally disoriented. In many cases, it is difficult for the affected person to seek and obtain counsel, and to decide a course of action within two weeks. By contrast, there are few valid reasons why the medical director or certifying EMS agency cannot accommodate a late request for a hearing. In any legal challenge that may occur, the certifying agency and medical director will be better served by examples of lenient process than by strict insistence on arbitrary deadlines. Return to Q.20

Note H

Where the certificate holder specifies in writing that he or she does not want a further review of all the facts of his/her case, no further action by the certifying agency or medical director is required (except to monitor any conditions of suspension, retraining, etc., which may have been imposed, and to notify the certificate holder when the period of discipline ends).

It is important for the certifying agency to maintain in its files the certificate holder's written communication (rejecting a further review). Also, if the written communication is at all inconclusive, the certifying agency or medical director should make additional contact with the certificate holder and remind him of his right to a (post-action) hearing of all the facts of the case.

32

Leadership and Team Building

Mike Taigman, EMT-P

The essence of leadership and team building lies in the formation of strong relationships with the team members. There are several strategies for building strong relationships with the people who practice medicine under the medical director's license. Time and energy are required to build a strong team. By investing in people, a strong team can be built.

The real work of an EMS system is providing quality care to the sick and injured. The challenge of being an EMS medical director is to create, facilitate, and choreograph a group of independent operators to practice high quality emergency medical care. The real test of a leader is how the team performs when no authority is present.

Reward the Positive

In relationships and team building one does not get what one wishes for, asks for, or begs for; rather, one gets what one rewards and expects. Blanchard, author of the *One Minute Manager* series, encourages people to use the three Rs for maintaining leadership and building strong relationships; these are recognition, reward and reinforcement. Recognize good performance, good behavior, and progress toward better performance. Reward outstanding performance, and reinforce whatever one wants to see more of. One medical director wanted all paramedics to contact medical control before releasing patients who refused transport. He had all the medical control physicians positively reinforce paramedics on the radio every time they called-in a refusal. He rewarded those paramedics who called-in every time; and used encouragement while those who needed to improve made progress. This approach had a greater impact on the problem than the method of his predecessor, which was to discipline those paramedics who failed to call and issue stern memos to everyone.

Many systems of medical direction are designed to discover mistakes and problems. When problems are searched for, they are found, focused on, talked about, and fretted over to the exclusion of strong performance. Whatever is focused on tends to grow. If one develops a systematic way of identifying strong performances, one will also see more of them.

The educational quality feedback loop is often programmed to find mistakes. The majority of tests handed back have only the wrong answers marked; it takes more effort to find things done well. It helps to establish a structured system to identify, recognize, and reward those who provide the best care to patients. In Kansas City, Missouri, a team including emergency medical technicians-ambulance (EMT-As), paramedics, managers, and the medical director was established to "catch" people providing good care. All their observations generated letters of commendation. The letters were mailed to the homes of the providers, and a copy was included in their personnel files. Every other week a "Quality Bulletin" full of anecdotes describing the star performers and their actions was distributed.

In New York City the medical director awarded small but distinctive shield citations to providers who were exceptionally kind, considerate, polite or helpful. It was not long before such attributes were recognized as important.

Positive expectations are the seeds of good results. Prehospital providers often rise to the level of their medical directors' expectations. Wherever pockets of clinically superb paramedics provide great care, there is generally an energetic medical director who expects nothing less than outstanding clinical performance. Conversely, areas with weak paramedic performance are frequently attended to by medical directors who function primarily on paper, lack vision, or resign themselves to mediocre field performance.

In his audio tape program *The Psychology of Achievement,* Brian Tracy discusses "expectation theory." He describes Dr. Robert Rosenthal of Harvard University who has conducted many experiments on expectation theory. In a classic case he went to a school district and randomly selected three teachers. He told them that they had been identified as the best teachers in the school district. As a reward for their teaching excellence, they would each be assigned select groups of students for the coming year. These students had the highest intelligence, the best behavior, and the strongest academic achievement scores in the district. "You should have a wonderful year; we expect dramatic results," he told them. To protect the children from harassment, they decided not to tell them that they had been specially selected. To prevent other problems, none of the parents were told, and to make it easier on the three teachers, this special reward was kept a secret.

At the end of the school year the students in these three classes finished with spectacular success. Their academic achievement scores were 22% higher than the rest of the school district. After the teachers were congratulated on their results, Dr. Rosenthal informed them that this had been an experiment. The children had been selected at random; he had no idea what their IQ or academic achievement scores were at the beginning of the school year. The amazed teachers wondered, "But how could this be? They were so easy to teach; they were excited and attentive." The teachers thought that it must have been their teaching ability. Only then did Rosenthal reveal to them the other half of the experiment. He said, "At the beginning of the school year we put all the teachers names into a hat and yours were the first three names that were drawn." This experiment reduced the variables to only expectations. Most of Rosenthal's work seems to indicate that if expectations are enthusiastically high, people will rise to meet them.

Develop a Flexible Response

How is a leadership style that enables the team to perform at its very best developed? Is one leadership style appropriate for all situations and all people?

Several years ago two general types of management styles were hypothesized—X and Y. The X leaders tend to be more autocratic, using their position power to achieve results. Ninety percent of their time and energy is directed toward the bottom 10% of their people. They often have a cynical view of employees and generally distrust them. These X type organizations invariably have a large membership in their "Ain't it Awful Club."

Conversely, Y leaders generally believe that their people are good and trustworthy. They construct systems to catch their people doing things right. Ninety percent of their time and energy is spent helping the top 50% get better. The concept is that employees perform well if they are provided with the tools and information to make good decisions. The leaders care most about how their people perform when they are not being observed.

Almost everyone wants to be a Y leader or a "good manager." This classification system is probably too simplistic for the real world. The most effective leaders have a variety of leadership styles. They are not always participatory or always autocratic; flexibility and adaptability are the keys to their success.

In his book *Leadership and the One Minute Manager,* Blanchard describes "situational leadership." In this system one of four different management styles is used based on what is most appropriate for the situation. No one style works in all situations; there is no best leadership style. The strong leader has access to each and knows which style applies to a situation.

Directing—This style is high on autocracy and low on participation; it is particularly useful for leading individuals with little experience or education in the current situation. For example, if one is introducing nasal intubation to paramedics for the first time, it is appropriate to direct their every move as they experiment with this new technique.

Coaching—In this leadership style leaders act like a sports coach. They direct the play, let the team members run it, watch carefully and critique their performances. EMS disaster exercise could benefit from this leadership style.

Supporting—With this leadership style the team members fully participate and rely on the leader only to support or to steer them back on the right track when they waver. Team members use the leader as a source of guidance. A medical director, interacting on the radio with a relatively experienced paramedic who is managing a complex patient, may use the supporting style.

Delegating—This style is reserved for very strong performers. Well-educated and experienced providers who have proven themselves over time respond well to being given the full responsibility of a situation or project.

In his book *The Greatest Management Principle in the World,* Leboeuf points out that trust and commitment are like sex. "Everybody wants more of it. Those who are talking the most about it are usually getting the least of it, and you can't get it without giving it."

Every interaction with or near anyone in an organization is an opportunity to make a lasting impression. In business circles, these impression opportunities are called "moments of truth." In these moments, reputations and abilities to influence are built or destroyed. It is amazing how the old management guidelines of "praise in public and reprimand in private" are disregarded. One of the fastest ways to strengthen your abilities to influence team members is to praise one of them in front of their peers; conversely, public reprimand leaves no path for the accused to "save face."

Be Creative

Listed here are some strategies to create positive, motivational, and effective moments of truth.

No matter how scientific and academic the conversation, the vast majority of a message that is received during an interaction with another human being is emotional. Albert Marabian researched interpersonal communications at UCLA. He found that of messages people receive 7% are made up of the words they use, 38% of their tone of voice, and 55% of their body language. Therefore, how one communicates has a greater impact than what is actually said. The phrase, "I love you," leaves one impression when it is delivered from a sarcastic angry person and another when it is shared in loving passion. When kindness and caring are communicated, even negative feedback is perceived positively by the receiver.

Replace "constructive criticism" with "useful feedback." The term constructive criticism is an oxymoron. Construct means to build; criticize means to tear down. When constructive criticism is provided, receivers are torn down; when that happens, they are not likely to improve performance. It is very difficult to improve effectiveness when one is feeling down. Also, people react to criticism by becoming defensive and are likely to become more firmly entrenched in their belief system. On the other hand, useful feedback is like a gift that can be used to improve the future. Useful feedback is a powerful relationship-building tool.

When providing useful feedback, replace *but* with *and*. Do not try to soften negative feedback, greasing up the target first by saying, "You are a really good paramedic but...." When most people hear *but* used like this, two things occur. First, they get the message that everything said before the "but" is a lie and second, it alerts them to an impending attack. Immediately a psychological defensive wall flies up. Of course, what is blocked by this wall is the very message that was to be delivered in the first place. It would be much better to say, "You are really a good paramedic *and* if you were more aggressive on your airway management your patients would be less likely to become hypoxic." When people hear a compliment followed by *and*, their ears perk up. They listen more attentively for the second half of the compliment. Then when they hear the useful feedback, it is emotionally tied to the compliment, and they feel good about putting the message into use.

It is a challenge to deal with things that have been labeled problems, failures, or screw-ups. Unlike the business world, in EMS each mistake is often viewed as a life or death issue. This approach creates anxiety that is counterproductive. Even if it is a life or death issue, rarely does the situation improve by making people feel bad while addressing it. It is much better to approach the problem as an opportunity for improvement. People work more diligently on opportunities than they do on problems; for most paramedics, mistakes and problems are mentally linked to punishment. Paramedics who feel punished when they have been "constructively criticized" have a hard time being caring and empathetic to patients.

Most customer service literature suggests that people treat others the way they have been treated. Medical directors who are kind and caring in their interaction with paramedics are likely to have paramedics who are kind and caring toward their patients. Conversely, paramedics who have been abused are more likely to become abusive. How paramedics feel when they leave an interaction with the medical director has a direct impact on the way they care for patients.

Similarly, meaningful feedback should be provided in private. Even if the feedback is not likely to embarrass or stress the receiver, it should be given in private. This approach increases respect for the leader; it also is more effective as demonstrated in the following case. A medical director dressed-down a paramedic in front of the emergency department staff and the patient; the paramedic had made a potentially dangerous mistake. Following the interaction, the physician felt that he had been effective in his communication. He also felt that it was an added benefit for the rest of the staff to hear the feedback so they would not make the same mistake. However, all the paramedic and the staff that witnessed the event could focus on was what a jerk the medical director was. They felt that he acted inappropriately, and they totally missed the feedback he provided. The general consensus was that in the future they needed to be more careful not to get caught.

A similar situation occurred in another city. However, this medical director chose to wait until the patient was cared for and his anger had dispatched. He then asked the paramedic to step into a private room to discuss what had happened. The paramedic was asked how he perceived the situation, and he was allowed to explain his thought process and decision-making. Only then did the medical director point out the cognitive flaws and provide remedial education. After the interaction, the medical director felt that he had been effective in communicating his message; more important, the paramedic felt the medical director really cared about the treatment that patients received. Feeling supported, the paramedic provided as many of his peers who would listen with the details so they would not make the same mistake. Now, paramedics in this system bring their mistakes to their medical director before he hears about them from another source. In addition, he is regularly sought out as a consultant for retrospective review and advice about challenging calls.

Both of these situations were dealt with by medical directors who in retrospect felt that they had been effective. It is important that the field personnel provide a reality check for the medical director. The reality that medical directors care enough to ask how they are doing and then listen to the feedback builds both their position and the team.

EMS team members generally have positive intentions; however, they may be difficult to discern. Few EMTs or paramedics wake up in the morning thinking, "I wonder how many patients I can harm today?" If the provider has a positive intent during a discussion, education and information will probably solve the problem. If providers do not have a beneficial motive for their incorrect actions, they may have chosen the wrong profession.

For the mental health of the providers and the medical director, severe discipline or feedback should be arranged both early in the day and early in the week. Often managers *avoid* difficult interactions by postponing them until the end of the workday or workweek. Predictably the pressure builds for both of the players and tensions rise in the organization. In addition, when the feedback is unavoidably punitive or handled poorly, providers must immediately take the burden home, if it is delivered at the end of the day or just before the weekend. Of course, this concept can be taken to extremes; in 1988 (at least two administrations ago at New York City EMS) no one ever wanted to be invited to Monday morning breakfast with the new administrator.

Making Rules

Protocols have strengths and limitations. Very little of the strength of a good protocol resides in the written document. The ability of a protocol to guide and improve care comes from the process of their preparation, implementation, and daily use. Protocols need to be flexible and dynamic in their ability to evolve and adapt with the changing needs of the system. Ideally, changes in the protocols should be driven by scientific research and choreographed by the local practice of medicine. Provider involvement in the development of protocols is essential. Protocols are best followed when they are well-understood; one of the best ways to understand them is to participate in their creation.

The education and implementation phases of protocol revisions are critical to the success of that protocol in field practice. Sufficient information, training, and understanding must be communicated to the providers. It is an absolute mistake to deliver a new protocol in every mailbox and expect instantaneous compliance.

The primary weakness of protocols is the inability of anyone to write a protocol for good judgement. Systems attempting to promulgate protocols that account for every variable of the EMS equation have paradoxically produced huge monoliths that are essentially incomprehensible. The key is to use protocols as guidelines thus everyone in the system is playing variations from the same sheet of music.

A "values-based" leadership style is more effective than a "rules-based" style. Most prehospital providers have at least three sources of information and guidance that govern their professional lives. The protocols guide the actual care of patients. The policy manual covers everything from uniforms and driving to shift times and workers compensation. National, state, or local rules cover the maintenance of their certifications. Additionally, union contracts, provider contracts, municipal policies, and who knows what else must be followed. From the perspective of the field providers, the only time a rule is used is when someone is in trouble. Medical direction never checks the policy and protocol manuals to find a way to reward someone for successfully managing a difficult airway.

A core problem with management by rules is that it allows people to quit thinking. All providers know of cases in which the supervisor intensely looks through the rule book until something that fits the situation at hand is found. Instantly, the supervisor relaxes when the rule that applies is located. If unsuccessful in the search for a rule, the supervisor quickly begins the process of writing. The results of these endeavors in reactionary rulemaking are often ridiculous. The following are a few real-life examples: "Starting June 15th there will be no slouching in the ambulance," and, "Forthwith employees are required to follow the following eight (8) step process for washing their hands after every patient contact or handling of equipment. Violators will be subject to the progressive disciplinary process." EMS administrators and medical directors who rely only on memos and addenda to the protocol manual for leadership rarely get their messages to the team.

Some rules help lead and build the EMS team. The key to effectively developing a new rule is to avoid overreacting to the current situation. A good strategy is to write the protocol, lock it away in a drawer for 30 days, and if it still makes sense to activate when it is revisited, then it is implemented. Most medical directors who use this technique find that they initiate far fewer protocols; however, because The Kuehl Rule states that a specific EMS problem always occurs in groups of three, there are times when a new protocol must be immediately introduced. The real secret of being a successful medical director is knowing which problems need immediate protocol revision and which do not.

Prehospital Care Report Review

Where does prehospital care report (PCR) review fit into the leadership system for a medical director? Some systems rely on "punitive" PCR review to monitor and improve quality. A PCR is like a resume; it is not a picture of reality, rather it is a skewed view of reality designed to achieve a desired perception in the mind of the reviewer. A positively oriented peer-based PCR review program is a great method to improve documentation; however, the process should also improve the actual care delivered.

In one system a red pen-wielding nurse reviewer boldly emphasized each time epinephrine was not given every 5 minutes on the dot during cardiac arrests. Within a month every single cardiac arrest had successive doses of epinephrine recorded at exactly 5-minute intervals. The nurse reported the dramatic effect the chart review process was having on patient care. Of course the physician realized that the paramedics simply knew what to do to stay out of trouble; they recorded the first time accurately then added five minutes to each successive time regardless of actual administration time. The PCR review of the previous example might improve patient care; however, PCR review that is punitive and is not performed by peers often results in survival adaptation.

Star Care

An organization should be lead with a simple set of values and principles, that is, a shared paradigm. Paramedic and author Thom Dick wrote such a set of guiding principles that has been adapted widely since its introduction at BayStar Medical Services in San Mateo County, California. Personnel at BayStar use this "Star Care" checklist to ensure they cover all aspects of each call. Medical directors and system administrators use the checklist to evaluate programs, policies, protocols, and improvements in their systems.

Safe—Were my actions *safe* for me, my colleagues, other professionals, and the public?

Team-based—Were my actions taken with due regard for the opinions and feelings of my *co-workers* including those from other agencies?

Attentive—Did I treat my patient as a *person?* Did I keep the patient warm? Was I gentle? Did I use the individual's name throughout the call? Did I tell the patient what to expect in advance? Did I treat family and friends with similar respect?

Respectful—Did I act toward my patient, colleagues, First Responders, hospital staff, and public with the kind of *respect* that I would have wanted to receive myself?

Customer Accountable—If I were face-to-face right now with the *customers* I dealt with on this response, could I look them in the eye and say, "I did my very best for you."

Reasonable—Did my actions *make sense*? Would a reasonable colleague of my experience have acted similarly under the same circumstances?

Ethical—Were my actions *fair and honest* in every way? Are my answers to these questions?

This Star Care checklist is printed on wallet-size cards and carried by everyone in the BayStar system. It provides a very simple yet powerful method to recognize, reward, and reinforce strong performance. It also provides a template to work through any improvement opportunities. Incidentally, this checklist may be reprinted if credit is given to Thom Dick and BayStar.

Summary

Building a strong team is the best way for medical directors to ensure that their patients and their license are cared for appropriately. During the 10 years that Norm Dinerman served as medical director of the Denver Paramedic Division, he regularly threatened to enlarge a copy of his medical license so that a 20 feet long and 10 feet tall rendition would hang on the wall of the paramedic day room. Displayed boldly on top of this unusual piece of twentieth century art would be the following words: "This rides with you today, take care of it!"

SUGGESTED READINGS

Blanchard K: *Leadership and the one minute manager,* New York, 1985, William Morrow & Co Inc.

Leboeuf M: *The greatest management principle in the world,* New York, 1985, Berkley Publishing Group.

McCormack MH: *What they still don't teach you at Harvard business school,* New York, 1989, Bantam Books.

33

Critical Incident Stress Management

Jeffrey T. Mitchell, Ph.D.

The United Nations International Labor Organization recently issued a report that calls job stress a worldwide plague and one of the most serious health issues of this century.[1] Human stress, which is a predictable byproduct of job conflict, job ambiguity, unrelenting pressures, shrinking support resources, and stressful contacts with people in need, is associated with illness, increased sick leave, changes in personality, marital and relationship discord, premature retirement, lowered job performance, injury on the job, disability claims against the employer, and early death.

Work-related stress claims represent the fastest growing and most costly (per incident) type of worker's compensation affecting American commerce. The National Council on Compensation Insurance notes that about 14% of all "occupational disease" worker's compensation claims are for excessive stress. The average medical and other benefit payments total $15,000, which is twice the average amount per paid claim for workers with physical injuries.[7] The estimated overall costs of stress in the U.S. economy is as high as $150 billion per year.[8]

Managers of EMS organizations would be accused of incompetence if they ignored the growing body of evidence that indicates that the United Nations report is accurate in its evaluation of global job stress. Ignoring the obvious places the employer and employees at grave risk of mistakes on the job, injuries, and stress-related disabilities. The cost of not responding appropriately to growing job stress is extreme in both financial and human terms.

Critical Incident Stress

One of the most serious forms of stress is traumatic stress or critical incident stress. It occurs when people are exposed to horrific, overwhelming, threatening, disgusting, grotesque, demanding, or shocking events that are beyond the range of normal human experience. These events are so unusual that they tax the coping abilities of those who experience them. Any mentally healthy person can experience this powerful and normal emotional response to a traumatic event (critical incident). Critical incident stress is a normal response of normal people to abnormal events. Although it is painful and distressing, most people recover from the experience.[9]

The great majority of people who experience a highly traumatic event recover from the experience in a reasonable time, but a small number are so seriously affected that they later develop a more serious condition called post traumatic stress disorder (PTSD), which is the most severe and incapacitating stress-related disorder. PTSD changes the way a person thinks, feels, and behaves. It also manifests itself in a wide range of physical symptoms. PTSD is so disruptive that it can effectively end a person's functional life and have severe negative effects on the person's family.[4] Becoming a victim of PTSD is a function of being exposed to a high-risk, potentially traumatizing situation or experience. It is not a result of poor training, inadequate moral fiber, physical or emotional weakness, or any other personal or job condition. It is not possible to predict PTSD, and there is no way to screen potential employees during the application process because everyone is vulnerable.[4,9]

Because PTSD is directly related to the exposure to highly traumatic events or experiences, providers of EMS are at a higher than normal risk. The prevalence of PTSD in the general population of the United States is less than 2%.[5] Emergency personnel have a higher prevalence of PTSD of about 4%.[9] At least one researcher has found sufficient symptoms to diagnose PTSD in 16% of fire fighters in a large Canadian city.[2]

It is clear from the discussion thus far that critical incident stress and its consequences (PTSD) endanger the health and survival of emergency personnel. Critical incident stress is also a significant problem for organizations, which risk legal, financial, and operational catastrophies, if they ignore this job stress problem.

Comprehensive Critical Incident Stress Management

Critical incident stress reactions can be lessened and PTSD can be prevented. Critical incident stress is positively responsive to early intervention by both professional and peer support personnel specially trained to manage traumatic stress and employ an established set of stress intervention techniques. Cost-effective programs have been developed and implemented to reduce stress and accelerate the recovery process. At present, 350 communities throughout the world have comprehensive critical incident stress management (CISM) programs, which have already proven their value in mitigating the effects of traumatic stress in emergency personnel and other groups. The comprehensiveness of these programs, however, must be recognized as the key to success.

EMS systems that attempt to deal with traumatic stress by using a single focused strategy such as the development of only an educational program are doomed to fail. A more sensible approach to traumatic stress management is a multifocal or comprehensive approach that includes a strategic plan for a wide spectrum of stress control programs.

A truly comprehensive CISM program has at least the following components:

- Extensive basic and continuing education program
- Critical incident stress team
- Significant other support programs
- Family support projects
- Administrator and supervisor education and support programs
- Peer support programs
- Mutual aid and community outreach programs
- Wide range of flexible intervention techniques such as:
    - mid-action support ("on-scene")
    - individual consults with peers
    - defusings
    - demobilizations
    - debriefings
    - follow-up services
    - informal discussions
    - chaplain services
    - professional counseling services
    - mutual aid programs with other organizations
    - community education programs

Building a comprehensive CISM program does not have to be an overwhelming and extremely expensive task, if it is done properly by combining resources with other emergency services in the community. It is not necessary for each organization to create its own comprehensive program to manage traumatic stress. A much more efficient and effective approach is to become a part of an extensive network of CISM services.

Practically every CISM team is a "combined emergency services" team that serves hospitals, fire services, law enforcement agencies, EMS programs, communications personnel, search and rescue groups, ski patrols, military services, and other primary response organizations.

These combined CISM teams work quite well. Because fire fighters serve fire fighters best, when an event predominantly affects fire service personnel, fire service peers are chosen to assist the affected fire fighters. When the event is more clearly defined as an EMS event, EMS peers are chosen to assist their peers. Similarly, law enforcement personnel are chosen from a CISM team to work with law enforcement personnel, and nurses are chosen to work with nurses.

All of these organizations feed members to the CISM team, and they all benefit from each other's experiences. They share in training the team, they use the same mental health professionals, and they rely on each other in a disaster. Other benefits of working together are that the various groups develop respect and understanding for the other professions, and they learn that there are many similarities among the various emergency service professions. Most important, combined CISM teams have a major advantage of being able to emotionally support one another in the difficult work of traumatic stress management.[10]

The combined CISM team makes sense on several points. It saves money, effectively uses resources, improves the breadth of the experience, and enhances training efforts. One service may contribute a clergyperson to the team, another may have a mental health professional, and yet another may provide the medical director. EMS providers, nurses, fire fighters, and police officers are usually drawn from the local services.

There are also serious psychological reasons why a broad spectrum team is more efficient and effective than a CISM team that is developed to serve only one emergency service. It is psychologically unsound for the providers of critical incident stress services and the recipients of those services to know one another well. Every medically trained person recognizes the inherent psychological dangers of providing medical treatment to seriously ill relatives or friends. Similar dangers exist for those who serve on CISM teams, and they often arise when supervisors try to provide support services for workers. Close association between those who give help and those who receive it causes emotional distress. The natural boundaries between work and personal feelings are threatened, and unnecessary anxieties are stirred on both sides.[9]

A combined emergency services CISM team is one situation in which competition between organizations is decreased and an atmosphere of mutual cooperation and support is enhanced. It is clearly a recommended course of action.

Traumatic Stress Education

Prospective traumatic stress education is one of the most essential keys in the prevention and reduction of critical incident stress in emergency services. Personnel forewarned about stress reactions tend to recognize the signs of distress earlier, and early recognition of stress symptoms leads to an earlier call for help. Prospective education enhances the potential that the help will be accepted and the recovery will be faster. Educated personnel take less time off of work, and their positive morale is maintained.

Ideally, every provider should be given prospective training. The general outline for critical incident stress education is as follows:

- Nature of ordinary stress (definitions, stress process)
- Stress in emergency services (cumulative, traumatic)
- Typical critical incidents (children, threats of violence, injuries to nurses)
- Immediate and long-range effects of traumatic stress
- Signs and symptoms of CIS
- Survival techniques for emergency personnel
- The CISM team
- Calling for help
- What the CISM team does (defusings, debriefings, one-on-one contacts, significant other support, follow-up services)

The properly trained CISM team members, when not involved in direct support services, spend most of their time teaching emergency personnel about traumatic stress.

Mid-action Support

On occasion a critical incident is so distressing that personnel have immediate reactions to it, showing signs of dysfunction while performing their duties. Such a situation demands immediate intervention by a trained CISM team member.

The immediate intervention is emotional first aid. It usually consists of a practical, common sense action that removes the distressed individuals from the immediate area and either gives them an alternate task or a few moments to recover before returning to work. Breaks, changing the tasks, redirecting attention, an understanding nod, and a variety of other supportive techniques are ways in which mid-action or on-scene support services are applied.[9]

Defusings

Defusings are one of the most frequently employed CISM techniques. They are short versions of the more formal debriefing process. Defusings are usually led by two CISM-trained peer support personnel. Although they are not time consuming, the results are often powerful.

For small groups, defusings are applied within hours of a highly traumatic event. The group is defused in a private setting before they are released to go home or back to their normal duties. Defusings last less than 1 hour and are best described as a conversation about a particularly distressing event. They consist of three main segments. First, there is a brief introduction in which the guidelines for the meeting are described and the personnel are motivated to participate actively. The second segment is the exploration of the incident. Descriptions of the specific incident are presented by those who were involved, and the leader may ask guiding questions. The defusing ends with a set of instructions and important pieces of information that may protect the staff from further harmful effects of the traumatic incident. If necessary a formal debriefing is arranged a few days after the defusing.[10]

Demobilizations

Demobilizations are rare occurrences in EMS because they are always associated with large scale or catastrophic incidents. They are used only when a large group of providers have been exposed to a highly distressing event.

Demobilizations consist of two parts. In the first part a small group of personnel who ordinarily work as a team are brought together after their work in an incident is complete. The team is then demobilized; they are given a 10-minute talk by a trained CISM team member on the potential stress effects of an exposure and the steps they can take to lessen the impact of the stress reaction. No one has to speak during the demobilization, and no questions are asked of those who are being demobilized. After the 10-minute talk, the listeners are asked if they need to say anything or if they have any questions. Usually the group being demobilized is so fatigued and numbed by their work that they do not have anything to say. The small group is then sent to another room where nutritious foods and fruit juices are available. Demobilizations are continued with additional groups until every group involved in the event is processed.[10]

Debriefings

A debriefing is the most complex and difficult of the stress mitigation and recovery processes. It can be provided only by a properly trained CISM team, consisting of a mental health professional and a few Critical Incident Stress Debriefing (CISD) trained peers.

A debriefing is a 2- or 3-hour group discussion of the traumatic incident, and it is made up of seven phases. The first phase of the CISD is the introduction phase, which concentrates on motivating the participants to actively participate in the process and informs them of the guidelines for the smooth conduct of the session.

The second phase is the fact phase. Personnel are asked to briefly describe their role and experiences during the situation.

The third phase is the thought segment of the debriefing. The participants describe their first thought or the most prominent thought after they came off of auto pilot during the incident.

The fourth phase of the CISD is the reaction phase, and it is considered the most emotionally powerful. The group members discuss the elements of the situation that caused them the most distress and have been the most difficult to cope with since the situation.

The fifth phase of the debriefing is the symptom phase. The participants are asked about the signs and symptoms of distress that they encountered during and after the incident, as well as how they are doing at the time of the debriefing.

The descriptions of the symptoms are an excellent jumping-off point for the CISD team to move into the sixth debriefing phase, which is the teaching phase. The CISD team teaches the members of the group helpful concepts related to stress mitigation and stress recovery. The participants are encouraged to ask any questions they may have.

The final phase of the CISD is the reentry phase in which the participants ask any remaining questions they may have and make any additional comments. The CISD team makes summary comments and the group is released.[10]

Individual Consultations

When only one or two providers are distressed by a situation and the remainder are not affected, a trained member of the CISM team can work independently with those affected. There is no need to bring together an entire group, if few are affected by an incident. Focused individual support can be applied when an individual requests help with a job-related or personal problem.

Guidelines for Effective Critical Incident Stress Management

Effective CISM programs are never an accident; they are carefully planned and managed efforts. EMS organizations, if they are going to provide the services that will preserve their personnel in their careers, must first make a proactive commitment to the appropriate development of a CISM program.

The first commitment is to find an appropriate person to chair the development committee. A major mistake emergency services make is assuming that CISM is a task for a mental health professional. No one denies that mental health professionals play a highly significant role in a comprehensive CISM program and are vital to program success. They are, however, generally very busy people with many conflicting duties and no time to develop, coordinate, and administer an entire CISM program. CISM is an emergency services function and is not the responsibility of mental health services.

Prehospital providers know that stress in the emergency setting is neither new nor unusual. They tend to trust and listen to one of their own who has expertise in CISM and EMS. Individual providers tend to be charged up about their stress, and they can channel all of that energy into effective stress prevention and mitigation programs if led by another provider with firsthand knowledge of the severe stress of emergency services.

Once an enthusiastic individual is chosen to head the development committee, arrangements should be made to coordinate efforts with a CISM team that may already exist in the area. Every effort should be made to join resources rather than set up a competitive team.

The emergency service should then develop a steering committee under the direction of the person selected to coordinate CISM efforts. The steering committee usually consists of representatives from the various groups participating in the CISM team and selected mental health professionals interested in establishing the team. The tasks assigned to the steering committee include selection of staff to serve on the team and the establishment of a policy and procedures committee to develop appropriate written operating procedures. Most steering committees have a subcommittee to assure close coordination with the local CISD team and with the International Critical Incident Stress Foundation, which serves as a coordinating, standard setting, and education body for CISM teams. The steering committee also must provide appropriate training and education opportunities for the CISM team members.

The CISM team should be a peer-focused support service that uses mental health professionals and chaplains as consultants. When effectively trained, led, and allowed to do its work, a CISM team is a powerful force in maintaining healthy and happy personnel. Therefore the next commitment the administration of the agency has to make is to trust the members of the CISM team to carry out their mission without threatening the operation of the agency.

CISM teams can only function if they have an open network of communication. There must exist an effective means for emergency providers to call for CISM team assistance. In addition, there should be consistent and frequent communication with the local, regional, and national CISM networks for information exchange and mutual aid.

An important guideline is to never assume that every mental health professional is equally trained and capable of dealing appropriately with emotional trauma. Few mental health professionals receive the appropriate training to manage critical incident stress reactions; many do not have the personality necessary to manage traumatic stress. Critical incident stress management is a specialty field, and only those with the appropriate training and experience should attempt to provide it. Services by well-meaning but untrained and inexperienced individuals are inherently dangerous and seriously jeopardize the recovery of providers in the midst of traumatic stress.

Proper training cannot be overemphasized. Every member of a CISM team, regardless of previous experience and education, should go through a specialized course of education and training in CISM and PTSD management provided by a skilled and experienced critical incident stress trainer. Exceptions lead to confusion in the provision of services, misrepresentation of expertise, misunderstanding and resentment among CISM members, and poor performance in the delivery of appropriate CISM services. Inadequately trained CISM personnel are prescriptions for disaster. Team member education should be viewed as a mechanism to assure quality services, as well as an opportunity to enhance the cohesiveness of the CISM team.

Effectiveness of Critical Incident Stress Management Services

The CISM field is only a little more than a decade old, but it has already made significant progress in assisting distressed emergency providers recover and continue to function in EMS. Emergency workers who went through debriefings show less signs of distress and feel less unique in their experience. They also recover faster and experience less long-range symptoms.[3,11,12] In addition, there is a considerable volume of anecdotal information that indicates that the CISM services have positive effects. Some of the factors that make CISM service effective are listed here:

- Early Intervention—CISM services are provided when people are ready for help because their natural guards are down.
- Opportunity for emotional ventilation—Expressing emotions lowers the level of stress arousal.[6]
- Structured approach—Providing structure when a group is facing chaos is reassuring and helps people recover.
- Enhances the person's ability to form concepts—The brain's ability to categorize experiences is vital to recovery from trauma. The debriefing process urges this type of concept formation.
- Group support—It is easier for people to recover from traumatic stress if they realize that they are not alone and not unusual in their reactions to the traumatic event.
- Peer support—It is easier to recover when the process is guided by people experienced in emergency services.
- Allows for follow-up—Much of the actual support work associated with CISM services is accomplished after initial services such as defusings and debriefings have been provided. The first contacts with the personnel can be used to make appropriate referrals to psychological services when individuals in need of specialized help have been identified.

Summary

The world experienced by EMS personnel is often threatening, violent, grotesque, shocking, and demanding. It is not likely that this grim picture will change in the near future. Therefore EMS agencies face either the task of developing and implementing a comprehensive CISM program or the potential of a costly deterioration of their personnel. The medical directors of those agencies will hopefully choose a proactive stance in regard to traumatic stress; what is at stake is the most valuable resource of any organization—its people.

REFERENCES

1. Bonderoff V: Epidemic for our times: stress, *Vancouver Sun,* p. B1, B9, March 27, 1993.
2. Corneil W: Personal communication, 1992.
3. Dyregrov A: Personal communication, 1992.
4. Everly G: *A clinical guide to the treatment of the human stress response,* New York, 1989, Plenum Publishing Corp.
5. Helzer J, Robins L, and McEvoy L: Post traumatic stress disorder in the general population, *N Eng J Med* 317:1630-1634, 1987.
6. Lang P: *The application of psycho physiological methods to the study of psychotherapy and behavior modification.* In: A Bergin and Garfield S: *Handbook of psychotherapy and behavior change,* New York, 1971, John Wiley & Sons Inc.
7. McCarthy M: Stressed employees look for relief in worker's compensation claims, *Wall Street Journal,* p. 34, April 7, 1989.
8. Miller A et al: Stress on the job, *Newsweek,* p. 40-41, April 25, 1988.
9. Mitchell J and Bray G: *Emergency services stress: guidelines for preserving the health and careers of emergency personnel,* Englewood Cliffs, NJ, 1990, Brady Publishing-Prentice Hall.
10. Mitchell JT and Everly GS: *Critical incident stress debriefing: an operations manual for the prevention of traumatic stress among emergency services and disaster workers,* Ellicott City, Md, 1993, Chevron Publishing Corporation.
11. Robinson R: Personal communication, 1992.
12. Wee D: Personal communication, 1993.

Further information about a comprehensive CISM program can be obtained from the Critical Incident Stress Foundation, 5018 Dorsey Hall Drive, Suite 104, Ellicott City, MD 21042, (410)730-4311.

34

Political Survival

Norm Dinerman, M.D., FACEP

The emergence and maturation of the specialty of emergency medicine has spawned and nurtured the development of prehospital care. In turn, prehospital care has become a subspecialty itself, attracting a subset of emergency and acute care physicians whose focus of technical expertise and clinical acumen has been directed toward the provision of care from the moment of system access until the arrival of the patient at the emergency department. Original EMS medical directors were those individuals fascinated by the possibility of extending "sophisticated" methodology to the patient at the scene. Equally intriguing to them was the opportunity to provide this technical sophistication by allowing individuals to operate under the broad-based concept of "licensure-extension" of the physician. Not surprisingly, by the very nature of prehospital care itself, those physicians attracted to this specialty were captivated by the eclectic and unique attributes of medical practice in this complex arena. They were soon faced, however, with daunting challenges concerning their own creativity in the equally complex arena of politics. The multiple interfaces required of the medical director inside and outside the medical community have created an especially challenging practice in which technical expertise by itself proves insufficient in creating a workable system. Although the magnitude of this challenge is attractive to some physicians, the emotional energy required and the intense continuous interaction in the political arena may cause an abbreviated career for even the most innately passionate physicians. As with most areas of medicine and like life itself, an "apprenticeship" is the means of conveying a "practice" from veteran to neophyte. The growth and development of training programs in emergency medicine have been slow to develop "fellowships" in prehospital care, however, and our literature contains few citations on formalized approaches.[1,4,6,8,9,10]

Structure, Force, and Climate

Although there are numerous structures the medical director may work in (full-time academic, full-time public safety with academic affiliation, part-time volunteer, etc.), none guarantees success. The skillful political behavior of physicians in their role ultimately determines the success of system function and may even alter the administrative structure in which the physician resides.

Politics and economics are omnipresent forces that medical directors must interact with as they attempt to craft and manage a prehospital care system. These "forces" are usually neither familiar, understood, or embraced by individuals who originally entered the field of medicine in pursuit of the satisfaction derived from patient care. Many opportunities for frustration and disappointment thus await the unwary and idealistic physician who fails to acknowledge these forces or is unable to master their elements. Similarly, physicians who appreciate the "leverage" gained from an understanding of politics and economics are rewarded by the growth and development of their systems. Some thoughts and perspectives are herein shared to enable creative employment of these forces for the ultimate benefit of the patient and the community.

For most physicians, the difficulty and resistance to comprehending the political climate in which prehospital care activities are crafted is deeply seated. How many physicians entered medicine because of a love of politics and economics? These are not motivating factors identified on a frequent basis by anyone in medicine. In addition, few individuals are able to provide an apprenticeship for aspiring medical directors that addresses the political realities requiring mastery. Fewer still are the institutions that have committed to providing a formalized experience in prehospital care, not to mention a fellowship. The attempted metamorphosis of clinicians into political "statespersons" more often than not results in their transmogrification into a political dyslexic. The technical dexterity and intellectual prowess of the physician do not readily provide the interpersonal skills and tools for triumphing in the political arena. Furthermore the frequently misperceived position of physicians as superior to other members of the health care team seduces them into behaving as such with nonmedical individuals; this behavior produces predictable and disastrous results. Political acumen must be forged slowly over time with a mentor who nurtures the individual physician.

The disaffection for politics inherent in most health care providers accrues perhaps because of the physician's affiliation with the precepts of the "craftsman." As one of four "corporate types" defined by Maccoby in his book, *The Gamesman,* craftsman experience perhaps the greatest disparity between the reality and the ideal. It is difficult for this individual to juxtapose the desired medical goals of a "perfect" prehospital care system with the political realities in any community. Friction between value systems surface. For most the emotional cost produced by this paradigm discordance is high, and for some, it is too great to sustain a career of permanence in this aspect of emergency medicine practice. In the pursuit of quality, however, the craftsperson is handicapped by the lack of a definition easily communicated to the political veterans in the community. Quality, like style, class, poise, and pornography, tends to be an attribute of human behavior that is recognizable but poorly articulated. Political awareness is not usually imbedded in the "genetic code" of the health care practitioner. At most, it remains a gene that needs to be "turned on."

Many definitions of politics abound, but it is based on an attempt to engender, gather, manufacture, or express consensus. The relationship to the technically "ideal" system at best is viewed as oblique from the perspective of the scientifically forged physician.

The genesis of EMS systems is not founded on logic and ration. These attributes are not the legal tender in the political community. They who possess the power and the money and who "sleeps" with whom are more often the determining factors.

Although the medical director may desire an arena devoid of political influences, this is as impossible to achieve as eliminating the vagaries of human behavior itself.

Case studies

Examples of the influence of politics in medicine are ubiquitous yet often subtle. Even in the most academic aspects of prehospital care such as the creation of medical protocols for providers (for example, ACLS), the political process is operative. Most obviously, legislation to enact seat belt, helmet, and drunk driving laws must enlist widespread public support in the very citadel of the political process—the statehouse. Between these two extremes, examples of political processes such as the following operate to varying degrees.

1. Determination of hospital destination policy for ambulances
2. Designation of trauma centers
3. Creation of a unified communications center
4. Participation of a hospital in the 9-1-1 system, emergency medicine residency, or helicopter program

Other examples of the use of the political process abound but are difficult to scrutinize from a distance. They are known only by those involved in the creation of a specific program and are shared infrequently and usually in confidence. Yet it is only through the process of sharing that the "apprenticeship" process is actualized. Clearly, forums to achieve this are necessary on local and national scales. For example, the unification of the Denver prehospital care system lacked the formalized participation of the fire department in 1979. A plan was drawn up to achieve such formalized control and assure the competence of the fire fighters, serving as First Responders. When presented to the fire chief, the plan was found unacceptable for a variety of reasons not the least of which was the perception of power ceding to physicians at Denver General Hospital. The medical director then donned fire fighter's clothes, and after direct observation and participation with firefighters in the provision of emergency medical care, designed a curriculum for First Responders. This was combined with the DOT course and gained acceptance by the fire service. More important, the educational process and the creation of a more formal involvement of the fire service was embraced by a sufficient number of city officials to encourage a "reevaluation" of the position taken by the fire chief. Ultimately a document prepared by the physician emergency medicine staff and accepted by the fire service was issued as an executive order by the mayor. The process took 2 years. Although the process was cumbersome, the outcome has proven durable.

The emplacement of paramedics at Stapleton International Airport provides another example of the political process in prehospital care systems design.[3] The growth of the population in Denver at the periphery of the city (the social epiphyseal plates of the community) produced an area of increasing demand for prehospital care services. As response times increased, complaints were heard from members of the city council representing these areas. The support of councilmembers for funding a paramedic response unit on a golf cart at the airport was obtained by a citizen over sight council. The site was chosen because of its identified volume of calls (approximately 5% of the system total) and the large number that were fraudulent, canceled, or refused. By providing paramedic presence at the airport, triage could be accomplished by system paramedics, reserving the use of ambulances for those who were both ill and willing to be transported. By encouraging the airport to financially support the endeavor, a public relations benefit could be realized and the overall system performance improved without additional cost to the fiscally strapped municipal hospital. The citizen oversight council and the city council were publicly praised for their insightful and creative address of a technically complex, operationally driven solution to the problem. The paramedic presence has increased consonant with growth of the airport facility. By avoiding the obvious solution of increasing the number of ambulances serving the entire system, the overall number of paramedics remained small (maximizing individual experience rate) and increased efficiency was gained. City ambulances were available for more calls because a unique solution for the airport had been created. A byproduct of the new system was the more rapid availability of advanced life support care for airport passengers and employees. If this were the initial objective of the project, it is highly unlikely that the Stapleton International Airport Mobile Paramedic Unit (SIAMPER) would have been emplaced simply because most passengers at Stapleton Airport do not vote in Denver.

Specific Pressure Points

The approach of the medical director who is new to the community must be one of openness and great caution. While espousing an "ideal" system, the physician should identify the power blocks, which typically consist of a bouillabaisse of the following:

- Mayor, council, manager
- Fire chief
- Line fire fighter
- Prehospital care providers
- Patients
- Taxpayers
- City attorney
- Regional EMS council
- State health department

Fundamental to appreciating the appropriate movement of a system is the physician's understanding of the pressure points within it. This knowledge requires patience, a willingness to invest time in each of the aforementioned principals, and an ability to discern the history of the present situation. A pivotal mission for physician advisers is to reframe, refocus, and redefine the agendas of others. Clearly, they must become intimate with the capabilities and desires of each provider group and the position of government leaders before choreographing a new system of prehospital care for the community.

Principles of Philosophy, Perspective, and Bias

The following five political senses require mastery.

A sense of mission—Your mission, that of the specialty, and that of the institution should first be defined then amalgamated. It also helps to frame the efforts of the medical director not only as a practice champion and political choreographer but as a genetic engineer as well. Indeed the manipulation of the system is analogous to skillfully revising the "genetic code" of the prehospital care system in the community. Although the object is to create a "superior species" of system that is more resistant to the onslaught of political viruses, one never knows what will crawl out of the petri dish 5 years from now. The mission of the EMS medical director is also that of a "steward" of the system. It is in this role as a "trustee" with a fundamental, medical, fiduciary responsibility to the patient that the physician must speak most directly.

A sense of tradition—The history of the community and its service should be studied. This provides guidance in maneuvering around the political obstacles that are barriers toward development.

A sense of position—The position of the medical director in the organization and the community, as well as the position of the service agency should be acknowledged. In addition, prehospital care (EMS) may be "positioned" technically in the practice of emergency medicine, operationally in public safety, and philosophically in public health. The ability of the medical director to articulate this categorization and relate to the individuals who inhabit these three worlds is important in determining overall success.

A sense of humor—A cheerful disposition is invaluable and should be perfected throughout the professional lifespan.

A sense of timing—The introduction of new ideas and programs should take advantage of other changes being made in the institution, community, or agency.

Principles of Planning

Goals of the organization and the individual require the achievement of excellence in five spheres—academic, operational, administrative, clinical, and community relations. The latter should be defined in the broadest possible context, including the health care provider, citizen, and every other "customer" medical directors and their agencies touch.

Understand the concept of "Political Darwinism." The political and economic topography define "reality." As the topography changes, individuals either adapt or perish. In other words, "mutate or die." Individuals that seize new and innovative management and communication styles and are alert to changes in the "big picture" can adapt the needs of the agency to the vicissitudes of politics. Always keep reality squarely in sight. Sadly, Darwinism isn't pretty.

Distinguish between politicians and those who are "political." Politicians are loyal to their constituency. Medical directors are free to be loyal to the principles of sound clinical practice. Directors' demonstrated "awareness" of the political climate in which they must work does not impugn their motives; however, they should not be apologists for their insight.

Systems evolve. The goal of system excellence is well-served and the sanity of the medical directors preserved if they appreciate the glacial time frame in which change is accomplished. Perhaps the most any one individual can hope for is to refine the system, preparing for a successor to refine it further. Yet another analogy is the "river" concept of individual efforts. Acute diversion of a river in one direction may beget spontaneous direction changes downstream for miles to come. Many if not most of these changes are unforseen.

Nurture colleagues. Patients and issues come and go. Long after colleagues have forgotten reasons for anger, they recall the unpleasantness of an interaction. Expressed alternatively, friends may come and go, but enemies accumulate. Colleagues outlast the issues and should be respected. Technical errors are more easily forgiven than those that are normative or behavioral.

Attempt to create win-win solutions to every problem. If this is impossible, ensure that both sides appreciate compromise.

Be the source, and become the force. Too often the goal of the medical director is to become the power broker in the community. By striving to become the "source" (that is, the consultative resource people turn to for guidance), medical directors soon become the force for change.

Define quality in meaningful terms. Because the definition of quality is so elusive, choose measurement parameters that are meaningful to the intended audience.

Choose realistic mentors. Mentors who are great and flawed are more likely to be emulated than those who are perceived as great and perfect. The former are seen as "human," the latter "god-like." There is hope of improving on the former but one can never reach the standards of the latter.

Observe why others fail. To be effective, one must have a good engine (innate talent), a good transmission (personality and communication skills), plenty of fuel in the tank (endurance), and a good set of windshield wipers (clear vision). It also helps to be on the most appropriate road. It is a waste to drive a Ferrari on a trail and dangerous to run a Jeep on the autobahn. When colleagues fail, observe the reasons.

Develop a shared paradigm for the staff. Stress the provision of agency services with competence, compassion, class, creativity, and credibility.

Strive to develop a demeanor and countenance that reflects an academic, intellectual and collegial approach to solving problems.

Principles of Action

Unlike the provision of police or fire suppression services, prehospital care is inextricably tethered to hospital health care politics and economics. Every transport of a patient is thus a political and economic statement. Institutional paranoia dictates that whoever controls ambulances controls the patients and the revenue. Ambulances thus become economically charged particles to be gathered by some institutions and repelled by others, depending on their fiscal "force fields." Stereotypically the trauma center may desire critically injured patients regardless of insurance status (or despite the absence of third-party coverage), but the suburban community hospital may avoid these patients in favor of the medically ill and third-party reimbursed clientele. In this economic maelstrom are medical directors, for whom none of this fiscal agenda is inherently germane, but the service they provide exists within it. Is it any wonder that such an individual perceives the political and economic topography as foreign if not hostile?

To steer an academically neutral course is an ordeal that has daunted many. No wonder the physician adviser feels like Harrison Ford, slashing through the political and economic vegetation! The following principles may aid physicians in their task.

An understanding if not a mastery of political judo is encouraged. As with their physical counterpart, politically diminutive physicians must understand the simple but effective maneuvers necessary to tumble opponents in the desired direction. The political agility of medical directors accrues from their allegiance to principles of medicine, not to a political constituency or the egomaniacal forces of their opponent.

Before pushing the first domino, know where the last one falls. Do not be tempted by the seductively easy "win," unless all the political connections of opponents are known. It is better to be the one who sets up the dominoes than one who pushes them. Natural political forces will cause one to fall eventually. Wise medical directors spend years establishing the desired directions they should fall, content that fate or circumstance will eventually tumble the first one.

The movements of the chess game are instructive. The pawn that slowly moves ahead can be as effective as any other "chesspiece." At any moment in time, the chessboard can be upset, moving all the pieces in different and unpredictable directions. For example, the regulatory bureaucracy may decree new and innovative torment for all or a new mayor may be elected. Public officials rapidly acquire a global perspective of each piece on the chessboard as well. As with the professional tournament athlete, consistent performance over time usually creates substantial success.

Covet identified problems. Complaints may be seen as "opportunities in drag." They permit creative manipulation of the system and insight into behavioral issues that must be addressed. The medical director plays the role of "problem-solver" as much as any other single role.

Identify the relationships between people. The prehospital care system in the community is a complex political ecosystem with myriad political connections between even the most far-flung members. A movement of alteration of the power at any end of the "pond" moves the "lily pads" at the other.

Become dispensable but not openly so. As a wise physician administrator once demonstrated, place a finger in the middle of a glass of water. The finger represents the director's presence in the system or institution. Remove the finger; notice the hole that is left.

Learn to swim with sharks.[2]

- If bitten, do not bleed.
- Before recognizing another individual as a nonshark, witness docile behavior on more than one occasion.
- Rescue an injured swimmer with due regard for external and internal reasons for the individual's incapacity lest you succumb during the effort.
- Periodically give sharks a forceful punch in the nose to remind them who has power.

Stage a crisis on your own terms. When a crisis looms, ensure that it occurs at an optimal time. For example, when funding for a poison center in the community was threatened by legislative inaction, the administrator notified the press that this clinical facility was about to lose its WATS line. This was timed for release shortly before Christmas, coincident with public safety messages to parents concerning the potential poisonous nature of Christmas foliage. The legislature authorized the funding before the holiday recess.

Be a political chameleon. It helps to have a full set of costumes for the projection of a panoply of images, depending on the political moment.

Identify all the customers. Too frequently, only the patient is identified as the customer. In any organization, however, internal and external customers must be satisfied, and they are not necessarily direct supervisors of the medical director. Every individual in the system who must be satisfied or at least acknowledged should be identified and never ignored.

Understand the business you are really in.[7] The medical director is a choreographer of care. The challenge is to rise above the technical image of the physician as a provider of care for only a single patient. In providing the choreography for the entire system, one cares for thousands of people and influences the well-being of people far beyond the limits of a single individual. This becomes one of the strongest motivating factors for the craftsman to continue system improvement.

Project academic passion with political neutrality. In other words, craft the system to enable acknowledgment and allegiance to medical imperatives while achieving political equanimity.

Visible power is vulnerable power. The final decision-maker enjoys the most ego-gratification and the least potential for long-term survival. The individual who is invisible and informal in the use of power is most insulated from assault but will not enjoy public adoration or recognition. Strive for a position between these two extremes, enabling a "low-profile" with a somewhat formalized power base.

Never satisfy a bureaucratic need completely, doing so causes them to forget. Partial solutions are occasional reminders to the bureaucracy of the importance of problem-solvers and the inadequacy of funding.

Control the key factors but not all. For example, medical directors must retain the power to sign-off the eligibility of each paramedic to sit for recertification. The power to "hire and fire" is thus focused on an academic arena rather than a political one.

Avoid the use of fear, embarrassment, anger, frustration, intimidation, and guilt. They are transparent and managerially myopic means of motivating behavior. They are also anti academic, anti intellectual, and anti collegial.

Survival alone defines a certain success of design and merits respect. Individuals who have existed within a system for some time have evolved successful forms of adaptation. Do not ignore what may appear to be conservative postures or clever camouflage.

Remain vigilant but not suspicious. The latter is an emotionally draining posture for confronting life.

Subject projects to the OREO analysis.

- Identify Opportunities
- Identify Resources
- Identify Expectations
- Identify Obstructions

Summary

History belongs to the person of letters, the student of language, and most of all to the master of synthesis. The individual who can amalgamate the various resources of the community and weave a tapestry involving many threads will be the individual who contributes the most to a system. Remember that institutions, professions, and communities are platforms for creativity. Respect them and ensure that they are used wisely.

Medical directors must consider their own personal evolution. The goal should be to leverage creativity at every opportunity. Assist not only a limited population of patients but an entire community. In the process, contribute to the knowledge base of the specialty and assist an entire nation. Key to this personal evolution is the need to become "more than a physician."

The EMS medical director must be a seasoned clinician (practice champion) able to move beyond the bedside and choreograph the system. The choreographers need not be the best dancers, but they must recognize who those individuals are.

Though politics and economics may appear abrasive to the physician, they are the grain of sand in the oyster that produces the pearl.

Remain professionally satisfied by performing meaningful work, identifying and placing yourself proximate to role models, keeping things eclectic, and capturing a childhood fantasy on a daily basis. Most of all, identify a vision of the medical director to enable all of the above.

REFERENCES

1. Boyle MF et al: Objectives to direct the training of emergency medicine residents on off-service rotations: emergency medical services, *J Emerg Med* 8(6):791-5, Nov-Dec 1990.
2. Cousteau V: How to swim with sharks: a primer, *Perspect Biol Med* 16(4):525-528, Summer 1973; and *Am J Nurs* 1960, Oct 1981.
3. Cwinn AA, Dinerman N, and Pons PT: Prehospital care at a major international airport, *Ann Emerg Med* 17:1042-1048, Oct 1988.
4. Dinerman N, Pons PT, and Markovchick V: The emergency medicine resident as paramedic: a prehospital in-field rotation, *J Emerg Med* 8(4):507-11, Jul-Aug 1990.
5. Maccoby M: *The gamesman: the new corporate leaders,* New York, 1976, Simon and Schuster Inc.
6. Otten EJ et al: A 4-year program to train residents in emergency medical services, *Acad Med* 64(5):275-6, May 1989.
7. Peters TJ and Waterman RH Jr: *In search of excellence: lessons from America's best run companies,* New York, 1982, Harper Collins.
8. Stewart RD, Paris PM, and Heller MB: Design of a resident in-field experience for an emergency medicine residency curriculum, *Ann Emerg Med* 16(2):175-9, Feb 1987.
9. Swor RA, Chisholm C, and Krohmer J: Model curriculum in emergency medical services for emergency medicine residencies, *Ann Emerg Med* 18(4):418-21, Apr 1989.
10. Valenzuela TD et al: Evaluation of EMS management training offered during emergency medicine residency training, *Ann Emerg Med* 18(8):812-4, Aug 1989.

Section Four

Specific Operational Problems

This penultimate section focuses on specific operational problems that every medical director will be expected to recognize and to solve, usually sooner rather than later.

The first five chapters of Section Four address infectious disease precautions and procedures, strategies to prevent inappropriate EMS utilization, protocols to safely resolve those situations when patients refuse medical assistance, interventions by nonsystem physicians and logical approaches to the cessation of resuscitation in the field.

The chapters on the medical aspects of automated external defibrillation, aeromedical responses, interfacility transports, pediatric patients, and hazardous material incidents provide even the neophyte medical director with the intellectual and philosophical tools to confidently develop authoritative and comprehensive system policies concerning these medically and politically controversial issues.

The final chapters lead the reader through some of the nuances of the undulating interfaces that exist among medical oversight, health care institutions, field care and the public, including diversions, designations, and both the local and national aspects of disaster medicine.

35

Infectious Diseases

Katherine H. West, B.S.N, M.S.Ed., CIC
Steven J. Rottman, M.D., FACEP

This chapter reviews communicable diseases that pose a risk to EMS personnel, measures for self-protection, and clinical management. Prehospital providers assume considerable personal risks that include exposures to toxic materials, burning structures, hazardous extrications, and daily "light and siren" responses. Often these hazards are visible; but all too often there is an additional risk of contracting a communicable disease because many infected patients are undiagnosed or unrecognized at the time of their EMS contact. In the past, prehospital personnel often viewed their blood splattered clothing as a symbol of being in action; however, with recent knowledge of communicable diseases, safer practice must be stressed. Each day additional unprotected communicable disease exposures are reported, and the number of occupationally acquired communicable diseases continues to grow in the health care worker community.

HIV Infection

The spread of human immunodeficiency virus (HIV) has resulted in the development of serious infection control measures for the EMS community. However, there is still a need for education about the facts and the myths concerning this virus, particularly when the many persons infected with HIV either are not aware of their infection or if they are may not be forthcoming.

Since 1981, when the Centers for Disease Control (CDC) began keeping track, nearly 300,000 cases of acquired immunodeficiency syndrome (AIDS) have been reported in the United States. It is estimated that 1.5 million Americans are infected. CDC continues to monitor, report, and make predictions regarding this disease. The most current trend noted is an increase of HIV infection in children, adolescents, and women. This trend is in direct contrast to the previously recognized high risk groups such as male homosexuals and intravenous (IV) drug abusers. There has been a rapid decline in the proportion of new AIDS cases among the gay population, from 75% of the total number in 1990 to 53% in 1991. An increase in the proportion of new cases from 15% to 24% has been noted in the IV drug user group, with a smaller increase in the proportion of new cases from 3% to 6% in the heterosexual population.[1]

In June 1988, after reviewing 10 years of study about HIV and hepatitis B virus (HBV) transmission, the CDC stated that blood, semen, and vaginal secretions posed a risk for transmission. Although not found to pose a risk, it was recommended that additional study be conducted on pericardial fluid, synovial fluid, cerebrospinal fluid, and amniotic fluid. It was additionally stated that the following bodily fluids did not pose a risk for transmission unless they contained visible blood: tears, sweat, saliva, urine, feces, vomitus, nasal secretions, and sputum.[2]

Based on that 1988 assessment, EMS providers are at risk of becoming infected with HIV by exposure resulting from a contaminated needlestick injury; splash of blood or body fluid into the eye, nose, or mouth; blood or body fluids in contact with an opening in the skin; and cuts with sharp objects covered with blood or body fluids.[3]

Since there has not been a nationally established network or protocol for the collection of information on cases of HIV exposure in the EMS community, it is difficult to document risk factors for exposure. In attempting to do so, hospital models are most frequently used, but these are not indicative of prehospital practice because they reflect a more controlled work environment. The number of cases of needlestick injury and subsequent seroconversion in the health care population reported in the literature remains low. The CDC currently reports the risk as being 0.32% for exposures.[4,5,6] Although this risk is relatively small, all members of the health care community should follow the recommended measures for self-protection. Medical directors and EMS supervisors must set the example and demonstrate ongoing support for aggressive infection control practices. In fact, monitoring for compliance is required under the Occupational Safety and Health Administration (OSHA) blood-borne pathogens standard published in December 1991.

The CDC is currently evaluating the risk of health care worker transmission of HIV to patients. Health care personnel identified as HIV positive should be handled on an individual basis with regard to their ability to function on the job.[7] The Americans With Disabilities Act should be reviewed by each medical director to ensure that policies and procedures are handled in an appropriate manner. This law has brought significant change in hiring practices. For example, no medical questions can be asked or physical examination given before offering an individual a position.[8] Areas that need to be addressed specifically in written policy format include postexposure notification, counseling, testing, postexposure prophylaxis, documentation of follow-up, and record keeping. Along with these, the maintenance of confidentiality of the information by both the physician and the employer must be ensured. It must be made clear that the employee should hold his exposure in confidence.[9,10]

As means and strategies for treatment develop, patients with AIDS are living longer. New medications have been released for the treatment of the various manifestations of this disease, and additional drugs are under investigation. However, the epidemic continues, with larger numbers of cases expected in the next few years. Education will remain the key factor in preparing personnel to optimally treat HIV-infected patients. Yet health care workers remain undereducated, and in many cases, are either careless or resistant to the use of personal protective measures. A study conducted at The Johns Hopkins Hospital in 1989, demonstrated that protective measures were used only 19% of the time and mostly with minor rather than major cases.[11] Another report showed that the implementation of universal precautions decreased exposure incidents from 5.07 to 2.66 exposures per physician per patient-care month, leading to both reduction in exposures and medical costs.[12] It must be understood that the creation of a totally risk-free environment is not possible. Thus in addition to enforcing compliance with policies and procedures for individual safety, medical directors and field supervisors should collaborate with equipment manufacturers in redesigning medical equipment with the aim of reducing exposures.[6]

Hepatitis Viruses

Since the 1950s, when the only recognized forms of hepatitis were A and B, researchers have discovered types C, D, and E, with additional viruses likely to be identified.[13] Of these viruses, hepatitis B and hepatitis C present the greatest risk for EMS workers.[13]

Hepatitis B

Hepatitis B has long been identified as a great risk to health care personnel. But the risk specifically for EMS personnel was only first assessed in 1983. In that Boston study, it was determined that EMS personnel were at 3 to 5 times greater risk than the general public for acquiring HBV occupationally.[14] Other studies from Seattle and Houston document similar degrees of risk.[15,16] The risk of acquiring HBV from an infected patient via a needlestick injury has been reported at between 6% and 30%.[1,16] Since up to 60% of infected patients do not exhibit any signs or symptoms, protective measures must be mandatory with all patients in the uncontrolled emergency environment.[17] HBV is much more hardy than HIV. It can survive on a surface for days and still pose a risk of transmission, whereas this does not pose a risk for HIV transmission. A history of HBV has also been linked to a high incidence of liver cancer. It has been estimated that each year approximately 8,900 health care workers become infected with HBV and that more than 250 die as a result of this disease.

Vaccination effectively prevents HBV infection. OSHA has mandated that hepatitis B vaccine be offered free to EMS personnel. Recommended immunizations for emergency personnel are the following:

1. Hepatitis B vaccine
2. Tetanus-diphtheria boosters every 10 years
3. Measles, mumps, rubella vaccine
4. PPD TB skin testing
5. Yearly flu vaccine[10,22]

This rule was put into effect via a Compliance Directive (CPL 202.44B) issued February 27, 1990 and became law with publication of the final rule on December 6, 1991. Vaccine must be offered within days of assignment to a position that would place the individual at risk. Every EMS service must have a vaccine program in place. Participation in the program is voluntary on the part of EMS personnel. Each service must also have a protocol for medical follow-up for exposure to HBV (Figure 35-1), and each member of the department should be familiar with it. Failure to comply with these regulations subjects the service to fines up to $70,000. A hepatitis vaccine program has four important aspects: education regarding both the vaccine and the disease, informed consent or documented nonparticipation, voluntary participation, and adequate record keeping. The medical director must ensure that a program is in operation and must evaluate employee participation. If low participation is noted, additional education to increase compliance must be provided. OSHA requires documentation of all these activities.[18]

Non-A/Non-B Hepatitis

Three distinct viruses, hepatitis C, hepatitis D, and hepatitis E, have been identified. Two additional viruses are expected to be identified in the near future. Hepatitis C virus (HCV) poses a risk to emergency personnel. It is transmitted in much the same way as HBV.[17] Identification of this virus has recently lead to availability of a screening test. It is estimated that 150,000 cases of this disease are reported each year in the United States. EMS medical directors should develop a protocol for exposure follow-up, which provides for screening emergency patients who are possible sources of the infection. The medication of choice for postexposure prophylaxis against HCV is immune serum globulin. Dosage is based on body weight.

Airborne Diseases

The Federal AIDS Prevention Act of 1990, often called the Ryan White Law, contains a provision for mandatory notification for emergency response personnel who are exposed to either airborne or bloodborne diseases. Medical directors must insure that the staff of EMS agencies under their direction be made aware of the very specific steps in the notification process.[19] The responsibility to report airborne disease exposures to EMS personnel and to track them falls on the receiving hospital since providers may not be aware of the airborne exposure.

Tuberculosis

The worst outbreak of tuberculosis (TB) in over 40 years was reported by CDC in 1990. It includes cases of antibiotic-resistant strains of the disease previously not seen. Groups at high risk include the homeless, nursing home residents, Asian immigrants, inmates, and the HIV-infected population.[1]

The differences between TB and atypical TB are unfamiliar to most prehospital EMS personnel. Education is important to help workers take rational steps to avoid infection. Measures for self-protection must be explained, especially in areas where TB is prevalent. Medical directors should keep abreast of the number of cases reported in their given areas and insure that local protocols for postexposure follow-up are current. INH remains the current drug for prophylaxis. However, with the incidence of drug resistant strains of TB, prophylaxis must be evaluated on an individual basis. All emergency personnel should be screened for TB and then tested on a routine basis.[20,21] For individuals who previously tested positive, a follow-up chest x-ray is not required unless symptoms develop. OSHA requires annual chest x-rays for employees such as firefighters who use self-contained breathing apparatus. The National Fire Protection Association (NFPA) has published standards addressing this area. Each service should obtain a copy.[22]

All TB exposures must be reported promptly and medical follow-up should be in accordance with the current CDC recommendations. The CDC guidelines published in December 1990 list many new considerations and should be reviewed and updated to ensure compliance. For example, specific guidelines exist for ventilation and mask usage. The CDC recommends the use of particulate filter respirator (PR) style masks, although no data supports the effectiveness of PR masks over that of molded masks. To be most effective, the PR mask should be placed on the patient.[20,21]

Meningitis

Meningitis has two major forms, viral and bacterial. When an employee is exposed to meningitis, a gram stain of the spinal fluid should be ordered to provide an indication of the type of causal agent. Because of the short incubation period for some forms of meningitis (1 to 3 days), time is of the essence in providing adequate prophylaxis. Notification, documentation, and medical follow-up are requirements under the law. An infection control officer should be designated to ensure that these requirements are met. The role of this individual is outlined in the Ryan White Law.[19] Although the actual law states that the public health officer should appoint this person, it is probably more practically done by the medical director. Of special note, OSHA requires that records with specific information including the date and time of exposure, job duty being performed during exposure, details of exposure, description of source of exposure, and details on counselling and follow-up treatment be maintained for the duration of employment plus thirty years.[19,26]

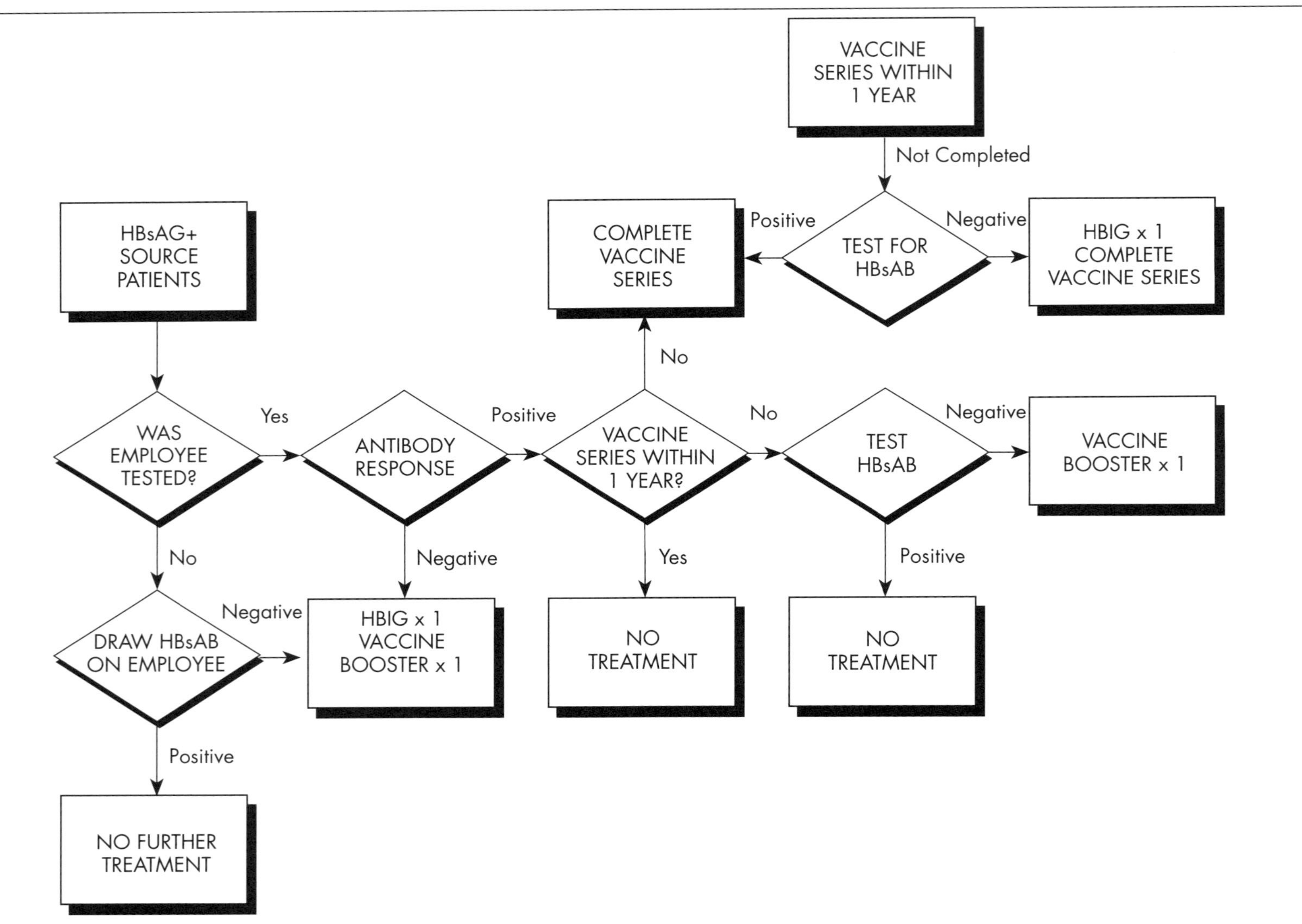

Figure 35-1. Post vaccine needlestick protocol. Modified from West K: *Infection control,* Springfield, Va, Emerging Concepts Inc.)

OSHA also requires that each agency have an exposure control program. The components of this program shall include: health records for each member, education regarding infection control and bloodborne pathogens. Blood-borne pathogens to be included in the training are HBV, HCV, HIV, and syphillis. This should be provided on hire and on a yearly basis, an immunization program for HBV, a notification process, medical follow-up protocols, compliance monitoring and engineering controls to reduce risk.[18] Figure 35-2 illustrates a form for documenting these activities.

Under NFPA guidelines, fire and rescue personnel should have HBV vaccinations, a tetanus-diphtheria booster, TB skin testing in addition to measles, mumps, rubella and yearly flu vaccine offerings. Fire departments have the option of using NFPA standards. However, such "standard of care" guidelines may have an influence in legal cases as they set a national standard.

Body Substance Isolation

The CDC and OSHA have published formal guidelines and regulations outlining measures for self-protection of emergency response personnel. These measures are also NFPA guidelines. In defining universal precautions "all blood and *certain* body fluids are to be considered infectious."[2] However, since the working conditions in the field make it difficult to ascertain if there is blood contamination of a fluid, emergency personnel should treat all body fluids as infectious. The terminology for this broader approach is body substance isolation (BSI) and this is an acceptable practice under the final OSHA regulations.[10]

OSHA requires that employers must furnish and make readily available personal protective equipment (PPE). As defined, PPE includes the following items: masks, protective eyewear, protective clothing and equipment, disposable gloves, heavy duty utility gloves for cleaning, firefighter gloves for handling sharp items, surfaces, cover gowns or a change of uniform, and waterless handwash solutions.[6,19,22,23] The box on p. 359 gives a comprehensive listing of appropriate personal protection equipment and practices.

The OSHA rules have brought many everyday practices into question. For example, can uniforms serve as PPE? If the employer determines that uniforms are PPE, then cleaning must be under the employer's "control."[24] This means that fire stations must either contract a laundry service or place washers and dryers in stations in order to avoid the cost of purchasing large numbers of cover gowns. While cover gowns should be available for potential large splash situations, reality is that the opportunity for their use is small.

Under the final OSHA rules, eating is not permitted in the vehicle if there is either body fluid present or if clothing is contaminated. Once the unit has been cleaned or clothing changed then you can eat there. A unit can carry scrubs in case a uniform is soiled and there is no time to return to the station before meal time.[24] The cleaning of contaminated vehicles and equipment should be performed immediately after patient transport, ideally at the hospital. Cleaning, disinfecting, and sterilizing of equipment is best done through an exchange program with the receiving medical facility, since most EMS stations do not have the proper equipment, training or controls to effectively monitor reprocessing of patient care equipment.[23] The boxes on p. 360 and 361 give recommendations for cleaning and disinfection.

Summary

Emergency care personnel commonly encounter patients with communicable diseases. The risk for acquiring an infection from these patients is real and has been documented. Because of the current epidemics of measles and TB, it is as important to follow up exposures to airborne diseases as to bloodborne diseases. Medical directors must remain current with the CDC, OSHA, and NFPA recommendations on infectious exposures and should assist in the development and management of the agency's exposure control plan, especially the notification and medical follow-up of exposures. The interaction between the medical director, the hospital, and the designated infection control officer is critical for the proper functioning of the plan. The measures outlined in this chapter will assist in reducing both exposures and liability. A strong exposure control program assists in the recruitment and the retention of employees by demonstrating concern for the provider in the current health care work place.

REFERENCES

1. HIV/AIDS Surveillance: *AIDS ALERT* 6(11):223, 1991.
2. Universal precautions for prevention of transmission of human immunodeficiency virus, hepatitis b virus, and other bloodborne pathogens in health-care settings, *MMWR* 37(24):377, 1988.
3. Joint Advisory Notice: Protection against occupational exposure to hepatitis b virus (HBV) and human immunodeficiency virus (HIV), October 19, 1987, Department of Labor/Department of Health and Human Services.
4. Gerberding JL: HIV transmission to providers and their patients, *The medical management of AIDS,* ed 3, Philadelphia, 1992, W. B. Saunders.

Text continued on p. 362.

EMPLOYEE-REPORTED EXPOSURE TO INFECTIOUS DISEASE
SCREENING/FOLLOW-UP PROCEDURE

S.S. # ____________________ Time ____________________

Employee's name ____________________ Position ____________________

Occurrence date ____________________ Reported date ____________________

Employee's reported description of the exposure:

____

____

____

Follow-up:
Contact source [ ] Chart reviewed: ____________ No contact source [ ]

Contact source laboratory test results:
SGOT ________ HBsAG________ STS________ HIV________ Other____________________

Employee's health file reviewed ____________________ Results____________________

Laboratory test ordered ____________________

Immunizations offered/recommended:
ISG [ ] HBIG [ ] Hepatitis [ ] Diptheria/Tetanus [ ] PPD [ ]

Other____________________

Attending physician's comments:

____

____

____

Signature ____________________ Date ____________________

Hospital Infection Control nurse notified of the exposure ____________________

Comments:

____

____

____

Signature ____________________ Date____________________

Referred to Infectious Disease physician: Yes [ ] No [ ] Appointment____________________

Recommendations:

____

____

____

Figure 35-2. Employee-reported exposure to infectious disease screening follow-up procedure. (Modified from Infection Control in the Emergency Department, West, KH, 1987.)

Examples of Recommended Personal Protection for Worker Protection Against HIV and HBV Transmission in Prehospital Settings*

Task or activity	Disposable gloves	Gown	Mask	Protective eyewear
Bleeding control with spurting blood	Yes	Yes	Yes	Yes
Bleeding control with minimal bleeding	Yes	No	No	No
Emergency childbirth	Yes	Yes	Yes, if splashing is likely	Yes, if splashing is likely
Blood drawing	At certain times[†]	No	No	No
Starting an intravenous (IV) line	Yes	No	No	No
Endotracheal intubation, esophageal obturator use	Yes	No	No, unless splashing is likely	No, unless splashing is likely
Oral/nasal suctioning, manually clearing airway	Yes[‡]	No	No, unless splashing is likely	No, unless splashing is likely
Handling and cleaning instruments with microbial contamination	Yes	No, unless soiling is likely	No	No
Measuring blood pressure	No	No	No	No
Measuring temperature	No	No	No	No
Giving an injection	No	No	No	No

*The examples provided in this table are based on application of universal precautions. Universal precautions are intended to supplement rather than replace recommendations for routine infection control, such as handwashing and using gloves to prevent gross microbial contamination of hands (e.g., contact with urine or feces).

[†]Gloves should be worn for phlebotomy if cuts, scratches or other breaks in the skin are present on the worker's hands, if the worker is inexperienced, or the situation suggests a greater possibility of bleeding.

[‡]While not clearly necessary to prevent HIV or HBV transmission unless blood is present, gloves are recommended to prevent transmission of other agents (e.g., Herpes simplex).

From *Centers for Disease Control, February 1989.*

Reprocessing Methods for Equipment Used in the Prehospital Health-Care Setting

Sterilization

Destroys: All forms of microbial life including high numbers of bacterial spores.

Methods: Steam under pressure (autoclave), gas (ethylene oxide), dry heat, or immersion in EPA-approved chemical "sterilant" for prolonged period of time, e.g., 6-10 hours or according to manufacturers' instructions. Note: liquid chemical "sterilants" should be used only on those instruments that are impossible to sterilize or disinfect with heat.

Use: For those instruments or devices that penetrate skin or contact normally sterile areas of the body, e.g., scalpels, needles, etc. Disposable invasive equipment eliminates the need to reprocess these types of items. When indicated, however, arrangements should be made with a health-care facility for reprocessing of reusable invasive instruments.

High-level disinfection

Destroys: All forms of microbial life except high numbers of bacterial spores.

Methods: Hot water pasteurization (80-100° C, 30 minutes) or exposure to an EPA-registered chemical "sterilant" as above, except for a short exposure time (10-45 minutes or as directed by the manufacturer).

Use: For reusable instruments or devices that come into contact with mucous membranes (e.g., laryngoscope blades, endotracheal tubes, etc.).

Intermediate-level disinfection

Destroys: *Mycobacterium tuberculosis,* vegetative bacteria, most viruses, and most fungi, but does not kill bacterial spores.

Methods: EPA-registered "hospital disinfectant" chemical germicides that have a label claim for tuberculocidal activity; commercially available hard-surface germicides or solutions containing at least 500 ppm free-available chlorine (a 1:100 dilution of common household bleach—approximately 1/4 cup bleach per gallon of tap water).

Use: For those surfaces that come into contact only with intact skin, e.g., stethoscopes, blood pressure cuffs, splints, etc., and have been visibly contaminated with blood or bloody body fluids. Surfaces must be precleaned of visible material before the germicidal chemical is applied for disinfection.

Low-level disinfection

Destroys: Most bacteria, some viruses, some fungi, but not *Mycobacterium tuberculosis* or bacterial spores.

Methods: EPA-registered "hospital disinfectants" (no label claim for tuberculocidal activity).

Use: These agents are excellent cleaners and can be used for routine housekeeping or removal of soiling in the absence of visible blood contamination.

Environmental Disinfection: Environmental surfaces which have become soiled should be cleaned and disinfected using any cleaner or disinfectant agent which is intended for environmental use. Such surfaces include floors, woodwork, ambulance seats, countertops, etc.

IMPORTANT: To assure the effectiveness of any sterilization or disinfection process, equipment and instruments must first be thoroughly cleaned of all visible soil.

From *Centers for Disease Control, February 1989.*

Recommendations for Decontamination and Cleaning of Rescue Vehicles

Clean-Up kit

Household utility gloves
Plastic spray bottle with cleaning agent
Plastic spray bottle with disinfectant solution or bottle with concentrated household bleach to be diluted with water (1:100 dilution approximates 1/4 cup bleach per gallon of water)
Disposable toweling
Plastic bags (hospital red bags, household plastic bags)
Basket/carrier to hold cleaning supplies

Clean-Up procedure for after each call

1. **Prepare vehicle for cleaning/decontamination**
   a. Always wear utility gloves throughout clean-up procedure.
   b. Remove used or soiled linen and place in designated bag for laundering. Either leave laundry at the hospital or reprocess in the EMS laundry using warm water, detergent, and bleach as recommended on the product labels.
   c. Discard any soiled dressings, bloody materials, and other contaminated, non-sharps waste in a red bag and leave at the hospital.
   d. Place reusable equipment which needs reprocessing in plastic bag (any color other than red).
   e. Check the vehicle for any needles or other sharps which may have been left and carefully dispose in a sharps container.
2. **Check for areas soiled with blood and other visible body substances and remove.**
   a. Remove moist blood and other body substances with paper toweling and discard in a red bag.
   b. Spray cleaner on affected area and remove any remaining blood or body substance. Dispose of towels in red bag.
   c. Spray disinfectant on affected area, wipe over the surface, and allow to air dry. Dispose of towels in red bag.
3. **Spray cleaner on remaining surfaces with which the patient had contact as well as surfaces which were used in the course of providing prehospital care. Wipe the surface with toweling and allow to air dry.**

Periodic Cleaning of Rescue Vehicles

On a regular basis (e.g., weekly, monthly), as determined by the frequency of vehicle use and obvious need, the floors, walls, interior and exterior of cabinets and drawers, benches, and other surfaces, should be thoroughly cleaned. The same cleaning agent used between cases can be used for this more extensive cleaning. A supply kit should be kept in a central location for this purpose (e.g., pail, reusable cleaning cloths that are laundered after use, supply of cleaning agents). Wipe with toweling and allow to air dry.
Since carpeting and permeable seat cover in the patient compartment of ambulances are more difficult to clean than non-permeable surfaces, their use is not recommended.
NOTE: Bleach solution should be made up fresh at the time of use or daily.

5. Guidelines for prevention of transmission of human immunodeficiency virus and hepatitis b virus to health-care and public safety workers, US Department of Health and Human Services, February, 1989.
6. Jagger J, Hunt EH, and Pearson RD: Estimated cost of needlestick injuries for six major needled devices, *Am J Infection Control* 11(11):584, 1992.
7. Recommendations for preventing transmission of human immunodeficiency virus and hepatitis b virus to patients during exposure-prone invasive procedures, *MMWR* 40:1992.
8. Americans With Disabilities Act, 1993.
9. Estimates of the risk of endemic transmission of hepatitis b virus and human immunodeficiency virus to patients by the Percutaneous Route During Invasive Surgical and Dental Procedures, (draft), January 30, 1991, Atlanta, Centers for Disease Control.
10. Occupational exposure to bloodborne pathogens, Proposed rule and notice of hearing, *Federal Register,* May 30, 1989.
11. Kelen GD et al: Human immunodeficiency virus infection in emergency department patients; epidemiology, clinical presentations, and risk to health care workers: The Johns Hopkin's Experience, *JAMA,* 262(4):516, 1989.
12. Wong ES et al: Are universal precautions effective in reducing the number of occupational exposures among health care workers? *JAMA,* 265(9):1123, 1991.
13. Lever AM: Non A/non B hepatitis: *J Hosp Infect* supplement A: 150, 1988.
14. Kunches LM et al: Hepatitis B exposures in emergency medical personnel: prevalence of serologic markers and need for immunization, *Am J Med* 75:269, 1983.
15. Pepe PE et al: Viral hepatitis risk in urban emergency medical services personnel, *Ann Emerg Med,* 15:454, 1986.
16. Valenzuela TD et al: Occupational exposure to hepatitis B in paramedics, *Arch Internal Med,* 145, 1985.
17. Protection against viral Hepatitis: Recommendations of the immunization practices advisory committee (ACIP), *MMWR,* 39(RR–2):1990.
18. 29 CFR Part 1910.1030: Occupational exposure to bloodborne pathogens, final rule, December 6, 1992. Department of Labor.
19. Public Law 101–381: Ryan White comprehensive AIDS resources Emergency Act of 1990.
20. West KH: A new epidemic: tuberculosis, *Rescue-EMS,* May/June 24–27, 1991.
21. Guidelines for preventing the transmission of tuberculosis in health-care settings with special focus on HIV-related issues, *MMWR,* 39(RR–17):1990.
22. National Fire Protection Association (NFPA–1581): Voted May 1991.
23. West KH: *Infectious disease handbook for emergency care personnel,* Philadelphia, 1987, JB Lippincott.
24. Compliance Directive CPL 2–2.44C: Occupational Safety and Health Administration, 1992, Department of Labor.
25. 29 CFR Part 1910.20: Access to medical records, 1990.

36

Inappropriate Use

Laurie Ann Otto, M.D.

Inappropriate use of the EMS system constitutes a large percentage of the calls in many systems. Not only are these calls expensive but since most systems have limited resources inappropriate usage of the system decreases the number of responding units available for true emergencies.

The term EMS misuse is preferred over EMS abuse. In most systems, inappropriate 9-1-1 calling is attributed more to the lack of public education regarding the purpose of EMS systems than it is to malicious intent. Blatant abuse is a small portion of the problem.

Causes of Abuse

Numerous reasons can be cited for why EMS is summoned for nonemergent problems. The following causes blend together to help explain why misuse is so rampant.

Ignorance

Many persons lack a fundamental understanding of what constitutes a true medical emergency. The caller's definition of an emergency is frequently not equivalent to that of a health care worker's. In the medical literature, an emergency is defined as a clinical condition which is life-threatening (requires immediate intervention to prevent death) or urgent (poses a threat to life and/or risk of disability without timely treatment).[15,18]

Transportation

All too frequently the EMS system is viewed as a free taxi service to the medical center. This attitude especially prevails in urban areas where large numbers of people do not have access to private vehicles and cannot afford alternative transportation which requires payment at time of transport.

Facilitation

Arriving at the hospital by ambulance frequently provides one with more expedient service than arriving by alternative means. Frequent users of emergency services quickly recognize this fact. Occasionally a patient who tires of sitting in the emergency department waiting room leaves the hospital and calls EMS from a few blocks away for transport back to the emergency department with the hope of obtaining quicker service.

Advice

Many people believe EMS provide "house calls." Persons placing such calls may have no desire for conveyance to a hospital but rather seek a medical opinion or want basic first aid.

Secondary Gain

Often persons who call EMS do not require emergency treatment but desire the attention the EMS crew and hospital personnel provide. This is frequently observed in patients who have stable chronic medical conditions or who have personality disorders.

Scope

The misuse of EMS systems is a widespread and longstanding problem. Estimates of inappropriate EMS use range from 31% to 66%.* In Erie County,

*References 8,9,14,15,18

New York, 1787 patients received ambulance transport during four weeks in 1972–1973. Following a retrospective chart review, a nurse categorized 563 (31%) of the patients as clinically not requiring an ambulance.[9]

In 1978, Morris and Cross analyzed 1000 consecutive patients who called for help and were transported by ambulance to a busy British emergency department. Patients were categorized according to their need for ambulance transport based on discharge diagnosis, age, and social state. They found 51.7% of the ambulance transports were unnecessary and that medical cases accounted for a greater percentage of necessary calls than did trauma and surgical cases.[14]

In 1987, O'Leary published an overall ambulance justification rate of 66% for a 2 month period in Dublin, Ireland. Ambulance need decisions were based on a retrospective chart review looking at condition severity and emergency department disposition.[15]

Gerson and Skvarch analyzed 1980 data from the Akron EMS system and reported that approximately one third of both patient groups who called for an ambulance, those 65 years of age and older and those under 65 years of age, did not require immediate ambulance transport to the hospital.[8]

In four Canadian cities between November 1980 and November 1981, 6405 patients who presented to emergency departments were categorized by a nurse as either needing or not needing an ambulance. The assessment was made after patient observation and chart review. Patients were divided by condition severity into emergent, urgent A (urgent and in need of ambulance transport), urgent B (urgent but not requiring ambulance transport), and routine. Patients in the emergent and urgent A categories were considered to need an ambulance. Out of the 6405 total patients, 518 (8%) arrived by ambulance of which 217 (42%) were considered to have used the ambulance inappropriately.[18]

Prevention

Since each EMS system is unique with its own set of problems and available resources, no single approach to confronting misuse fits all situations. There is a general consensus, however, that educating the public and health care community is crucial in combatting EMS misuse.[7,14,25]

Kerr and Byrd's study of nursing home patients transferred to the Veteran's Administration emergency department by ambulance found nearly half the study group could have been treated at the nursing home by a visiting physician with minimal medical equipment. Ambulance transport was used not only for patients with emergent conditions but also for patients who were difficult to transport sitting, patients who required supervision because of disruptive behavior, and for inexplicable reasons in patients with minor complaints.[12]

Many cities have undertaken multi-media campaigns in an attempt to educate people regarding appropriate 9-1-1 usage. These campaigns have included nightly news segments, cable TV videos, public service announcements, newspaper articles, and presentations to community group gatherings. Some cities have also sent informational letters to nursing homes and physicians describing when and when not to access 9-1-1. There is always the danger that public education will increase the call volume of both appropriate and inappropriate calls.

Beneficial results are difficult to measure with public education campaigns. Many of the cities which employed the education campaigns felt they were useful but did not formally study their effectiveness. For two months in 1987, an intense education campaign targeted at patients who were at risk for coronary artery disease was undertaken in King County, Washington. The campaign stressed the symptoms of an acute myocardial infarction along with the importance of acting quickly and calling 9-1-1. The study groups consisted of patients who consented to a telephone interview four to eight weeks following discharge from an intensive or coronary care unit for chest pain in the pre-message time period (401 patients) and the post-message time period (489 patients). Significantly more patients in the post-message time period heard new information about acute myocardial infarction than patients in the pre-message time period. However, there was no significant change in the proportion of patients who reported hearing the importance of early treatment or calling 9-1-1. The time delay in seeking treatment and the usage of 9-1-1 did not change significantly between the two groups.[11]

Transport Policies

Besides decreasing inappropriate 9-1-1 utilization through better education each EMS system has the option of setting transport policies. Most systems do not have such formal protocols in place and when a policy to refuse transport does exist it is usually done on a case by case basis rather than by general guidelines.[19]

Denying transport significantly increases system liability.* The concern exists that if a formal policy to

*References 8,9,14,15,18

combat frequent misuse is not implemented field personnel will informally "triage-out" patients without authorization or may convince patients that they do not need to be transported.[4] Such cases are frequently documented by the crew as "patient refuses transport."[22] The medical director may remain unaware of this practice until problems arise.

Once a provider "suggests" that the ambulance is not necessary, it is inappropriate for the system to treat the call as a refusal of medical assistance since the legal risks are as great as when a patient is left against their will. This aspect of the topic is further discussed in the chapter on refusal of medical assistance.

If a refusal policy is to be established there are two periods when formal guidelines or algorithms can be applied: call screening and scene triage. Call screening is riskier because no face-to-face patient assessment has occurred. The decision to deny service is based only on the telephone interview. Criteria for refusal at this stage needs to be well defined. Types of calls that may be considered for refusal to send during call screening include: (1) the desire to have a prescription filled, (2) the desire to be taken to a clinic appointment, and (3) the desire to have a nonemergent chronic condition evaluated. Scene triage is more common but can be more complex and may involve contact with a physician for approval. It is less risky because it allows for a decision to be made after an actual patient assessment.

Specific Approaches

Most cities in the United States do not have specific protocols in place for confronting EMS misuse; however, some have established extensive guidelines. Milwaukee, New York, Pittsburgh, St. Louis, and Salt Lake City all have very different written, predetermined approaches to deal with the problem.

Milwaukee

Milwaukee has a two-tiered system. All calls are triaged using a computer-aided dispatch system. All nonemergency calls are assigned to private EMT-A ambulance companies. If a complaint is deemed to require paramedic care or if the level of care is undetermined, a fire engine company and a paramedic ambulance are dispatched. The fire engine company, staffed by EMT-A's almost always arrives on the scene first. If the engine company does not feel that paramedics are required, the ambulance is canceled and a private ambulance is summoned. Paramedic transportation is provided free of charge by the city whereas the private ambulance companies bill for their services.

Milwaukee's triage and transport policy identifies patients in whom the circumstances are believed to present a high potential for serious injury or illness and, as such, require paramedic care and transport. The policy does not delineate types of patients who should be transferred to the private EMT-A units. Milwaukee's policy identifies the following patients as requiring a paramedic transport[13]:

> (1) individuals who have fallen a vertical distance of 15 or more feet, (2) those in whom there is a high degree of suspicion of cervical injury, (3) any patient who is in the care of his medical doctor and the physician requests paramedic transport, (4) tricyclic overdoses regardless of presenting symptoms, (5) individuals with abnormal vital signs, (6) any individual whose history or physical exam indicates a potentially life-threatening problem and (7) any individual who has been involved in trauma and has required prolonged or complicated extrication.

Questions on specific cases are addressed at monthly quality management meetings involving the private companies, the fire departments, and the paramedic staff. Although this system may not be a strong deterrent for 9-1-1 misuse, it does keep the paramedic ambulances available for persons who truly do require their services.

New York

New York City has had a scene triage system in effect since 1985. If field personnel, after completing a history, a physical exam, and treatment, believe a patient does not require emergency direct medical care or is not sufficiently ill or injured to necessitate emergency transport to a hospital, the field team contacts and discusses the situation with direct medical control. If the physician agrees that the person does not require transport, the patient is so informed. The patient is also given a document which explains that if his condition changes he is to call medical control directly, not 9-1-1. Field personnel cannot refuse transport without physician contact.[16] This system is seldom used. Many field personnel maintain they are at risk when asking the physician for a triage decision and that it does not save time. Even if transport is denied, a complete patient evaluation and all the normal paperwork plus the forms must be completed along with contacting a physician. Frequent-ly it is easier to transport the patient than go through the entire procedure. (see Appendix I.) The full value of this law and the procedure will be as an adjunct to "treat and release" EMS primary care.

Pittsburgh

To combat EMS misuse, Pittsburgh implemented a multiphase plan. The plan started with an extensive multimedia campaign aimed at educating the population on appropriate usage of 9-1-1. The campaign included numerous press releases and half-hour television programs on the three government cable channels. In addition, information letters were sent to physicians and nursing homes. To keep down costs, the use of press releases and free advertising was maximized. The remainder of the program was funded with budgeted city tax dollars. In August 1990, following the education campaign, crews began to identify runs that did not require prehospital treatment or where alternative means of transportation could have been utilized. During this phase, patients were transported as usual. A letter explaining when to call 9-1-1 was sent to all individuals who were identified as inappropriately using the system.[1] The third phase of the plan started in January 1991. It allowed denial of transport after evaluation. In some circumstances, physician consultation was not required.

A physician contact was needed to deny treatment or transport for the following[2]:

> (1) history of loss of consciousness, current mental status changes, slurred speech, evidence for illicit drug intoxication, (2) any complaint related to the cardiovascular system (shortness of breath, chest pain, dizziness, syncope, abnormal heart rate, abnormal blood pressure), (3) patients in which there is either a mechanism of injury or physical signs that suggest possible head or neck injury and (4) any abnormal vital signs.

Without physician contact, the crew could refuse treatment or transport for[2]:

> (1) patients with no indication of immediate significant illness or injury, (2) patients who have had no recent change in a chronic condition . . . (3) a child with a fever without evidence for altered mental status, seizure activity, airway compromise and who is in the presence of an adult caregiver, (4) routine transfers to hospitals for elective admission or evaluation (5) pregnant patients who are primigravida and whose contractions are greater than ten minutes apart, (6) patients with isolated small (less than one inch) distal extremity lacerations without evidence for arterial bleeding or motor dysfunction and (7) patients without a medical complaint.

Salt Lake City

In June 1979, Salt Lake City officials passed an EMS Abuse Ordinance stating that any person who makes an unlawful request of service by summoning the Salt Lake City Fire Department EMS system to "respond unnecessarily, falsely, capriciously or for non-emergent situations" shall be guilty of a misdemeanor and may be punished by a fine up to $299 and/or 6 months in jail. The EMS Abuse Ordinance defines nonemergency situations as[20]:

> alcohol intoxication, minor lacerations, minor contusion and sprains, minor illnesses, insect and animal bites not deemed emergencies, rash and skin disorders, hives without dyspnea (difficulty breathing), home delivery to avoid doctor and hospital services, venereal disease, patients seeking non-emergency transportation, forehead and scalp lacerations only, cold syndrome, sore throat, earache, hiccough, nervousness, anxiety, toothache, minor bruises, non-life–threatening overdoses, and non-life–threatening self-inflicted injuries.

All sworn members of the fire department have the legal authority to issue misdemeanor citations and can directly cite violators of the EMS Abuse Ordinance. If the abuse is only suggested and it is a minor or first offense a warning may be issued. The offender is read the entire ordinance and an EMS abuse report filed. If there is blatant or repeated abuse, a copy of the ordinance is given to the person and a citation issued. By signing the citation, the offender agrees to appear in court. If the offender refuses to sign, the police are summoned and the offender arrested. Salt Lake City EMS officials estimate thirty to forty arrests are made per year. EMS personnel are subpoenaed to court only if the person pleads "not guilty."[21]

Public service announcements combined with the EMS Abuse Ordinance did have a positive impact in decreasing inappropriate use of 9-1-1 in Salt Lake City. The ordinance was designed to discourage inappropriate 9-1-1 use and was not specifically intended to punish misuse.

St. Louis

St. Louis is an EMS system with each ambulance staffed by a paramedic and an EMT-A. The city has a high volume of 9-1-1 calls considering its size and population. At the communication center, calls are triaged and prioritized by paramedics and EMT-As using a priority dispatch system. No caller is denied a response, but low-priority callers are advised to anticipate a long wait for the ambulance when the system is busy. If a potentially life-threatening call is triaged when no ambulance is available, an ambulance transporting a low-priority patient may be diverted. The low-priority patient remains in the ambulance with the EMT-A while the paramedic evaluates the patient with the potentially life-threatening complaint. If the paramedic requires assistance, another unit is summoned; otherwise the ambulance transports both of the patients.

In mid-1988, a thorough review of 9-1-1 calls was conducted and a plan to combat misuse initiated.

Following a public education campaign, field personnel flagged 9-1-1 misuse charts. These charts were reviewed by the EMS training officer and/or the medical director. If they confirmed it was a misuse case, an informational mailing was sent to the patient or party requesting the ambulance. This letter informed the patient that their ambulance request was felt to be unnecessary and explained the appropriate usage of the 9-1-1 system, including why it is so important that the system be used correctly. The letter also explained that patients are charged for EMS service and described the patient's forthcoming bill. The business office expedited billing of these calls.[24]

The program did decrease 9-1-1 usage, but because St Louis still has a large amount of inappropriate 9-1-1 use, the city is considering expanding the program further to include (1) charging individuals identified as using the EMS for "house calls," (2) initiation of a scene triage program consisting of medically-equipped minivans staffed by one paramedic, and (3) operation of EMT-A units to handle low-priority calls that would possibly pick up multiple patients before proceeding to the hospital.[5]

Florida

The state of Florida recently amended its statutes to include penalties for EMS misuse. The statues now state,[6] . . .

> (3) Whoever willfully and with intent to defraud obtains or attempts to obtain services from a licensee is guilty of: (a) A misdemeanor of the second degree... (b) A misdemeanor of the first degree... (4) Whoever summons any emergency medical services vehicle pursuant to this part or reports that an emergency medical services vehicle is needed when he knows or has reason to know that the services of the vehicle are not needed is guilty of: (a) A misdemeanor of the second degree... (b) A misdemeanor of the first degree....

These new statutes became effective October 1992. What affect these changes will have on Florida's EMS systems is unknown.

Summary

Inappropriate usage continues to plague most EMS systems. The problem needs to be further addressed and acceptable solutions derived. Six different approaches have been outlined in this chapter revealing the wide spectrum of possible solutions to the problem. By decreasing EMS misuse, the likelihood of prehospital personnel and resources being available to expedite care of patients with true emergencies increases.

REFERENCES

1. City of Pittsburgh Department of Public Safety, Bureau of Emergency Medical Services, Memo: Inappropriate use of EMS services, August 1990.
2. City of Pittsburgh Department of Public Safety, Bureau of Emergency Medical Services, Memo: Protocol—Patients that can be refused treatment or transport, January 1991.
3. City of St Louis, Department of Health and Hospitals, Emergency Medical Services: Procedure for identification of 9-1-1 ambulance misuser, 1988.
4. Dernocoeur J: Pitfalls of refusals, *JEMS* 9:79-83, 1982.
5. Dreifuss R: 911 misuse, *EMS* 18:43-45, 1989.
6. Florida State Statutes: Section 20, Section 401.41.
7. Gardner GJ and The use and abuse of the emergency ambulance service: Some of the factors affecting the decision whether to call an emergency ambulance, *Arch Emerg Med* 7:81-89, 1990.
8. Gerson LW and Skvarch L: Emergency medical service utilization by the elderly, *Ann Emerg Med* 11:610-612, 1982.
9. Gibson G: Measures of emergency ambulance effectiveness: Unmet need and inappropriate use, *JACEP* 6:389-392, 1977.
10. Goldberg RJ et al: A review of prehospital care litigation in a large metropolitan EMS system, *Ann Emerg Med* 19:557-561, 1990.
11. Ho MT et al: Delay between onset of chest pain and seeking medical care: The effect of public education, *Ann Emerg Med* 18:727-731, 1990.
12. Kerr HD and Byrd JC: Nursing home patients transferred by ambulance to a VA emergency department, *J Am Geriatr Soc* 39:132-136, 1991.
13. Milwaukee County Paramedic Program Policy and Procedure Section s.10. *Transport/Triage Policy,* effective date, September 1990.
14. Morris DL and Cross AB: Is the emergency ambulance service abused? *Brit Med J* 281:121-123, 1980.
15. O'Leary C et al: Ambulance-user analysis in an accident and emergency department, *Irish Med J* 80:422-423, 1987.
16. Operating Guide for New York City EMS: *On-Scene Triage Procedure,* New York, 1985.
17. Page JO: Refusal to transport: The legal backlash, *Emergency* 12:47-51, 1978.
18. Rademaker AW, Powell DG, and Read JH: Inappropriate use and unmet need in paramedic and nonparamedic ambulance systems, *Ann Emerg Med* 16:553-556, 1987.
19. Results of Pittsburgh's EMS Patient Refusal Survey, (unpublished).
20. Salt Lake City Emergency Medical Services Abuse Ordinance, Chapter 2, Title 14, Sections 14-2-8.
21. Salt Lake City EMS District Protocol No. 30: EMS abuse ordinance enforcement, March 1988.
22. Seldon BS, Schnitzer PG, and Nolan FX: Medicolegal documentation of prehospital triage, *Ann Emerg Med* 19:547-551, 1990.
23. Shanaberger CJ: Protect yourself, avoiding the claim of abandonment, *JEMS* 1:143-145, 1990.
24. Soler JM et al: The ten-year malpractice experience of a large urban EMS system, *Ann Emerg Med* 14:982-985, 1985.
25. Webb SB and Christoforo J: The use and mis-use of ambulance services by the population using the emergency department at the hospital of St. Raphael, *Conn Med* 34:107-114, 1970.

Appendix I

Operating Guide for NYCEMS: On-Scene Triage Procedure

PURPOSE: To establish policy and provide on-scene triage of patients.

SCOPE: This procedure applies to the Emergency Medical System physicians who provide medical control system and to personnel who provide prehospital medical care through the NYCEMS dispatch system, as indicated by an asterisk (*).

BACKGROUND:

*A. The New York State Legislature's On-Scene Triage Bill recently became effective. The legislation allows a physician to refuse transport of patients not in need of emergency medical care or neither sufficiently ill nor injured to necessitate transportation to a hospital by means of an ambulance, upon consultation with EMTs or paramedics on the scene after they have physically examined such patients. Such determination shall be based solely upon the medical condition of the person being considered for ambulance transportation.

*B: On-Scene Triage Program will be conducted under stringent medical control and subject to extensive evaluation by the Vice-President of HHC for EMS. Members of the Service shall understand fully the necessity for obtaining complete and accurate documentation for all patients who are denied transport at the scene.

POLICY:

*A. All members of the Service and employees of voluntary hospitals who provide prehospital emergency care through the NYCEMS dispatch system shall:

*1. Continue to provide care to all persons in need of such care in accordance with existing EMS patient-care protocols and operating procedures.

*2. Perform complete patient assessments for all patients in accordance with existing EMS procedures.

*3. Obtain complete and accurate documentation on the PCR. PCRs must be completed for all patients regardless of patient disposition.

*B. Requests for ambulance transportation which, in the opinion of the member(s) of the Service are felt not to require emergency medical care nor necessitate transportation to a hospital by means of an ambulance, based upon physical examination of the patient and accompanying history, shall be denied by the resource physician, pursuant to the procedure described below.

PROCEDURE:

*A. Upon responding on an assignment, if a member of the Service encounters a person whom he/she feels does not require emergency transportation to a medical facility, the member(s) of the Service shall:

*1. Obtain a complete patient history, documenting all pertinent findings clearly on the PCR.

*2. Perform a physical examination of the patient, in accordance with EMS patient-care protocols, recording all pertinent findings accurately on the PCR.

*3. Obtain at least two (2) sets of vital signs for the patient and record the times that they were obtained in the appropriate sections of the PCR.

*4. Upon completion of the patient history and physical examination, if the member(s) of the Service still feel that such person either is not in need of emergency medical care or is not sufficiently ill or injured to necessitate transportation to a hospital by means of an emergency ambulance, the member(s) shall:
   *a) Contact the EMS Telemetry Matrix via landline at (718) 326-9090. Units which have telemetry capability should utilize the landline number in order to save telemetry contact for emergencies. However, contact with the Matrix may be made via telemetry, when necessary.
*5. Relay the following patient information to the resource physician on duty:
   *a) Vital signs
   *b) Chief complaint
   *c) Physical examination findings
   *d) Pertinent history
   *e) Message ID number
*6. If, for any reason, a resource physician is unavailable to answer the call, or if contact with the resource physician cannot be made within five (5) minutes or, if permission to deny ambulance transportation is not granted by the resource physician, the member(s) of the Service shall:
   *a) Provide prehospital care and transport the patient to a 911 receiving hospital unless the patient decides to refuse medical assistance.
   NOTE: NO PATIENTS SHALL BE DENIED AMBULANCE TRANSPORTATION UNLESS APPROVAL HAS BEEN RECEIVED FROM THE RESOURCE PHYSICIAN.
   *b) Obtain a signed RMA from the patient should he/she refuse medical assistance.
*7. If the resource physician approves the request to deny ambulance transportation:
   *a) Inform the patient that his/her condition does not require emergency ambulance transportation to a 911 receiving hospital and that they have been instructed by a physician not to provide ambulance transportation.
   *b) Advise the patient that this denial of ambulance transportation will in no way prejudice future requests via 911 for ambulance service for true medical emergencies.
   *c) Encourage the patient to seek alternative means of transportation to a medical facility (i.e., private car, public transportation, taxi, private ambulance service) if the patient still desires to go to a medical facility.
   *d) If the patient insists that the members of the Service provide transportation to a medical facility, the patient shall be allowed to speak directly with the resource physician.
   *e) Provide the patient with the patient copy of EMS Form 10-95 (top portion of form—see Appendix II) which shall be signed by the crew members on the scene, indicating their unit number, the message ID number for the assignment and their shield numbers. The medical control copy (last page) of the PCR shall be attached to this form and given to the patient.
   *f) Request that the patient sign the acknowledgment portion (bottom portion) of EMS Form 10-95 and attach the signed acknowledgment form to the hospital copy of the PCR. One of the crew members shall sign as witness in the appropriate space.

g) As indicated on EMS Form 10-95, should the patient require emergency ambulance transportation within 24 hours of denial of service, they should contact the EMS Telemetry Matrix at (718) 386-5094 for assistance. Patients should also be informed that requests for ambulance service can only be processed via the above-listed telephone number within the 24-hour period as described above. After 24 hours, the patient's chart number and complaint history will be deleted from the computer and subsequent requests for emergency ambulance service must be routed via 911.
NOTE: When revised PCRs become available, the information as described in items "e," "f," and "g" above will be incorporated into the PCR. Members of the Service shall then attempt to have the patient sign the 10-95 section of the PCR, located on the back of the hospital copy of the PCR. Crew members shall sign the appropriate section of the PCR, located on the back of the medical control copy of the PCR. All sections shall be completed, including: date, unit's radio designation, message ID number, call type, sex/age of patient, chief complaint, presenting problem, time of contact with physician, crew members, shield numbers, vital signs, history, medications, allergies, and presumptive diagnosis. This copy of the PCR shall be given to the patient.

*h) Complete any other documentation required for the PCR, indicating clearly in the disposition section of the PCR, the code 10-95.

*i) Transmit a signal 10-95, using modat and/or verbal signals as necessary, and return to available status.

*j) Turn in the hospital copy of the PCR to the tour supervisor at the conclusion of the tour of duty.

B. The Resource Physician shall:

1. Record all information received from field personnel on the Triage Checklist (copy included in Appendix III).
2. Review all checklist items with field personnel, ensuring that all sections of the checklist and appropriate sections of the PCR are completed before making a determination regarding denial of ambulance transportation.
3. Upon satisfactory completion of the checklist, make a determination regarding approval or disapproval of ambulance transportation, relaying this determination to the EMS personnel on the scene.
4. Forward completed triage checklists to the office of the Chief of Operations by the end of his/her tour of duty for incorporation with other documentation (i.e., print-out and PCR copy). Completed documentation will be collated by the Chief of Operations for submission through the Executive Director to the Vice-President of HHC for EMS for review and evaluation of the on-scene triage program.
   a) Resource physicians who provide medical control for the on-scene triage program at a location other than the EMS Telemetry Center (e.g. base stations or medical control facilities) shall submit completed triage checklists to the EMS Tour Supervisor at the completion of the tour.
   b) EMS Tour Supervisors at these locations shall ensure that completed checklists are retrieved from medical control facilities in a timely fashion for submission to the Vice-President of HHC for EMS as described above.

5. Upon receiving a call-back from a patient who has been denied ambulance transportation within the past 24 hours, instruct the Telemetry Operator to forward the job to the appropriate borough dispatcher for assignment.

C. EMS Telemetry Center Operators shall:
   1. When resource physicians are unavailable at the Telemetry Center, forward requests for denial of transportation to the resource physician on-duty at the alternate medical control facility for on-scene triage (e.g., Queens Hospital Center). If a resource physician is unavailable at the alternate medical control facility, advise the crew to transport the patient to a 911 receiving hospital.
   2. When resource physicians are unavailable at the Telemetry Center and a call-back is received from a patient who has been denied ambulance transportation within the past 24 hours and who is now requesting ambulance transportation to the hospital, re-open the job and forward it to the appropriate borough dispatcher for assignment.

D. EMS Tour Supervisors shall:
   1. Collate all hospital copies of PCRs received for 10-95 dispositions, recording the PCR numbers of these copies in the station log.
   2. Forward these copies of the PCR and any other accompanying documentation to the Borough Command Office by the end of his/her tour of duty.

E. The Borough Commander or his/her designee shall assume responsibility for ensuring that copies of the PCRs and any accompanying documentation are collated for submission through the chain of command to the Vice-President of HHC for EMS within 24 hours.

F. Communications Tour Commanders shall ensure that print-outs are obtained for all assignments with a 10-95 disposition during their tour of duty. These print-outs shall be forwarded through the chain of command to the Office of the Chief of Operations at the end of the tour commander's tour of duty.

G. The Chief of Operations shall ensure that all documentation received regarding the on-scene triage program (i.e., print-outs, PCRs, triage checklists) are collated on a daily basis for submission through the Executive Director to the Vice-President of HHC for EMS.

Appendix II

EMS Form 10-95

YOUR CONDITION DOES NOT REQUIRE TRANSPORTATION BY AMBULANCE TO A MEDICAL FACILITY. YOU HAVE BEEN EXAMINED BY THE EMERGENCY MEDICAL SERVICE SPECIALISTS WHOSE SHIELD NUMBERS ARE INDICATED BELOW AND THEY HAVE COMMUNICATED WITH A PHYSICIAN WHO HAS DETERMINED, IN ACCORDANCE WITH STATE LAW, THAT YOU DO NOT REQUIRE EMERGENCY VEHICLE TRANSPORTATION EITHER BECAUSE YOU ARE NOT IN NEED OF EMERGENCY MEDICAL CARE OR BECAUSE YOU ARE NEITHER SUFFICIENTLY ILL NOR INJURED TO REQUIRE TRANSPORTATION BY AMBULANCE TO A HOSPITAL. IF YOU FEEL A MISTAKE HAS BEEN MADE, ASK THE CREW TO LET YOU SPEAK TO THE PHYSICIAN.

SHOULD YOUR MEDICAL CONDITION CHANGE AFTER THE UNIT HAS LEFT, YOU MAY CONTACT MEDICAL CONTROL AT (718) 386-5094 AND EXPLAIN THE SITUATION. WHEN THE PHONE IS ANSWERED, GIVE YOUR MESSAGE ID NUMBER. THIS NUMBER (INDICATED BELOW) AND YOUR EXAM HISTORY REMAIN IN THE COMPUTER FOR 24 HOURS. AFTER THAT TIME, OR, IF YOU CANNOT GET THROUGH AT THE NUMBER LISTED ABOVE, YOU MUST CALL 911 FOR ASSISTANCE. CALLS RECEIVED AT THE MEDICAL CONTROL PHONE NUMBER LISTED ABOVE CAN ONLY BE PROCESSED WITHIN THE 24-HOUR PERIOD AND WITH AN ACCOMPANYING MESSAGE ID NUMBER.

PLEASE ONLY CALL 911 FOR REAL EMERGENCIES; OTHERWISE USE OTHER MEANS TO REACH THE HOSPITAL, THE PHARMACY OR THE DOCTOR'S OFFICE. THANK YOU.

Message ID # _______________ Date __________________ Unit # _________________

Crew members' shield #s________________ ____________________

(Attach to the Medical Control Copy of the PCR. To be retained by the patient.)

ACKNOWLEDGMENT

"I hereby acknowledge that I have been informed that I do not require transportation by ambulance to a medical facility. I have been examined by the Emergency Medical Service Specialist who has communicated with a physician who has determined in accordance with State Law that I do not require emergency vehicle transportation either because I am not in need of emergency medical care or because I am neither sufficiently ill nor injured to require transportation by ambulance to a hospital."

Date ___________________ Patient Signature ____

Witnessed by ____

Message ID # ___________

(Attach to the Hospital Copy of the PCR and forward copies to the Tour Supervisor at the end of your tour of duty.)

Appendix III

On-Scene Triage Checklist

TRANSPORT APPROVED ☐

TRANSPORT DENIED ☐

DOCTOR'S SIGNATURE ______________________

DOCTOR'S NAME & ID NO.____________________

UNIT NO.______________________

MESSAGE ID NO. ______________________

CALL TYPE ______________________

PATIENT'S AGE _________ PATIENT'S SEX _____

FACILITY _______________ DATE ______________

CALL REC'VD VIA TELEMETRY CHANNEL NO. __

CALL REC'VD VIA TELEPHONE ☐

SPECIALISTS NAME & SHIELD NO.____________

____

PATIENT'S/NEIGHBOR'S/NEXT OF KIN'S TELEPHONE NO. ________________________

PRIORITY OF CALL ___________________________

CHIEF COMPLAINT ___________________________

<u>VITAL SIGNS</u>

TIME	BP	PULSE	RESP	SKIN MOISTURE	SKIN TEMP	SKIN COLOR	PUPILS	MENTAL STATUS

A. ACUTE SYMPTOMS — SIGNIFICANT? YES ☐ NO ☐

B. HISTORY & MEDICATIONS — SIGNIFICANT? YES ☐ NO ☐

C. ABNORMAL PHYSICAL FINDINGS — SIGNIFICANT? YES ☐ NO ☐

D. PATIENT'S REASON FOR REQUESTING AMBULANCE TRANSPORT — REASONABLE? YES ☐ NO ☐

ITEMS A - D ON THE REVERSE SIDE MUST BE CHECKED "NO" AND A SECOND SET OF VITAL SIGNS MUST BE TAKEN BEFORE YOU CAN DENY TRANSPORT.

<u>VITAL SIGNS</u>

TIME	BP	PULSE	RESP	SKIN MOISTURE	SKIN TEMP	SKIN COLOR	PUPILS	MENTAL STATUS

DID YOU SPEAK WITH THE PATIENT? YES ☐ NO ☐

TRANSPORT APPROVED ☐

DENIED ☐

EXPLANATION - AS NECESSARY ____________________

____

____

____

DATE CASE REVIEWED ____________ REVIEWED BY ____________

ALL FORMS WILL BE DUPLICATED AND SUBMITTED THROUGH THE CHAIN-OF-COMMAND TO THE OFFICE OF THE CHIEF OF OPERATIONS FOR FORWARDING TO THE EXECUTIVE DIRECTOR AND TO THE VICE-PRESIDENT OF THE NEW YORK CITY HEALTH AND HOSPITALS CORPORATION FOR THE EMERGENCY MEDICAL SERVICE, WITHIN 24 HOURS.

37

Refusal of Prehospital Care

Lawrence Mottley, M.D., M.H.S.A. FACEP

Only within the past 15 years has the medical literature focused on the patient's need for and the right to informed consent for medical treatment. As late as 1976, this concept was derided in the medical community as "a legislative fiction that destroys good patient care and paralyzes the conscientious physician. . . . It is not applicable, even by definition, to a large segment of the involved population. *The term has no place in the lexicon of medicine.*"[4] With 15 years of hindsight, such a statement appears ludicrous. The rapid adaptation of this doctrine is perhaps the most eloquent testimony of its inherent correctness.

The nonpsychiatric literature deals almost entirely with the inpatient who cannot consent yet requires emergency medical treatment. Although some articles touch on the issue of consent in the emergency department, a search of literature for the past 15 years revealed no articles focusing on the issue of those patients who refuse medical treatment in the emergency department, much less in the prehospital arena. There is, however, a small body of literature concerning patient refusal of psychiatric treatment that is peripherally analogous to this discussion. This area is uncharted territory previously defined by prehospital care providers. There is little case law or regulatory action addressing this problem.

This chapter discusses the application of the informed consent process to a subset of emergency patients: those patients treated by EMS providers who are not yet physically at the hospital and hence not yet evaluated by a physician. The role of the concept of "informed refusal" as an integral part of informed consent is discussed and applied. "Denial of aid" and "no transport" are briefly discussed, and "refusal of medical assistance" is discussed at length, since it is the essence of the application of informed consent in the prehospital theatre. Finally, this theoretical discussion is translated into a policy statement addressing one group of such patients, whose prehospital treatment has been the focus of increasing debate (see Appendix).

Informed Consent

The origins of the doctrine of informed consent can be found as far back as 1914, when Justice Cardoza stated "every human being of adult years and sound mind has a right to determine what shall be done with his own body.* This was further expanded in Natanson *v.* Kline (1960), who ruled that physicians had an "obligation to disclose and explain in simple language" the risks and complications of a procedure.

The amount of time in provider training allocated to important issues of consent, patient autonomy, and decision making is slight and barely enough for the responsibility routinely thrust on prehospital personnel. To legal authorities, prehospital personnel have a limited scope of training traditionally restricted by the following underlying assumptions: the prehospital care provider responds to, assesses, and stabilizes to the extent possible in the prehospital phase, then transports the patient to a higher level of medical care, specifically a physician. State laws and court rulings have generally failed to address the nature of the relationship between the patient and prehospital provider. By analogy, in some states, the professional registered nurse (RN) may have an independent relationship with a patient; in other states, the relationship depends on and is by virtue of the attending or personal physician of the patient. This can be an important issue

*Schloendorff *v.* Society of New York Hospital, 211 NY 125, 1 29-30, 105 N.E. 92, 93(1914).

when evaluating termination of the relationship in the field and the patient's refusal of medical assistance. At least one federal court ruling held that a physician's assistant who treated and discharged a patient without the patient or patient's chart ever having been reviewed by a physician was below the standard of care.*

An implicit assumption exists that all patients coming into contact with prehospital care providers will be seen by a physician before being released. Clearly this does not occur in practice. While there are innumerable factors and circumstances in patient encounters in the field, there are essentially three types of no-transport situations (quadrants B, C, and D of Table 37-1). Each has its own underlying or contributing factors, and each has its own legal implications. Similarly, each may have a different remedy to be summarized by the medical director in a protocol for the prehospital providers. As seen in Table 37-1, only the patients in quadrant A fit the underlying assumption; that is, those patients who desire to be transported to the hospital and whom EMS desires to transport to the hospital.

Patient Refuses Transport and EMS Disagrees (B)

The most complex quadrant of the matrix (Table 37-1) is quadrant B. This is the true *refusal of medical assistance* (RMA). In these instances, the EMS providers believe the patient has or may have a medical problem that requires immediate evaluation or treatment and that may be immediately or potentially life-threatening without definitive care. The patient, however, refuses to go to the hospital. This area is fraught with danger to both the patient and the prehospital care provider.

Table 37-1. Matrix of Patient Transportation Decision

	Patient desires transport?	
	Yes	No
EMS desires to transport?		
Yes	A*: Transport	B: Refusal of medical assistance
No	C: Denial of aid	D: No transport

*The patient desires transport and EMS agrees. Obviously, there is neither a medical nor a legal issue.

*Polischeck *v.* United States, 535 F. Supp. 1261 (1982).

The RMA form typically contains language indicating that the patient was advised to go to the hospital and that he understands the consequences of the decision not to go to the hospital, which may include a more severe illness or death. A key statement in such a document is the explicit assertion that the EMS provider did advise the patient to go to the hospital and that the patient understands the risks of serious complication if he does not go to the hospital.

Desire for a Specific Hospital

Patients often request transport to a particular hospital, such as the hospital of their personal physician. It is equally common for EMS provider agencies to have a policy requiring transport to the closest hospital. Two good reasons for such a policy include keeping units within their service districts and the importance of transporting critical patients to the nearest appropriate hospital. However, there are also valid reasons to comply with the desires of the patient. It is usually in the best interest of an individual patient if the continuity of care can be maintained by a physician who knows the patient and who has ready access to the patient's prior records.

A reasonable compromise can often be reached between these two alternatives. Some large EMS providers have adopted two rules. The first rule often is known as the *10-minute rule* and allows the prehospital providers to transport a stable patient to the hospital of patient choice if it is no more than 10 minutes further than the nearest hospital. This eliminates the vast majority of complaints, since most patients are reasonable and do not request transportation long distances in an acute situation. However, this is not always the case. Under the second rule, in the instance where the prehospital care providers feel that there is a potentially life-threatening problem, the direct medical control physician is contacted, advised of the patient's condition, and may authorize the patient to be transported anywhere in the city *if* the patient would otherwise refuse EMS transport.

Specialty Referral Center Candidates

Trauma and other specialty referral centers present a special problem. When field personnel identify a specialty referral candidate, such as a trauma patient, who expresses a desire to go to a hospital other than the designated trauma center, the situation becomes a conflict between the best medical judgment of the provider and the desires of the patient. A strong case can be made that the trauma patient cannot make an informed judgment in the prehospital setting. If the patient is brought to a nontrauma center and dies at the hospital, the case could be made that the patient was not legally competent to make such a decision and that the provider should not have complied with the patient's wishes. If, on the other hand, a patient is brought to a trauma center against his will and does survive, the patient would be filing suit against EMS for saving his life. The provider should act as would a reasonable and prudent provider in that community; that is, to act in the best medical interests of the patient, reflected in written trauma treatment protocols.[*] Therefore it is a reasonable course of action to transport defined trauma patients to trauma centers even though the patient may object, as long as he does not physically resist (see Appendix). Caroline also emphasizes the necessity of both informed consent and informed refusal.[1]

The leading case addressing the issue of informed refusal is the California case of Truman *v.* Thomas.[†] In that case the California Supreme Court held that a physician had a duty to warn a patient of the dangers involved in refusing to undergo a diagnostic test. In the Truman case, a physician had repeatedly requested his patient submit to a diagnostic test. The patient had refused, to the point that the physician ultimately refused to prescribe any further medication until she underwent the test. The physician went as far as informing the patient's pharmacist of his decision, but because he had not specifically delineated to the patient the risks of refusing the test, the physician was held liable when the patient was ultimately found to have inoperable cancer.

Before Truman *v.* Thomas, the controlling doctrine had been Cobb *v.* Grant, which required that a physician divulge "to his patient all information relevant to a meaningful decision process."[‡] The interpretation in the Cobb case and subsequent cases applied only to patient consent for a procedure. If the patient did not undergo the procedure, the assumption—until Truman—was that the doctrine did not apply. Subsequently, a New York court delineated the decision rule that the law would assume that the patient would have acted "as a reasonable person would have acted if he knew all pertinent information."[§] A California court further extended the liability to physicians who simply refer a patient to a specialist for possible treatment.;[||]

All these cases refer to Cobb for its seminal elucidation of this doctrine. Cobb has the following four essential postulates:

- The knowledge of the physician and the knowledge of the patient are not in parity.
- Adults exercise control over their own body with the right to determine what treatment is acceptable.
- Consent to treatment must be informed.
- Because of the nature of the physician-patient relationship, the physician has a special obligation to the patient.

In Truman, the court found the concepts of 'informed consent' and "informed refusal" to be "indistinguishable."

The courts have recognized certain exceptions to the rule of informed consent. One of the principal exceptions is the emergency situation when the patient lacks capacity. Rozovsky delineates two conditions for such an exception to apply.[5] First, the patient must be incapacitated and unable to reach an informed judgment. This limitation "may be attributable to an injury . . . shock, or trauma . . ." Second, "a life-threatening or health-threatening disease or injury that requires immediate treatment is present," where delay would mean death or impairment.[¶]

Patient Refuses Transport

In some instances a family member or concerned bystander calls EMS, but the patient does not share the concern and refuses transportation to the hospital. This is a classic double bind. If there is a bad outcome, the family may sue if the patient is not transported, yet the patient may sue if he is transported against his will.

If in the judgment of the crew there is no evidence of acute or life-threatening problems, then they may explain the situation to the caller and utilize an RMA form (preferably witnessed by the caller and the police), while offering to return should the patient change his or her mind.

If there is a substantial risk of further deterioration, the situation becomes much more complex. In such an instance, EMS providers should take some or all of the following steps:

*Barber: Informed consent in medical therapy and Research, 1980: "If the patient lacks capacity to make an informed judgment in an emergency situation, the physician should act as would a reasonable provider."

†Truman *v.* Thomas 27 Cal 3d 285 P2d 902, 165 Cal Rptr 308(1980).

‡Cobb *v.* Grant 8 Cal 3d 229, 502 P.2d 1, 104 Cal Rptr 505(1972).

§Crisher *v.* Spak 471 NYS 2d 741.

||Moore *v.* Preventive Medicine Medical Group, Inc. 223 CaR[3] 859: In this case, a physician referred a patient to a dermatologist for evaluation of a skin mole found on routine examination. He was held liable for failing to explain the risks of not going to the dermatologist as suggested.

¶Codified e.g. in Ga. 88-2905 (1971).

1. The EMS crew attempts to persuade the patient to accept transportation
2. The EMS crew enlists the aid of the family in persuading the patient.
3. The EMS crew asks the Police Department's assistance in persuading the patient to voluntarily go to the hospital.
4. An EMS supervisor responds to the scene in an additional attempt to persuade the patient as well as to provide documentation by a person of supervisory rank.
5. The EMS crew calls direct medical control and, preferably on a tape-recorded line, the direct medical control physician talks directly to the patient. One study has shown that, even if the patient has resisted all entreaties up to this point, 40% of the patients acquiesce and accept transportation to the hospital when the direct medical control physician so requests.[3]

If the patient continues to refuse, the physician will have the opportunity to determine if the patient is alert, oriented and has the "capacity" to make a reasonable and knowledgeable RMA. The physician can then reasonably authorize the prehospital care providers to discontinue their efforts, if all reasonable steps in the interest of patient care have been taken. On the other hand, if in the physician's judgment, the patient does *not* have the capacity to make such a decision, the physician should enlist the aid of the Police Department to involuntarily remove the patient to the hospital. In most jurisdictions, only a police officer may legally do this.

A tape-recorded system provides positive documentation of the number of times that the patient was requested to go to the hospital and that the patient knowingly chose not to be transported. It may also provide documentation that the patient refused to speak to the physician or EMS crew, and of the patient's mental status and capacity to make an informed judgment.

Patient Desires Transport and EMS Disagrees (C)

The magnitude of misuse of ambulance resources for medically unnecessary ambulance transport varies widely. It appears to be greatest in the larger cities and least in the rural areas:[2] "The refusal to transport is the single most common complaint." Attempts to rectify this situation by refusing ambulance transportation on the basis of provider assessment at the scene are fraught with liability. Publicly owned or operated EMS services, including contracted services, have a duty to aid victims of accidents or other emergencies.[5] It is likely that private and volunteer services have a similar duty, once they have responded. Should the patient have an adverse outcome it would become virtually impossible to justify the failure to treat and transport the patient.* Additionally, the argument can be made that the failure to treat and transport the patient constitutes a diagnosis by a prehospital provider that is more properly reserved for a physician (see Chapter 36).

Therefore if a disagreement about the necessity for transport arises between the patient and the providers, the direct medical control physician should decide whether the patient requires transport. Although this leads to overuse of the ambulance and even tolerates abuse of the system, it minimizes the risk of inappropriately denying ambulance transport to an ill patient. It is clear that such a system of medical decision making is more practical in a paramedic system with direct medical control than in a system that commonly does not have a mechanism for EMT-A personnel to contact the direct medical control physician. Nevertheless, when there is direct medical control, as there is in virtually all paramedic systems, it is clear that the failure to transport a patient is a potentially serious liability for the direct medical control physician and the system.

Patient Refuses Transport and EMS Agrees (D)

Assume that EMS is called to the scene of an automobile accident where the person involved in the accident does not initiate the call. Neither the victim nor the EMS crew identifies a serious injury or any injury at all and the victim refuses transportation to the hospital. The EMS crew may ask the patient to sign a statement on the prehospital care report (PCR) indicating that the patient does not wish to be transported to the hospital. However, the only printed form for the patient to sign when he declines transportation to the hospital is the RMA form.

Often, because of misplaced faith in the value of an RMA, the result is that the patient is asked to sign a statement that neither the patient nor the prehospital care provider believes is true. Should this patient have problems subsequently it would be difficult to reconcile the findings on the PCR (which should indicate no injury) with the statement on the RMA that indicates that the patient is at risk by not going to the hospital. Similarly, if the patient *was* advised to go to the hospital, then the legal counsel might ask why more aggressive procedures were not put into effect. Clearly, if neither the patient nor the EMS providers believe the

*Green *v.* City of Dallas, 545 SW 2nd 284 (Tex Civ App Amarillo

patient is in need of immediate transportation to the hospital, the patient should be asked to sign a statement to that effect *rather* than an RMA statement. It may be appropriate to provide such patients with follow-up care sheets in the event signs or symptoms do present.

Summary

Although the concept of informed consent is well established in medicine, the concept of informed refusal is often more germane to EMS.

When there is disagreement between patient and crew over the need to transport, access to direct medical control is essential. Should a field unit agree with the patient that transport is not required the "traditional" RMA form is *not* appropriate.

The medical director should ensure that both the EMS personnel and direct medical control physicians have an understanding of their duties and obligations in the various nontransport situations. This includes a familiarity with the assessment abilities of the prehospital providers, applicable state and local laws, transport times, call volume, and number of available ambulances and supervisors.

Patients whose medical condition is immediately life-threatening should be taken to a medically appropriate treatment facility, even if they express a desire to be treated elsewhere.

The Appendix contains a sample destination policy for trauma patients.

REFERENCES

1. Caroline N: *Emergency medical treatment: a text for EMT-As and EMT-Is,* ed 3, 1991.
2. Proceedings of the first national conference on the medical-legal implications of emergency medical care, 1976.
3. Kuehl A: Personal communication, New York, 1986.
4. Laforet: *JAMA* 1582, 1976.
5. Rozovsky F: *Defense Law Journal* 33:579, 1984.
6. Southwick A: *The law of hospital and health care administration,* 1988.

Appendix

Trauma Destination Policy for the New York State Department of Health

As always, the Department's first concern is to ensure the best care for each patient while protecting the right of the patient to choose the provider of that care, or indeed, to choose not to accept care at all.

It is essential that such a decision by a patient be an informed decision. Informed consent is a guiding ethical and legal principle of medical care that the Department vigorously supports.

It is axiomatic that a patient cannot make an informed judgment unless he fully understands the risks and benefits of the course of treatment suggested by the provider. In the major trauma patient, this is often not possible. A number of factors interfere with the normal process of informed consent. First, the patient's injuries may result in an alteration of the patient's mental status. Such an alteration may result either directly from an injury to the head, or indirectly due to injury to other areas of the body resulting, for example, in shock or extreme pain. Obviously, a patient with an altered mental status is unable to make an informed judgment, nor is the prehospital provider trained to determine the patient's capacity to do so.

Secondly, the time constraints required to effectively treat trauma patients are extreme. Effective trauma care is measured in minutes. The nationally recognized principle of the "golden hour" of trauma care requires that optimum patient care can be achieved if the patient reaches definitive trauma center care as expeditiously as possible. The time required to list and explain the risks and benefits of the various transport alternatives in a meaningful manner would prevent the patient from receiving this optimal care.

Third, and perhaps most important, informed consent requires that the patient be informed of the suggested and alternative courses of action, and the risks and benefits of each. Yet, in the prehospital setting, the provider is a certified EMT not a licensed physician. The scope of training of an EMT does not include knowledge of the complications, alternatives, or even the likely outcome of a particular course of action, much less the range and likelihood of reasonably known complications. Thus, since the information needed to make an informed judgment in the prehospital setting is unavailable, an informed judgment—by definition—cannot be made.

In the absence of informed consent, the provider should follow the course of action of a reasonable and prudent EMT. Such course of action is clearly laid out in the New York State Emergency Medical Service BLS protocols. All EMTs are required to follow these protocols.

Finally, it is important to remember that the decision made by the EMT is the hospital destination. Once at the appropriate hospital, the patient will be cared for by a licensed physician, who can accurately determine the capacity of the patient to make an informed judgment and provide the information necessary for that informed judgment to be made.

For these reasons, it is the position of the Department that trauma patients, as defined in the New York State Emergency Medical Service BLS protocols, be transported in accordance with those protocols, even if the patient objects.

38

Bystander Physicians

Sam Senturia, M.D.
Robert Bass, M.D.

It is not uncommon for EMS personnel to encounter physicians in the field. These physicians may be bystanders who come on an incident or private physicians with an established relationship to the patient. The interaction of physicians in the field with EMS personnel can create a great deal of confusion when trying to define medical authority and responsibility for patient care. If a patient is seriously injured or ill, this confusion, coupled with the stress of the situation, can lead to emotionally charged confrontations. Such confrontations rarely benefit patient care.[1] For this reason, it is important that prehospital care systems prospectively develop policies that address the interaction of field providers with bystander or private physicians who are at the scene. Several EMS systems have implemented specific protocols for managing these problems.

Defining the Problem

Although there are no clear data that describe the incidence of such encounters, they are not infrequent. In one survey in 1991, paramedics from five urban areas reported an average of 3.4 encounters within the previous year.[2] Likewise, although it would seem self-evident that the expertise of a physician present at the scene would improve the quality of field management, there are no empirical data demonstrating such a benefit. There are data available to suggest that direct medical control is of benefit in certain groups of patients who are critically ill or injured and who require treatment beyond or in deviation from protocols.[3] At the present time, it can only be assumed that field physician intervention might have similar benefits.

Field personnel generally have a negative perception of their interaction with physicians in the field, and believe that such encounters benefit patient care in relatively few cases. A number of factors contribute to those perceptions, including a feeling by paramedics that physicians do not understand them or their roles. According to paramedics, some physicians in the field insist on intervening because they assume that current providers have little if any training.[2]

There are a number of reasons why a bystander physician may benefit patient care. Physicians may have greater training and medical knowledge or may be able to perform procedures that the providers can not. This is particularly likely in a rural environment where provider training is often more limited. Depending on his specialty training and experience, the physician may be more skilled in a particular intervention. Of course, if the physician has an established relationship with the patient, his knowledge of the patient's history and problems may be invaluable. And, field expertise aside, physicians have a legitimate interest in the management of patients transported from their offices.

On the other hand, there are times when the physician may be a significant liability. Unless he is trained or experienced in prehospital care, critical care medicine or emergency medicine, he may not, in fact, be as knowledgeable or as skilled as the providers. In addition, he may be unfamiliar with unique prehospital interventions such as the pneumatic antishock garment, the principles of evacuation and transport, or the unique legal issues of the prehospital environment. For example, an internist or cardiologist might be alarmed by the immediate transport of a hypotensive blunt trauma victim before the placement of intravenous (IV) lines, since this is contrary to the management of medical cardiopulmonary emergencies, although justified in the prehospital management of trauma. In one dispute over this issue, a persistent physician was handcuffed by police to keep him away from the resuscitation area. At scenes where safety is an issue, physicians who are not familiar with field hazards may detract from patient care by distracting field providers who must ensure that the physician does not become a victim.

Other times at issue is the assumption of responsibility for patient care. This is implicit whenever the physician uses a particular skill or intervention not used by the local EMS. For example, EMS providers responding to an office call may encounter a physician who wants to use a non-EMS formulary drug such as procainamide. Although the physician has the drug readily at hand, if the providers are unfamiliar with the medicine, he will place the patient, the providers, and himself in a precarious position if he decides to administer IV procainamide but then relinquishes further care to the providers.

Defining the Varieties of Interactions

The role and responsibility of a physician at the scene is not easy to define and may vary greatly depending on the circumstances. In general, the following three varieties of interaction between bystander physicians and EMS providers can be described:

1. The physician turns over responsibility for the care of the patient completely, and the EMS system handles all further care. This accounts for the majority of physician and EMS interactions.
2. The physician turns over the responsibility for the care of the patient to the EMS system but offers advice and assistance.
3. The physician assumes full responsibility for patient care.

Most bystander physician encounters result in the physician turning over the patient to the EMS providers with perhaps some assistance offered. In such circumstances the providers proceed with their evaluation and treatment according to their protocols. If the physician decides to intervene and to deviate from the protocols, he should first request and receive full medical authority from direct medical control. In such circumstances the physician assumes responsibility for patient care and must accompany the patient to the hospital.

The opportunity for significant intervention by bystander physicians in the case of minor injuries and, in particular, at the site of major trauma is generally limited. In such cases, physicians usually do little more than an assessment and provide first aid; the patient is turned over to EMS personnel for further care and transportation. Unless the physician has performed an invasive procedure or is needed for care beyond the scope of the EMS providers, the physician acting in such a manner does not need to accompany a patient to the hospital.

Often, while EMS personnel are assessing the patient and initiating care, a physician will offer advice and suggestions for continued care. This type of intervention potentially benefits the patient in need of more sophisticated care. In such cases, knowledgeable physicians and EMS personnel working as a team can provide the best outcome for the patient.

Problems may arise when the intervening physician is not familiar with prehospital care or deviates from either established protocols or recognized standards of care. Whether intentional or inadvertent, a deviation from protocol creates a potential legal problem that must be resolved by direct medical control, who should have the authority to decide if it is appropriate. Medical authority and responsibility may then be granted or withheld. The position statement of the American College of Emergency Physicians (ACEP) suggests that even if a bystander physician is present, direct medical control remains responsible for patient care.[4] In the event of a disagreement between the two physicians, the provider should take orders from direct medical control. In the case of a private physician, the ACEP position is that providers should defer to the orders of the private physician who assumes responsibility for the patient's care; responsibility reverts to direct medical control when the private physician is no longer in attendance. Nevertheless, communication between the physician and direct medical control is essential in such circumstances. When direct medical control disapproves of a private physician's interventions, a mutually agreed on compromise that does no harm to the patient is usually better than invoking a hard line approach.

At the Physician's Office

Patients who are in a physician's office frequently have had diagnostic procedures and therapeutic interventions initiated before the arrival of EMS. In such cases, everything possible should be done to maintain the appropriate continuity of care. This usually involves the physician or members of his staff accompanying the patient during transport to the hospital, particularly if the EMS system is not capable of providing the same level of care that the patient received in the office.

At the other extreme, EMS providers often find patients in the office who require critical interventions that have not even begun. This situation is worsened when the providers are "ordered" by the physician or his staff to do nothing but transport the patient. In such cases, a rapid evacuation to a more neutral environment where protocols can be initiated and a direct medical control consultation can be obtained is in order. Confrontations rarely improve the outcome. The best approach often is to maintain a professional and composed attitude and to exit the office as quickly as possible. Incident reports, if necessary, can be followed up by the system medical director. Obviously careful documentation in the prehospital care report (PCR) after such encounters is mandatory.

Office calls can be expedited by developing office response protocols, which specify office addresses and any other idiosyncracies of access, the entrance at which an employee will be awaiting the crew, and the arrangements that will be made for clinical management in the office. These protocols are stored in the computer database at dispatch and are immediately available. The New York Hospital Paramedic Service has avoided many problems by developing such a protocol with each affiliated physician. This has improved not only response time and access but also the relationship among physicians and paramedics. Such office response protocols are applicable to larger EMS systems.

Medical Authority

In developing guidelines that deal with physicians at the scene, EMS agencies must consider any relevant state laws that define the authority of such physicians, whether private or bystander. In a few states, regulations may provide that the ultimate responsibility is the bystander physician. However, the authority for medical care delivered by the EMS agency rests with the medical director. Since prehospital care is viewed as the delivery of health care by the medical director through EMS provider intermediaries, the EMS providers should be viewed as agents of the medical director rather than of the physician at the scene. Medical directors (the physicians with medical oversight responsibility) may delegate direct medical control to other physicians, who therefore also have the authority to override bystander physicians. The potential liability to the system, the medical director and direct medical control physicians, must be considered before allowing any bystander physician to direct care using agency resources.

Guidelines

In developing guidelines, it is important to consider all the potential roles that a physician at the scene may assume. When the physician is a bystander who does nothing more than either transfer care of the patient to EMS or offer advice and assistance, patient care continues as with any other call. Any further active assistance should be authorized only by direct medical control.

Physicians who give orders or perform procedures should be properly identified since EMS incidents have attracted individuals posing as physicians. If the physician is not known to the EMS providers, he should be asked to provide both proof of his state medical licensure and appropriate identification. In some circumstances, it may be helpful to know the physician's specialty certification, as well as his prehospital and critical care experience. When relevant, such information should be relayed to direct medical control to assist with decision making.

Whenever possible, direct medical control and the physician at the scene should speak with one another. The physician should be told that he will be required to document any orders given or procedures performed and that it may be necessary for him to accompany the patient to the hospital; this communication process must not delay assessment and care of the patient by the EMS providers.

When direct medical control approves the physician, the field personnel should be notified. Such notification should delineate the degree of authority that has been delegated by direct medical control. At any point that the providers feel that the care deviates from standards, is not appropriate, or goes beyond what was authorized, direct medical control should be notified. Physicians who give orders, perform procedures, or assume full medical responsibility generally should accompany the patient to the hospital; however, this decision is ultimately the responsibility of direct medical control. Physicians who offer only assistance with the implementation of protocols need not necessarily accompany the patient. In those cases, to avoid a potential claim of physician abandonment, the patient should be stable and in no obvious need of further physician intervention. In cases where a physician has assumed full medical responsibility, especially where interventions have been initiated, the physician should be required to accompany the patient to the hospital. Physicians who refuse to do so should speak to direct medical control and should be warned that refusal to accompany the patient might be interpreted as abandonment.

When physicians give orders or perform procedures, they must provide written documentation on the PCR, including their name, license number, office address, and telephone number. In fact, whenever a physician is at the scene of a prehospital encounter, this information should be obtained.

Guidelines should also address the procedure to be followed when EMS providers are unable to establish contact with direct medical control. In such cases, state laws and the best interests of the patient should be considered. In a rural environment with limited provider capability, when a physician who is well known to the EMS providers offers assistance it would be unreasonable to deny the patient such an intervention. In contrast is the urban situation where sophisticated prehospital care is routinely available. EMS providers without communications, when confronted with an unknown bystander physician intervening in a potentially harmful way, may have to politely decline his offer of assistance and expeditiously place the patient in the unit for transport. Occasionally police assistance will be necessary. Guidelines governing such situations should be prospectively issued by medical oversight and must take into consideration local circumstances, as well as all applicable laws and regulations.

Several EMS agencies have developed information cards for bystander physicians that delineate important points for the physician contemplating intervention (Appendix I). In addition to thanking the physician for volunteering assistance, they briefly summarize the legal authority directing the EMS providers and list the options for intervention. There should be a clear indication that assumption of responsibility for patient care or use of special expertise will either probably or definitely require a commitment to accompany the patient to the hospital.[6] In New York City, physicians wishing to assume management of patient care must also sign a separate document (see Appendix II). The information cards may be intimidating and should not be used simply to deter or delay physician intervention, especially when it would be beneficial. In actual practice the cards are not frequently employed when the providers welcome assistance.

Summary

Bystander physicians may fulfill various roles in conjunction with EMS providers. Any involvement beyond first aid level assistance should be approved by direct medical control. The need for bystander physicians to assume responsibility for patient care should be rare in urban EMS systems but not uncommon in rural districts. With the exception of a few states, the ultimate medical authority in the field is the EMS medical director, who may delegate responsibility to the direct control physician. EMS agencies should develop guidelines to manage the various scenarios of field cooperation, including the distinctive concerns of private physicians and office calls. The potential liability to the EMS agency should be considered before allowing bystander physicians to direct patient care.

REFERENCES

1. Vost A: Physician intervention at the scene: Another point of view, *JEMS* 14:60-67, 1989.
2. Mellick LB et al: Paramedic perceptions of the on-scene physician, *Prehospital and Disaster Medicine* 6:331-334, 1991.
3. Erder MH, Davidson SJ, and Cheney RA: On-line medical command in theory and practice, *Ann Emerg Med* 18:261-268, 1989.
4. American College of Emergency Physicians: Control of advanced life support at the scene of medical emergencies, *Ann Emerg Med* 13:547-548, 1984.
5. Pepe PE and Stewart RD: Role of the physician in the prehospital setting, *Ann Emerg Med* 15:1480-1483, 1986.
6. Smith M: Hello . . . I'm a Doctor, *JEMS* 17(5):37-38, 1992.

Appendix I

Non-solicited Medical Intervention Protocol Card

NON-SOLICITED MEDICAL INTERVENTION PROTOCOL

Thank you for your offer of assistance.

Please be advised that these Emergency Medical Technicians are operating under the authority of the State of New York and under protocols established by the NYC 911 Emergency Medical Service System. These EMTs may also be New York City certified Paramedics who are operating under the authority of a medical control physician and standing medical orders.

To avoid confusion and to expedite patient care, no individual should intervene in the care of this patient unless the individual is:

1) requested to by the attending New York City Emergency Medical Service Personnel, or
2) authorized by the medical control physician, or
3) is capable of delivering more extensive emergency medical care at the scene.

HHC 614 (R Jan 85)

IF YOU ASSUME PATIENT MANAGEMENT, YOU ACCEPT RESPONSIBILITY FOR PATIENT CARE UNTIL THE ATTENDING NEW YORK CITY EMERGENCY MEDICAL SERVICE PERSONNEL OR MEDICAL CONTROL PHYSICIAN ACCEPTS THAT RESPONSIBILITY. THIS WILL REQUIRE THAT YOU ACCOMPANY THE PATIENT TO THE EMERGENCY DEPARTMENT.

Your cooperation is appreciated.

James T. Kerr *Executive Director*	Alexander E. Kuehl, M.D., M.P.H. *Vice President*

Physician Information Card

THANK YOU FOR YOUR OFFER OF ASSISTANCE
This EMERGENCY MEDICAL SERVICES team is operating under Washington law and policy established jointly by the EMS Medical Director of Pierce County and the Tacoma-Pierce County Health Department. The EMS team is functioning under the command of the base-hospital physician. If you wish to assist, please see other side for options.

Tacoma-Pierce County
Health Department
Emergency Medical
Services Division

____
Emergency Medical Services Medical Director

In general, the physician who has the most expertise in the management of the emergency should take control. This is usually the base-hospital physician. You may: (1) Request to talk directly to the base-hospital physician to offer your advice and assistance; (2) Offer your assistance with another pair of eyes, hands or suggestions, but let the EMS team remain under base-hospital physician control; or (3) If you have an area of special expertise for the patient's problem, you may take total responsibility, if delegated by the base physician, and accompany the patient to the hospital.

Appendix II

Assumption of Patient Management Statement

"I,________________________, license #________________________, have assumed authority and responsibility for patient management in the case to which this document refers.

I understand that in order to do this I must accompany the patient, in the ambulance, to the Emergency Department. I further understand that all EMS patient-care protocols must still be followed."

____

Signature

________________ ________________

Date Time

____

Witness: EMS Member

____

Witness: NYPD Officer, if present

39

Resuscitation Issues

Paul Pepe, M.D., FACEP, FCCP, FCCM, FACP

Most resuscitation efforts are initiated at a moment's notice, usually unexpectedly, and often with very little or no knowledge whatsoever about the patient involved. This scenario is particularly true in the out-of-hospital setting where most resuscitations are now initiated. The very nature of the typical situation seldom lends itself to a calm, rational, or informed decision-making process. Because any delay in resuscitation uniformly worsens the chance of successful outcome and because irreversible damage to the brain and other key organs can occur within minutes, most patients are resuscitated without discrimination but not always without question. The true difficulty generally occurs subsequent to the initiation of resuscitative measures.

There are very few circumstances in medicine that can evoke as much emotion and anxiety as aggressive, unconditional decisions to resuscitate. EMS practitioners routinely initiate and conduct certain resuscitations with much reluctance. Their emotions tell them that resuscitation of an asystolic jaundiced 90-year-old man reported to have metastatic cancer is a fruitless endeavor. Furthermore, it can be rationalized that allowing that person to die from a sudden cardiac arrest is more humane than attempting to prolong a life that may only be a painful, bedridden existence. Beyond this is the consideration that intervention interferes with a natural process and that the waiving of resuscitative efforts is not an active act of negligence but rather a realistic acceptance of the human condition. In essence, this line of thinking would constitute a general recognition of the well-known concept of "the right to die with dignity."

On the other hand, there are arguments that any attempts to discriminate between those who should and should not be aggressively resuscitated is the first step on the road to genocide.[21] How old is "too old?" Where does one draw the line? Who will decide such criteria for waiving resuscitation? In this line of thinking, failure to attempt resuscitation not only defies the Hippocratic oath, it neglects the patient's ultimate right—the right to live.

No matter what rationalizations and arguments one uses, be they internalized or openly expressed, heartfelt or rhetorical, they are not always clear-cut. Decisions concerning who should be resuscitated involve multifactorial issues ranging from religious, moral, ethical, legal, humanistic, and medical factors to considerations of patient rights, the effects on family, and even the availability of medical and financial resources.[2]

Regardless of these issues, the worst place in the world for self-fulfilling prophecy is in the arena of resuscitation medicine. To date, however, decisions not to initiate resuscitative efforts or, by the same token, decisions to discontinue them, have been based on probabilities of success.[5,12,31] Therefore the ultimate decisions must be based on sound medical data, an open mind, and experienced judgment.

As an example, a physician's decision to discontinue resuscitation efforts and pronounce the patient as "dead" is usually based on medical knowledge of established outcome statistics. Take the case of a patient who has presented to paramedics with asystole and who is flaccid and without neurologic response. Bystanders report that they found him "not breathing" and called for help. In addition, there was a known response time for medical rescuers of 10 minutes and no basic cardiopulmonary resuscitation (CPR) was performed during that period. This presentation was subsequently followed by a failure to develop any electrical complex on the electrocardiogram (ECG), or any other clinical response whatsoever, after the provision of basic CPR (chest compressions), endotracheal intubation, proper ventilatory techniques with 100% O_2, "three rounds" of standard intravenous (IV) drug therapy, and even an attempt at transcutaneous pacing.[13,14] In such a scenario, most physicians would feel entirely comfortable with stopping subsequent efforts. Since there is now an enormous collective experience that provides us with a well-established general knowledge base that under these circumstances and despite further efforts at resuscitation, no one has been known to survive.[4,5,16,31] But clearly, our collective medical experience also tells us that on occasion a patient presenting with asystole, and even the long response time, has been known to survive, neurologically intact because such resuscitation attempts were initiated.[12] In a recent study of 193 survivors of out-of-hospital cardiac arrest in Houston, more than 20% of these patients (successfully discharged from the hospital) presented with ECG rhythms other than ventricular fibrillation (e.g., asystole, idioventricular, or a normal-appearing complex).[26] Therefore it may be inappropriate to waive initial efforts despite the apparent bleak probabilities of survival indicated by a presenting ECG rhythm.

This section examines the various arguments concerning universal resuscitation and, whenever possible, examine the validity and caveats of medical and scientific data influencing these positions. And since, in most circumstances, almost all patients will at least receive an initial resuscitation attempt, it will also examine the decision to discontinue, which is really "at the heart" of the discussion. In the end, even after extensive, consensual discussions with family, the accountable EMS physician will effectively be responsible for the actual orders to waive resuscitation attempts or, if initiated, to discontinue any resuscitation efforts.[2] Such decisions, as complex as they are, should be based on a sound understanding of the concepts and data supporting them. The following discussion will attempt to update the EMS physician with regard to the latest information and rationales influencing these decisions.[4,14,26]

Resuscitation Decision

There are two major issues that EMS physicians and their surrogates must face: (1) Should resuscitation attempts be initiated in all patients? and (2) When should the resuscitation attempt be terminated? The following discussion will look at the pros and cons of these two issues.

Rationales Against Universal Resuscitation

There are four key problems with unconditional resuscitation attempts:

1. Some patients have an obvious irreversible/irreparable condition, the treatment for which is beyond the current capabilities of any available medical resources (for example, rigor mortis, incineration, and decapitation).[13]
2. It is unrealistic, extraordinarily expensive, and occasionally dangerous to respond to and treat all victims of cardiopulmonary arrest or severe injury, particularly since most will die without certain unique conditions being present (for example, it is unlikely that anyone will survive untreated cardiopulmonary arrest in a rural setting where the closest rescue personnel are a half hour away).[21]
3. The patient involved expressly did not wish to have any "heroic measures" implemented because he had a documented, terminal, irreversible process.[15,19,28,29]
4. Brains are permanently damaged sooner than are cardiovascular systems; therefore there is a certain risk of creating a population of neurologic cripples when the number of cardiovascular resuscitations regularly exceed the number of salvaged nervous systems.[21,33]

Definition of Death

Although religious definitions may vary, most scientists would define death as a somewhat progressive process that involves an ongoing continuum of events usually beginning with oxygen deprivation to certain critical tissues, subsequently followed by adenosine triphosphate (ATP) depletion in others such as rigor mortis, and finally the decay process. In other words, a finite point in time at which death is present is an oversimplified view of the process. Since no one has the capability of seeing "a soul leave the body," of clinical significance for the EMS practitioner is somehow identifying that point in time beyond which this process or certain key elements of this process (e.g., permanent cognitive brain tissue injury) are irreversible.[13,19]

In that respect, notwithstanding the perfunctory caveats about hypothermia ("the patient is dead only when he is warm and dead") and certain drug overdoses, it is generally accepted that a patient is in an absolutely irreversible condition when found to be cold, stiff with rigor mortis, and/or marked with dependent lividity.[2,13] The same applies for those with transected torsos, complete incineration, decapitation, or decomposition.[2,13,16] However, in many situations, there are no clear-cut clinical signs that tell the would-be rescuer if that critical point has occurred.[2,13]

Pupils may fixate in dilation as early as 90 seconds of anoxia or because of some ophthalmological or pharmacological reason. Therefore a lack of initial pupillary response is not a definitive indicator of potential outcome. In addition, individual patients have different responses and tolerances for those processes which cause irreversible states. While age and previous state of health both correlate with outcome, they are only modest correlations in comparison to the elapsed time interval after arrest (downtime) and the time of initiation of basic and advanced life support.*

Elapsed Interval of Arrest

While the interval before therapy has often been shown to be a clear key element in survival rates, the reported time intervals from collapse to intervention are not always accurate, nor are they always a totally reliable indicator of outcome in individual cases. Permanent, significant brain injury can occur within 3 to 4 minutes after sudden complete cessation of breathing or heartbeat, but some can tolerate twice that time or even longer under certain circumstances. And what about those who do not have sudden and complete cessation of cardiopulmonary function? Some patients have ill-defined intervals of arrest such as those who started out with a gradual depression of cardiovascular function that occurs in various shock states (for example, severe hemorrhage, cardiogenic shock, gradual respiratory arrest, rapid ventricular tachycardias). They may have permanent or severe damage of critical organs even before complete clinical cessation of cardiopulmonary function.

Even when breathing and heartbeat are initially present, certain traumatic injuries are clearly irreparable in terms of current capabilities to deal with them. For example, conditions such as decapitation, anatomical decerebration, transected torsos, and massive, explosive penetration across the midline of the brain are currently considered to be beyond our ability to salvage. Other types of physical damage, such as certain types of injuries to the heart or great vessels, not easily apparent from external inspection, are often beyond repair as well. However, as technology and medical discoveries evolve, these injuries, that often we glibly call "lethal" injuries, may eventually be within our ability to treat.

So, outside of these anatomical limitations, how long is too long? Even when the collapse is witnessed, time estimates are fairly inaccurate. Minutes may have "seemed like hours" to those distraught relatives in the home or in the hospital to roommates who are anxiously awaiting help. By the same token, even when response times are documented by rescuers to be quite long (a dispatch to patient contact interval of greater than 10 minutes), patients occasionally are resuscitated successfully and even achieve long-term survival. Furthermore, although witnesses report that the patient "fell out" right at the time of the initial call for her help, on closer questioning, it may be revealed that the patient "was still breathing a little" just up to the time of arrival of the rescuers. Therefore some limited spontaneous circulation may have been present as in some cases of ventricular tachycardia.

*References 2,10,11,13,14,34,35.

Initial Cardiac Rhythm

The presenting ECG rhythm, though somewhat indicative, is not always useful in predicting downtime.† While "coarse" ventricular fibrillation (VF) may predict a better outcome than "fine" VF, neither EKG interpretation is an absolute guarantee of the arrest interval nor the patient's eventual outcome.[34] In addition, technological, physiological, and anatomical variations may alter our perception and ECG interpretation of heart activities.[22] Likewise, while those presenting with asystole or a pulseless idioventricular rhythm have a much bleaker chance of surviving relative to those presenting with coarse VF, some still survive despite this initial picture of apparent cardiac standstill.[8,26,34,35]

Certainly those patients who receive defibrillation, but have no residual rhythm despite several minutes of good oxygenation, basic CPR, and adrenalin administration, have been down without adequate coronary artery circulation for a significant period of time (Figure 39-1). Occasionally, some patients respond well to initial therapeutic interventions, but their hemodynamics eventually

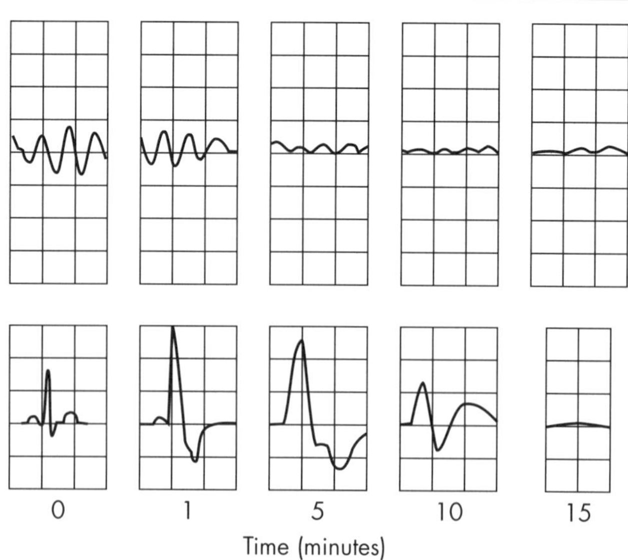

Figure 39-1. A sample time course of the ventricular fibrillation waveform *(top)* demonstrating a deterioration of coarse to fine fibrillation. The lower panel shows samples of the conversion rhythms one might expect as time elapses.

†References 2,12,21,26,31,35.

dwindle. Presumably, this might occur because of a significant coronary artery occlusion that may have precipitated the event or because of a state of refractory peripheral vascular "paralysis." On the other hand, a few patients who have a poor initial response may still go on to do well after persistent efforts.[12]

But these cases usually are the exception to the rule. While not absolute, the response to initial therapy is one of the more reliable indications of the elapsed time interval of arrest as well as prognosis in the patient with VF. Although an initial presenting rhythm of coarse VF is more apt to be converted to an organized rhythm associated with spontaneous circulation than fine VF, this observation is much less reliable than the actual response to initial therapeutic interventions.[4,22,34]

Similarly, with a "dwindling heart" presentation (pulseless idioventricular rhythm or asystole) similar to that pictured electrocardiographically in Figure 39-2, the response to initial therapy is the key. Many patients with a simple respiratory arrest, even when pulseless, apneic, and asystolic, will respond and recover fully intact if they receive immediate aggressive therapy. Often oxygenation with a brief period of basic CPR will be the only necessary procedures, particularly if aggressive endotracheal intubation is readily performed. Again, reported "downtime" alone is not a good indicator of whether or not to start the resuscitation. On the other hand, failure to respond to the initial therapy, particularly after IV epinephrine infusion, predicts an extremely bleak outcome.[4,35] Because the majority of patients presenting with a dwindling heart syndrome probably have nonhypoxemic myocardial hypoxia (before arrest) such as that resulting from obstruction of a major coronary artery, correction of respiratory and peripheral circulatory impairments are usually fruitless if the compromised heart still fails to beat as a result of nonperfusion in the coronaries. Therefore since the cardiovascular response to initial therapy is one of the best indicators of the arrest interval, resuscitation should generally be initiated to gain this prognostic insight.[24]

Time to Advanced Life Support

On occasion, an emergency medical dispatcher may get a clear-cut report such as "my husband, John, just stopped breathing." Rescue personnel arrive 15 minutes later (time documented) and find the patient to be asystolic. It would seem almost straightforward that the situation is futile and brain death is virtually guaranteed.[5,31,35] However, it still behooves the physician responsible for "pronouncing" death to be absolutely certain that all of those reported conditions were, in fact, all true, present, and documentable before declaring that there is irreversible death. In the prehospital setting, where most arrests occur, the rescuers are basic level emergency medical technicians (EMT-Bs) who, in most states, legally cannot pronounce patients dead unless acting under the orders of a physician.[2,18,21] Failure to initiate the resuscitation while evaluating the situation or contacting the direct medical control physician would obviously cause a critical period of time to elapse, most likely resulting in irrevocable outcome.[13]

Data from the best EMS systems have indicated that, without advanced life support (ALS), patients uncommonly survive beyond fifteen minutes of arrest despite basic CPR.[5,10,11,34,35] This has led many to believe that such cases are hopeless and that if ALS is not initiated within 10 to 12 minutes of a witnessed arrest, survival is unlikely. However, many clinicians have had experiences with patients who survived despite lengthy delays in ALS (>30 min) or even despite hours of on-going CPR when ALS was initiated immediately after collapse.[12] One major problem is defining what the authors actually mean by ALS; future studies must evaluate specific interventions. Except in certain environments, time limits should generally be disregarded when deciding whether or not to initiate resuscitation in an individual case.[8,11,21]

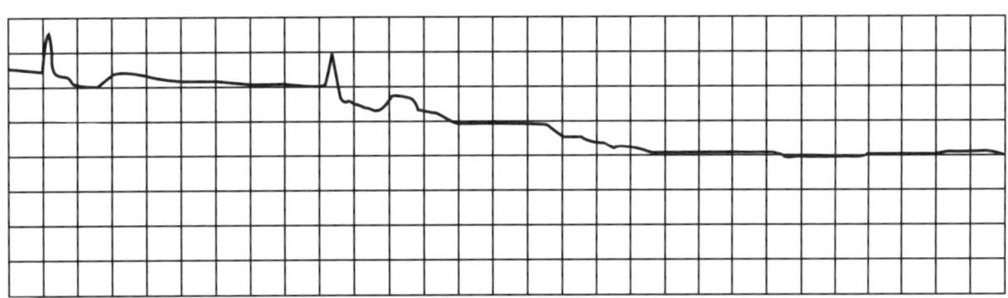

Figure 39-2. The typical electrocardiograph tracing seen in the "dwindling heart" scenario as it deteriorates from pulseless idioventricular to asystole.

Waiving Resuscitation Because of Hearsay

All of the previous considerations essentially argue in favor of the current standard that, in the absence of rigor mortis, lividity, or decapitation, resuscitation efforts should always be initiated in the prehospital setting whenever rescuers are asked to respond.[2,13,18,21] Those personnel are therefore compelled to initiate the resuscitation attempt despite protests from family, bystanders, or self-proclaimed authorities such as lawyers or even "doctors" on the phone.[2] However, this becomes difficult when EMS crews arrive and a family member says, "Papa has cancer and this is his doctor on the phone and he says not to do anything." Even with a "Living Will" or a "Durable Powers of Attorney" in hand (assuming prehospital care personnel are familiar with them), without documented medical records, or without the unfamiliar physician on the phone being able to provide evidence that he is the patient's physician, the medical care provider still may be at medical-legal risk when waiving resuscitation. Although recent expert medical consensus supports a more liberal attitude toward waiver of resuscitation efforts in reportedly terminal patients, the chance of making a "mistake" remains worrisome.[14] "Living Wills" and "Advanced Directives" usually require physician interpretation and formulation into a treatment plan (e.g., No CPR). They do not necessarily indicate "No CPR" by themselves.[14] So for the most part, in the absence of decapitation, incineration, lividity, or rigor mortis, the prehospital providers take a degree of risk when waiving resuscitation without bonafide physician directive. Ideally, the pronouncing physician should be well-known to the EMS providers and a well-defined, well-clarified, well-accepted prospective decision should have been reached. This may require initiation of efforts until that physician directive can be obtained. Nevertheless, common sense and compassion should always take major roles in the decision process.

Better yet, if the family or legal guardians wished no resuscitation, they should not have activated the EMS system. For example, in hospice programs, if it is the well-established and accepted will of the patient to die of his terminal illness, the program caretakers or family should not call the EMS system to "pronounce" or evaluate patients. Nevertheless, families may still call for help or a medical examiner may contact the police who inadvertently calls EMS. Therefore it would be better that such patients be registered with the medical examiner's office or other appropriate authorities and they be notified accordingly. To that end, recent programs have been established in which certain persons with terminal disease can be pre-registered with the EMS program as having a Do Not Resuscitate (DNR) disposition.[14,20] With official documents and identification mechanisms (photo identifications, wristbands) being part of the "system", such approaches can work to avoid difficult scenarios. Such programs are already beginning to work well in several communities.

Traumatic Arrest

Decisions regarding the waiver of resuscitation efforts for those situations involving apparent circulatory arrest in trauma victims also pose some tough problems. Although the term *traumatic cardiac arrest* is often used, it is not always exactly clear as to when the patient "arrested." Apnea is a fairly reasonable sign of true respiratory arrest. However, "pulselessness" may be a lack of perceived pulses. Often a heartbeat can be auscultated or a good sinus rhythm recorded on the ECG monitor in a "pulseless" patient, so the moment of true cardiac arrest (total nonperfusion) is not always clear. This is best exemplified by the scenario of pericardial tamponade. Therefore trauma indices, while useful for comparative studies, may be inappropriate for waiving resuscitation.[6] Granted the initial presence of asystole usually predicts nonviability. However, some trauma victims have been known to survive.[12] On the other hand, asystole on arrival at the hospital after prehospital endotracheal intubation is probably a sign of irreversibility.

While most victims of injury will not be resuscitated when there is circulatory arrest, there are clear exceptions. In fact, the term *DOA* may in some circumstances be a dangerous anachronism. For example, in the Seattle study of trauma victims receiving CPR, 25% of the group did survive.[7] The survivors usually were those who were "young, intubated, and penetrated."[7] Also, almost all survivors were responded to and transported to a surgically aggressive trauma center within 15 minutes. As a result, nearly 70% of all those with penetrating injury survived. Only 10% of the blunt trauma patients survived despite similar therapy. However, this study demonstrated that under certain conditions, apparent circulatory arrest is not necessarily a futile situation for all trauma patients, even those victims of blunt injury. Similar results have been currently achieved in the Houston EMS system and in Washington, DC, with respect to penetrating injures.[9,30]

There are cases for which resuscitation is not reasonable. Take the example of a large gunshot wound into the center of the left chest or through the head (temple to temple) in an apneic, pulseless, asystolic patient who is found with fixed and dilated pupils and who has no audible heart beat. This generally indicates a nonsalvageable patient, especially when surgical intervention is more than 10 to 15 minutes away.[7,9] Looking at the collective statistics, there are probably no reported survivors of such conditions. Nevertheless, there are some empiric (although arbitrary and not entirely proven) rationales for initiating resuscitation in penetrating injury patients who have apparent circulatory arrest. These include (1) a monitored arrest and there is close availability of emergency thoracotomy by expert physicians with expert surgical back-up; (2) the wound is localized (to the head) and the patient is a potential transplant donor; (3) the presence of either an organized rhythm on ECG or an audible heart beat, or (4) suspicion of a reversible process such as tension pneumothorax, open pneumothorax, upper airway obstruction, or pericardial tamponade and EMS personnel are trained to manage such cases.[9,24,25]

As discussed, in blunt trauma, the salvage rate for patients with circulatory arrest is almost negligible.[7,30] It is probably only possible to save these patients in settings when a single organ injury is involved (which is difficult to predict in the prehospital setting) and when thoracotomy is immediately available.[7] It could be argued that without clearer scientific studies to prove the futility of resuscitation attempts under specific circumstances, the same caveats given for penetrating injury probably could still apply. Nevertheless, EMS medical directors must also weigh the hazards of emergency transport (collisions and communicable disease exposures) before committing EMS personnel to universal resuscitation efforts in victims of blunt injury who have circulatory arrest. Victims of blunt injury who have agonal or asystolic ECG presentations and do not immediately respond to airway and respiratory procedures are candidates for field termination of efforts and pronouncement of death. In general, if the airway is intact and no reversible process is apparent, resuscitation efforts and transport are futile when there is cardiopulmonary arrest in a patient with blunt trauma at any distance from the trauma center.

Whatever policy is used, one must always consider the presence of a potentially reversible underlying medical condition that led to the patient's fall or motor vehicle collision. For example, an occasional patient with ventricular tachycardia may be involved in an automobile wreck and be found "dead" by EMS crews. It is possible that ventricular tachycardia was initially sustained with some minimal perfusion and then evolved into a ventricular fibrillation just before the arrival of EMS personnel.

Therefore aggressive therapy for the medical condition is still warranted. Likewise, even an asystolic patient may be the victim of a sudden hypoxic event (seizure or choking) that is still potentially reversible. Placement of an endotracheal tube would help to clarify this issue. If severe injuries are apparent and airway/respiratory procedures do not improve the situation, the blunt injury patient with asystole is a clear candidate for termination of efforts.

Testing Responsiveness

As portrayed, with certain exceptions, aggressive initiation of resuscitation should be undertaken for most cardiac arrest cases, despite initial appearances. Therefore the response to initial therapy is the key issue. This philosophy would be shared by most medical and legal organizations.[13] The Uniform Determination of Death Act, which has been adopted by some states and which is endorsed by the American Bar Association and the American Medical Association, states that

> An individual who has sustained either 1) irreversible cessation of circulatory and respiratory functions or 2) irreversible cessation of all functions of the entire brain, including the brain stem, is dead. A determination of death must be made in accordance with accepted medical standards.

What this means is that resuscitative efforts should begin in almost all cases where there has been no prospective agreement (for example, specialized EMS DNR identification or other appropriately charted DNR consensus).[14] Without testing the responsiveness of the circulatory system through attempts at resuscitation, one cannot determine the true irreversibility of circulatory and respiratory function.[13] Likewise, one cannot state whether brain function is irreversibly lost without reestablishing circulation. Therefore no matter where the resuscitation is conducted and no matter who is conducting it, it is critical that the trial of both resuscitative measures is carefully detailed and chronologically recorded to validate the hopelessness of the case. By documenting the failure to respond to resuscitative efforts, the criterion of irreversibility of the cessation of circulatory and respiratory function can be established. This will help to end any speculation as to the recoverability of the brain. Without circulation, the brain will not survive.

Family Protest

Often, EMS personnel are called but are told on arrival, that "the family wants nothing done." It is quite common for paramedical personnel to be called to a residence where they find an elderly person in cardiopulmonary arrest. Despite family protests that the patient "has cancer" and should be left alone, the rescue personnel should usually initiate the resuscitation.[2,14,18] As stated previously, despite threats of legal action, under such circumstances the providers and their base-station physicians actually would be ill-advised to stop or waive resuscitation without better documentation. Commonly it is the stated wish of the family that no "heroic" or "extraordinary" measures be taken and that they do not want their loved one "kept alive" by artificial means. Often they are reflecting the patient's own statements from some previous occasion . . . or so they say. While it is becoming more and more acceptable among lay persons to let their loved ones "die with dignity," it must be clear in the responsible physician's mind that there is no hope of survival when "following the family's wishes." Unfortunately, selfish motivations can exist, especially when elderly sick patients create a financial and emotional burden for the family or when inheritance is a concern. Therefore without prior knowledge of circumstances and prospective decisions, the EMS personnel should generally provide aggressive resuscitation. On the other hand, they should also attempt to aggressively resolve the situation by acquiring pertinent confirmation of an irreversible condition if at all possible. Again, common sense and compassion are still two of the physician's most important tools under such difficult circumstances. Such traits must be passed on to the EMS personnel representing the EMS physician by constant example and day-to-day role-modeling.

Impaired Person

Resuscitation of an already neurologically impaired patient is another difficult area, but is akin to the approach used in terminally ill patients with malignancies. Like the oncologist who can render a prognostic opinion concerning the type of malignancy with and without therapy, the neurologist or neurosurgeon may be able to provide similar documentation. But outcome is often more difficult to define with severe neurological impairment, and surprises are known to occur.

Even for previously healthy persons, the argument exists that there is a potential for creating a population of neurological cripples by overzealous resuscitation efforts. Perhaps two or three in a hundred of those patients who survive long-term may enter a limbo of severe neurological impairment following "successful" cardiac arrest resuscitation.[17,26] Generally, patients either survive and eventually become awake and neurologically intact or they go on to have progressive cerebral edema and systemic deterioration with ensuing death over the next 48 to 72 hours. Collective experience suggests therefore that the odds are overwhelmingly in favor of surviving with a reasonably intact neurological state and not a state of vegetation.[2,26] The major exceptions are the premature infant, the severe head-injured patient, or the cerebral vascular accident patient whose outlooks are much harder to predict at the time of initial resuscitation.[33]

Age

Although resuscitation of the elderly has been discouraged in certain in-hospital cases, the experience from Belgium, as well as the Seattle, Houston, and Milwaukee EMS systems, favors aggressive resuscitative efforts, particularly those presenting with VF. Although survival rates are slightly lower and life expectancy shorter, functional survivors can be common.[3,17,32]

Summary on Initiation of Resuscitation

Without a clear-cut DNR status, resuscitation should probably be initiated in any victim of cardiopulmonary arrest who is not in a state of rigor mortis or who does not have dependent lividity, regardless of the presenting ECG. Even when it seems "hopeless," there are rare anecdotes that vindicate initiation of aggressive resuscitation efforts. Beyond this is the usually unspoken issue that the more EMS providers perform their skills, the better they are able to handle the next case. Although it may appear a little irreverent, there is almost a social obligation to perform one's resuscitation skills as often as possible so that subsequent patients get even better care. So even the elderly, asystolic patient with an unknown elapsed interval of arrest should receive aggressive resuscitative attempts, not only because of the occasional "surprises," but also because every resuscitation attempt improves the subsequent performance of practitioners in terms of both skills and experience. This philosophy can be viewed as one that is life saving in the long run. Rather than an invasion of an individual's right, it is more of a method to better guarantee the ultimate right of others and occasionally that very individual the right to live.

Rationales for Stopping Resuscitation

Termination of Efforts

Since it is the rare occasion in which the initiation of resuscitations are waived, the real decision comes after the resuscitation effort has begun. The issue becomes "How far do we go?" There are several arguments in favor of stopping a resuscitation effort. For example, documentation may become available that the patient has a terminal process with an imminent death. Another example would be a situation in which there is no response to therapy and the chances of hurting rescuers far outweigh the chances of patient survival.[14,16]

Caveats

All of these arguments sound reasonable, but they also deserve close scrutiny and understanding on the part of the accountable EMS physician before they are accepted. While a person with diagnosed acquired immunodeficiency syndrome (AIDS) or small-cell carcinoma of the lung may be dead within 2 years, it must be recognized that any given individual may return to a reasonable lifestyle for at least several months if resuscitated early in the course of the disease. Therefore the statement that "the patient has lung cancer" should not be considered an absolute rationale, particularly when the condition is generically classified as "lung cancer" and reported as hearsay. Therefore in the absence of a documented DNR status the most reasonable rationale for stopping a resuscitation is the lack of response to initial resuscitative measures.

Criteria for Termination

As stated before, the patient who has had an unwitnessed arrest and who remains in asystole despite aggressive initial therapy will not be salvaged.[4,16,31,35] Furthermore, recent data have now provided fairly discrete criteria for terminating resuscitative efforts at the scene for all other cases of arrest. Specifically, adult patients will not survive an out-of-hospital arrest if all of the following criteria are present: (1) unmonitored arrest (not associated with trauma, primary respiratory etiology, drug overdose or temperature aberration); (2) absence of spontaneous circulation within 25 minutes of the initiation of standard advanced cardiac life support (ACLS) techniques; (3) absence of persistently recurring/refractory VF; and (4) absence of any neurological signs.[4] These criteria are applicable independently of the reported "downtime" or basic CPR interval. Although there are no guarantees for survival, those with monitored arrest, persistently recurring VF, or even a transient return of pulses may occasionally survive despite more than 25 minutes of ACLS. Therefore continued in-hospital efforts could be argued in such cases. However, using today's state-of-the-art approaches, there are no other apparent exceptions.[13,22,35] Obviously, if future therapeutic advances are to be tested, these criteria should be modified. Again, resuscitation medicine is the last place for self-fulfilling prophecies.

Scene Pronouncements

If efforts are to be terminated at the scene, it is advisable for the patient to be pronounced dead by the direct medical control physician who is in contact with the EMS personnel.[12,14] As stated before, this may obviate the dangers of racing through busy traffic with the unlikely to-be-saved patient, a situation which may endanger the lives of both the rescuers and other innocent bystanders. In addition, it avoids the distraction of emergency department personnel and resources from other serious cases, and it circumvents the expense of the emergency department billings for the family and the health care system as a whole.

This practice is already in effect in many EMS systems.[32] But while this practice seems logical, there are several caveats to be considered. First, the physician is not truly present to pronounce the patient as "dead" even though the intermediaries are legally considered "the eyes and ears of the physician." Second, many families are emotionally attached to the concept of taking the patient "to the hospital" as providing the "ultimate" in care. Alternatives to on-scene termination would then be hospital transport without lights and siren (nonemergency mode) when further efforts appear futile. Local medical direction, in conjunction with governmental authorities, should determine the best policy for the local community.

Pronouncements in the prehospital setting can be acceptable as long as the responsible physician meticulously trains the personnel and has extreme confidence in their abilities and judgment, both medically and interpersonally with families.[11,21] As with other EMS medical care, the physician may delegate an act of medical practice to the EMS personnel, as long as the physician involved is willing to take responsibility for that decision.[24,30] It is therefore a good practice that pronouncements be confirmed after consultation with a direct medical control physician or responsible medical director.[12] This practice also should be considered in EMS systems with EMT-A providers as well, particularly when lengthy transports are involved.[14] Otherwise, state and local authorities should be encouraged to develop protocols for the initiation and discontinuation of CPR in areas where more advanced care is not available. Prospective training is a must. More importantly, the example of the physician role model who is compassionate and professional is a key element to success of such a policy.[24]

Subtle Values of Resuscitation Efforts

Positive communications from families of cardiac arrest victims have not only come from the survivors, but more often from the families of those patients who died. Most of the time these families are grateful for their impressions that the EMS system and the receiving hospital did "everything possible" and that they were given the satisfaction that their loved one got "the best shot he could have had." In addition, they also mention the perspective that even the 2 or 3 days of transient "survival" gave the family members a better chance to adjust and come to terms with the loved one's demise. In essence, the aggressive resuscitation efforts made the transition easier for them, and the hospital costs were not so much a major burden in their minds. Perhaps the insurance company actually relieves the burden, and this approach translates into higher medical costs for us all. For now though, the sociological consensus appears to be that when there is any question or possibility of salvage, one should always provide initial aggressive care. In fact, asking families at the time of a failing resuscitation attempt whether or not they feel that the patient should receive further care is usually unfair and a difficult burden to place on them.[2] This does not preclude informing them or discussing options, but in most cases, they will avoid having the overwhelming responsibility of "ending it all." Therefore termination policies set in place by medical community consensus should be established to take this burden off of the family. Again, termination policies should still be considered a tool not a shackle for the online EMS physician.

Unusual Circumstances

Pregnancy

If witnesses report that a pregnant woman lost respirations 10 minutes ago and that they had been doing basic CPR somewhat ineffectively because the mother is trapped in a car and the witnesses appear reliable about their timing and CPR performance, it is unlikely that any intervention will be successful. While there exists enough oxygen in the placental intervillous space to support fetal metabolism for 8 minutes or more after sudden arrest in the mother,[33] 5 minutes of fetal distress will usually result in an Apgar score of 5 under the best of circumstances. In a premature infant, the prognosis would be more dismal and if the fetus is less than 32 to 33 weeks old, survival is probably unlikely. In addition, in trauma cases, the circulatory compromise is progressive, indicating the probability of even more compromise. So we need to try to obtain a history of when the baby is due.

However, these data, while helpful, usually are not available nor completely reliable and one must pragmatically approach the situation with a clinical guess at fetal age. A fundus that is round and the size of a large bowling ball is probably reflective of a 6-month-old fetus and survival is unlikely, even in the hospital setting. On the other hand, a football-shaped fundus half way between the umbilicus and xiphoid process probably reflects a 32-week-old or older fetus and there is an outside chance of success in a witnessed arrest. If the mother decompensates in front of the EMS personnel, they should treat the mother as usual, which would most likely mean provision of airway and rapid transport to a definitive care-providing facility. If the time elements are still reasonable, resuscitation of the baby still may be appropriate.

Multiple Casualties

Triage decisions at the multiple casualty incident (MCI) are often difficult and probably only 80% accurate even when the most experienced medical personnel make the priority judgments.[27] The standard approach is not to become preoccupied with pulseless patients if there are multiple patients with serious injuries. Of course, if there are 40 patients, 39 of whom are "walking wounded" and the other one is in a state of cardiopulmonary arrest, the resuscitation is quite appropriate. But in circumstances where life-threatening but reparable injuries are present in several patients and available personnel resources are limited, waiving resuscitation for a pulseless, apneic patient is probably appropriate.

The best guideline is to do what will save most lives long-term.[27] For example, even if there are critically ill or injured patients, the "walking-wounded" or "normals" should be evacuated first if hazards still exist. They are more apt to survive long-term, unless they become injured by ongoing hazards. When hazards are not present, then the usual triage routine of "sickest first" applies. Among those whose state is immediately life-threatening, who should be the first resuscitated? Again, who is more apt to survive long-term? The severe head-injured patient (unconscious and barely responsive to anything but deep painful stimuli) who has a blood pressure of 85 mm Hg has a much poorer prognosis than the nearby "shocky appearing" patient with abdominal trauma, also with a blood pressure of 85 mm Hg but who is very lucid. Therefore the second patient should receive priority for evacuation as the probability of long-term survival is greater despite a similar degree of hypotension.

The patient with a femur fracture, although it is a potentially life-threatening injury, is unlikely to die immediately and evacuation/treatment can be delayed even though the patient has an even better chance of long-term survival than the abdominal trauma case. All things considered, both patients can be salvaged, especially if other assistance will be shortly available. Within the group of patients who are determined to be the most serious because of immediately life-threatening injuries, one should consider the resources available and then triage according to best chances of long-term survival.

Summary

Universal attempts at resuscitation will probably continue to be questioned, particularly as resources decrease.[2] The great majority of patients who are victims of cardiac arrest will die, even under the most optimum circumstances. But the collective body of knowledge that we now have compels us to at least try an initial attempt at resuscitation in almost all cases in which there are no documented, prospective determinations of DNR status. The issue of when to stop these initial attempts has become less difficult to pinpoint. Recent data have provided us with better guidelines and criteria for aggressive termination of efforts. But such decisions usually depend on the ultimate decision of an accountable physician. It is that physician who must directly or through EMS personnel pronounce death and inform family and friends that their loved one is gone forever. The Golden Rule may well apply. If it was a member of the physician's family, how would he decide? The decision is not one that should be mandated by some law or protocol, but rather by sound, informed medical judgment and, most importantly, a little wisdom.

"Wisdom" is most often defined as accumulated philosophic or scientific learning, meaning that research efforts and improved methods of identifying those who will or will not be salvaged must be continually sought. In addition, it means that we should search for better resuscitation techniques and technologies, particularly those applied in the out-of-hospital setting.[23] Furthermore, it means that this seeking must also be combined with humanity and compassion.

REFERENCES

1. Bergner L et al: Service factors and health status of survivors of out-of-hospital cardiac arrest, *Am J Emerg Med* 3:259-263, 1983.
2. Bioethics Committee, American College of Emergency Physicians: Medical moral, legal and ethical aspects of resuscitation for the patient who will have minimal ability to ultimately survive, *Ann Emerg Med* 14:919-926, 1985.
3. Bonnin MJ, Pepe PE, and Clark PS: Survival prognosis for the elderly after out-of-hospital cardiac arrest (abstract), *Ann Emerg Med* 18:189, 1989.
4. Bonnin MJ, Pepe PE, and Clark PS: Key role of prehospital resuscitation in survival from out-of-hospital cardiac arrest (abstract). *Ann Emerg Med* 19:466, 1990.
5. Brain Resuscitation Clinical Trial I Study Group: Neurologic recovery after cardiac arrest: The effect of ischemia, *Crit Care Med* 13:930-931, 1985.
6. Champion HR, Gainer PS, and Yackee E: A progress preport on the trauma score in predicting a fatal outcome, *J Trauma* 26:927-931, 1986.
7. Copass MK et al: Prehospital cardiopulmonary resuscitation of the critically injured patient, *Am J Surg* 148:19-26, 1984.
8. Cummins RO et al: State-of-the-art review—Improving survival from sudden cardiac arrest: the "chain of survival" concept. Statement for Health Professionals from the Advanced Cardiac Life Support Subcommittee and the Emergency Cardiac Care Committee, American Heart Association, *Circulation* 83:1832-1847, 1991.
9. Durham LA et al: Emergency center thoracotomy: Impact of prehospital resuscitation, *J Trauma* 32(6):1-5, June 1992.
10. Eisenberg MS, Bergner L, and Hallstrom A: Cardiac resuscitation in the community—importance of rapid provision and implications for program planning, *JAMA* 241:1905-1907, 1979.
11. Eisenberg MS, Bergner L, and Hallstrom A: Paramedic programs and out-of-hospital cardiac arrest. I. Factors associated with successful resuscitation, *Am J Public Health* 69:30-38, 1979.
12. Eisenberg MS and Cummins RO: Termination of CPR in the prehospital arena, *Ann Emerg Med* 14:1106-1107, 1985.
13. Emergency Cardiac Care Committee, American Heart Association: Standards and guidelines for cardiopulmonary resuscitation and emergency cardiac care, *JAMA* 255:2841-3044, 1986.
14. Emergency Cardiac Care Committee, American Heart Association: Standards and guidelines for cardiopulmonary resuscitation and emergency cardiac care, *JAMA* 261:2171-2299, October 28, 1992.
15. Haber JG: The living will and the directive to provide maximum care—the scope of autonomy, *Chest* 90:442-444, 1986.
16. Kellermann AL, Staves DR, and Hackman BB: In-hospital resuscitation following unsuccessful prehospital advanced cardiac life support: 'Heroic efforts' or an exercise in futility? *Ann Emerg Med* 17:589-594, 1988.
17. Longstreth WT et al: Does age affect outcomes of out-of-hospital cardiopulmonary resuscitation? *JAMA* 264:2109-2110, 1990.
18. McCarthy P: Do not resuscitate: Administrative and ethical considerations in prehospital arrests, *J Emerg Med Services* 9:26-30, 1983.
19. McIntyre KM: *Medicolegal considerations in cardiopulmonary resuscitation and emergency cardiac care.* In Medical Control in Emergency Medical Services Systems, 1981, Washington, DC, National Academy Press.
20. Miles SH and Crimmins TJ: Orders to limit emergency treatment for an ambulance service in a large metropolitan area, *JAMA* 254:525-527, 1985.
21. Page JO, Pepe PE, and Ayres RJ: *Resuscitation in the prehospital setting—when to start, when to stop.* From the Proceedings of the second annual meeting of the National Association of Emergency Medical Services Physicians, August 19, 1986, San Diego, Calif.
22. Pepe PE: *Advanced cardiac life support: state of the art.* In Vincent JL, editor: Emergency and intensive care, Berlin, 1990, Springer-Verlag, pp. 565-585, 1990.

23. Pepe PE: Out-of-hospital resuscitation research: rationale and strategies for the evaluation of basic and advanced life support interventions. Special Symposium Issue on Methodology in Cardiac Arrest Research. *Ann Emerg Med* 22 (special supplement):1993.
24. Pepe PE, Bonnin MJ, and Mattox KL: Regulating the scope of EMS, *Prehosp Disast Med* 5:59-63, 1990.
25. Pepe PE, and Copass MK: Prehospital care. In Moore EE, editor: The American College of Surgeons committee on trauma—*Early Care of the Injured,* ed 4, Philadelphia, 1990, BC Decker.
26. Pepe PE et al: Out-of-hospital cardiac arrest presenting with rhythms other than ventricular fibrillation (abstract), *Crit Care Med* 20:585, 1992.
27. Pepe PE, Stewart RD, and Copass MK: Ten golden rules for urban multiple casualty incident management, *Prehosp Disast Med* 4:131-134, 1989.
28. Raffin TA: Value of the living will, *Chest* 90:444-446, 1986.
29. Rosner F: The living will, *Chest* 90:441-442, 1986.
30. Rozycki GS et al: Resuscitative thoracotomy—trends in outcome, *Ann Emerg Med* 19:462, 1990.
31. Smith JP and Bodai BI: Guidelines for discontinuing prehospital CPR in the emergency department, *Ann Emerg Med* 14:1093-1098, 1985.
32. Tresch DD et al: Should the elderly be resuscitated following out-of-hospital cardiac arrest? *Am J Med* 86:145-150, 1989.
33. Turkel SB, Sims ME, and Guttenberg ME: Postponed neonatal death in the premature infant, *Am J Dis Child* 140:576-579, 1986.
34. Weaver WD et al: Amplitude of ventricular fibrillation waveform and outcome after cardiac arrest, *Ann Intern Med* 102:53-55, 1985.
35. Weaver WD et al: Considerations for improving survival from out-of-hospital cardiac arrest, *Ann Emerg Med* 15:1181-1186, 1986.

SUGGESTED READINGS

Bedell SE et al: Do-not-resuscitate orders for critically ill patients in the hospital: How are they used and what is their impact? *JAMA* 256:233-237.

Brennan TA: Do-not-resuscitate orders for the incompetent patient in the absence of family consent, *Law, Medicine and Health Care* 14(1):9-19, 1986.

Buchsbaum HJ, Clapp JF, and Crosby WM: Trauma in pregnancy. *American College of Obstetrics and Gynecology Continuing Medical Education Program* 12:1-9, 1986.

Charlson ME et al: Resuscitation: How do we decide? *JAMA* 255:1316-1322, 1986

Iserson KV: Forgoing prehospital care: Should ambulance staff always resuscitate? *J Med Ethics* 1991;17:19-24.

Lipton HL: Do-not-resuscitate decisions in a community hospital: Incidence, implications and outcomes. *JAMA* 256:1164-1169, 1986.

Maggiore WA: Withholding resuscitation. The medical, legal and ethical concerns. *J Emerg Med Services* 1991;16:94-98.

Roth R et al: Out-of-hospital cardiac arrest: Factors associated with survival. *Ann Emerg Med* 13:237-243, 1984.

Understanding the living will, *Senior Medical Review* 1:4-6, 1986.

40

Automated External Defibrillation

James Atkins, M.D., FACP

The development of sophisticated microprocessors has allowed the development of automated defibrillators. These automated defibrillators either can be implanted permanently or used as external devices similar to a standard defibrillator. The implanted forms are called automatic internal cardiovertors (AICD). The AICD usually has a battery/circuitry box in the abdomen. These devices will give a limited number of shocks. If a patient has an AICD in place, the prehospital personnel should still treat the patient like any other patient, including defibrillation if needed. The only concern with the AICD is to make sure that the defibrillator electrodes are least 2 inches away from the battery/circuitry box. If an AICD should fire while someone is touching the patient, the person might feel a small jolt but this should not cause harm. The focus of this chapter is on the external form of automated defibrillators, commonly called automated external defibrillators (AED).

Background

There has been a renewed emphasis on early defibrillation over the past several years. The 1986 *JAMA* guidelines on cardiac resuscitation gave emphasis to the importance of time to defibrillation as a key determinate of success in resuscitation of individuals having suffered a cardiac arrest.[23] This importance was reemphasized with a high priority in the 1992 *JAMA* guidelines.[1] The importance of early defibrillation has been emphasized in a number of publications.*

Initially, early defibrillation was performed by paramedics, nurses, or physicians. However, there were extreme logistical problems in the rapid delivery of defibrillation because of the limited number of these types of personnel in the pre-hospital environment. Both in King County, Washington, and in the state of Iowa, it was shown that EMT-B trained personnel could perform defibrillation with a minimum amount of training.[8,25] As there were 40 times as many EMT-Bs in the United States as paramedics, this allowed an expansion of the concept of early defibrillation. With AEDs this concept can be further expanded. Recently, the American Heart Association (AHA) has added AED material to its *Textbook of Advanced Cardiac Life Support,* along with an instructor guide and slides, which include the concept of automated defibrillation.[2,16] The AHA in its guidelines emphasizes the chain of survival (Figure 40-1).[2] This chain includes four basic links: early access, early CPR, early defibrillation, and early advanced cardiac life support. Early access means prompt recognition of the problem and activation of EMS through 9-1-1. Early CPR encourages the bystander to perform CPR and recommends that first responders should also begin CPR. Early defibrillation includes automated defibrillation by the First Responders.

AEDs have been shown to be an effective way of defibrillating patients.[8,25] Several EMS systems have pointed out the critical nature of time in determining patient survival from cardiac arrest. Eisenberg showed that the survival was 43% in witnessed cardiac arrests when CPR was begun within 4 minutes and defibrillation occurred within 8 minutes.[12] However, if CPR and defibrillation were delayed for 12 and 16 minutes, respectively, survival was 0%. Most unwitnessed arrests are not discovered for several minutes. For these reasons, witnessed cardiac arrests have a significantly better survival rate than unwitnessed cardiac arrests. The shorter the response time, the greater is the chance of long-term survival. Weaver showed early defibrillation in VF was an important determinate of success.[26] Long-term survival from VF was

*References 1-4,6,7,10,11,14,18,19,22,29.

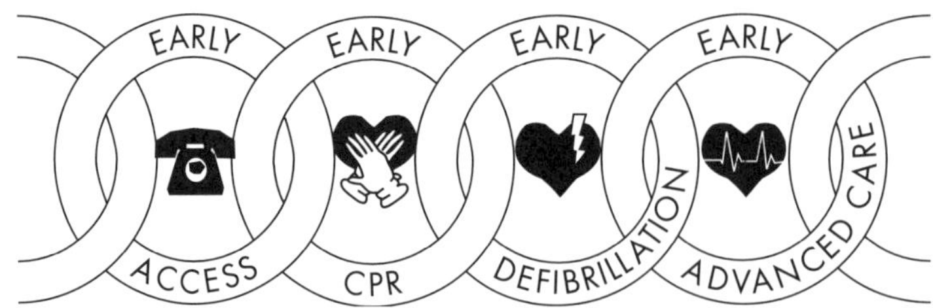

Figure 40-1. The emergency cardiac care system's concept is displayed schematically by the "chain of survival" metaphor. (From *Textbook of advanced cardiac life support,* 1990, American Heart Association.)

related to response time of a team with a defibrillator. Long-term survival was 37% for a 1 to 3 minute response time, 31% for a 4 to 6 minute response, 23% for a 7 to 10 minute response, and 14% for a greater than 10 minute response for patients in witnessed ventricular fibrillation. Kuehl demonstrated an improvement in long-term survival following all pre-hospital cardiac arrests from 2.2% to 7.1% when defibrillation occurred within 6 minutes of 9-1-1 notification.[17] With these parameters in mind, AEDs have been developed that can accurately analyze the rhythm, charge the device, and deliver a shock to the patient. These automated devices have been used in a number of studies with both EMT-Bs and First Responders. The pilot studies have shown that, with a minimal amount of training (4 to 10 hours), patients can be reliably defibrillated with these devices.

Devices

There are several different variations of AEDs available. Some are fully automatic. When the "on" button is pressed the device will analyze the ECG, arm itself, shock, and then reanalyze and repeat the sequence if indicated. Other devices have additional features, making them more operator dependent. Semi-automatic defibrillators have an "analysis button" that starts the process. The machine will then have a visual or auditory signal suggesting the patient be shocked. The operator then presses a "shock" button to defibrillate the patient. These latter machines are usually called semi-automatic or shock advisory types of AEDs. Some devices also have the ability to change the energy delivered by pressing a button, while others do this automatically.

All of these devices have paste-on electrodes, which must be applied before use. Once the electrodes are in place, the device is activated. The device will then check the electrode resistance. If the electrodes are not making good contact, the device will give a visual or verbal signal to check the electrodes, and the machine will be disabled from analyzing or shocking the patient until the electrodes are making satisfactory contact. Some devices will also look for variations in resistance as a result patient movement or breathing; these devices will not activate if there are major variations in resistance. Once the machine has checked the electrode contact, the ECG will be analyzed. The machines can reliably tell the difference between medium to coarse VF and other cardiac rhythms. Once the machine has determined VF, the defibrillator will be armed or charged. After charging the defibrillator, some machines will automatically discharge, while others will give a visual or verbal signal to press a button to shock. Algorithms can be programmed into some AEDs, for example, some will automatically shock using an algorithm chosen by the medical director such as first shock 200J, second shock 200J, and third and subsequent shocks 360J. The machines will either continuously record the timing of events and ECG strips or simply before and after the defibrillation. The reliability of the machines is very high; They are more reliable at determining VF than most human operators. Human operators may not always shock the patient in VF or may delay shocking because they are unsure. Human operators occasionally shock artifacts. Studies in the past have shown that 10% of shocks by human operators are improper, a result of misinterpretation of information. The reliability of AEDs is greater than 96%.*

These devices have been shown to increase resuscitation rates both in rural areas and urban areas. Both the King County data and the Iowa data have shown improvement in resuscitation rates.† In Dallas, the resuscitation rates in some fire districts tripled, to greater than 10% survival for all cardiac arrests and greater than 21% for ventricular fibrillation patients.[28]

The cost effectiveness in various applications has not been determined. For example, placing these devices in low risk areas such as a small office may

*References 8,9,13,15,20,24,25,27.

†References 9,13,15,20,24,25,27.

not be cost effective, since only one in several hundred such offices may ever have a cardiac arrest.

Other applications may prove more cost effective, such as on a first responding fire engine that annually handles 10 to 20 cardiac arrests. The physician director should look at the potential use of the device and the expected survival, estimated from previous studies.* For example, in a given community the ambulance takes 7 minutes to get to an area of town while the fire engine arrives in 3.5 minutes. This area averages nine cardiac arrests per year. Using the data from Seattle and King County, if paramedic ambulance defibrillation only were used, the expected survival would be one patient. The expected survival, if First Responder defibrillation were used, would be two patients. Hence, an automated defibrillation program would be expected to save one additional life per year. Since the devices will be used over 7 years, the cost per year would be $1,000, and the incremental cost of such a program would be $1,000 per life saved. Thus this would be a cost effective program. In another scenario, a similar area has a cardiac arrest every 7 years. That would mean that an additional life would be saved every 63 years. The cost of such a program might be $63,000 per life saved. This calculation does not consider ongoing educational costs or liability costs; these latter costs appear to be minimal in most systems.

It may also be cost-effective to place these types of devices in shopping malls, security offices, and elderly care facilities. However, the costs of training and supervision, issues of medical oversight, liability, and cost effectiveness must be determined before these programs begin.

Medical Oversight

If a program appears to be feasible and has the potential of financial support from the host agency, the physician director must carefully plan how medical oversight will be provided. Medical oversight normally has three temporal elements: prospective, concurrent, and retrospective. Prospective and retrospective medical oversight are usually elements of indirect medical control. Direct medical control by radio, telephone, or physician presence is not necessary with these devices. The device is making the decision; therefore the physician cannot see how the device is making that decision and cannot reasonably determine whether or not to override the decision. Thus good prospective and retrospective medical oversight must be established.

Medical oversight starts with legislation. The use of these devices is controlled or restricted in many states by the various medical practice acts. The physician must comply with these laws. In many states, the law will have to be changed or new state regulations will have to be written. Once the legislative and/or regulatory authorizations are in place, the physician director must ensure that the proposed plan is in accordance with those laws and/or regulations.

After obtaining the legislative approval, the physician director must then develop policies, procedures, and protocols. Automated defibrillator programs must have rigid protocols and policies in place. These devices must be used only in patients with a cardiac arrest. The safety of the device can be improved by making sure the device is only attached after it has been determined that there is a cardiac arrest. The protocols must consider all potential outcomes. For example, the patient may be defibrillated after the first, second, or third shock. The protocol must address what should be done in each eventuality. The protocols and procedures must address what is to happen if the device recommends no shock. If an error message is given by the machine, then the protocol must address how to handle the problem. Therefore, great care must be given in developing the protocol. If the personnel using the AED turns over care to a different set of personnel for transport, policies must be in place for how these two teams interface. Weigel et al have performed a thorough study of automatic defibrillator policies.[28]

Another major area of prospective indirect medical control is training and certification. The physician director must be actively involved in setting up the training and certification of the personnel using the device. These devices are very simple to learn to use. The important lessons to teach are safety and the fact that errors can be made. Safety must be a major portion of the training. To ensure that the device does not inappropriately shock someone with a perfusing rhythm (the chance is very remote with these devices), the operator must understand that the device is never to be used except in cardiac arrest. The other major area of safety is to make sure that no one is touching the patient or anything that can conduct electricity from the patient, such as metal or water. Since the devices are very quick, the operator must insure that everyone is clear of hazard before the device is activated. The operator must insure that everyone stays clear until the device has finished the cycle and is in a safe mode.

The major difference between traditional defibrillators and AEDs in VF algorithms is the pulse check. There are no pulse checks between shocks with an AED (Figure 40-2). A pulse check is not needed. During defibrillation with a manual defibrillator, the electrodes may come loose, causing an artifact to appear on the screen that can be misinterpreted as

*References 8,9,13,15,20,24,25,27.

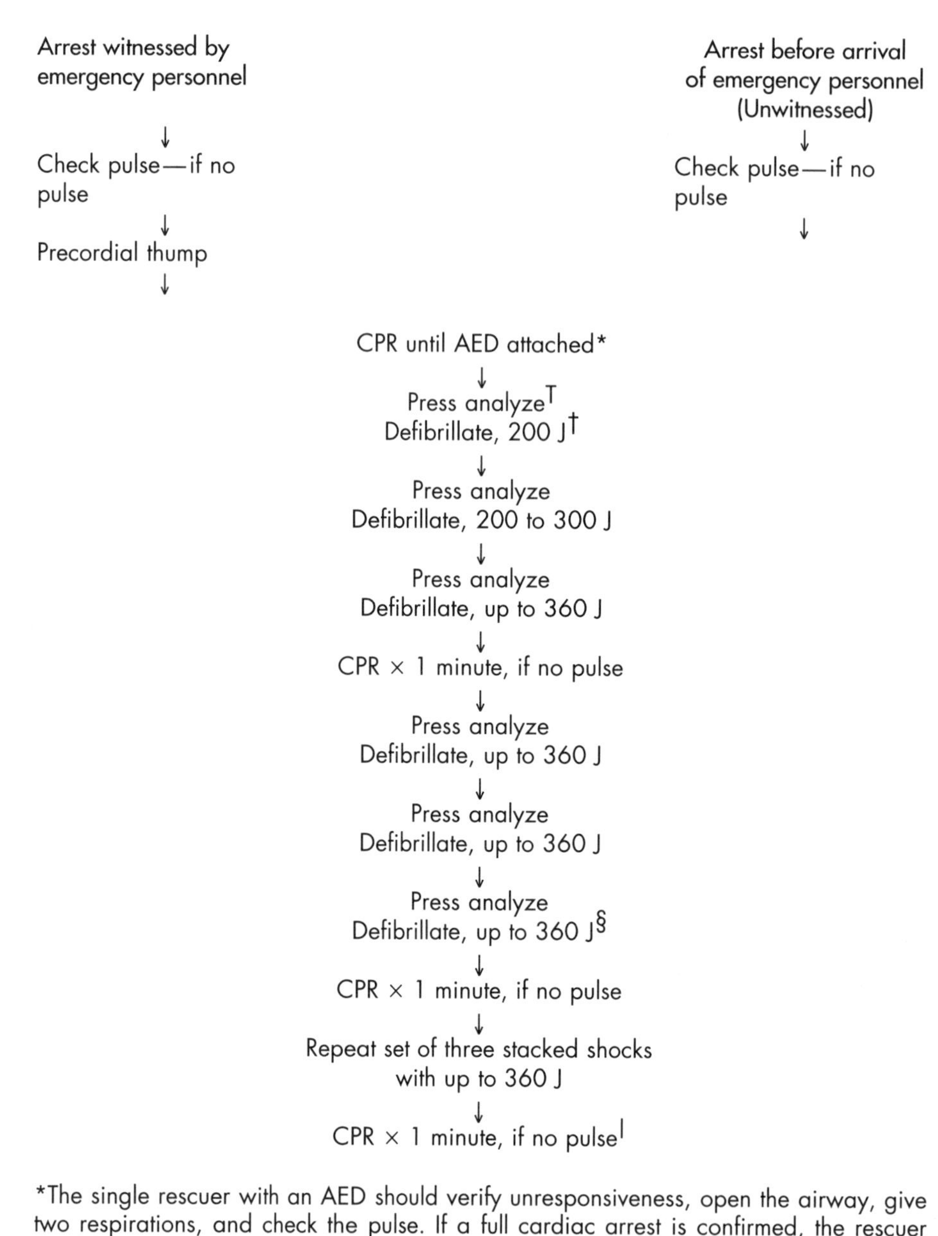

*The single rescuer with an AED should verify unresponsiveness, open the airway, give two respirations, and check the pulse. If a full cardiac arrest is confirmed, the rescuer should attach the AED and proceed with the algorithm.

[T] If "no shock indicated" appears, check pulse, repeat 1 minute of CPR then reanalyze. After three "no shock indicated" messages, repeat analyze period every 1 to 2 minutes.

[†] Pulse check is not required after shocks 1, 2, 4, and 5 unless the "no shock indicated" message appears.

[§] If ventricular fibrillation recurs after transiently converting (rather than persists without converting), restart the treatment algorithm from the top.

[|] In the unlikely event that ventricular fibrillation persists after nine shocks, repeat sets of three stacked shocks with 1 minute of CPR between each set.

Figure 40-2. Algorithm protocol for using an automated defibrillator in ventricular fibrillation and pulseless ventricular tachycardia. (From *Textbook of advanced cardiac life support,* 1990, American Heart Association.)

VF. A pulse check is a method of determining effectiveness of a shock should the electrodes become dislodged (or there is patient movement artifact), and this artifact is not recognized. With an AED, analysis will not begin if the electrodes are loose; an error message will be given. Safety is a second reason not to perform pulse checks between shocks. Automated defibrillators may recharge and shock a second time within five to ten seconds; it is possible that a person doing a pulse check might get shocked. Another major difference with automated defibrillators is that shocks are given in stacks of three shocks. Figure 40-2 contains the AHA's recommended algorithm for use of an automated defibrillator.[2] A sample course outline is also provided in the AHA instructors guide.[12]

Training should address all of the potential outcomes that can occur and also should teach all of the problems that can arise. These devices give error messages such as "check electrodes," "tape inoperative," "no memory module," or "maintenance required." The student must know the appropriate actions to respond to each of these warnings or error messages. Once the training is complete, the students must be certified in accordance with the state laws and regulations. Retraining is also needed. If the device is not used within 3 months, a 1-hour refresher in-service course improves performance.

Retrospective review is the other major area of indirect medical control. Retrospective indirect medical control includes review of the prehospital care report (PCR), review of the voice and ECG recordings, and statistical review. The PCR can give the major times involved. The primary goal is to have the patient defibrillated as quickly as possible. The secondary goal is to deliver the first three shocks within 1 minute, if appropriate. Therefore the PCRs need to be reviewed to see what time delays occurred and to determine if the time delays were appropriate. Sometimes there are logical and acceptable reasons for delays, such as the patient could not be found or the patient did not have an arrest until the team had been on site for a period of time.

Review of voice and ECG tapes is another major method of retrospective medical control. Safety and timing can be determined from the memory cartridge. The time delays may be quite different than what was reported on the PCR. Figure 40-3 shows an automated form of a PCR. Reasons for time delays may be determined by listening to what was actually happening. Safety also can be analyzed. For example, if cardiopulmonary resuscitation is identified on the ECG or voice tapes while the automated defibrillator is in an analysis, charging, or defibrillation mode, the team clearly needs reeducation. These logs also can determine whether the device did its job appropriately. Rarely in our experience has the tape or module found a device error; frequently it finds an operator error.

Statistical records are another key area of retrospective analysis. It is essential that the medical director knows whether the program is doing an acceptable job as compared to what other programs are doing nationally. Only by comparing local statistics to national statistics can the local program improve. All programs can be improved; it is the statistical comparisons that tell a program how.

The operators must check the device on a routine basis. Daily or shift checks of the device and its ancillary equipment are needed. Figure 40-4 shows a check form that was developed by the Federal Drug Administration.

Summary

An early defibrillation program with AEDs can greatly improve the potential survival from cardiac arrest. In order to be effective, it must be well planned with effective indirect medical control. The AHA has recommended that every ambulance should be equipped with a defibrillator and that the personnel should be trained to perform defibrillation.[1] Scotland has recognized the importance of early defibrillation by placing an AED on every ambulance; they have reported improved survival.[5] Both the AHA and the National Heart, Lung, and Blood Institute's National Heart Attack Alert Program have recommended that this should be done.[1,21] With the widespread availability of AEDs, this recommendation should become a reality.

REFERENCES

1. Adult advanced cardiac life support, *JAMA* 268:2199-2241, 1992.
2. Anderson M, Atkins JM, Austin D et al: Automated external defibrillation. In *Textbook of advanced cardiac life support,* Dallas, 1990, American Heart Association.
3. Atkins JM: Emergency medical service systems in acute cardiac care: state of the art, *Circulation* 74 (suppl IV):IV4-8, 1986.
4. Atkins JM et al: Toward earlier defibrillation, *Emerg Med Serv* 11:70, 1986.
5. Cobbe SM et al: Heartstart Scotland—initial experience of a national scheme for out of hospital defibrillation, *British Med J* 302:1517-1520, 1991.
6. Cummins RO and Eisenberg MS: EMT defibrillation: A proven concept, *American Heart Association Emergency Cardiac Care National Faculty Newsletter* 1:1-3, 1984.
7. Cummins RO: EMT defibrillation: National guidelines for implementation, *Am J Emerg Med* 5:254-257, 1987.
8. Cummins RO et al: Automatic external defibrillation: Evaluations of its role in the home and in emergency medical services, *Ann Emerg Med* 13:798-801, 1984.

Text continued on p. 406.

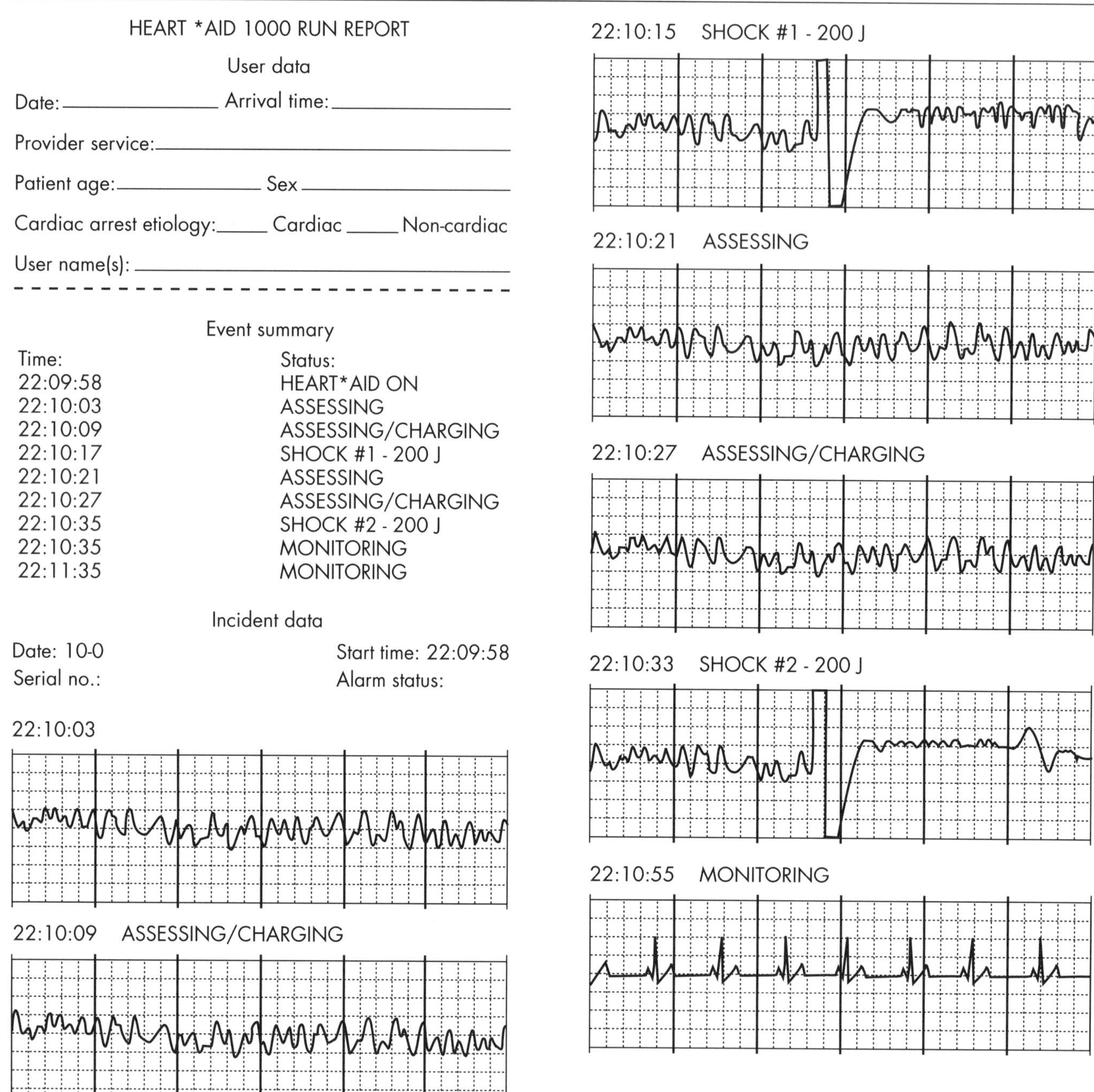
HEART *AID 1000 RUN REPORT

User data

Date: ______ Arrival time: ______

Provider service: ______

Patient age: ______ Sex ______

Cardiac arrest etiology: ____ Cardiac ____ Non-cardiac

User name(s): ______

Event summary

Time:	Status:
22:09:58	HEART*AID ON
22:10:03	ASSESSING
22:10:09	ASSESSING/CHARGING
22:10:17	SHOCK #1 - 200 J
22:10:21	ASSESSING
22:10:27	ASSESSING/CHARGING
22:10:35	SHOCK #2 - 200 J
22:10:35	MONITORING
22:11:35	MONITORING

Incident data

Date: 10-0 Start time: 22:09:58

Serial no.: Alarm status:

22:10:03

22:10:09 ASSESSING/CHARGING

22:10:15 SHOCK #1 - 200 J

22:10:21 ASSESSING

22:10:27 ASSESSING/CHARGING

22:10:33 SHOCK #2 - 200 J

22:10:55 MONITORING

Figure 40-3. Sample of an automated patient case record form the module of a Heart Aid 1000 defibrillator. (Modified from Weigel et al: *Automated defibrillation,* Englewood, Colo., 1988, Morton Publishing.)

Operator's Shift Checklist for Automated Defibrillators

Date: ______________________ Mfr/Model no.: ______________________ Location: ______________________

Serial no. or Facility ID no.: ______________________

DIRECTIONS: At the beginning of each shift, inspect the unit carefully. If problems are noted, place an "R" (to refer to the "Remarks/Corrective Action" section) in the correct column. Note any problems or corrective action taken. Sign the form.

	1st Shift	2nd Shift	3rd Shift	Remarks/Corrective Actions
1. Defibrillator unit				
a. Clean, no spills, clear of objects on top				
2. Defibrillator pads				
a. Set of two present? b. Package sealed and ready for use? c. Expiration date appropriate?				
3. Cables				
a. Inspect for cracks, frays, broken wire (1) Defibrillator-to-pads cables (2) Defibrillator monitor leads, if applicable (3) Defibrillator-to-charger cables				
4. Supplies				
a. Carrying case b. Cassette tape c. Monitoring electrodes d. Alcohol wipes e. Razors f. Spare pads g. ECG paper h. Spare battery i. Manual override key j. Memory module, event card plus spare				
5. Battery				
a. Plugged into live outlet b. Spare batteries charging c. Full charge checked				
6. Indicators				
a. Monitor working b. Energy select working c. Charge light working d. Power-on display working e. Tape recorder working f. Memory module in/out g. Audible alarms: disconnected cables, charging, shock				
7. Charge/Display cycle				
a. Unit detects connected and disconnected electrodes b. Unit detects, charges, and delivers shock for "VF" x 3 c. Unit increases energy level for 3rd shock d. Unit responds appropriately to non-shockable rhythms e. Manual override capability operable				
Directions: Please check the appropriate box below after each use of the checklist.				
1. No action required				
2. Minor problem(s) corrected				
3. Disposable supplies replaced				
4. Major problem(s) identified (OUT OF SERVICE)				

Signatures: 1 ______________________ 2 ______________________ 3 ______________________

Figure 40-4. Sample of an operator's checklist for automated defibrillators. (Modified from Defibrillator Working Group of the Center for Devices and Radiological Health, Food and Drug Administration.)

9. Cummins RO et al: Sensitivity, accuracy and safety of an automatic external defibrillator: report of a field evaluation, *Lancet* 11:318-320, 1984.
10. Cummins RO et al: Automatic external defibrillators: clinic, training, psychological, and public health issues, *Ann Emerg Med* 14:755-760, 1985.
11. Cummins RO, Eisenberg MS, and Stults KR: Automated external defibrillators: Clinical issues for cardiology, *Circulation* 73:381-385, 1986.
12. Eisenberg MS, Bergner L, and Hallstrom A: Cardiac resuscitation in the community. Importance of rapid provision and implications for program planning, *JAMA* 241:1905-1907, 1979.
13. Eisenberg MS et al: Treatment of out-of-hospital cardiac arrest with rapid defibrillation by emergency medical technicians, *N Engl J Med* 302:1379-1383, 1980.
14. Eisenberg MS and Cummins RO: Defibrillation performed by the emergency medical technician, *Circulation* 74 (suppl IV):IV9-12, 1986.
15. Eisenberg MS et al: Treatment of ventricular fibrillation: Emergency medical technician defibrillation and paramedic services, *JAMA* 251:1723-1726, 1984.
16. Instructor's Manual for Advanced Cardiac Life Support: Early Defibrillation, 1990, *American Heart Association.*
17. Kuehl AE: Survival rates following cardiac arrest in a two tiered urban EMS system (abstract), *Clinical Scholars Program,* Princeton, 1990, The Robert Wood Johnson Foundation.
18. Newman MM: National EMT-D study, *J Emerg Med Serv* 11:70-72, 1986.
19. Newman MM: The survival advantage: Early defibrillation programs in the fire service, *J Emerg Med Serv* 12:20-46, 1987.
20. Ornato JP et al: Limitation on effectiveness of rapid defibrillation by emergency medical technicians in a rural setting, *Ann Emerg Med* 13:1096-1099, 1984.
21. Proceedings of the National Heart, Lung, and Blood Institute Symposium on Rapid Identification and Treatment of Acute Myocardial Infarction: *Issues and Answers,* Washington, DC, 1991, National Heart, Lung, and Blood Institute, US Department of Health and Human Services, Public Health Service, National Institutes of Health.
22. Ruskin JN: Automatic external defibrillators and sudden cardiac death (editorial). *N Engl J Med* 319:713-715, 1988.
23. Standards and guidelines for cardiopulmonary resuscitation and emergency cardiac care, *JAMA* 255:2841-3044, 1986.
24. Stults KR: Planning, implementing and evaluating a successful EMT-D program. In *EMT-D: Prehospital defibrillation,* Bowie, Md, 1985, Brady Communications.
25. Stults KR et al: Prehospital defibrillation performed by emergency medical technicians in rural communities, *N Eng J Med* 310:219-233, 1984.
26. Weaver WD et al: Factors influencing survival after out-of-hospital cardiac arrest, *J Am Coll Cardiol* 7:752-757, 1986.
27. Weaver WD et al: Improved neurologic recovery and survival after early defibrillation, *Circulation* 69:943-948, 1984.
28. Weigel A, Atkins JM, and Taylor J: In *Automated defibrillation,* Englewood, Colo, 1988, Morton Publishing.
29. White RD: EMT-defibrillation: Time for controlled implementation of effective treatment, *American Heart Association Cardiac Care National Faculty Newsletter* 8:1-3, 1986.

41

Air Medical Transport

Steven Meador, M.D.
Ronald Low, M.D., M.S.

The U.S. military first used helicopters extensively for the transportation of severely injured patients during the Korean War, and their use was refined during the Vietnam War.[26,27] Investigators felt that helicopter evacuation was a major factor in reducing mortality from severe battlefield injuries. The National Academy of Science's 1966 report on accidental death and disability revealed the lack of civilian air medical services, despite the apparent efficacy of these services in military trauma.[25] Maryland State Police began transporting trauma victims to the University of Maryland with helicopters in 1969.[14] The first U.S. hospital-based helicopter service began in 1972 at St. Anthony's Hospital in Denver. The Military Assistance to Safety and Traffic (MAST) program began as a pilot program in San Antonio, Texas, during 1970 and subsequently became available in many areas of the country.[31,36] Initially, areas of sparse population or difficult terrain benefited most from Helicopter Emergency Medical Services (HEMS). Their number rose slowly during the following decade but has increased significantly since then.[12] The rapid expansion has stopped; the use of HEMS has been stable at approximately 220 helicopters for the past 3 years. Most regions of the country have access to HEMS. Interestingly, use is dropping in the two largest cities. New York City has one part-time service now based in the suburbs, and the one helicopter in Los Angeles ceased operation in the summer of 1991. Current system planners see EMS helicopters as useful for rapid patient transport or transporting patients in need of special equipment or personnel that are unavailable in the regular emergency medical system.

Many controversies surround the use of HEMS; some argue that these aircraft are expensive and ineffective, yet others argue that helicopters save lives.[5,9,13,18,35] Serious flaws in past research of helicopter effectiveness have only added to the controversy. Patients seldom require a fixed-wing ambulance unless they need a long transport (usually greater than 150 miles). This occurs either in areas of low population density such as the Southwest or when patients require highly specialized and distant medical resources such as liver transplantation.

Regulatory Authority and Standards

Regulation of the operation of EMS aircraft is complex, although some experts argue that regulations originally designed to cover helicopter taxis do not adequately govern helicopter ambulances.[33,34] There are three categories of regulation that cover the operation of HEMS.

1. Federal Air Regulations (FARS), which govern all civilian air operations in the United States, govern most EMS aircraft. The Federal Aviation Administration (FAA) administers these regulations.
2. Military regulations govern military (primarily Army and Coast Guard) helicopters even when used to transport civilian patients. For the purposes of transporting civilian EMS patients, military operations resemble the FARS.
3. Federal air regulations also do not have jurisdiction over public service agencies (state and local police, fire, or EMS departments) who can establish their own rules. These agencies often operate helicopters in ways prohibited under FARS.

Except for the designation of "lifeguard" status (see p. 409) and a few other specific regulations, the regulations governing HEMS are the same rules that govern all "air taxis." There have been calls for developing more specific FAR's to apply to EMS operations, but the FAA has yet to develop such rules.[9,33]

The EMS helicopter industry has made attempts to establish voluntary guidelines that go beyond the minimum standards of the FAA. Following a series of EMS helicopter accidents in the mid 1980s, the National EMS Pilots Association and the American Society of Hospital Based Emergency Air Medical Services (ASHBEAMS), which is now called the Association of Air Medical Services (AAMS), recommended that flight programs increase pilot staffing from an average of two pilots per helicopter to four. They also recommended the restriction of EMS missions under visual flight rules. Air Regulations allow helicopters to fly under visual flight rules, if the pilot can see 1/2 mile through fog or haze and there is at least 300 feet between the ground and overlaying clouds. The voluntary guidelines increase the restrictions to at least 1-mile visibility and a cloud layer no lower than 500 feet. At night the guidelines recommend against flight when visibility is less than 3 miles or the clouds are less than 1000 feet above the ground. EMS programs around the United States have generally adopted these guidelines, and the accident rate has subsequently dropped.

An offshoot of AAMS, the Commission for the Accreditation of Air Medical Services (CAAMS) proposed a longer list of guidelines. These guidelines extend beyond air operations to cover medical direction, administration, and nursing operations. Programs that meet these guidelines are eligible for inspection and possible accreditation similar to JCAHO accreditation of hospitals. The CAAMS accreditation process is in its infancy. It is not yet known if the many HEMS programs will seek CAAMS accreditation, or how the CAAMS guidelines will evolve.

Air Ambulances as Part of the Health Care System

The use of helicopter ambulances is widespread. Unfortunately, their use has overtaken the limited research on when and how they improve patient outcome. EMS systems use HEMS for a variety of missions; each program usually defines its role. There are three main sponsoring groups—hospitals, military, and public service (state and local fire, ambulance, or police). For hospital-based aircraft, most flights transfer patients from smaller to larger facilities. Some programs, however, transport patients directly from the accident scene to the hospital, and a few have this service as their major mission. Military helicopters can be used for interhospital transfer or accident scene pickup. These services also commonly transfer patients following search and rescue missions. The role of public service air ambulances varies greatly from system to system. Some helicopters used primarily for police surveillance work must be quickly diverted for ambulance work; others have EMS as their primary mission.

Safety

Flight safety has been a major concern in the operation of HEMS. EMS airplanes do not appear to pose particular safety risks. Experience suggests that EMS helicopters crash at twice the rate of other civilian helicopters. This accident rate has been the topic of reports of the National Transportation Safety Commission, the aviation press, the medical press, prime time television, and other "lay" media. These sources suggest the following possible reasons for this accident rate:

1. Pressure to complete a potentially lifesaving mission, even if the mission seems hazardous.
2. Requests occur at any time, and flights can rarely be scheduled for ideal conditions.
3. Flight crews must remain "on call" for long periods of time before flying and may not be well-rested when they take off.

Recent research has thrown additional light onto the subject of EMS helicopter crashes. The ability to navigate "on instruments" without reference to ground landmarks is one element of safe HEMS operation.[21] The FAA has required commercial airlines to have this capability for years, but it is not required of civilian HEMS. Programs that fly frequently have lower accident rates than programs that fly infrequently. Reasons for this difference are not clearly identified, but possible explanations include the following:

1. These helicopters may be more extensively maintained, because most EMS helicopters must have an inspection after every 100 hours of flight time.
2. Pilots of these programs may have more recent flight experience and familiarity with local terrain and weather patterns.
3. More ancillary support may be available in terms of administrators, dedicated communications personnel, mechanics, ground facilities, etc.

4. There are mechanical advantages (for example, lubricating seals) to flying a helicopter often.

Pilot work load appeared to be a major source of safety problems in the mid-1980s. At that time, HEMS staffing typically included two pilots per helicopter. Since then the ratio of pilots has increased to about four pilots per helicopter and the accident rate has dropped slightly. The improvement cannot clearly be ascribed to the increased level of staffing, because several other changes occurred simultaneously. Limited analysis of recent flights has not shown pilot staffing to be a statistically significant independent predictor of EMS helicopter accidents.[34]

Besides increased pilot staffing, changes made in the mid-1980s include

1. More conservative limits for accepting flights to be conducted in poor weather,
2. Isolating the pilot from patient information to eliminate psychological pressure to complete a mission, and
3. Stricter limits on the number of consecutive hours that a pilot can work.

EMS safety interest has primarily focused on preventing accidents but has also made some effort to minimize morbidity and mortality should an accident occur. Studies of military accidents have shown increased survival from the use of helmets and fire resistant clothing; some HEMS have adopted these measures for their crews.[16] Additionally, almost all EMS helicopter programs include recurrent safety training that teaches crew members the use of survival gear and emergency procedures. If an emergency landing becomes necessary, the entire crew must be aware of aircraft emergency procedures. Through flight orientation and regular updates they must maintain knowledge of how to jettison the doors, exit the helicopter, turn off the fuel and electrical supply, and operate the Emergency Locator Transponder. If an emergency landing occurs in a remote area, the crew will rely on survival training and equipment. When an emergency has resulted in an accident, there has been more than a 50% survival rate.[11] Although the actual accident risk is small, emergency and survival training can minimize losses.

Aviation Aspects

Typically a company (vendor) rents a helicopter ambulance to a hospital or other agency. Pilots and mechanics work for the vendor; medical personnel work for the hospital. The vendor is responsible to the FAA for the operation of the helicopter. Some hospitals own helicopters and may be directly responsible to the FAA for the operation of their aircraft. Regardless the pilot is ultimately responsible for any decision involving the flight of the aircraft.

The aircraft equivalent of "lights-and-siren" priority over other traffic occurs when a pilot announces "lifeguard" status. Air traffic controllers and other pilots then give the lifeguard aircraft routing priority over all other aircraft. Rerouting other aircraft, particularly large commercial jetliners, is very expensive. Regulations limit "lifeguard" status to cases in which there is an immediate threat to the patient.

Helicopters used for EMS vary in price, size, and speed. Price varies from $1 million to $4 million; they cost between $400 per hour to more than $3000 per hour to fly. Flight speed in still air runs between about 110 miles per hour to 190 miles per hour. Winds usually slow an aircraft down, but a tail wind speeds up that leg of a trip. Lifting capability varies. Some helicopters with medical equipment and necessary fuel aboard can only lift the pilot, one or two medical personnel, and a moderately heavy patient. Programs use larger helicopters to carry standard equipment, extra supplies, nurses, and physicians to the scene of a disaster. Helicopters with only one engine tend to be cheaper, slower, and have less lifting capability compared with twin engine helicopters.

Helicopter blades and airplane propellers work most efficiently in dense air. Air becomes less dense with increases in altitude, temperature, and humidity. Operation around high mountains or in hot, muggy weather requires the use of more powerful helicopters.

Patient illumination is a particular problem with smaller EMS helicopters such as twin engine helicopters. The patient care area of these smaller helicopters cannot be separated from the pilot. At night the pilot must use dark-adapted vision. The cabin must be kept dark or only faintly illuminated with red light. Patients may be brightly illuminated in separate areas aboard the larger aircraft. Smaller aircraft can only carry limited equipment. Noise is a problem on all aircraft; auscultation provides limited information about a patient.[19]

All EMS helicopters have the basic equipment the pilot would need to fly "on instruments" in an emergency. The FAA permits intentional instrument flight only if the aircraft has certain redundant systems and the pilot has specified training and recent experience. This instrument capability has an improved safety record and a slightly improved ability to complete missions that would otherwise be canceled. The aircraft and pilot requirements for instrument flight can substantially increase operating costs.

Dispatching and Communications

Various air-medical standards require 24-hour service access, continuous flight following, and communication of pertinent data between requesting agencies, flight crew, and recipient agencies.[1,2,4] Such demands require a full-time dedicated dispatch center.[10]

The dispatcher or Air Medical Communication Specialist (AMCS) receives the request for transport, notifies the crew, determines navigation coordinates, identifies known hazards, arranges patient acceptance, relays patient information, coordinates operations, and maintains communications.[1,4] This list of duties usually precludes regional ground EMS dispatch centers from performing HEMS dispatch.

Communication specialists should be capable of communicating with prehospital providers, other service dispatchers, and physicians. CAAMS has suggested standards for AMCS training.[1] AAMS has developed a communication specialist training program for air medical services.[4] Beyond a general knowledge of the prehospital environment, personnel should be specifically trained to enhance integration into the EMS system. Training should include the following: the prehospital system, procedures for placement of a helicopter at a scene, prehospital communication centers, all communications used in the prehospital environment, and all procedures for scene safety.

The Federal Communications Commission has allocated portions of the very high frequency (VHF) low, VHF high, and ultrahigh frequency radio bands for use of public safety and EMS services. Some jurisdictions also operate equipment in the band range above 800 MHz. HEMS communication equipment must be able to transmit and receive (transceive) on any of the above frequencies used by agencies interacting with the service.[1] It is essential that the staff of HEMS programs is able to communicate with all outside agencies. Equipment also must comply with FAA communication requirements for flight operations and air traffic control.

Medical Staffing

There are many different approaches to air medical crew staffing.[15] Training programs exist for physicians, nurses, paramedics, and basic providers.[3] Staffing selection depends on factors such as economics, marketing, public relations, competition, personnel availability, patient mix, crew capacity, and state practice acts. No one staffing choice is necessarily superior to another.

CAAMS classifies air medical services as either critical care, advanced life support (ALS), or basic life support (BLS), based on the highest level of provider administering patient care.[1] While a patient is on board, all levels of service should have at least two air medical team members. Critical care services must have either an appropriately trained physician or registered nurse. ALS services must have at least one certified paramedic, and BLS services must have at least one Emergency Medical Technician (EMT). Air medical services should not transport patients whose requirements exceed the capabilities of its crew members. If physicians are used to meet minimum staffing requirements, they must be trained as any other air medical crew member and have experience and familiarity with EMS.

Flight nurses should be selected for both experience with critical patients and interest if not experience in prehospital care. Nurses with experience in critical care units or emergency departments are used most often. For credibility and good patient care, it is important that flight nurses become familiar with the prehospital environment. In addition to flight and safety orientation, instruction should include training to qualify for EMS provider status in the local prehospital system. Requirements vary from state to state and are usually satisfied either by demonstrating advanced cardiac life support (ACLS) certification and proficiency as an EMT or completing a specific prehospital nurse course. Some state and local practice acts may require full paramedic certification to qualify as an EMS provider. In situations where EMS provider capability is impractical for nursing personnel, nurses must receive equivalent training to enable them to function in the prehospital environment.

If the flight nurse staff qualifies for EMS status in the local EMS system, all such personnel should be provided experience on ground EMS units. Such experience enhances credibility and cooperation with the EMS system. Ground EMS experience also may enhance staff skill use, particularly for low-volume HEMS.

Paramedic presence in the crew may enhance acceptance of the program by the prehospital community. Many programs have used alternative crew staffing patterns, apparently without diminishing their use.

Flight paramedics should be selected from local EMS services when possible. Selection of individuals with leadership, experience, and rapport in their system promotes acceptance of the service. Providers with firsthand experience in the local system have greater confidence in leading prehospital incidents. Their background can be a valuable resource when introducing other crew members to the local EMS system. Take care not to deplete the community of experienced providers to avoid unnecessary resentment. Besides flight and safety orientation, flight paramedic instruction should increase clinical experience through in-hospital rotations in the emergency department and the medical, surgical, and neonatal intensive care units.

Other non-physician medical staff should be selected according to the specific needs of the program. If staff are to function in the prehospital environment, certification as an EMT-B should be a minimum requirement, and experience is desirable. It is important that programs adequately train all medical staff for safe and appropriate prehospital patient management.

Direct Medical Control

Physicians used as crew for prehospital missions should meet local requirements for direct medical control. Physicians are not uniformly trained for the prehospital environment, they require specific training to participate in and supervise prehospital care. In some regions, prehospital providers are forbidden by law to take orders from other than approved direct medical control physicians. A physician with such approval can interface with the prehospital system without question of authority. Physician qualifications for medical control are discussed elsewhere in this text. Physician crew must have a thorough knowledge of the local prehospital system and are ultimately responsible to the EMS system medical director.

Debate concerning physician appropriateness or necessity as part of the flight crew continues. The cost-effectiveness of attending-level staff and appropriateness of resident-level staffing continue to be questioned.[6,23,29]

With the development of EMS systems in the 1970s, the concept of direct medical control to supervise prehospital care emerged. Most EMS systems use direct medical control for part if not all of prehospital ALS care. Direct medical control must be considered when integrating flight services into EMS services. The presence or absence of flight physician staff influences the approach to system coordination.

The use of non-physician flight staffing can raise questions over continuation of care during ground and flight service interactions. Physicians supplying medical direction for ground prehospital care have valid concerns about the liability of releasing patients to HEMS providers. The HEMS service must establish policies regarding patient transfer from ground to flight service. Alternatives include continuation of direct medical control, transfer of control to flight service associated physicians, and the exclusive use of standing orders for HEMS care. The first option allows for greater consistency in ground and flight therapy, whereas the latter options allow for greater consistency in air medical service. If flight service physicians are to administer direct medical control, they should meet local EMS requirements. Whichever method is used, a policy should be approved and endorsed by the prehospital system governing body. Such policy also should define procedures for non-transfer of patients to reduce potential liability.

The use of flight physicians for HEMS staffing can remove questions over continuation of care as the flight physician would assume full responsibility upon patient transfer. Physician staffing does create questions regarding the interaction of the physician with ground providers. In most situations, flight physicians should only give direction for patients identified for the air medical service. Medical direction for other patients should be conducted through normal operations. Procedures for non-transport of patients should be established through approved EMS system policy.

Indirect Medical Control

All prehospital response by HEMS should be audited to at least the standards of the local EMS system and should include chart or tape critiques. Ideal flight and ground service integration requires review and monitoring of the entire EMS response, including dispatch, ground service, air medical transport, and receiving hospital. In 1990 AAMS published an in-depth discussion of quality assurance for air medical transport.[17]

If different medical directors audit ground and flight services, there should be a free exchange of chart records so each director can evaluate the effectiveness of system integration. Simultaneous review of both charts is important for evaluation of both dispatch appropriateness and the quality of patient care. This is particularly important following an incident report or complaint.

The performance, supervision, and use of skills by non-physicians in the prehospital environment is unique. Skill performance must be monitored to assure quality patient care. Non-physician flight staff skills should be monitored at the same level as those of ground EMS personnel. Monitoring may require a record of invasive and diagnostic skills for each provider. Provision should be made for retraining personnel when skill frequency or skill performance is inadequate.

Case review and continuing education sessions are important mechanisms for maintaining and improving the quality of patient care. To maintain EMS status and increase credibility, non-physician flight staff should meet or exceed the requirements for ground EMS services. When possible, joint sessions between ground and flight services enhance system integration.

Dispatch, Loading, and Destination Selection

The EMS system must establish policies governing the dispatch, loading, and destination of patients. Such policies must define who is authorized to make decisions and provide guidelines. Policies must cover the selection and use of multiple air medical services. Destination selection for flight services should respect local categorization of emergency services, trauma, burns, reimplantation, and neonates. HEMS should not be used to bypass local facilities unless appropriate to advance the level of care. The procedures for destination selection should be established and regionally approved.

Documentation

Complete and accurate medical care records are important to HEMS. Although air medical services often require more extensive documentation than ground EMS services, standard prehospital forms should be incorporated into the flight service record. Such forms should be supplemented as needed to satisfy the requirements of the service. Standardization allows for continuity in prehospital data collection and efficient EMS system auditing. As mentioned, there should be free exchange of ground and flight records within the EMS system.

Education

The integration of air medical transport into an EMS system requires systemwide education that includes hospitals, dispatch centers, and prehospital providers.

All medical facilities in the local EMS system that interact with prehospital providers should be informed of the capabilities and operation of HEMS. When feasible, there should be on-site demonstrations of the craft. Each facility should receive information on staffing, dispatch procedures, indications for use, operational policies, and restrictions. Direct medical control facilities need to understand EMS system policies for air medical transport and how to access the flight service.

Safe and efficient HEMS responses to the prehospital environment require thorough coordination with ground EMS dispatching. Procedures for relaying the exact location of prehospital incidents must be established between all ground dispatch facilities and the flight operations center. Ground EMS dispatch centers must understand the requirements of the flight service, including landing zone, ground personnel (landing officers), and ground communications. Instruction of all dispatch centers must occur before the flight service begins prehospital operation.

Prehospital providers such as EMTs, fire service, rescue, and police require orientation to HEMS. Practical, instructive presentations should be offered to all emergency providers in the range of prehospital response. These orientations should cover dispatch criteria, dispatch procedures, landing zone guidelines, and safety. In addition to improving the effectiveness of prehospital response, these presentations provide good public relations for the program and parent institution.

As for interfacility transport, appropriateness of transport is a concern of all participants in prehospital response. Sophisticated, expensive HEMS should be reserved for the critically ill or injured person, unless mitigating factors such as ground inaccessibility are present. Overuse must be modified, but underuse restricts potential patient benefit. Services should use nationally accepted indications as criteria for transport, whether in the hospital or prehospital arena.[22] Controversies such as how effectiveness is measured, whether patients with acute myocardial infarction should be placed in this high-stress environment, and what scoring system is most accurate in deciding the need for transport remain concerning HEMS transport.[5,7,8,20,28,30,32,37] Ongoing studies may eventually settle these issues, but acceptance of HEMS for transport of the critically ill or injured appears well-established.

Multi-casualty Incidents and Disasters

A disaster is an event that requires a response that exceeds the resources of the community. HEMS could be an important resource in major incidents and disasters. Its role in disasters may differ from the usual scene response and patient transport, and therefore must be planned and tested if it is to be used safely and effectively. Disaster planning also should address internal disasters in preparation for potential aviation mishaps involving the medical helicopter.

Local hazards-assessment studies should be conducted, and the potential for air medical assistance should be considered. HEMS are of primary use in disasters that produce life-threatening medical emergencies. However, use for aerial surveillance, search and rescue, and transport of personnel and supplies to the disaster scene represent realistic alternatives.[24] Disasters may produce conditions that compromise flight safety. These situations are to be avoided. Careful preplanning can prevent dangerous and inappropriate use.

Emergency management officials must be appraised of the capabilities and limitations of the flight service. These officials should be encouraged to include HEMS in their disaster plans with guidelines for use. Necessary guidelines include use, dispatch, safety, use of multiple services, and destination selection. These policies must be established before disaster occurrence and should require flight program participation in appropriate disaster exercises. Despite the cost, such participation produces greater understanding of effective use and establishes safe procedures.

Summary

HEMS have rapidly become the standard of care for transport of the critically ill or injured patient. The potential for interaction with ground EMS is significant. Full system integration improves patient care, enhances efficiency, and maintains safety as a top priority.

REFERENCES

1. Accreditation standards of the commission on accreditation of air medical services, Anderson, SC, 1991.
2. American Society of Hospital Based Emergency Air Medical Services (ASHBEAMS): *Minimum quality standards,* current revision, 1987, The Society.
3. ASHBEAMS: *Air medical crew national standard curriculum: instructor manual,* Pasadena, Calif, 1988, The Society.
4. Association of Air Medical Services: *Manual for air medical communications operations: rotorcraft/fixed wing,* Pasadena, Calif, 1989, The Association.
5. Baxt WG and Moody P: The impact of rotorcraft aeromedical emergency care service on trauma mortality, *JAMA* 249(22):3047-3051, 1983.
6. Baxt WG and Moody P: The impact of a physician as part of the aeromedical prehospital team in patients with blunt trauma, *JAMA* 257(23):3246-3250, 1987.
7. Baxt WG et al: Hospital based rotorcraft aeromedical emergency care services and trauma mortality: a multicenter study, *Ann Emerg Med* 14:859-864, 1985.
8. Baxt WG et al: The failure of prehospital trauma prediction rules to classify trauma patients accurately, *Ann Emerg Med* 18:1-8, 1989.
9. Campbell J, Low RB, and Bowman D: The efficacy of ground versus air transport in patient outcome. *J Okla State Med Assoc* 82(7):311-314, 1989.
10. Collett HM: Dispatch and communications survey, *Hospital Aviation* 6:5-5, 1987.
11. Collett HM: Aeromedical accident trends, *Hospital Aviation* 7:10-15, 1988.
12. Collett HM: Mid-year report, *J Air Med Trans* 10(7):25-26, 1991.
13. Cowart VS: Helicopter, other "air ambulances": time to assess effectiveness? *JAMA* 253(17):2469-2477, 1985.
14. Cowley RA et al: An economical and proved helicopter program for transporting the emergency critically ill and injured patient in Maryland, *J Trauma* 13(12):1029-1038, 1973.
15. Crew mix: a survey of programs shows a variety of working models, *Aeromedical Journal* 1:12-15, 1986.
16. Crowley JS: Helicopter aircrew helmets and head injury. USACS Tech Rep 90-1, US Army Safety Center, Systems Engineering Division, Fort Rucker, Ala.
17. Eastes L and Jacobson J, editors: *Quality assurance in air medical services,* Orem, Ut, 1990, WordPerfect Publishing.
18. Fromm RE et al: Utilization of specialized services by air transported cardiac patients: an indicator of appropriate use, *Aviat Space Environ Med* 63(1):52-55, 1992.
19. Hunt RC et al: Inability to assess breath sounds during air medical transport, *JAMA* 265:(15):1982-1984, 1991.
20. Kaplan CR, Walsh D, and Burney RE: Emergency aeromedical transport of patients with acute myocardial infarction, *Ann Emerg Med* 16:55-57, 1987.
21. Low RB et al: Operational safety of helicopter ambulances: beneficial effect of instrument flight capability and frequent flights, Submitted for publication.
22. Macione AR and Wilcox DE: Appropriateness of utilization: a method of assessment, *Hospital Aviation* 4:37-38, 1985.
23. MacNab AJ: Optimal escort for interhospital transport of pediatric emergencies, *J Trauma* 31(2):205-209, 1991.
24. Morris G: *Mass casuality response.* In: *Air-medical crew national standard curriculum,* Pasadena, Calif, 1988, ASHBEAMS.
25. National Academy of Sciences, National Research Council: *Accidental death and disability: the neglected disease of modern society,* Washington, DC, 1966, The Academy.
26. Neel SH Jr: Helicopter evacuation in Korea, *US Armed Forces Medical Journal* 6:691-702, 1955.
27. Neel SH Jr: Army aeromedical evacuation procedures in Vietnam: implications for rural America, *JAMA* 204(4):309-313, 1968.
28. Ornato J et al: Ineffectiveness of the trauma score and the CRAMS scale for accurately triaging patients to trauma centers, *Ann Emerg Med* 14:1061-1064, 1985.
29. Rhee KJ et al: Is the flight physician needed for helicopter emergency medical services, *Ann Emerg Med* 15(2):174-177, 1986.
30. Rhee KJ et al: Therapeutic intervention scoring as a measure of performance in a helicopter emergency medical services program, *Ann Emerg Med* 15:40-43, 1986.
31. Scheib BT: MAST: A decade of service, *JEMS* 8:38-45, 1983.
32. Schneider S et al: Critical cardiac transport: air versus ground, *Am J Emerg Med* 6:449-482, 1988.
33. Thomas F, Gibbons H, and Clemmer TP: Air ambulance regulations: a model, *Aviat Space Environ Med* 57(7):699-705, 1986.
34. Thomas F et al: A nationwide survey of civilian air ambulance services, *Aviat Space Environ Med* 56(6):547-552, 1985.
35. Urdaneta LF et al: Evaluation of an emergency air transport service as a component of a rural EMS system, *Am Surg* 50(4):183-188.
36. US Department of Health and Human Resources: *Military assistance to safety and traffic: report of test program,* Washington, DC, 1971, The Department.
37. Wilcox DE and Macione AR: A comparison of the ability of six severity-of-illness scales to predict mortality and health care expenditures, *Ann Emerg Med* 15:497-498, 1986.

42

Interfacility Transports

Steve Meador, M.D.
Ronald Low, M.D., M.S.

EMS leaders have long recognized the importance of regional planning for the transport of patients between facilities. Patient transfer for specialized care and rehabilitation is one of the original 15 mandatory EMS system components.[2,13] In addition to tertiary referral, there are other demands for interfacility transport. Patients may request transfer to maintain continuity of care or to conform to the requirements of third-party payers such as health maintenance organizations (HMOs). Transfer may be used in cases of bed shortages to improve resource use or patient care. In some areas, hospitals transfer patients to shift the costs of uninsured care to government hospitals or "public facilities." This chapter presents the perspective of both regional EMS systems and individual prehospital EMS units. It does not attempt to provide a detailed description of specialty transport; this is well-described elsewhere.[5,7-9]

Level of Care

In EMS systems, transfer occurs through three methods—private vehicle, prehospital service, or dedicated interfacility service. The EMS system has little interaction with private vehicles, unless private transport results in the need to dispatch prehospital services for untoward events. EMS systems with inadequate resources for the performance of interfacility transport may rely on private vehicles more often than systems with adequate resources.

Various levels of prehospital service may be used for interfacility transport. Many patients require no medical care en route. Such patients may require only elective diagnostic procedures or transfer to or from rehabilitative or chronic care institutions. This medically limited service often known as an "invalid coach" functions as a taxicab. These patients require a driver and an attendant with modest skills, possibly only first aid training.

Transport services staffed by basic level emergency medical technicians (EMT-Bs) provide noninvasive support. Facilities use these services for stable patients when they do not anticipate an intratransport need for drug or other invasive treatments. They also may select non-paramedic services if no other service is available or other health care providers such as nurses will accompany the patient.

Ambulance services using EMT intermediates, paramedics, or nurses commonly perform transfers. Although often pressed into serving as a critical care team, the training, experience, and scope of practice of prehospital services limit their critical care capabilities. Overuse of field units for interfacility transfers also makes them unavailable for prehospital responses.

Dedicated services can be either a general critical care or specialty transport. General services can respond to a large variety of patient problems; the training, experience, and scope of practice is often greater than that of prehospital services.[4] They are likely to be better equipped for critical care monitoring and use of a wider variety of medications. For example, general transport services are usually more familiar with the cardiovascular medications and infusion pumps required to support patients with myocardial infarction. In addition, many dedicated services provide an accompanying physician.

Facilities use specialty transport services for neonatal, pediatric, and cardiac patients. Specialty services have become a standard of care for critical neonates requiring specific equipment and specially trained providers.[8] The use of other specialty services is less well-defined, and their function is frequently filled by dedicated general transport or prehospital services. When assessing the need for specialty services, one should match the anticipated needs of the patient with the training, experience, and capabilities of the transport team.

Personnel

Any discussion of staffing decisions for interfacility transport must begin with the question of physician versus non-physician staffing. Although several authors have attempted to define the need for physicians, the question hinges on the training and experience of the alternative non-physician staff, as well as individual patient needs.[3,14,15,20] No data exist that define which patients require a physician. The benefits of physicians on interhospital transport can be viewed as either an increase in the level of procedure capability or an improvement in treatment decision-making. Concerning procedure skill level, service directors can project the need for physicians by assessing whether patients require skills beyond the proficiency of the non-physician staff. Anticipating the need for en route physician judgment is more difficult. En route decision-making can be supplied through direct radio or telephone communications. Although prehospital care often relies on this methodology, its appropriateness for long interhospital transports of critical care patients is not proven. Unfortunately, decisions to include physician staffing are based on the availability of adequately trained and experienced physicians. Although many programs use rotating residents as transport physicians, a trained and dedicated physician group provides a higher and more consistent level of care.

Non-physician staffing can include providers trained at many levels. Providers trained at the advanced first aid or Certified First Responder level may be sufficient for stable patients with no anticipated need for medical treatment (for example, patients requiring transport to a rehabilitation facility). Although one may question the need for any training for routine transports, providers should have enough training to quickly recognize an emergency and have experience in lifting and moving patients.

Emergency medical technicians-Ambulance (EMT-As) are a minimum staffing requirement for medical treatment or monitoring. The choice between EMT-As, paramedics, nurses, or respiratory therapists is complex and depends on the system and the patient. The first axiom is that no providers should be allowed to exceed their scope of practice. For instance, EMT-As or EMT-Bs trained only within the current United States Department of Transportation National Standard Curriculum are not trained in invasive procedures and have no experience in the monitoring of intravenous (IV) fluids or the administration of medications. Use of EMT-B level care may necessitate conversion of IV lines to a heparin lock that requires neither monitoring nor maintenance. Another factor to consider is that prehospital personnel are often unfamiliar with the disease spectrum of many interfacility transport patients. When deciding whether it is appropriate to use EMT-As or paramedics, one must consider whether the patient's illnesses are within the experience of the prehospital providers. Nurses may often appear to be a superior choice for transport personnel because of greater training and experience. Nurses, however, often lack specific experience in airway management and use of ambulance equipment. Respiratory therapists may be considered as supplemental crew to improve airway management or ventilator capabilities.

EMS systems can solve many crew staffing and training problems by developing interhospital transport protocols. Prehospital responders use protocols such as standing orders with great success.[18] Similarly, interhospital transport protocols should be employed to define staffing, equipment, and treatment. Such protocols are the basis for education of all staff participating in interfacility services.

Transport Vehicles

Any vehicle may perform transfers, but ground ambulances, rotor wing, and fixed wing aircraft are most common. An EMS system must always anticipate a need for ground ambulance transfers. The need varies according to the types, numbers, and accessibilities of health facilities and the availability of other specialized transport services. Air transport is often considered superior solely because of a reduction in transport time; however, because of the time required for lift-off and landing, it is rarely an advantage over ground transport for short distances (20 miles or less). Air transport is also subject to weather limitations that frequently make it unavailable. In situations where time is unimportant, ground ambulances offer the advantages of a lower cost and a lower accident rate.[1,17] For example, during neonatal transports, specialty teams are more concerned with providing a high level of care than reducing transport time.[16]

Rotor wing services offer the advantages of a dedicated team, general availability (during good weather conditions), and uninterrupted transfer from hospital to hospital. A discussion of standards for air medical transport is found in Chapter 41. For distances greater than 100 miles, a fixed wing service is usually more practical. Selection and evaluation of a fixed wing service should be done before the transport is needed because the quality and experience of fixed wing services vary greatly. It is easier to accomplish an appropriate fixed wing transport when facilities make standing arrangements before the actual need arises.

Origin and Destination

Interhospital transfer may require more than one service and may involve the exchange of patient and information several times. From an EMS system perspective an interhospital transport may be from hospital to hospital, hospital to transport service, transport service to transport service, or transport service to hospital. Obviously, adequate and consistent medical care must be provided to the patient at all stages. Planning and protocols must consider the process for exchange of patient and information. The need to transfer a patient from one service to another is common, especially when using aircraft. The use of a fixed wing service often requires shuttling a patient from the hospital to the airport and from the receiving airport to the receiving hospital. In the interest of shortening time to definitive care the fixed wing transport personnel may receive the patient at the airfield rather than at the hospital. An EMS system that anticipates the need for such interservice transfers must plan and develop protocols; without such preplanning, confusion and poor communications may result in less than optimal patient care.

Spectrum of Care

Interfacility transport may be accessed to provide scheduled diagnostic or rehabilitative services or to shift the costs of uninsured care to public facilities. An EMS planner must develop standards for such interfacility transports to control both medical and legal liability and to improve system efficiency. The top priority of EMS systems must be emergency interhospital transports. At a minimum, system planning should address the specialty areas of systems care—trauma, burn, spinal cord injury, acute coronary and acute medical, poisoning, obstetrical, neonatal and pediatric and behavioral and psychiatric. The demand and use in each of these areas should be monitored and directed by the medical director.

Trauma

The interhospital transfer of trauma patients is common. Although trauma centers may be designated and protocols for the diversion of patients may be in place, prehospital trauma triage is imperfect; it often results in mistriage of some severely injured patients to non-trauma centers.[11] Trauma centers are not distributed uniformly, and some patients may first be stabilized at a local hospital. The American College of Surgeons has produced guidelines for the indications of transferring patients to trauma centers.[10]

Non-trauma facilities frequently transfer patients in unstable or partially stabilized conditions. Such patients require definitive and timely surgical intervention at the trauma center to lower morbidity and mortality. Time of transport is a critical element in the patient's survival. The transferring facility must consider service availability and speed to minimize time to definitive care, choosing the program that will accomplish the transfer quickest. Ground and air medical vehicles should be adequately equipped for the immobilization and management of trauma victims. Although EMT-As are well-trained in the initial management of trauma patients, it is likely that a patient requiring transport to a trauma center will require advanced airway and monitoring techniques beyond the skills of EMT-As. Prehospital paramedic services usually adequately meet the demands of the trauma patient. It is rare, but occasionally higher training or physician staffing is required.

Burns

Burn patients frequently require interhospital transfer. Burn patients are often taken from the place of injury to acute care facilities or trauma centers that are not burn centers. Patients with greater than 20% body surface area burns benefit from care in a burn center. Extremes of age, location of burns, and the presence of other illness influence the likelihood of benefit from treatment in a burn center.[19] Burn patients must be stabilized if possible at the initial receiving institution. This treatment should include adequate fluid resuscitation and attention to other traumatic injuries. Once stabilization is accomplished or at least approached the speed with which burn patients are transported to burn centers is not as important as the speed with which trauma patients are transported to trauma centers. The primary concern with burn patients is the continuance of fluid resuscitation and airway management. Such needs require advanced care but allow choice in vehicle and staffing. Decisions can be primarily based on cost, convenience, and safety when there is a lower emphasis on speed.

Spinal Trauma

Spinal cord injuries are frequently associated with additional trauma, and such patients are initially managed as are other trauma victims. Following stabilization, these patients benefit from the experienced treatment and rehabilitative services available at spinal cord centers. Transfer is rarely time critical and as with burn patients should be influenced by factors of safety, convenience, and cost. In cases of high cervical lesions the transport team should be proficient in airway management, but most spinal injured patients may be adequately managed with EMT-As.

Coronary and Medical

Many indications exist for the transfer of acute coronary or acute medical patients. For example, patients may be transferred for acute subspecialty care, for diagnostic procedures, or because of a lack of appropriate inpatient beds. Because prehospital paramedic services commonly treat cardiac and other types of acute medical patients, they may be used for interhospital transfer as well. The potential treatment requirements of the patient during transport must be identified to ensure that they are within the scope of practice of the staff. Rapid transport primarily depends on the stability of the patient. For stable patients, time is a noncritical factor. Patients requiring definitive care demand immediate transport by the fastest appropriate method. Most patients require a degree of advanced care, and some patients may require nurse or physician staff during the transport.

Poisoning

A need for complex management or a specific antidote may necessitate the transfer of poisoning or venomous bite victims to designated toxicology centers. These patients frequently have multisystem compromise, requiring both respiratory and hemodynamic support. Time to definitive therapy is often critical, and the complexity of these patients frequently requires an experienced and sophisticated team. Patients require a sophisticated provider at a minimum and frequently need nursing and physician attendance as well.

Obstetrical

High-risk obstetrical patients may benefit from treatment in a tertiary care center. Federal law that defines any woman in active labor as unstable complicates transfer of these patients.[12] Such patients may be transported before delivery only when there is a clear and obvious benefit. Because of the potential of delivery, all obstetrical transports should be made by experienced and well-trained teams. Physician staffing may not be mandatory, but it is highly desirable. Any personnel replacing physician staff must be able to conduct a delivery and manage anticipated complications in the mother or neonate. Obviously, time is critical; therefore air medical services need to be considered for long distances.

Pediatric and Neonatal

The need for pediatric and neonatal interfacility transport evolved with the development and enhancement of pediatric tertiary care centers.[16] Many acute care hospitals lack inpatient pediatric capabilities; many more lack sophisticated pediatric or neonatal ICUs. It is common for a child to present to an acute care facility that does not have the capability to provide definitive care. Critically ill or premature neonates may be delivered at hospitals that lack sophisticated neonatal intensive care. It is not only the lack of facilities but often the lack of training and experience of the staff that motivates an institution to transfer children. Ideally a specially trained team will bring the appropriate clinical expertise to the institution and stabilize the patient before transport.[16] For these difficult pediatric patients, transfer of the patient to definitive care is not nearly as important as transport of definitive care to the patient. This fact alone often requires that systems use specialty services. Many children requiring transfer have organ system failure, and personnel with the appropriate training and equipment provide better patient care.[5,8,16]

The American Academy of Pediatrics published guidelines for the transportation of pediatric patients.[8] These guidelines recommend that medical transport team members are formally trained and competent in pediatric transport and experienced in pediatric critical care. Specific needs for patient stabilization define the requirements for equipment and drugs. Such guidelines can usually be met only by pediatric specialty or select general transport services.

Behavioral and Psychiatric

Patients with behavioral or psychiatric diseases commonly require interfacility transport because many acute care medical facilities do not provide inpatient psychiatric services. Even those hospitals with inpatient psychiatric beds may not have the capacity to treat all patients that present to their facility with psychiatric disorders. Some states encourage hospitalization at specific institutions. Once stabilized and medically cleared at the transferring facility, patients should not require treatment during transport and no specific equipment should be required. Use of restraints during transport should be defined by written policy. Transport by EMT-As or EMT-Bs is adequate to fulfill most medical needs. Paramedic providers should not be required; their scope of practice does not add any additional benefit to these patients. Some states require the presence of an individual with police power.

Medical Oversight

As in prehospital care, indirect medical control has an important role in the interfacility transfer process. Indirect medical control should include the development of policies and protocols for transfer, the development of training programs for providers, and the retrospective review of transports to provide quality assurance. All transfers should be retrospectively evaluated for appropriateness of the service and treatment provided. Adherence to system policies and protocols must be monitored, and any discrepancies should be analyzed, concerning the need for remedial training, discipline, or policy modification.

Direct medical control may have a role in interfacility transfers. The physical presence of a transport physician may improve treatment decisions and patient care.[14,15,20] Decisions may be supplied through direct radio or telephone communications. If providers involve direct medical control before initiating any transport, the en route physician can ensure the use of an appropriate level of service. Without access to direct and indirect medical control, prehospital providers may accept patients beyond their scope of practice. When providers give an adequate assessment before transfer, direct medical control can be a useful resource for managing unanticipated patient problems.

Legal Issues

No patient transport should occur without consideration of legal implications. The Emergency Medical Treatment and Active Labor Act (also known as COBRA) mandated specific procedures for interfacility transfer.[6,12,22] The law permits patient transfer only when the patient requests transfer, when it can be demonstrated that the benefits of transfer outweigh the risks, or after stabilization of the patient's emergency condition. Any consent or refusal by the patient concerning a transfer must be in writing and must document a full disclosure of federal requirements and the risks and benefits to the patient. There must be communication with the receiving institution before the transfer that verifies the acceptance of the patient and the capability to provide appropriate medical treatment. The transferring institution must provide all records concerning the patient's examination and treatment. Federal legislation is directed at institutions and does not specify requirements for transport services.[21] It is in the interest of all transport providers to ensure that they are not the agent of an inappropriate transfer. Interfacility transport services should require before initiation of transport a copy of any appropriate patient consents or refusals, the name of the accepting physician at the receiving institution, and a general inventory of all records provided. When possible, EMS providers should clear interfacility transports with direct and indirect medical control and verify that the level of care is appropriate. Following these procedures demonstrates a good faith effort by the service to ensure an appropriate transfer.

Beyond legal requirements, providers should never exceed their scope of practice during an interfacility transfer. Every patient must be carefully evaluated before transfer to ensure that training or skills beyond those of the providers are not required. Providers should be encouraged to challenge the transfer process. Any concerns should be voiced to the transferring physician and be well-documented in the patient's record. When there is a difference of opinion between the transferring physician and the transfer service, direct and indirect medical control should be used to resolve conflicts and full documentation should occur. All conflicts resolved or unresolved should be reviewed by indirect medical control so proper education and policy can be made.

Summary

The interfacility transport of patients is a crucial component of any EMS system. Because transfers involve multiple institutions and potentially multiple services, it is only through careful planning, adherence to system protocol, and ongoing system evaluation that systems can ensure appropriate patient care. Policies and protocols must be formulated to anticipate patient demand and system problems.

REFERENCES

1. Auerbach PS et al: An analysis of ambulance accidents in Tennessee, *JAMA* 258:1487-1490, 1987.
2. Boyd DR et al: Medical control and accountability of emergency medical services (EMS) systems, *IEE Transactions on Vehicular Technology* 28(4):249-262, 1979.
3. Burney RE et al: Comparison of aeromedical crew performance by patient severity and outcome, *Ann Emerg Med* 21:375-378, 1992.
4. Ehrenwerth I, Sorbo S, and Hackel A: Transport of critically ill adults, *Crit Care Med* 14(6):543-547, 1986.

5. Frankel LR: The evaluation, stabilization, and transport of the critically ill child, *Int Anesthesiol Clin* 25:77-103, 1987.
6. Frew SA: *Patient stabilization.* In: Dehart KL, editor: *Patient transfers: how to comply with the law,* Dallas, 1991, American College of Emergency Physicians.
7. Gore JM et al: Evaluation of an emergency cardiac transport system, *Ann Emerg Med* 12(11):675-678, 1983.
8. Hackel A et al: Guidelines for air and ground transportation of pediatric patients, *Pediatrics* 78(5):943-950, 1986.
9. Icenogle TB et al: Long distance transport of cardiac patients in extremis: the mobile intensive care (MOBI) concept, *Aviat Space Environ Med* 59:571-574, 1988.
10. *Interhospital transfer of patients.* In: *Resources for optimal care of the injured patient,* 1990, The American College of Surgeons.
11. Knopp R et al: Mechanism of injury and anatomic injury as criteria for prehospital trauma triage, *Ann Emerg Med* 17(9):895-902, 1988.
12. Krugh TD: Is COBRA poised to strike? a critical analysis of medical COBRA, *J Health Hospital Law* 23(6):161-175, 1990.
13. Law of the 93rd Congress, Emergency Medical Services Systems Act of 1973, Public Law 93-154, Washington, DC, Nov 16, 1973.
14. MacNab AJ: Optimal escort for interhospital transport of pediatric emergencies, *J Trauma* 31(2):205-209, 1991.
15. McCloskey KA and Johnston C: Pediatric critical care transport survey: team composition and training, mobilization time, and mode of transportation, *Ped Emerg Care* 6(1):1-3, 1990.
16. McCloskey KA and Orr RA: Pediatric transport issues in emergency medicine, *Emerg Med Clin North Am* 9(3):475-489, 1991.
17. National Transportation Safety Board Safety Study: *Commercial emergency medical service helicopter operations,* NTSB/SS-88/01, Washington, DC.
18. Pointer JE and Osur MA: Effect of standing orders on field times, *Ann Emerg Med* 18:1119-1121, 1989.
19. *Resources for optimal care of patients with burn injury.* In: *Resources for optimal care of the injured patient,* 1990, The American College of Surgeons.
20. Rhee KJ et al: Is the flight physician needed for helicopter emergency medical services, *Ann Emerg Med* 15(2):174-177, 1986.
21. Shanaberger CJ: Understanding COBRA's twists and turns, *JEMS* 101-103, 1991.
22. Strobos J: Tightening the screw: statutory and legal supervision of interhospital patient transfers, *Ann Emerg Med* 20(3):302-310, 1991.

43

Pediatric Issues

George L. Foltin, M.D., FAAP, FACEP
Arthur Cooper, M.D., FACS, FAAP, FCCM

Modern EMS evolved in the 1970s because of the recognition in the 1960s that (1) trauma and sudden cardiac emergencies were the leading causes of death in this nation and (2) largely volunteer, fire company-based rescue squads were not by themselves optimally prepared to meet this challenge. The physicians who first created EMS were trained chiefly in the adult-oriented specialties of surgery, internal medicine, cardiology, and anesthesiology.[4] Infants and children were cared for in the EMS system, but their needs were not specifically addressed and deficiencies in their care were not recognized.[10] Yet pediatric patients comprise some 5% to 10% of prehospital transports, 30% of emergency department visits, 21% of all prehospital trauma care, and 12% of all in-hospital trauma care.[19]

Although the EMS system itself did not develop with a focus on the special needs of infants and children, the health care system in its entirety obviously did. Centers of excellence in pediatrics dedicated to the tertiary care of children with infectious, metabolic, and developmental diseases, cancer, congenital anomalies, and multiple trauma have always existed. The current emphasis on critical management of serious childhood illness, however, has led to increasing reliance on transport of sick and injured children to these centers, particularly in urban environments where access to primary care is shrinking.[31] Moreover, there is growing recognition that trauma, especially preventable injury, is the leading public health problem for children.[51] Together, these factors fostered the development of Emergency Medical Services for Children (EMSC) in many parts of this country. The EMS medical director therefore should be aware of this new component of the system including the need, the cost, the sources for funding, and directions for further improvement.

History

Government Discovers EMS

Before the 1960s, prehospital emergency care was neglected in the United States. Individuals with little if any formal training in trauma care provided emergency treatment. Although professional organizations such as the American College of Surgeons and the American Academy of Orthopaedic Surgeons were beginning to address this problem, ambulances were rarely if ever properly equipped or staffed to handle even simple prehospital emergencies, involving adults or children.

The revolutionary changes in EMS systems following the 1966 publication of the National Academy of Sciences (NAS) report, *Accidental Death and Disability: The Neglected Disease of Modern Society,* are now well-known to the public who has come to expect high quality prehospital emergency care as a basic health right.[7] What is rarely noted is that neither this landmark report nor the key legislative initiatives that resulted from it such as the Highway Safety Act of 1966, the Emergency Medical Service Systems Act of 1973 and the Preventive Health and Health Services Block Grant Program of 1982 that ultimately replaced the EMS Systems Act made special mention of the unique needs of infants and children in the emergency care system. However, Neonatal care was regionalized under the EMS Systems Act. As late as 1986, reviews describing the enormous progress made in EMS during the past two decades failed to mention pediatrics as a specific component of EMS.[73]

EMS Discovers Pediatrics

Review of early efforts by EMS planners to address pediatrics reveals a well-meaning but inaccurate needs assessment. The special needs of infants and children were simply not appreciated. This is not to say that their needs were intentionally overlooked; literature identifying that the epidemiology of prehospital problems of children are different than those of adults had not yet been published. However, this lack of knowledge gave rise to the false notion that children could be treated as little adults.

As a result the original Department of Transportation (DOT) curriculum did not adequately reflect the pediatric emergencies commonly encountered in the field or emphasize the necessary skills. Instead the didactic pediatric component focused on illnesses and injuries that were irrelevant to field care and did not focus on recognition of conditions that prehospital interventions would affect. Another area that most training programs still lack is clinical time spent evaluating children in an emergency department or on a pediatric unit. Such "hands-on" experience allows the trainee to learn assessment of the pediatric patient from experienced child health professionals.

Pediatrics Discovers EMS

The process of improving the pediatric components of systems was initiated at the local and state levels in various regions by interested members of the pediatric, surgical, and emergency medical communities during the late 1970s and early 1980s.[10] In 1978 the pediatric community of Los Angeles noticed that EMS was not fully meeting the needs of children. This recognition resulted in the formation of a multidisciplinary committee with representatives from regional pediatric organizations, the regional EMS agency, and the county Health Department. The committee developed guidelines for prehospital care of pediatric emergencies, a pediatric equipment list for prehospital care providers, a curriculum for the education of paramedics in pediatric emergencies, and a plan for integration of EMSC into the existing EMS system.[63] The Maryland Institute for Emergency Medical Service Systems (MIEMSS) is a model for a successful and fully integrated system, and was one of the first systems to incorporate pediatric trauma receiving hospitals.[26] Others have also been active in incorporating EMSC in their regions through a systems approach, notably Mobile, Alabama, New York, and Milwaukee.[20,34,59]

Recent literature describes the unique epidemiology of pediatric prehospital care and documents deficiencies in the approach to children in the accessing, education, equipping, and medical control of prehospital personnel. Although the acuity level of pediatric prehospital problems is lower than that of adults (approximately 0.5% of transported children require tertiary care and 5% involve life-threatening or limb-threatening problems) children account for 5% to 10% of all ambulance runs.* The result is that the average EMT or paramedic rarely cares for critically ill or injured children; thus their pediatric skills are difficult to maintain. Although constant retraining could improve skill and knowledge retention, in most communities prehospital providers do not yet receive even the appropriate training needed to care for children. Moreover, the appropriate array of equipment sizes is often not available. In many communities specific protocols do not exist for pediatric prehospital care, reflecting a lack of pediatric expertise in both direct and indirect medical control. It is therefore hardly surprising that prehospital providers and medical control physicians rate critical pediatric calls among their most stressful encounters.[8]

Government Discovers EMSC

Federal funding has been available for EMSC system development since 1985, through the EMSC Demonstration Grant Program. Projects were originally set up in Alabama, California, New York and Oregon to improve EMSC and integrate this care into existing EMS systems. Since that time, 23 additional states have received funding for EMSC. The EMSC projects have developed strategies, programs, and resources that are shared nationally and have provided expertise and outreach for surrounding states and regions through knowledge transfer and use (KTU) programs.[29,38] In 1991 National EMSC Resource Centers were established in Torrence, California, (The National EMSC Resource Alliance: NERA) and Washington, D.C., (The EMSC National Resource Center: NRC), vastly increasing access by the rest of the nation to educational material, recent advances and expertise in medicine, legislation, and data collection.

The current program is administered jointly by the Office of Maternal and Child Health (OMCH) and the EMS Division of the DOT National Highway Traffic Safety Administration (NHTSA). EMSC consists of six phases of care, containing several of the elements addressed in the EMS Systems Act of 1973 (see box on p. 422). It encompasses the entire spectrum of care for a child requiring emergency services and exists within the established EMS System. These phases of care may reside in one or more of the multiple independent agencies that comprise the EMS system.

*References 13,20,28,37,44,55,62,63,65,66,72.

Participants in Federal EMSC Demonstration Grant Program

Alabama	New Hampshire
Alaska	New Jersey
Arkansas	New Mexico
California	New York
District of Columbia	North Carolina
Florida	Ohio
Hawaii	Oklahoma
Idaho	Oregon
Louisiana	Texas
Maine	Vermont
Maryland	Washington
Michigan	Wisconsin
Missouri	Utah
Nevada	

Components of EMS versus Phases of EMSC

EMS Component	EMSC phase
Manpower	Prevention
Training	System access
Communications	Field treatment
Transportation	Emergency department
Treatment	Inpatient treatment
Facilities	Rehabilitation
Critical care units	
Public safety agencies	
Consumer participation	
Access to care	
Patient transfer	
Coordinated patient recordkeeping	
Public information and education	
Review and evaluation	
Disaster plan	
Mutual aid	

Emergency Medical Services for Children System Development

Improved outcome from prehospital intervention following cardiac arrest is an EMS success for adults but not for children.[14] It has been suggested that because cardiac arrest is rare in pediatrics, a more appropriate benchmark of success in the prehospital care of critically ill and injured children is intervention in pre-arrest respiratory failure and shock situations.[20] Bystander cardiopulmonary resuscitation (CPR) and prehospital intervention have proved effective in pediatric near-drowning and foreign body aspiration.[36,55] There is also evidence suggesting the importance of prehospital care in pediatric trauma management; 80% of childhood injury deaths occur before admission to the hospital, and EMS agencies are involved in the vast majority.[10,24]

Prevention and Access

Emergency and intensive care for critically ill and injured children is expensive in terms of personal anguish and societal cost.[12] Prevention has the best outcome and costs far less. The link between communities and EMS agencies can be strengthened by developing, improving, and supporting successful injury and illness prevention programs. Parents can also be taught CPR, recognition of serious injury and illness, when to call for help, and what to do until help arrives.

Field Care

Models for field treatment of pediatric patients should be based on the epidemiology of childhood illness and injury, using outcome data to support the interventions performed. Cardiac disease is rare in children, and evidence does not demonstrate an improved outcome that justifies the delay inherent in providing advanced cardiac life support (ACLS) to children in the field, whether for status epilepticus, poisoning, or vascular instability from dehydration. This is not to suggest that children should be categorically denied ACLS in the prehospital environment or that on-scene decisions regarding the need for ACLS are infrequently required, but rather that as for the adult trauma patient, priorities must be established.[54] Thus although the value of early prehospital advanced airway intervention in pediatric patients is clear, the majority of pediatric prehospital emergencies do not require ACLS interventions.[55]

The majority of pediatric patients require only short-term intervention, and prehospital care, usually at a basic level, is a single, crucial link. Although an investment is clearly required for manpower and training, the cost of an inadequate pediatric EMS response is much higher for the society and the family.[13] Yet at present, few prehospital personnel have adequate education and training in basic pediatric knowledge and skills, and fewer still have sufficient exposure to critically ill and injured children to retain these capabilities over time.[64,66,68] Many systems only recently started acquiring appropriate equipment for pediatric emergency care, despite the low cost.[11]

Systems in the process of developing their pediatric capabilities cannot expect field personnel to suddenly feel comfortable with pediatric patients. Rather, a system's pediatric capabilities evolve as field personnel gain experience with children. If EMS teachers impart a positive mindset, prehospital providers respond with an attitudinal change that persists even when technical skills do not. Constant reinforcement of pediatric skills, building on the similarity to adult skills while emphasizing the differences, is essential to this process; it is a necessity for any system that plans to deliver appropriate pediatric care.

Modern EMS planning has evolved to the point that field care is initiated at the moment the caller makes contact with the dispatcher, through the use of pre-arrival instructions. Very little work has been done examining the provision of appropriate care for children by dispatchers either in their triage role of deciding level and urgency of response or in their ability to provide pre-arrival instructions for pediatric emergencies. Anecdotal reports attest to successful outcomes in individual pediatric cases because of timely provision of pre-arrival instructions.[41] Obviously, these "saves" did not occur by chance. The dispatchers involved had to be sufficiently familiar with CPR and airway clearing techniques to be able to describe them over the telephone to distraught and untrained caretakers and convince the callers that they could actually perform them.

Hospital Care: Emergency Services

Seidel and associates suggest that the availability of a receiving hospital with expertise in pediatric care effects outcome as much if not more than the quality of the prehospital care.[65] This notion combined with the growing recognition by emergency physicians and pediatricians that the education they received in emergency pediatrics during residency training was inadequate has led to an increasing emphasis on pediatrics in emergency departments nationwide.[35] Guidelines both by the American College of Emergency Physicians (ACEP) and jointly by the American Medical Association and the American Academy of Pediatrics define a minimum standard of pediatric care for hospital emergency departments, including postgraduate training and continuing education requirements.[1,49] Experiments with voluntary consensus standards have also been successful in many locales, particularly southern California's Emergency Departments Approved for Pediatrics (EDAP) Program and New York City's 9-1-1 Receiving Hospitals System.[48,63]

Hospital Care: Critical Care and Trauma Centers

A statewide study of Oregon by Pollack and associates indicated that regionalization of care for critically ill and injured children can improve outcome, if they are properly triaged and quickly transferred to a tertiary pediatric center.[53] A population-based study by Cooper and associates in New York showed that outcome is better among injured children cared for in trauma centers with pediatric expertise than in other hospitals.[9] A review by Marganitt and others of the MIEMSS pediatric experience demonstrates that compliance with regionalization guidelines allows as many as 90% of children with potentially lethal injuries to be treated in a pediatric trauma center.[40] Still unresolved is the question of whether seriously injured children can be successfully managed in adult trauma centers. However, preliminary observations suggest that if the responsible surgeons (1) are experienced in pediatric trauma care, (2) are committed to providing this care, and (3) practice in an environment where appropriate pediatric emergency, critical, and acute medical-surgical and nursing care services are readily available, outcome may be as good as in comparable pediatric trauma centers.[22,32]

Systems Issues: Urban

Most large metropolitan areas possess adequate monetary and professional resources for pediatric prehospital care. The chief obstacle to the development of EMSC in most cities is that the systems developed without specific emphasis on pediatric illness and injury. Thus it has sometimes been difficult for child advocates to convince the administrative and medical leaders of the systems to invest in EMSC during an era of dwindling resources. Yet there are compelling reasons to do so. Proficiency in management of pediatric prehospital emergencies is increasingly becoming the standard of care in this nation, and those who ignore the special needs of infants and children expose the municipalities that they serve to the possibility of adverse legal judgments regarding the adequacy of their pediatric prehospital care. Such settlements often prove far more costly than additional pediatric protocol development, education, equipment, medications, and medical control.

Systems Issues: Rural

Children who are injured or become suddenly ill in rural areas are least likely to benefit from an adequate EMS response because of the large, sparsely populated areas that rural systems must cover. The result of long distances, difficult environmental conditions, and rough terrain is often prolonged response and transport times. Life-threatening injuries occur infrequently at any given location in rural areas, but 70% of all highway fatalities occur on rural roads. Prehospital and hospital personnel working in rural settings manage children with injuries as serious as any in a regional trauma center but far less frequently; and they are less likely to have adequate training in pediatric emergencies.[45]

Medical Oversight

Every EMS system has its strengths and weaknesses. The logical approach to system development is for the medical director to identify the latter and build upon the former. In this process, each component of the system is carefully reexamined, and its pediatric needs are fully assessed. Emphasis should be placed on basic skills, but the system should not deny any child advanced interventions if they are needed and can be provided.

Education and Training

Developing and maintaining the knowledge, skills, and attitudes necessary for pediatric resuscitation requires no reorientation with respect to basic management principles; however, it must be reassured that previously mastered adult knowledge and skills can be readily transferred to infants and children as long as differences in anatomy, physiology, disease spectrum, and patient assessment are understood and special techniques that have been mastered are constantly reinforced. Numerous educational packages that meet these objectives have been developed under the auspices of the federal EMSC Grant Program. Such programs are available through the National Resource Centers.[29] Many locales are also adapting the American Heart Association-American Academy of Pediatrics' Pediatric Advanced Life Support (PALS) course for prehospital personnel, which has been received enthusiastically by most paramedics.[5] Minimum standards for education and training of all prehospital emergency personnel, as defined by a consensus Task Force on Education and Training from the federal EMSC projects, are also available (see box at right).[13]

Courses that can be self-taught or separated into modules allow for wide dispersion of teaching materials. The latter approach has been successfully adopted by the New York State Pediatric Prehospital Care Course.[15] Greater use of modern telecommunications technologies has also been advocated to permit rural providers access to training traditionally centered at major teaching institutions. Such telecommunications can be used for dissemination via broadcast or mobile teaching stations such as the laser disc system developed by the Idaho EMSC Project.

Minimum Standards for Education and Training in EMSC

Basic

Knowledge
- Anatomic and physiological differences
- Psychological and developmental issues
- Pediatric physical assessment
- Pediatric vital signs
- Spectrum of pediatric illness or injury requiring emergency care
- Principles of neonatal and pediatric resuscitation
- Recognition and management of pediatric respiratory distress or failure
- Recognition and management of pediatric shock or trauma
- Treatment of pediatric medical-surgical emergencies
  - Burns
  - Near-drowning
  - Seizures
  - Poisoning
- Recognition and reporting of child abuse
- Recognition and management of SIDS
- Critical incident stress debriefing

Skills
- Infants and child CPR
- Infant and child obstructed airway clearing maneuvers
- Infant and child airway and ventilatory management
- Pediatric vital signs determination
- Pediatric pneumatic antishock garment use
- Pediatric extrication and spine immobilization

Advanced

Review and reinforcement of all basic requirements, plus . . .

Knowledge
- Need for endotracheal or nasogastric intubation in pediatrics
- Need for intravenous or intraosseus access in pediatrics
- Dosage and administration of drugs in pediatric emergencies
- Dosage and administration of fluid in pediatric emergencies

Skills
- Pediatric endotracheal and nasogastric intubation
- Pediatric intravenous and intraosseous access
- Pediatric defibrillation and cardioversion
- Pediatric needle thoracostomy and cricothyroidostomy

Education and training of professionals and the public. In: Seidel JS and Henderson DP, editions: *emergency medical services for children: a report to the nation,* Washington, DC, 1991, National Center for Education in Maternal and Child Health.

Direct Medical Control

Direct medical control may be provided by emergency department attendants, residents, or specially trained nurses and paramedics; large centralized systems may have a dedicated physician provide direct medical control for the entire system. In examining this component of EMS care, medical directors must ensure that training of direct medical control physicians is sufficient to provide sophisticated medical input for field personnel caring for infants and children. Incorporating physicians knowledgeable in pediatric telephone triage and transport medicine such as pediatric emergency and intensive care physicians proves especially useful in EMSC system development and operation. Finally, in developing protocols for direct medical control of pediatric emergencies, the crucial role of basic providers must not be neglected. The majority of the prehospital medical care, particularly in rural areas, is provided by basic providers with the most limited pediatric experience and therefore the most acute need for medical guidance.

Indirect Medical Control

Because of the maturation of the specialty of emergency medicine and the subspecialty of pediatric emergency medicine, every medical director should expect at least one member of the local physician advisory council to have pediatric expertise. In New York City, this individual is actually an appointed representative from a citywide committee on EMSC. Such an arrangement ensures that pediatric implications of policies and planning are consistently addressed. It also provides a liaison to the pediatric community that often has a fragmentary understanding of the system.

Because of the infrequency of serious pediatric illnesses in the field and the unique presentations in comparison with adult illnesses, New York City pediatric EMT-B protocols were developed for a core group of critical pediatric conditions, using directed assessments to facilitate timely interventions (see top box this page).[47] In spite of inadequate data to support prolonged scene time for pediatric prehospital interventions, numerous New York City paramedic protocols were developed using an approach termed "conservative yet permissive" (see bottom box this page).[10,47] The approach is conservative in that maintenance of airway, breathing, and circulation, rapid transport to an appropriate facility, and keeping the child warm are the primary priorities. It is permissive in that paramedics have standing orders that allow intubation based on their judgment and other paramedic interventions are permitted en route if there is unavoidable transport delay.

New York City Regional Emergency Medical Advisory Board Pediatric EMT-B Protocols

Pediatric respiratory distress or failure
Pediatric obstructed airway
Pediatric croup or epiglottitis
Pediatric non-traumatic cardiac arrest
Pediatric shock
Care of the newborn infant
Newborn resuscitation
Child abuse

From *New York City Regional Emergency Medical Advisory Board Prehospital Basic and Advanced Life Support Treatment Protocols,* New York, 1991, New York City EMS.

New York City Regional Emergency Medical Advisory Board Pediatric Paramedic Protocols

Pediatric respiratory arrest
Pediatric obstructed airway
Pediatric croup or epiglottitis
Pediatric non-traumatic cardiac arrest
Pediatric asthma
Pediatric anaphylaxis
Pediatric altered mental status
Pediatric status epilepticus
Pediatric traumatic or hypovolemic shock
Pediatric traumatic or hypovolemic arrest

From *New York City Regional Emergency Medical Advisory Board Prehospital Basic and Advanced Life Support Treatment Protocols,* New York, 1991, New York City EMS.

Modification of this paradigm may be necessary where lengthy transport times are anticipated because of great distance from the field to the receiving hospital. When a long ambulance run is anticipated, investment of valuable time to further stabilize the patient before transport is more justifiable than when transport time is short. Yet the vast majority of prehospital providers are basic providers based in rural and wilderness regions; advanced providers are concentrated in the urban and suburban communities. Protocols designed for remote areas may therefore require interface with sophisticated providers dispatched by helicopter, or specialized training in intermediate levels of care that permits providers with limited education in pediatrics to obtain definitive airway control and establish venous access before transport may be necessary.

Systems that perform more sophisticated interventions on children have a responsibility to study the effects of their efforts so optimal approaches can be developed.

Equipment-Medications List

ACEP recently developed guidelines of minimum equipment needs for pediatric prehospital care at both basic and advanced levels.[50] The Task Force on Education and Training of the Federal EMSC Grant Program has also written guidelines (see box this page).[16] Although medications required by children differ little from those needed by adults, drug dosages for the most part are determined on the basis of size. The use of color-coded tapes that key drug doses and equipment selection to body length has proved effective in the field and is now standard equipment in many agencies.[39]

The actual cost of equipping systems for pediatric resuscitation is remarkably low. Because many services already have some of the equipment, meeting current recommended standards is relatively inexpensive; for systems that do not already have equipment, comparing the actual costs of obtaining this equipment with other fixed expenses may be illuminating.[11] For example, a single vehicle can be fully outfitted for considerably less than the price of a single automatic external defibrillator.

Minimum Guidelines for Pediatric Equipment in Ambulances

Basic

Pediatric stethoscope, infant-child attachments
Pediatric blood pressure cuffs, infant-child sizes
Disposable humifidier(s)
Pediatric simple-nonrebreathing oxygen masks, all sizes
Pediatric face masks, all sizes
Pediatric bag-valve devices, infant-child sizes
Pediatric airway adjuncts, all sizes
Pediatric suction catheters, all sizes
Pediatric Yankauer device
Pediatric extrication collars, all sizes
Pediatric extrication equipment (including infant car seat)
Pediatric limb splints, all sizes
Pediatric traction splint
Pediatric pneumatic antishock garment

Advanced

All of the above, plus . . .
Pediatric endotracheal tubes, all sizes
Pediatric stylets, all sizes
Pediatric laryngoscope blades, all sizes
Pediatric Magill (Rovenstein) forceps
Pediatric intravenous catheters, all sizes
Pediatric intraosseous needs, all sizes
Pediatric nasograstric tubes, all sizes
Pediatric ECG electrodes
Pediatric defibrillator paddles, infant-child sizes
Pediatric dosage-packed medications or fluids
Pediatric dosage-volume wall chart
Mini-drip intravenous infusion sets

From Emergency Medical Services Education and Training Taskforce, Emergency Medical Services for Children Grant Program, Bureau of Maternal and Child Health Resources Development: *Summary of Education and Training Issues Survey Responses,* Rockville, Md, 1988, US Department of Health and Human Services.

Funding

There are 16 million children seen in the emergency departments of the nation each year. In 1985 the cost for children aged 0 to 14 years approximated $13.8 billion. From 1979 to 1987, there was a 25% increase in the number of children living in poverty, and from 1983 to 1988, there was a 13% decrease in the number of childern with health insurance. Moreover the death rate for children from preventable injuries is twice that of other industrialized countries; a significant proportion are due to violent crime.[18]

Certainly, public funds are best spent on prevention. However, when primary prevention fails, secondary prevention (the prompt recognition of a pediatric emergency, rapid response by trained emergency providers, and early provision of definitive care) is necessary to avoid further deterioration. Few children actually require critical interventions at the scene or during transport, but all children with potentially life-threatening illnesses or injuries deserve an assessment sophisticated enough to determine the need for such interventions. Thus the question is whether to expect the same level of system performance for children as is expected for adults; if so, the marginal cost of preparing providers to meet the needs of infants and children is an investment worth many times the initial down payment, especially when it is realized that the societal cost of a single childhood injury death is estimated at $250,000.[60]

Controversies

Regionalization

Data now exist attesting to the efficacy of pediatric intensive care unit and trauma center care in improving the outcome of combined system trauma victims with severe closed head, thoracoabdominal, and multiple skeletal injuries.[48,53] Yet for patients with life-threatening, non-traumatic illnesses, evidence demonstrating clear survival benefit from regionalization is lacking. Nonetheless, referral of critically ill and injured children to centers providing comprehensive pediatric care is well-established and has led such institutions to develop and extend their capabilities in pediatric critical care. Many centers have established teams for secondary transport of patients to such institutions. Such practices are costly but increasingly seen as an integral part of hospital-based pediatric critical care medicine, providing a decisive advantage in an increasingly competitive marketplace.

Because few institutions possess the monetary or professional resources to provide such a level of care to pediatric patients, the number of centers that participate is limited.[21] Only in larger metropolitan areas are a full range of pediatric specialty services available at more than one institution. If possible, critically ill or injured pediatric patients should undergo primary transport to these institutions. However, because many seriously ill or injured pediatric patients are transported by parents or police unaware of differences between hospitals with respect to the level of pediatric expertise, every receiving hospital must be capable of initiating resuscitation and stabilization of such children.

Triage Scores and Disaster Management

Triage scores are potentially an important tool in pediatric prehospital care, but they must be valid, reliable, and practical.[75] Both the Champion Trauma Score and Revised Trauma Score have been used in the pediatric population, but neither is ideal because they fail to account for the greater impact of severe closed head injury in children on ultimate outcome.[6,17] For this reason, the Pediatric Trauma Score (PTS) (Table 43-1) was developed and has been prospectively validated for field use.[2,58,71] Although its advantages have not consistently proved decisive in relation to other scores, it encourages safer triage practices, is acceptable for outcome assessment, as well as field use, and carries the endorsement of the ACS Committee on Trauma and the American Pediatric Surgical Association Committee on Trauma, which in addition to pediatric trauma center guidelines has published a list of possible indications for transfer to a pediatric trauma center (see box on p. 428).[27,30,46,51,70]

Disaster management in pediatrics is in its infancy, judging from the lack of published studies in this area. Review of the January 1989 Avianca plane crash in Nassau County, New York, provides valuable insight into the current state of ignorance. The Nassau County disaster plan, like most others nationwide, made no special provisions for triage and transport of critically injured children (PTS ≤ 8) to appropriate facilities, and more than half were not taken to pediatric critical care or trauma centers. Moreover, coordinated medical control was ineffective, transport times extended, and field documentation of the extent and severity of pediatric injuries by the 50-some volunteer ambulance squads that participated was extremely poor.[74]

Legal Issues

Refusal of medical assistance (RMA) is one of the most vexing legal problems confronting the medical director. In situations that pose an immediate threat to life, the doctrine of implied consent is the basis for medical intervention, and supersedes other concerns.[33] In less urgent situations, only those individuals with full parental rights may decline to accept prehospital emergency medical care for a child once requested. However, in most jurisdictions the law protects emergency providers that proceed in good faith to render medical assistance to a child if they perceive a potential threat to life or limb, even when permission is denied by the child's legal guardian.

Somewhat less clear is the prehospital provider's responsibility in cases of potential child abuse, including medical neglect. The prehospital provider of course is obligated to treat and transport any child

Table 43-1. Pediatric Trauma Score

	+2	+1	-1
Size (kg)	>20	10-20	<10
Airway	Normal	Maintained	Unmaintained
Systolic blood pressure (mm Hg)	>90	50-90	<50
Central nervous system	Awake	Obtunded	Coma
Open wound	None	Minor	Major
Skeletal trauma	None	Closed	Open-Multiple

From Tepas JJ et al: The pediatric trauma score as a predictor of injury severity in the injured child, *Pediatr Surg* 22:14-18, 1987.

Possible Indications for Transfer to a Pediatric Trauma Center

History of Injury

Patient thrown from a moving vehicle
Falls from > 15 feet
Extrication time > 20 minutes
Passenger cabin invaded > 12 inches
Death of another passenger
Accident in a hostile environment (heat, cold water, etc.)

Anatomic Injuries

Combined system injury
Penetrating injury of the groin or neck
Three or more long bone fractures
Fractures of the axial skeleton
Amputation (other than digits)
Persistent hypotension
Severe head trauma
Maxillofacial or upper airway injury
CNS injury with prolonged loss of consciousness, posturing, or paralysis
Spinal cord injury with neurologic deficit
Unstable chest injury
Blunt or penetrating trauma to the chest or abdomen
Burns, flame, or inhalation

System Considerations

Necessary service or specialist not available
No beds available
Need for pediatric ICU care
Multiple casualties
Family request
Paramedic judgment
Serverity scores: Trauma Score ≤12, Revised Trauma Score ≤11, or Pediatric Trauma Score ≤8

From Harris BH et al: American Pediatric Surgical Association: principles of pediatric trauma care, *Pediatr Surg* (in press).

whose life or limb may be in jeopardy. If no such emergency exists but abuse is judged likely, prehospital providers should request police assistance in consultation with a medical control physician, because in most jurisdictions, peace officers are vested with the final responsibility for public intervention in private matters. Regardless of the outcome of any particular event, however, the provider is obligated to perform a brief visual survey of the immediate surroundings for evidence of abuse, in addition to the usual patient assessment, to record all pertinent findings on the prehospital care report, and to verbally transmit this information to the physician or nurse on duty at the receiving hospital. In cases of RMA, the provider must communicate with other appropriate authorities, as well as the direct medical control physician.

Presumption of Death

CPR is indicated when the emergency provider encounters an unresponsive, pulseless, apneic patient. Prehospital providers often are permitted by protocol not to institute resuscitative measures in cases where there is rigor mortis, extreme dependent lividity, tissue decomposition, obvious mortal injury, or a properly executed Do Not Resuscitatate order that conforms to the local laws. None of these is typically present in the death of a child. By contrast the most common fatal illnesses encountered by prehospital providers in the field are sudden infant death syndrome and traumatic cardiac arrest following blunt injury.

It is well-recognized that the outcome following unwitnessed asystolic cardiac arrest, the dysrhythmia universally associated with both the above conditions, is abysmal. This has led some authorities to suggest that neither time nor effort should be expended in attempting to resuscitate such children. However, attempts at resuscitation of children are justified despite near-certain failure. Distraught parents know at least that everything possible was done to revive their child. Similarly, distressed prehospital providers will be reassured that their failure to intervene did not contribute to ultimate demise, thereby minimizing the psychic impact of the critical incident.

Summary

The current project to revise the EMT-A curriculum sponsored by NHTSA has a strong pediatric focus. A pediatric module is also being prepared for the EMS Medical Director's Course reflecting the newly appreciated need for focus on this special body of knowledge. Pioneering EMS-EMSC systems have already examined intubation, intraosseous infusion, defibrillation, and ability of dispatch operators to identify true pediatric emergencies.* There is evidence that resuscitation of children in the prehospital phase of care improves outcome. Separate works by Rivara and Quan demonstrate that control of the airway and provision of adequate ventilation are critical to survival of children suffering multiple trauma and near drowning.[55,61]

Even so, more extensive studies are needed to determine which interventions will result in the most benefit for children in the prehospital setting. For example, intraosseous infusion has been sug-

*References 23,34,49,52,54,67,69.

gested as a useful procedure in the prehospital phase of care to gain emergency vascular access to children. Studies demonstrate that this procedure can be successfully used in the prehospital setting.[23,42,69] However, studies demonstrating that intraosseous infusion improves outcome for children have not yet been performed.

The fact that EMSC is a new area of the EMS system makes it ideally suited to careful study. One must be careful not to deny advances in pediatric critical care to children such as intraosseous infusion only because their value in prehospital pediatric emergency medicine has not yet been unequivocally proven. Logical interventions must be tried and studied, because EMSC is still in the early stages. In these endeavors, the EMS medical director occupies the central role, when new treatments are developed and evaluated that ultimately may benefit adults, as well as children.

The promise EMSC holds as an integrating force for the EMS system as a whole may prove to be its most important future role. EMSC requires and typically commands the truly collegial participation of many providers from a broad range of medical, surgical, nursing, and prehospital disciplines. It cannot be separated from the system as a whole, and each component must work in concert with all other parts for the optimal outcome of the child and the family. In short, it is the ideal model for the comprehensive EMS and trauma care system envisioned by the EMS medical director.[3,25,56]

REFERENCES

1. American College of Emergency Physicians: *Pediatric equipment guidelines,* Dallas, 1990, American College of Emergency Physicians.
2. Aprahamian C et al: Pediatric trauma score, *Arch Surg* 125:1128-1131, 1990.
3. Barkin R: *The system and training.* In: Barkin R, editor: Pediatrics in the emergency medical services system, *Ped Emerg Care* 6:72-77, 1990.
4. Boyd DR: *The history of emergency medical services (EMS) systems in the United States of America.* In: Boyd DR, Edlich RF, and Micik S, editors: *Systems approach to emergency medical care,* Norwalk, Conn, 1983, Appleton and Company.
5. Chameides L, editor: *Textbook of pediatric advanced life support.* Dallas and Elk Grove Village, 1988, American Heart Association and American Academy of Pediatrics.
6. Champion HR et al: Trauma score, *Crit Care Med* 9:672-676, 1981.
7. Committee on Trauma and Committee on Shock, Division of Medical Sciences, National Research Council-National Academy of Sciences: *Accidental death and disability: the neglected disease of modern society,* Washington, DC, 1966, National Academy of Sciences.
8. Cooper A and Foltin G: *Education and training of prehospital personnel.* In: Dieckmann RE: *Planning and managing systems for pediatric emergency care,* Baltimore: Williams & Wilkins (in press).
9. Cooper A et al: Efficacy of pediatric trauma care: a population-based study, *J Pediatr Surg* (in press).
10. Cooper A et al: Epidemiology of pediatric trauma: importance of population-based statistics. *J Pediatr Surg* (in press).
11. Cooper A et al: Costs of equipping and training emergency personnel for pediatric resuscitation, *Ped Emerg Care* 7:385, 1991 (abstract).
12. Division of Injury Control, Centers for Disease Control: Childhood injuries in the United States, *Am J Dis Child* 144:627-644, 1990.
13. *Education and training of professionals and the public.* In: Seidel JS and Henderson DP, editors: *Emergency medical services for children: a report to the nation,* Washington, DC, 1991, National Center for Education in Maternal and Child Health.
14. Eisenberg MS, Bergner L, and Hallstrom A: Cardiac resuscitation for the community: importance of rapid provision and program planning, *JAMA* 241:1905-1907, 1979.
15. Elling R and Cooper A, editors: *Prehospital pediatric care course student manual,* Albany, NY, 1991, New York State Department of Health.
16. Emergency Medical Services Education and Training Task Force, Emergency Medical Services for Children Grant Program, Bureau of Maternal and Child Health Resources Development: *Summary of education and training issues survey responses,* Rockville, Md, 1988, US Department of Health and Human Services.
17. *Field categorization of trauma patients (field triage).* In: American College of Surgeons Committee on Trauma: *Hospital and prehospital resources for optimal care of the injured patient and appendices A through J,* Chicago, 1986, American College of Surgeons.
18. *Financing emergency medical services for children: identifying resources.* In: Seidel JS and Henderson DP, editors: *Emergency medical services for children: a report to the nation,* Washington, DC, 1991, National Center for Education in Maternal and Child Health.
19. Foltin G and Fuchs S: Advances in pediatric emergency medical service systems, *Emerg Med Clin North Am* 9:459-474, 1991.
20. Foltin G et al: Developing pediatric prehospital advanced life support: the New York City experience, *Ped Emerg Care* 6:141-144, 1990.
21. Foltin G et al: Regionalizing care for critically ill and injured children: coast to coast experience. Presented at the Annual Meeting of the Ambulatory Pediatric Association, Washington, DC, May 1989.
22. Fortune JM et al: A pediatric trauma center without a pediatric surgeon: a 4-year outcome analysis. Presented at the Annual Meeting of the Eastern Association for the Surgery of Trauma, Hamilton, Bermuda, Jan 1992.
23. Fuchs S et al: A prehospital model of intraosseous infusion, *Ann Emerg Med* 20:371-374, 1991.
24. Gausche M et al: Pediatric deaths and emergency medical services (EMS) in urban and rural areas, *Pediatr Emerg Care* 5:158-162, 1989.
25. Haller JA: Toward a comprehensive emergency medical system for children, *Pediatrics* 86:120-122, 1990.
26. Haller JA et al: Organization and function of a regional pediatric trauma center: does a system of management improve outcome? *J Trauma* 23:691-696, 1983.
27. Harris BH et al: American Pediatric Surgical Association: principles of pediatric trauma care, *J Pediatr Surg* (in press).
28. *History of emergency medical services for children.* In: Seidel JS and Henderson DP, editors: *Emergency medical services for children: a report to the nation.* Washington, DC, 1991, National Center for Education in Maternal and Child Health.
29. Human Interaction Research Institute: *Emergency medical services for children innovation bank, ed 3,* Washington, DC, 1991, National Center for Education in Maternal and Child Health.
30. Kaufmann CR et al: Evaluation of the pediatric trauma score, *JAMA* 263:69-72, 1990.
31. Knickman R, Smith D, and Berry C: *Improving ambulance use in New York City: a final report,* New York, 1989, The Commonwealth Fund.

32. Knudson MM, Lewis FR, and Shagoury C: Can adult trauma surgeons care for injured children? Presented at the Annual Meeting of the American Association for the Surgery of Trauma, Philadelphia, Sep 1991.
33. Lazar RA: *EMS law: a guide for EMS professionals,* Rockville, Md, 1989, Aspen Publications.
34. Losek JD et al: Prehospital care of the pulseless, nonbreathing pediatric patient, *Am J Emerg Med* 5:370-375, 1987.
35. Ludwig S et al: Pediatric training in emergency medicine residency programs, *Ann Emerg Med* 11:170-173, 1982.
36. Luten R: *Access to optimal care.* In: Luten R and Foltin G, editors: *Pediatric resources for prehospital care,* Elk Grove Village, 1990, American Academy of Pediatrics Committee of the Section on Emergency Medicine.
37. Luten R: *Educational overview.* In: Luten R and Foltin G, editors: *Pediatric resources for prehospital care,* Elk Grove Village, 1990, American Academy of Pediatrics Committee of the Section on Emergency Medicine.
38. Luten R: *Emergency medical services for children projects.* In: Luten R and Foltin G, editors: *Pediatric resources for prehospital care,* Elk Grove Village, 1990, American Academy of Pediatrics Committee of the Section on Emergency Medicine.
39. Luten RC et al: A rapid method for estimating resuscitation drug doses from length in the pediatric age group, *Ann Emerg Med* 17:576-581, 1988.
40. Marganitt B et al: Children hospitalized for traumatic injuries in Maryland: statewide epidemiologic trends over 8 years. Presented at the Third Pediatric Critical Care Colloquium, Santa Monica, Calif, Oct 1989.
41. Marzulli J: EMS phone turned into lifeline: operator helped save baby, *New York Daily News,* December 6, 1991.
42. Miner WF et al: Prehospital use of intraosseous infusion by paramedics, *Ped Emerg Care* 5:5-7, 1989.
43. Mustalish AC: Emergency medical services: twenty years of growth and development, *N Y State J Med* 86:414-420, 1986.
44. National Highway Traffic Safety Administration: *Summary of consensus workshop on EMS training programs,* Washington, DC, 1990, US Department of Transportation.
45. National Highway Traffic Safety Administration: *EMS services: program update,* Washington, DC, 1989, US Department of Transportation.
46. Nayduch DA et al: Comparison of the ability of adult and pediatric trauma scores to predict pediatric outcome following major trauma, *J Trauma* 31:452-458, 1991.
47. *New York City regional emergency medical advisory board prehospital basic and advanced life support treatment protocols,* New York, 1991, New York City Emergency Medical Service.
48. New York City 9-1-1 Receiving Hospitals Advisory Committee: *New York City 9-1-1 receiving hospitals emergency department standards, ed 5* (revised), New York, 1991, New York City Emergency Medical Service.
49. *Pediatric emergencies.* In: American Medical Association Commission on Emergency Medical Services: *Guidelines for the categorization of hospital emergency capabilities,* Chicago, 1989, American Medical Association.
50. Pediatric Emergency Medicine Committee and Emergency Medical Services Committee, American College of Emergency Physicians: *Minimum pediatric prehospital equipment guidelines,* Dallas: 1991, American College of Emergency Physicians.
51. *Planning pediatric trauma care.* In: American College of Surgeons Committee on Trauma: *Resources for optimal care of the injured patient,* Chicago, 1990, American College of Surgeons.
52. Pointer JE et al: Clinical characteristics of paramedics' performance of pediatric endotracheal intubation, *Am J Emerg Med* 7:364-366, 1987.
53. Pollack MM et al: Improved outcomes from tertiary center pediatric intensive care: a statewide comparison of tertiary and nontertiary care facilities, *Crit Care Med* 19:150-159, 1991.
54. Pon S et al: Utilization of prehospital care by pediatric patients in New York City, *Pediatr Emerg Care* 5:286, 1989 (abstract).
55. Quan L et al: Outcome and predictors of outcome in pediatric submersion victims receiving prehospital care in King County, Washington, *Pediatrics* 86:586-593, 1990.
56. Ramenofsky ML: Emergency medical services for children and pediatric trauma system components, *J Pediatr Surg* 24:153-155, 1989.
57. Ramenofsky ML: *How can we address the differences in trauma versus illness systems?* In: Haller JA, editor: *Emergency medical services for children: report of the 97th Ross Conference on Pediatric Research,* Columbus: 1989, Ross Laboratories.
58. Ramenofsky ML et al: The predictive validity of the pediatric trauma score, *J Trauma* 28:1038-1042, 1988.
59. Ramenofsky ML et al: EMS for pediatrics: optimum treatment or unnecessary delay? *J Pediatr Surg* 18:498-504, 1983.
60. Rice DP et al: *Cost of injury in the United States: a report to congress,* Atlanta, 1989, Centers for Disease Control.
61. Rivara FP et al: Evaluation of potentially preventable deaths among pedestrian and bicyclist fatalities, *JAMA* 261:566-570, 1989.
62. Seidel JS: The six *Ts* of emergency medical services for children: triage, time, treatment, transportation, tertiary care, and training. In: Barkin RM, editor: Pediatrics in the emergency medical services system, *Ped Emerg Care* 6:72-77, 1990.
63. Seidel JS: *EMS-C in urban and rural areas: the California experience.* In: Haller JA, editor: *Emergency medical services for children: report of the 97th Ross Conference on Pediatric Research.* Columbus, 1989, Ross Laboratories.
64. Seidel JS: Emergency medical services and the pediatric patient: are the needs being met? II. Training and equipping emergency medical services providers for pediatric emergencies, *Pediatrics* 78:808-812, 1986.
65. Seidel JS and Henderson DP, editor: *Prehospital care of pediatric emergencies,* Los Angeles, 1987, Los Angeles Pediatric Society.
66. Seidel JS et al: Emergency medical services and the pediatric patient: are the needs being met? *Pediatrics* 73:769-772, 1984.
67. Seigler RS, Tecklenburg FW, and Shealy R: Prehospital intraosseous infusion by emergency service personnel: a prospective study, *Pediatrics* 84:173-177, 1989.
68. Simon JE: *Current problems in the management of pediatric trauma.* In: Haller JA, editor: *Emergency medical services for children: report of the 97th Ross Conference on Pediatric Research,* Columbus: 1989, Ross Laboratories.
69. Smith RJ et al: Intraosseous infusion by prehospital personnel in critically ill pediatric patients, *Ann Emerg Med* 17:491-495, 1988.
70. Tepas JJ et al: The pediatric trauma score as a predictor of injury severity: an objective assessment, *J Trauma* 28:425-429, 1988.
71. Tepas JJ et al: The pediatric trauma score as a predictor of injury severity in the injured child, *J Pediatr Surg* 22:14-18, 1987.
72. Tsai A and Kallsen G: Epidemiology of pediatric prehospital care, *Ann Emerg Med* 16:284-292, 1987.
73. US Department of Transportation, National Highway Traffic Safety Administration: *Emergency medical technician: national standard curriculum, ed 3* Washington, DC, 1984, Department of Transportation.
74. VanAmerongen R et al: System response to a disaster: the pediatric perspective, *Ped Emerg Care* 6:234-235, 1990 (abstract).
75. Wesson DE et al: Injury scoring systems in children, *Can J Surg* 30:398-400, 1987.z

44

Hazardous Materials

Daniel Grant Hankins, M.D., FACEP

A hazardous material (HazMat) exposure in the prehospital phase can present many problems to an EMS medical director. The medical director must have a working knowledge of hazardous materials, the common toxicological exposure syndromes, and the appropriate responses.

At a minimum the EMS physician should be familiar with the information in Standard 472 of the National Fire Protection Association (NFPA). Many states offer courses based on this standard. The state of Minnesota, for instance, has a 4-hour course entitled Hazardous Material Awareness for Minnesota First Responders. (Table 44-1). This was developed by the State Fire Training Center and is presented by fire departments and vocational schools. EMS physicians taking this course or its equivalent would be able to work in the relatively safe areas of a HazMat incident and know how to protect themselves from injury. Medical directors should be able to obtain information on such HazMat awareness training from local fire authorities.

HazMat incidents may occur as part of an EMS incident or as an isolated problem without victims. Many disasters and multiple casualty incidents have a hazardous materials component. The presence of hazardous materials at an EMS scene can increase risk for EMS personnel, as well as for victims. Risk of EMS workers being injured or killed at any EMS scene is magnified when hazardous materials are present. Victims may also have increased morbidity or mortality from underlying injuries if hazardous materials are present. Recognition of the potential ill effects of chemicals at a scene is vital for EMS personnel and their medical director to prevent further injuries. Federal law mandates worker safety during HazMat responses. HazMat situations add industrial toxicology and decontamination problems to EMS responses. Treatment of specific exposures is not the purpose of this chapter but rather a consideration of the generic approach to such incidents.

Preparation

For a HazMat incident to be an emergency, all of the following must be present: (1) a bad chemical in (2) a bad container that is in (3) a bad location. If any of these three conditions are not present, then an emergent situation does not exist and an aggressive approach is not warranted. Each situation must be carefully evaluated individually to determine if active intervention is necessary and risk to personnel is warranted.

A uniform set of guidelines for personnel and apparatus must be developed to ensure safety and must be integrated into the local disaster plan (see Appendix). Matters are complicated by the variety of possible responders. Specific duties for responders must be spelled out in the plan along with the level of training required for each task such as decontamination, interdiction of the involved material, or care of already decontaminated victims. Different levels of training are necessary for workers in the HazMat situations, depending on where they are located. In general, there are three zones in HazMat events. The hot zone is the area most immediately dangerous to life and health. EMS personnel should not be in this area. Appropriately clothed fire personnel work in the hot zone. The warm zone has less contamination and contains the forward command area. Protective clothing is also required here, and decontamination occurs here. EMS workers usually do not operate in the warm zone, but fire fighters do. The cold zone is where all the normal EMS functions such as staging, triage and treatment occur. Personnel in the cold zone may only need a few hours training, but workers in the hot zone may have several hundred hours of hazardous materials training.

The Incident Command System (ICS) has evolved over the past 20 years as the best way to

Table 44-1. General Characteristics and Examples of Hazardous Materials

General Category DOT Classifications	Examples	General Hazardous Properties
Explosives and blasting agents		
Class A explosive	Dynamite, dry TNT, black powder	Sensitive to heat and shock
Class B explosive	Propellant explosives, rocket motors, special fireworks	Contamination could cause explosion Thermal and mechanical impact potential
Class C explosive	Common fireworks, small arms ammunition	
Blasting agent	Ammonium nitrate—fuel oil mixtures	
Gases (Compressed, Liquified or Dissolved under Pressure)		
Flammable gas	Liquefied petroleum gas, acetylene, hydrogen	Explosion potential BLEVE*
Nonflammable gas	Carbon dioxide, sulfur dioxide, anhydrous ammonia	Flammability hazard Vapor-air
Cryogenic	ethylene, nitrogen	Liquified gases—cold temperatures—frostbite-high expansion ratio
Flammable and Combustible Liquids		
Flammable liquid	Acetone, gasoline, methyl alcohol	Flammability hazard
Pyroforic liquid	aluminum, alkyls, alkyl boranes	Explosion potential
Combustible liquid	fuel oils, ethylene glycols	BLEVE Vapor-air Potentially corrosive, toxic, thermally unstable
Oxidizers and Organic Peroxides		
Oxidizer	Ammonium nitrate fertilizer, hydrogen peroxide solution	Supply oxygen to support combustion of nonflammable materials
Organic peroxide	Benzoyl peroxide, peracetic acid solution	Explosively sensitive to heat, shock, friction. Potentially toxic
Poisonous and Infectious Substances		
Poison A	Arsine, hydrocyanic acid, phosgene	Harm from inhalation, ingestion, absorption
Poison B	aniline, arsenic, methyl bromide	
Irritant	tear gas, xylyl bromide	
Etiologic agent	anthrax, botulism, rabies, tetanus	Flammability potential
Radioactive Substances		
Radioactive material	Plutonium, cobalt, uranium, uranium hexafluoride	Harm: Particulate—alpha and beta particles Radiation—gamma rays Internal and external
Corrosives		
Corrosive material	Acids—hydrochloric acid, oleum, sulfuric acid Bases—caustic soda, caustic potash	Harm: Disintegration of tissues, external Fuming potential Oxidizing effect Splatter potential
Other Regulated Materials		
ORM A	Dry ice, carbon tetrachloride	Toxic
ORM B	Quicklime, metallic mercury	Corrosive
ORM C	Oakum, bleaching powder	
ORM D	Consumer commodity	
ORM E	Hazardous substances—pentachlorophenol, adipic acid—and hazardous wastes	

*BLEVE=boiling liquid expanding vapor explosion.

manage complex emergency scenes when multiple agencies are responding. The presence of police, fire, and EMS at an incident can create jurisdictional and chain of command problems. The ICS is flexible and may be small or large, depending on the scope of the response. The ICS may be a single person for a small incident or a committee at a central command post for a large disaster. The ICS oversees the situation and determines priorities. The EMS medical director or a representative coordinates the EMS response with police and fire departments, state organizations (such as the pollution control and perhaps federal pollution agencies), and radiation agencies through the ICS. Usually at such HazMat scenes, police or fire commanders have overall control, but the medical director must have medical input with the ICS. Federal law mandates the ICS for all HazMat incidents.

Search and rescue is often conducted by different personnel than those that provide the initial emergency medical care. Fire fighters have a basic understanding of the response to HazMat and the use of protective gear; therefore when the prehospital EMS providers are fire fighters, the training task is easier. If the EMS providers are not fire fighters, they need additional education about how to protect themselves. Avoidance of contamination is the easiest course to minimize the creation of additional victims among EMS personnel. Therefore it is best not to allow untrained EMS crews into the contaminated zone but rather to bring decontaminated victims to the medical people. Because of the number or severity of victims, this may not always be possible. If a serious situation is at hand and an aggressive approach by EMS personnel is warranted, the workers still must be protected. Because special protective equipment is often not carried on ambulances, consideration must be given to stocking protective equipment for ambulance crews that may be exposed to HazMat situations (see box at right). The Federal Occupational Safety and Health Administration (OSHA) may levy large fines if workers have inadequate training or protection.

The NFPA has drafted standards for hazardous materials that are now in effect for EMS personnel. These guidelines establish minimal national standards in the training of EMS personnel for HazMat situations. Though different levels of HazMat skills are expected of various levels of EMS providers, this bulletin also describes a higher level of provider competent to direct and coordinate EMS activities at a HazMat incident. Leonard offers an excellent review of legislation and puts the complex relationships of HazMat response involving the federal, state, and local governments, EMS, and the EMS medical director in perspective.

Priorities

One of the most difficult concepts for prehospital personnel to understand in HazMat situations is the reversal of their usual inclination to rush in and help the victims. They are taught to act quickly in order to save victims, but in potential HazMat situations the priorities must be altered.

At potential HazMat sites the first priority is scene control to minimize both further injuries and spread of contamination. The scene must be isolated. Access by unnecessary or unauthorized emergency personnel, the news media, and all others must be restricted until the substance is contained. Because a cautious approach is necessary, ambulance units should establish themselves upwind at a safe distance. It is much easier to prevent contamination than to deal with even a minimal postcontamination situation.

The second priority is to identify the substances involved. Only then can a rational decision be made about whether a search for victims may be made by trained personnel with appropriate protection. The risk to rescuers must always be weighed against the likelihood of a successful rescue. Although it is difficult for EMS personnel to stand back and allow a victim to go without care, it is appropriate in some HazMat situations.

The operational decisions made at a scene are determined by the nature of the chemicals involved and usually are not medically driven. The person with the most HazMat experience (usually the senior fire official) should determine whether the material has risks such as a respiratory toxin, systemic toxin, or explosive. Only after specific identification is made can either the safe, appropriate rescue and treatment of the victims or the evacuation of

Equipment Items on Ambulance to Deal with a HazMat Incident

- Plastic trash bags 3 to 4 mil thick
- Plastic sheeting (6 mil) to cover doors, benches, windows, essential portable equipment, and perhaps to wrap patient
- Plastic body bag (alternative to wrap patient)
- Duct tape to seal cabinets
- Rubber boots
- Rubber gloves (neoprene is more resistant to chemicals than latex)
- Rubber aprons
- Disposable gowns or coveralls
- Reference books

the general population be initiated. Evacuation presents a difficult set of logistical and political problems that require implementation of a predetermined disaster plan.

The medical assessment of the situation from close range requires adequate protection and training for the involved personnel (see box below). At a minimum, initial survey of the site requires binoculars, protective gear, and self-contained breathing apparatus; this initial survey determines the extent of the problem and the type of material involved. If there is a suspicion that the material requires more than routine fire fighter protective clothing, then more sophisticated Tyvec, Butyl, or Polyvinyl Chloride suits are necessary (see box on following page). The EMS personnel must remain at a safe distance until

Levels of Protection

When response activities are conducted where atmospheric contamination is known or suspected to exist, personnel protective equipment must be worn. Personnel protective equipment is designed to prevent or reduce skin and eye contact, as well as inhalation or ingestion of the chemical substance.

Personnel equipment to protect the body against contact with known or anticipated chemical hazards has been divided into four categories.

1. Level A protection should be worn when the highest level of respiratory, skin, eye, and mucous membrane protection is needed.

   a. Personal Protective Equipment
   Positive-pressure (pressure demand), self-contained breathing apparatus (MSHA/NIOSH* approved).
   - Fully encapsulating chemical resistant suit.
   - Gloves, inner, chemical resistant
   - Gloves, outer, chemical resistant.
   - Boots, chemical resistant, steel toe and shank; (depending on suit boot construction, worn over or under suit boot.)
   - Underwear, cotton, long john type.*
   - Hard hat (under suit).*
   - Coveralls (under suit).*
   - Two-way radio communications (intrinsically safe).

   *Optional

2. Level B protection should be selected when the highest level of respiratory protection is needed, but a lesser level of skin and eye protection. Level B protection is the minimum level recommended on initial site entries until the hazards have been further identified and defined by monitoring, sampling, and other reliable methods of analysis, and personnel equipment corresponding with those findings utilized.

   a. Personal Protective Equipment
   - Positive-pressure (pressure-demand), self--contained breathing apparatus (MSHA/NIOSH approved).
   Chemical resistant clothing (overalls and long sleeved jacket, coveralls, hooded two piece chemical splash suit, disposable chemical resistant coveralls).
   - Coveralls (under splash suit).*
   - Gloves, outer, chemical resistant.
   - Gloves, inner, chemical resistant.
   - Boots, outer, chemical resistant, steel toe and shank.
   - Boots, outer, chemical resistant.*
   - Two-way radio communications (intrinsically safe).
   - Hard hat.*

   * Optional

3. Level C protection should be selected when the type of airborne substance is known, concentration measured, criteria for using air-purifying respirators met, and skin and eye exposure is unlikely. Periodic monitoring of the air must be performed.

   a. Personal Protective Equipment
   - Full-face, air-purifying respirator (MSHA/NIOSH approved).
   - Chemical resistant clothing (one piece coverall, hooded two piece chemical splash - suit, chemical resistant hood and apron, disposable chemical resistant coveralls).
   - Gloves, outer, chemical resistant.
   - Gloves, inner, chemical resistant.*
   - Boots, steel toe and shank, chemical resistant.
   - Boots, outer, chemical resistant.*
   - Cloth coveralls (inside chemical protective clothing).*
   - Two-way radio communications (intrinsically safe).
   - Hard hat.*
   - Escape mask.*

   * Optional

4. Level D is primarily a work uniform. It should not be worn on any site where respiratory or skin full details.

Refer to the Office of Emergency and Remedial Response, Environmental Response Division Interim Standard Operating Safety Procedures for full details.

From Lappe and Frederick: *Hazardous materials for EMS providers:* Minnesota State Board of Technical Colleges.

*Mine Safety Health Association/National Institute of Occupational Safety and Health

Protective Materials

A. Tyvek:	Product of DuPont, spun-bonded nonwoven polyethylene fibers, has reasonable tear, puncture, and abrasion resistance, provides excellent protection against particulate contaminates, inexpensive and suitable for disposable garments.
B. Nomex:	Product of DuPont, aromatic polyamide fiber, noncombustible and flame resistant up to 220;dgC, thus providing good thermal protection, very durable and acid resistant, used in fire fighters' turnout gear and some fully encapsulating suits.
C. Polyethylene:	Used as a coating on polyolefin material such as Tyvek, increasing resistance to acids, bases, and salts, good general purpose disposable product.
D. Saranex:	Made of Saran, a Dow product, coated on Tyvek, very good general purpose disposable material, better overall protection than polyethylene, resists chlorinated hydrocarbons.
E. Nitrile:	Also referred to as Buna-N, milled nitrile, nitrile latex, NBR, acrylonitrile, resists degradation by petroleum compounds, alcohols, acids, and caustics, used in boots and gloves, commonly available and inexpensive.
F. PVA:	Polyvinyl alcohol, resists degradation and permeation by aromatic and chlorinated hydrocarbons and petroleum compounds, major drawback is its solubility in water, used in gloves.

From Lappe and Frederick: *Hazardous materials for EMS providers*, Minnesota State Board of Technical Colleges.

the risk is fully assessed. HazMat incidents must be considered dangerous until proven otherwise.

The Chemical Manufacturers Association has a 30-minute video about HazMat responses called *First On the Scene: Hazardous Material Safety*. It describes the response to these situations, provides guidelines for hazardous material responses, and illustrates how to react. It is worthwhile for all EMS providers and physicians to view this tape.

Identification

Identification of most hazardous material substances is uncomplicated if one understands the labeling of the containers. Every medical director should be familiar with the *Emergency Response Handbook: Guidebook for Hazardous Material Incidents,* published by the Department of Transportation and every emergency vehicle should carry a copy. When hazardous materials are being transported, shipping papers that identify the substances should be located (1) in the cab of the motor vehicle, (2) in possession of a crew member on the train, (3) on the bridge of the vessel, or (4) in the aircraft pilot's possession. In addition, tank trucks must display placards (Figure 44-1) with the ID number of the hazardous material being transported. The guide book illustrates vehicle placards and how to interpret them. Once the material is identified, there is also a treatment guide that indicates the main hazards and emergency actions to deal with the toxic substance and the initial first aid for victims.

There may also be a telephone number on the shipping papers or cargo manifest so the manufacturer can be contacted for more information on handling the material and dealing with victims. Unfortunately, the placard system is not foolproof. There are many examples of emergency workers killed and injured during HazMat incidents involving improperly marked substances. Extreme caution is always warranted. There is a different marking system called NFPA 704 for HazMat fixed-facilities such as green oxygen tanks outside hospitals (see box on page 437 and 438).

Another important source of information about product identification is ChemTrec—the hot line of the chemical industry (1-800-424-9300). Although some help for victim management can be obtained from the specific chemical manufacturer or from ChemTrec, the best source of medical information may be the regional poison control center. Poison control centers have significant information on hazardous substances, in addition to the usual ingested toxins; the data are clinically helpful. Communication with the poison control center is an important part of the HazMat response plan. A mixture of hazardous substances that together produce unique and different toxicities, in addition to those caused by the individual materials, is a common problem. Poison control and ChemTrec should be able to assess possi-

UN Class Numbers

Class 1—Explosives
Class 2—Gases (compressed, liquified or dissolved under pressure)
Class 3—Flammable liquids
Class 4—Flammable solids or substances
Class 5—Oxidizing substances
    Division 5.1-Oxidizing substances or agents
    Division 5.2-Organic peroxides
Class 6—Poisonous and infectious substances
Class 7—Radioactive substances
Class 8—Corrosives
Class 9—Miscellaneous dangerous substances

- The four digit UN or NA numbers must be displayed on all hazardous materials packages for which identification numbers are assigned. Example: ACETONE UN 1090.
- UN (United Nations) or NA (North American) numbers are found in the Hazardous Materials Tables, Sec. 172.101 and 172.102 (CFR, Title 49, Parts 100-199)
- Identification numbers may not be displayed on "POISON GAS," "RADIOACTIVE" or "EXPLOSIVE" placards. (Sec. 172.334)
- UN numbers are displayed in the same manner for both Domestic and International shipments.
- NA numbers are used only in the USA and Canada.

When hazardous materials are transported in Tank Cars, Cargo Tanks and Portable Tanks, UN or NA numbers must be displayed on:

PLACARDS OR ORANGE PANELS

1090 and

Appropriate Placard must be used.

1090
3
FLAMMABLE
3

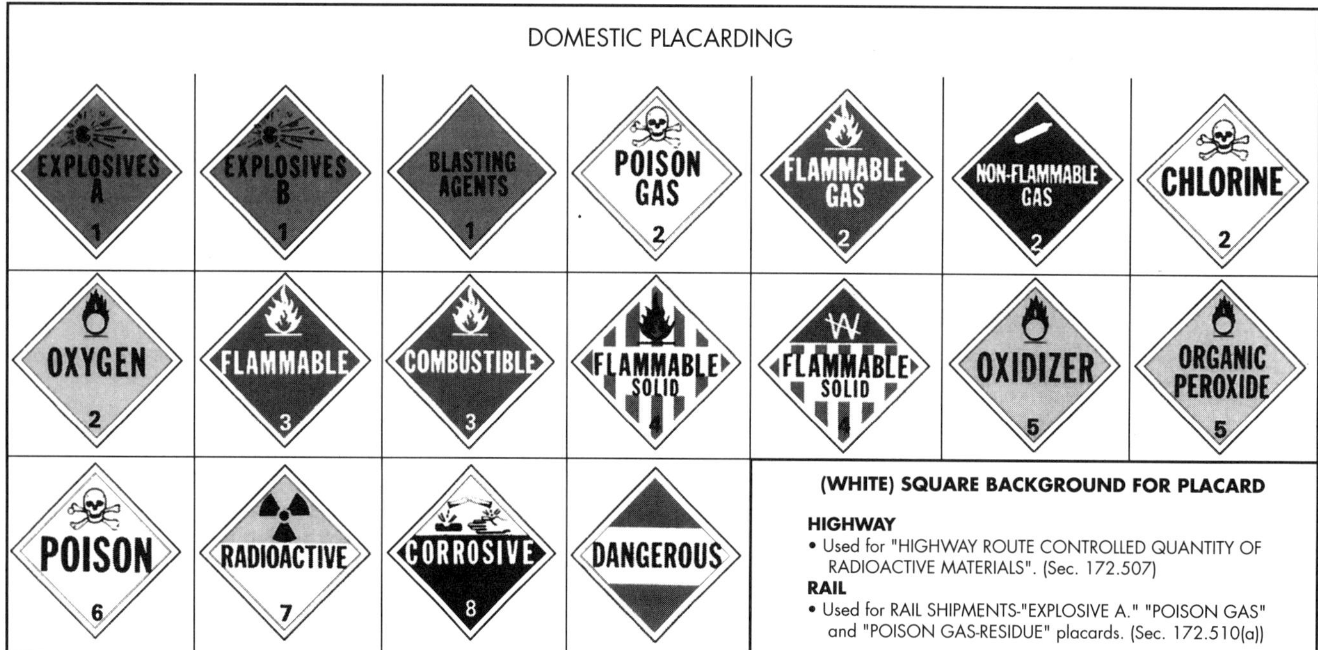

Figure 44-1. UN and NA identification numbers. Domestic placarding. (From Hazardous Material Awareness for Minnesota First Responders, Minnesota State Board of Technical Colleges.)

ble effects of various chemical mixtures and how best to treat victims. An aggressive treatment approach may not be necessary if the patient has no toxic signs; however, if the material cannot be identified, then the worst possible toxic scenario must be assumed. Safety of response personnel must be paramount.

Product control, confinement, and cleanup should only be performed by experienced personnel. Obviously, both prior planning with the responsible agencies and periodic testing of HazMat responses during disaster drills are necessary.

Decontamination

Once the victims are removed from danger, decontamination is a problem for patients, EMS personnel, and HazMat responders. In general, EMS personnel get involved only after decontamination, but for critically ill patients some medical intervention may be needed before decontamination is accomplished. Decontamination procedures vary with the nature of the chemical. In general, clothing and jewelry should be removed and the skin flushed with copious amounts of water for 20 minutes. Neutralization of acids and alkalis should not be attempted because of the possibility of further damage from the heat of reaction. Special irrigating solutions may be required (for example, Zephiran for hydrofluoric acid) but are often not available on the scene. The most readily available material for decontamination is water; the 20-minute flush will dilute most chemicals. Occasionally, chemicals are

NFPA 704 System

Health (Blue)

In general, health hazard in fire fighting is that of a single exposure which may vary from a few seconds up to an hour. The physical exertion demanded in fire fighting or other emergency conditions may be expected to intensify the effects of any exposure. Only hazards arising out of an inherent property of the material are considered. The following explanation is based upon protective equipment normally used by fire fighters.

4 Materials too dangerous to health to expose fire fighters. A few whiffs of the vapor could cause death or the vapor or liquid could be fatal on penetrating the fire fighter's normal full protective clothing. The normal full protective clothing and breathing apparatus available to the average fire department will not provide adequate protection against inhalation or skin contact with these materials.

3 Materials extremely hazardous to health but areas may be entered with extreme care. Full protective clothing, including self-contained breathing apparatus, coat, pants, gloves, boots, and bands around legs, arms and waist should be provided. No skin surface should be exposed.

2 Materials hazardous to health, but areas may be entered freely with full-faced mask self-contained breathing apparatus, which provides eye protection.

1 Materials only slightly hazardous to health. It may be desirable to wear self-contained breathing apparatus.

0 Materials which on exposure under fire conditions, would offer no hazard beyond that of ordinary combustible material.

Flammability (Red)

Susceptibility to burning is the basis for assigning degrees within this category. The method of attacking the fire is influenced by this susceptibility factor.

4 Very flammable gases or very volatile flammable liquids. Shut off flow and keep cooling water streams on exposed tanks or containers.

3 Materials which can be ignited under almost all normal temperature conditions. Water may be ineffective because of the low flash point.

2 Materials which must be moderately heated before ignition will occur. Water spray may be used to extinguish the fire because the material can be cooled below its flash point.

1 Materials that must be preheated before ignition can occur. Water may cause frothing if it gets below the surface of the liquid and turns to steam. However, water fog gently applied to the surface will cause a frothing which will extinguish the fire.

0 Materials that will not burn.

Reactivity (Stability) (Yellow)

The assignment of degrees in the reactivity category is based upon the susceptibility of materials to release energy either by themselves or in combination with water. Fire exposure was one of the factors considered along with conditions of shock and pressure.

4 Materials which (in themselves) are readily capable of detonation or of explosive decomposition or explosive reaction at normal temperatures and pressures. Includes materials which are sensitive to mechanical or localized thermal shock. If a chemical with this hazard rating is in an advanced or massive fire, the area should be evacuated.

3 Materials which (in themselves) are capable of detonation or of explosive decomposition or of explosive reaction which require a strong initiating source or which must be heated under confinement before initiation. Includes materials which are sensitive to thermal or mechanical shock at elevated temperatures and pressures or which react explosively with water without requiring heat or confinement. Fire fighting should be done from an explosive-resistant location.

2 Materials which (in themselves) are normally unstable and readily undergo violent chemical change but do not detonate. Includes materials which can undergo chemical change with rapid release of energy at normal

Continued.

NFPA 704 System—Cont'd

	temperatures and pressure or which can undergo violent chemical change at elevated temperatures and pressures. Also includes those materials which may react violently with water or which may form potentially explosive mixtures with water. In advance or massive fires, fire fighting should be done from a safe distance or from a protected location.
1	Materials which (in themselves) are normally stable but which may become unstable at elevated temperatures and pressures or which may react with water with some release of energy, but not violently. Caution must be used in approaching the fire and applying water.
0	Materials which (in themselves) are normally stable even under fire exposure conditions and which are not reactive with water. Normal fire fighting procedures may be used.

From *Hazardous Material Awareness for Minnesota First Responders* - Minnesota State Board of Technical Colleges.

encountered that react with water such as elemental sodium or white phosphorus. In such situations, the risk-benefit of water irrigation must be weighed. Brushing may be needed to remove particulate or adherent chemicals.

After decontamination the standard primary patient survey and initial clinical interventions should be performed. Airway, breathing, and circulatory supports are especially important in HazMat situations because the most common critical problems are cardiorespiratory and central nervous system in origin. The specific effects of the particular hazardous substance determine the initial medical approach and the expected complications. Because accurate information about the material may not be immediately available, it is best to transport the patient to a medical facility after a general decontamination without waiting for complete information. If the patient is critical and the hazard to EMS personnel is judged to be minimal, then transport before decontamination may be appropriate. This means that at a later time the personnel, the vehicles, and the victims will have to be decontaminated.

Radioactive material spills provide unique problems to responders, acting in both the rescue and EMS capacities. The threat of radiation induces a fearful response in prehospital personnel even when other hazards are more dangerous. On-site personnel should have specific training in dealing with radiation accidents and decontamination of victims. The prehospital providers may not be able to differentiate between a victim contaminated with radioactive material and one irradiated but not contaminated. The irradiated victim is not a hazard for the rescuer, but the contaminated person may be. A monitoring instrument such as a Geiger counter is needed to determine the need for particulite decontamination. If the device is not available, then the victim is assumed to be a hazard to others. Warning labels or placards assist in assessing the risks to both victims and prehospital workers.

Decontamination of patients exposed to radioactive material is somewhat different than routine chemical decontamination. The hot zone must be strictly isolated. Personnel entering the hot zone must wear protective disposable outerwear that is carefully removed and contained upon exit. Personnel exiting the hot zone must also be monitored for radioactive contamination. Clothing and other items removed from victims must be placed in containers to avoid contaminating others. Water used to irrigate must also be carefully contained to avoid groundwater contamination. In the unusual situation where the victims are too ill to undergo scene contamination, the best approach is to wrap them in body bags or sheets (including head cover) and then to transport to the local hospital designated to receive radiation victims. The patient's immediate medical needs should be met on-scene or in the ambulance. The receiving hospital can carry out decontamination while dealing more definitively with the patient's medical problems. After the incident the medical director in conjunction with state and federal radiation experts assesses the radiation risks that occurred.

Postincident Follow-up

The medical director should be involved in debriefing participants in the incident. This session should focus on how things could have gone better. Follow-up of possible toxic effect of the hazardous materials on workers and long-term occupational health surveillance may be necessary. The medical director should coordinate the input of toxicologists and occupational health specialists to prevent the prehospital providers from becoming long-term victims.

Summary

The priorities at a HazMat scene are different from most other EMS responses. They are as follows:

1. Secure area and deny access to nonessential personnel.
2. Identify the substances involved.
3. Assess the risks of conducting victim rescue in relationship to the protective gear available and the toxin present.
4. Decontaminate the victim.
5. Prevent the spread of contamination.
6. Evaluate, resuscitate, and treat the victim.
7. Decontaminate rescuers and vehicles.

Because caution is the best approach to these situations, balancing the risk to rescuers against the risk to victims is difficult. Medical directors may be asked to participate, and they must be prepared.

Suggested Readings

Bronstein AC and Currance PL: *Emergency care for hazardous materials exposure,* St. Louis, 1994, Mosby–Year Book.

Burton BT and Bayer MJ, editors: Hazardous materials, *Topics in Emergency Medicine* 7:1-70, 1985.

Cashman JR: Are we headed toward a Bhopal on wheels? *Emer Serv* 19:27-31, 1987.

Christen HT: Hazardous materials and the First Responder, *Firehouse* 63-71, Jul 1989.

Currance PL: EMS crosses hazmat lines, *JEMS* 58-64, Feb 1989.

Fawcett HH: *Hazardous and toxic materials: safe handling and disposal,* 1984, John Wiley & Sons Inc.

Goldfrank LR: *Toxicologic emergencies: a comprehensive handbook in problem solving,* 1982, Appleton-Century-Crofts.

Goldfrank LR et al: *Goldfrank's toxicologic emergencies,* 1986, Appleton-Century-Crofts.

Leonard RB et al: SARA (Superfund Amendments and Reauthorization Act), Title III: implications for emergency physicians, *Ann Emerg Med* 18:1212-1216, 1989.

National Fire Protection Association: *Standard for professional competence of responders to hazardous materials incidents, Bulletin 472,* 1989, The Association.

National Fire Protection Association: *Standard for emergency medical services for hazardous materials incident response, Bulletin 473,* 1991, The Association.

Noll GG and Hildebrand MS: Hazardous wastes operations and emergency response, *Firehouse* 54-58, Jul, and 79-83, Aug 1989.

Proctor NH and Hughes JP: *Chemical hazards of the workplace,* 1987, J B Lippincott Co.

Richter LL et al: A systems approach to the management of radiation accidents, *Ann Emerg Med* 9:303-309, 1980.

Staten C: Hazardous materials: the EMS response, *Emergency Medical Services* 18:34-41, 64, 1989.

Stutz DR, Ricks RC, and Olsen MF: *Hazardous materials injuries: a handbook for prehospital care,* 1988, Bradford Communications Corp.

Scott UL: *Hazardous material accidents and toxic exposures.* In: Nelson RN, Rund DA, and Keller MD, eds: *Environmental emergencies,* 1985, WB Saunders Co.

US Department of Transportation: *1990 Emergency resource guidebook: guidebook for hazardous material incidents,* Washington, DC, US Government Printing Office.

Appendix

Model Hazardous Material Protocol

Purpose

To establish a safe and uniform set of guidelines for personnel and apparatus while operating on the scene of a hazardous materials emergency.

Haz/Mat Response

All Haz/Mat emergency operations will be conducted at three levels of skill and equipment. These usually follow the order of the arrival of units at the scene, the First Responder, the rescue squad and the Haz/Mat response team.

All Haz/Mat operations shall be conducted in accordance with the following management procedures.

All Haz/Mat responses will be considered dangerous until confirmed otherwise.

To ensure maximum control and safety of personnel responding to hazardous materials incidents, all incoming units, with the exception of the first arriving company and the Haz/Mat unit, rescue squad and the Command Officer, shall stage upwind at a safe location away from the incident.

The following are the eight steps in controlling a hazardous materials incident:

Steps performed by the first arriving company. These are to be performed in full turn-out gear including the wearing of the S.C.B.A. (Self Contained Breathing Apparatus).

1. Site management. The area is to be isolated, and all unauthorized personnel must be denied entry and a perimeter established.
2. Identification of involved materials. Must be conducted in a safe manner without endangering personnel by checking placards, boxes, barrels, etc. to get a preliminary estimate of the materials involved.

The following steps are to be conducted by the Incident Commander using the rescue squads and the hazardous response units.

3. Hazard and risk assessment. The hazards and risks must be evaluated to determine what necessary procedures need to be taken; i.e., evacuation for 5,000 feet in all directions, high volume streams to cool tanks in a potential BLEVE condition, etc., or no risk at all. (BLEVE is Boiling Liquid Expanding Vapor Explosion.)
4. Select the proper protective suits and equipment, Tyvec, Butyl, P.V.C., etc., nonsparking tools, containment barrels, plug and dike, patches, plugs, sand, etc.
5. Information and resource coordination. Manuals, books, computer access to hazardline, where are needed materials such as sand, lime, acid or base foam, etc., and who can deliver them.
6. Product control and confinement. Actual hands-on application of plugs, patches, dikes, lime, foams, etc.
7. Decontamination. Cleaning of suits, tools, and personnel.

The last step in this procedure is performed by the Incident Commander and attended by all personnel involved.

8. Termination. Documentation of all activities. *Debrief all personnel. Hold a formal critique.*

From St. Paul Fire and Safety Services

45

Multiple Casualty Incidents

G. Patrick Lilja, M.D., FACEP
Michael A. Madsen, D.O.
Jerry Overton, M.P.A.

EMS medical directors must assure that medical protocols exist for both the daily treatment and transportation of patients and situations that place unexpected demands on the system. At times an event occurs that overloads the EMS system with a large influx of patients for a short period of time; though such events occur sporadically, the system must be prepared. Therefore development of a multiple casualty incident (MCI) plan is crucial. The plan should be as simple as possible. The plan must be flexible and follow normal operating conditions as closely as possible.

Definition of a Multiple Casualty Incident

Though a number of events may be called catastrophic events or disasters, there is no one agreed on definition. Natural events such as tornadoes, hurricanes, earthquakes, and floods, as well as man-made events such as large fires, explosions, or terrorist activities may cause large numbers of casualties. Disaster was the term used for an occurrence that disrupted the function or structure of a community with widespread injury or loss of property, but the EMS community now defines such an occurrence as a multiple casualty incident or if devastating a catastrophic event.

An MCI is a man-made or natural event that requires multiple responses in a timely manner to minimize injury and death. Depending on the size of the community, the MCI may or may not overwhelm existing resources and may or may not require outside assistance.

For large communities an apartment building fire producing 30 casualties represents an MCI that can be handled without outside assistance. In smaller communities, a two automobile collision may require mutual aid from adjoining EMS agencies. An agency often declares an MCI whenever the number of patients exceeds three or the number of ambulances required is more than two. Using this approach, a consistency in MCI response is established; responders and dispatchers do not have to ponder when the event will reach the level of activity needed for MCI plan implementation or, depending on that system's activity at that time, whether the system will be overwhelmed. Instead the first arriving personnel can concentrate on what is needed—triage, communication, and patient care. The adoption of a standard definition also increases cooperation among neighborhood systems and prevents systems from abusing mutual aid arrangements.

It is important to clarify that an MCI does not require the routine activation of mutual aid. The most frequent use of mutual aid is when the demand on a system outstrips its existing resources or the closest available unit to a specific patient is located in another community. Whether mutual aid agreements are formal or informal, they should be recognized in the MCI plan.

Planning

It does little good to begin the planning process after the MCI has occurred. The properly designed and implemented MCI plan is a complicated undertaking. Once completed and practiced, a smoothly functioning MCI plan provides the proper and effective response to incidents as varied as automobile accidents, the Kansas City Hyatt Regency Hotel skywalk collapse, or the World Trade Center bombing.

The properly constructed MCI plan is both general and expandable. Plans drafted for specific response to a specific event such as a tornado or train derailment are ineffective. As society has increased in complexity, the potential for the MCI has also increased. For every coal mine collapse there are many hazardous material accidents, and where many feared the widespread destruction of a hurricane many now fear the widespread contamination of a radiation accident.

Instead of concentrating on a specific event the MCI plan should concentrate on levels of response and resources. The rapid deployment of personnel, vehicles, equipment, and supplies may be necessary, and the source of each must be part of the plan.

Hospital resources must also be considered when preparing the plan. These considerations should take special note of any unique or specialized services such as a burn center that are available. Usually, it is not only the number of casualties that overwhelms a given medical facility but the type of injuries and the resources that the patients require as well. A large number of closed fractures not requiring operative reduction seldom overloads a community hospital; on the other hand, a large number of patients with penetrating thoracic or abdominal wounds may quickly outstrip the operative capacity of even a tertiary hospital.

In devising the plan, EMS physicians must coordinate with other agencies, including police departments, fire departments, and civil defense agencies. Each has a management responsibility and a role in the administration of the plan.

The scene management of an MCI site involves much more than the provision of care to the injured. This management process is called the Incident Command System (ICS). One agency, usually the fire department, establishes a unified, overall command and designates the incident commander (IC). If the fire department is not involved, command often falls to the highest ranking officer in the EMS agency. Other agencies assist the IC. In developing the EMS portion of the plan the system medical director must make sure that the EMS plan coordinates parallels and integrates with the other aspects of emergency preparedness. The individuals involved in overall scene management should function from the command post (CP). The CP should be near but not directly involved in the incident site. Physicians in the field must relate to and take direction from individuals more skilled in rescue situations. By planning ahead with the local hospitals, police, fire, and emergency management, the possibility of conflict can greatly be reduced. Unless the physician is the manager, EMS command is responsible for EMS operations at the incident and the physician's role is not incident management.

Communications

In reviewing previous MCIs, communications is the operational component most often overwhelmed. When possible, communications must be performed through normal EMS radio channels. A plan that relies on additional communication networks or changes the routine radio procedures leads to confusion. The use of cellular telephones also poses problems because the increased traffic ties up the available cells, especially in larger scale MCIs.

All EMS units responding to an MCI should be assigned to a single channel by dispatch for coordination. In addition, medical information transmitted to receiving facilities should be assigned a frequency. Radio communications among agencies is important, but this should occur between the MCI command post and the EMS dispatch center rather than at the responding unit level. Administrative communications between agencies is often unnecessary; however, in the rare instance that it is needed, it should be on a frequency separate from those of EMS dispatch and direct medical control.

The first arriving EMS unit at the scene of an MCI should immediately inform the dispatch center that the incident is indeed an MCI and approximate the number of casualties. This begins the dispatch of additional resources to the scene. It is imperative that the dispatch center immediately implement the MCI plan, alert command staff, and notify potential receiving hospitals. Obviously, as more information is gathered from the MCI site, hospitals and dispatch must be updated. In addition, the initial arriving unit also must survey the scene for any hazards and determine if there is a need for specialized equipment and personnel.

Once patient transport has been initiated, EMS personnel must be aware that they need to obtain and transmit abbreviated histories and physical exam data. During an MCI, there is not time to transmit complete reports on every patient or to expect lengthy radio orders for individual patients. Rather, EMS personnel continue to function under their protocol for standing orders and relay estimated arrival times, the number of patients, and the types of injuries to the receiving hospital. Additional information unnecessarily uses channels needed by other personnel.

In most MCIs, telephone communications are unreliable because telephone systems are unavailable at the site or overloaded. Cellular phones offer a great degree of flexibility, but are also dysfunctional because they ultimately use normal telephone circuits. A system of communication that depends on the local telephone service should not be developed. Rather a centralized control must be designated to assess receiving hospital capabilities and communicate those capabilities to the MCI site so victims can be appropriately distributed. This communication link assures quick mobilization and effective use of hospital resources.

This centralized control must be linked by appropriate dedicated communications to hospitals in the system and to the dispatch center. Operating under its auspices may be a field medical unit with an EMS physician, serving as the scene physician in charge. Ambulances, rescue units, and other public safety units function under the ICS and in conjunction with the field medical unit. This model provides for rapid augmentation of field support from available hospital resources and also allows the continuation of normal ongoing function of the hospitals. Finally, it can quickly be expanded without relying on new or different levels of commands or operation procedures.

Triage

Triage is an integral part of the MCI plan. It is not, however, mandatory that it occur at or even near the site of the MCI. Determining whether and where field triage should be initiated depends on three circumstances. The first is the number and type of casualties. The second is accessibility to the scene and the presence of ongoing hazards or dangers. Finally the number of casualties must be compared to the available transport vehicles. If transportation resources are able to immediately evacuate all casualties, then field triage can be expedited. Field triage is necessary mainly when the number of casualties overwhelms the capabilities of the immediately available transport units or the resources of the closest receiving hospital. When field triage is used, the most critically injured patients are transported first.

Triage is initiated by the first responding unit and performed by the most experienced personnel at the MCI site. It is imperative that the individual responsible for triage is specified by the plan. If the plan calls for a change in triage officer as the incident progresses, then this protocol must be clearly indicated.

At times, depending on the scope of the MCI, additional triage sites are necessary. Field triage functions most efficiently when victims are confined to a relatively small geographic area such as the site of a building collapse, fire, or explosion and when the triage site is centrally located. In certain types of catastrophic events such as earthquakes or hurricanes, victims may be spread over miles. In these situations, initial field triage is still necessary before the patients are transported to a central triage location called a casualty collection point, which may be the local hospital provided it is still functioning.

The system developed for initial triage is known as Simple Triage and Rapid Treatment (START). This system is based solely on clinical presentation and not type of injury. Patients are categorized as either high priority (immediate) or low priority (delayed) after three parameters have been evaluated. Level of consciousness, respiratory status, and perfusion status are all briefly examined, and if a deficit is found the patient is immediate. If all three conditions are within normal limits, the patient is delayed. Further triage is done by EMS personnel in the field or at the receiving hospital.

Another system, consisting of four categories, has been established for physicians or EMS personnel triaging patients. Category I patients require immediate care or transport. This category includes major injuries to the thorax, abdomen, or head for which surgical intervention or airway stabilization is immediately needed. Category II patients are less seriously injured but still require surgical care. The injuries are not immediately life-threatening. Category III includes patients with minor injuries that do not need immediate stabilization. Category IV includes dead victims. This category may also include patients who are not dead but have obvious fatal injuries.

The use of triage tags by field personnel remains controversial. Although many argue for triage tags in civilian MCIs, their use is not always effective. To be used efficiently, they must be implemented routinely for MCIs large and small.

Physicians at the Scene

Physicians, particularly the EMS medical director, may play an important role at a MCI. They have three functions, including (1) overall medical assessment of the situation with an evaluation of the scope of injuries and number of casualties, (2) triage, and (3) treatment.

Before providing overall medical assessment and establishing a relationship with EMS providers already on the scene, the physicians should ascertain the location of the CP and report to the IC. Should communication fall under their responsibility, physicians should update hospitals regarding the scope and number of casualties. Experienced physicians are best able to determine the degree and complexity of injuries and match them with the required hospital resources. They also must continually update hospitals with information. Critics cite numerous cases where hospitals either were not informed of a sudden influx of casualties or were waiting for patients long after the last victims were transported.

Physicians should perform triage at the request of triage teams and stand ready to assist in the decision-making process. Only in the rarest of circumstances should physicians render treatment at the scene, and they must never delay transportation to definitive care. Victims usually require specialized lifesaving medical procedures before transport, are trapped, or need ongoing life-sustaining medical care. Unless large numbers of physicians are available, their expertise at the scene of an MCI is most appropriately used in advising other providers rather than actually performing less than lifesaving procedures on individual patients. A single physician cannot function in all of the three positions—assessment, triage, and treatment.

Patients generally begin arriving at hospitals within 30 minutes, and another triage process occurs. Each hospital should have its own facility MCI plan, and the ultimate survival of a victim may be the result of quick action by the emergency department staff. EMS physician response to the hospital and the provision of definitive treatment is the final and sometimes most difficult phase of patient care and thus must not be overlooked.

Physicians should also be aware of relationships with the press. Physicians involved with MCIs are sought out by the media, but the assignment of the media to a public information officer (PIO) is the responsibility of the IC. If the physician is assigned the PIO responsibility, premature release of information or speculation on the cause of the event must never be provided.

Terrorist Activity

Organized terrorist actions have steadily increased in recent years, and U.S. interests have been the target of many of these attacks. Until the bombing of the World Trade Center, the continental United States had been largely spared. Because terrorist activities frequently include bombings, assassinations, hijackings, and hostage captures, large numbers of people may be injured. MCIs caused by terrorist actions can be linked to wartime conditions therefore EMS physicians should be aware of the fundamental differences in their management.

The most significant difference is the need for a heightened level of security. The injuries in a terrorist incident are the result of violence, and there is the distinct possibility that further violent acts will occur. A common terrorist tactic is to detonate a second device at the site where rescue workers are treating victims of the original incident. The IC at the scene of a suspected terrorist action is usually the senior law enforcement officer present. A hot zone or internal perimeter is established to keep unessential individuals a safe distance from potential dangers and to prevent terrorists from escaping. EMS or medical teams responding to a potential terrorist action should approach cautiously and check with law enforcement personnel before proceeding into the scene. Emergency vehicle staging areas should be decentralized, with vehicles well-dispersed to avoid becoming a secondary target. Communications can be monitored by terrorists, and care should be taken to avoid transmitting detailed locations of treatment sites or command posts.

Patient triage and treatment at the scene should be especially abbreviated to minimize the exposure of emergency crews and patients to gunfire or secondary explosive devices. In most cases, casualties can be quickly removed from the internal perimeter and transported immediately. If casualties exceed transportation resources and a triage and treatment area is needed, the site should be located in a protected location, and security personnel should be assigned to protect and monitor the area. Terrorists masquerading as victims may infiltrate treatment areas or hospitals. Therefore evaluation should be performed on all patients before they enter either the treatment area or the ambulance. The triage area should be closely monitored by armed security personnel to prevent weapons from entering the treatment chain.

The close liaison between EMS and law enforcement required at terrorist incidents is not well-developed in most systems. EMS medical directors should develop a relationship with local and regional law enforcement and assist with the development of terrorism contingency plans. Some systems have successfully developed special medical reaction teams that train with the police special operations teams to rapidly provide medical care and evacuation within the internal perimeter.

Mass Gatherings

Mass gatherings are special circumstances under which an MCI occasionally occurs. This type of event places an additional burden on the system. Large concerts, athletic contests, parades, or political rallies can attract thousands or even hundreds of thousands of individuals to a single location. Such events require special planning because they result in an increased number of patients and also disrupt transportation. For example, streets may be closed to ambulances by the sheer volume of people.

A plan for any mass gathering should include aid stations, appropriately staffed and geographically dispersed throughout the area and throughout the crowd. Several EMS systems have bicycle or scooter paramedic programs that can relatively quickly respond through a crowd. These events may require alternative forms of patient transport such as stretchers on golf carts. Ambulances should be stationed at the periphery of the event with routes to hospitals predesignated.

Debriefing

After every MCI, debriefing sessions for the EMS personnel must be provided. Debriefing is an essential psychological support for the involved personnel. When providers confront a large number of seriously injured or dead victims, there is a significant sometimes delayed psychological stress. A formal approach should be developed prospectively to deal with such stress. It is imperative to have professionals skilled in stress management lead discussion groups with all involved personnel. Mental health professionals should be included in the planning process and as part of the response team. The EMS agency should have critical incident stress debriefing teams that provide support for personnel that have experienced stressful incidents. Although it is not possible to entirely alleviate stress, individuals develop coping mechanisms that are greatly enhanced by appropriate therapeutic sessions. Should additional individual support be required by an individual rescuer, the mental health community should be educated to understand the special needs involved.

Summary

Preparing for an MCI requires a logical and tested plan based on the normal operation of the existing EMS system. The plan must allow both for rapid expansion and significant abbreviation of the routine treatment and communication procedures. If the plan is well-defined and well-rehearsed, then it is more likely to function satisfactorily when the MCI occurs. However, the first hurdle is to ensure that a well-designed and smoothly functioning EMS system has been established and serves as the foundation.

SUGGESTED READING

Aghababian RV: Hospital disaster planning, *Top Emerg Med* 7(4):46-54, 1986.

Aufder HE: Disaster response: principles of preparation and coordination, St. Louis, 1989, The CV Mosby Co.

Burkle FM, Sanner PH, and Wolcott BW, editors: Disaster medicine, New York, 1984, Examination Publishing Co.

Butman AE: Responding to the mass casualty incident: A guide for EMS personnel, Westport, Conn, 1982, Emergency Training.

Comfort LK: Managing disaster: strategies and rating perspectives, Durham, NC, 1988, Duke University Press.

Cooper GJ et al: Casualties from terrorist bombings, *J Trauma* 23:955-967, 1983.

Crowley RA, editor: Mass casualties: a lessons learned approach, DOT HS 806 302, 1982, US Department of Transportation, National Highway Traffic Safety Administration.

Cuny FC: Introduction to disaster management, lesson I: the scope of disaster management, *Prehospital and Disaster Medicine* 7:4, Oct-Dec 1992.

Cuny FC: Introduction to disaster management, lesson II: concepts and terms in disaster management, *Prehospital and Disaster Medicine* 8:1, Jan-Mar 1993.

Doyle CJ: Mass casualty incident: integration with prehospital care, *Emerg Med Clin North Am* 8:163-75, 1990.

Haynes BE and Freeman C, editors: Casualty collection point guidelines, Sacramento, Calif, 1989, Emergency Medical Services Authority.

Jones GW: *The Brighton bombing,* Orlando, Fla, Feb 1985, 1985 National Disaster Conference.

Kupperman RH: Conflict, terrorism, and civil unrest, *Journal of the World Association of Emergency and Disaster Medicine* 2:60-63, 1986.

Lauder P: San Ysidro slaughter: the EMS experience, *Emergency* 16:34-48, 1984.

Mahoney B: *Disaster planning.* In: Tintinalli J, Krome RE, and Ruiz E, editors: Emergency medicine: a comprehensive study guide, 1992, McGraw-Hill.

Mahoney LE and Reutershan TP: Catastrophic disasters and the design of disaster medical care systems, *Ann Emerg Med* 16:1085-1091, 1987.

Melton JR and Riner RM: Revising the rural hospital disaster plan: a role for the EMS system in managing the multiple casualty incident, *Ann Emerg Med* 10:39-44, 1981.

Mitchell JT and Grady B, editors: Emergency services stress: 444guidelines for preserving the health and careers of emergency services personnel, Englewood Cliffs NJ, 1990, Brady Communications.

Sidenberg BS: Medical consequences of conflict and civil unrest, *Journal of the World Association of Emergency and Disaster Medicine* 2:63-68, 1986.

START: *A triage method,* Newport Beach, Calif, 1989, Hoag Memorial Hospital Presbyterian.

Waeckerle JF: Disaster planning and response, *New Engl J Med* 324:815-821, 1991.

Appendix

Multiple Casualty Incident Protocol

A. Procedures for First Responding ambulance crew:

The first ambulance crew arriving on the scene will do the following:

1. Conduct incident communications on primary dispatch channel.
2. Quickly obtain information and *report back to the dispatcher:*
   - Nature and scope of incident
   - Number and type of casualties
   - Best route into the area
   - Possible ambulance staging area
   - Any possible hazards, including if decontamination of victims may be needed
3. Identify and establish contact with the Incident Command Post. Maintain communications throughout incident.
4. Establish EMS communications and triage station, close to patients but out of hazard zone:
   - Locate triage clear of hazards and obstructions;
   - Place flashing green light on top of ambulance;
   - Wear identifying vests:
     Orange—triage paramedic
     Blue—communications paramedic
5. Update dispatch on casualties, approach route, and the EMS staging area (other responding units *will not* drive into the immediate site).
6. Utilize "disaster tags" (triage paramedic and medical director only) at triage station.
7. Request additional help at triage from Fire/Police Command as needed.
8. Report to First Responding ambulance supervisor or medical director.

B. Procedures for other responding ambulance crews:

After being dispatched to incident location, all responding paramedic crews after the first paramedic crew will do the following:

1. Conduct incident communications on primary dispatch channel. Incident dispatching will be done by the primary service area dispatcher and all responding crews should communicate with this dispatcher. Non-incident communications should be done on regular business channels.
2. All ambulance movement to and from the scene of a multiple casualty situation will be on lights and siren.
3. Respond to ambulance staging area indicated by dispatcher. Specific on-site questions will be directed to the communications paramedic. Crews will remain at staging area until instructed by communications paramedic.
4. Receive patient assignment from triage paramedic (orange vest).
5. After receiving patient(s), ambulance crews will contact control hospital to report patient information and hospital destination. Relay minimal information regarding:
   - Number of patients
   - Critical or non-critical
   - General injury types

   Primary receiving hospital will advise crews when nearest medical control hospital can no longer receive patients. Ambulance crews should also report their status and destination to dispatcher.
6. If ordered by medical command authority, all medical interventions will be by standing orders; otherwise contact hospital physician control is needed.
7. After delivering patients to assigned hospital, all crews will contact dispatcher for ongoing assignment until relieved.

46

Catastrophic Events

Leo Bosner, M.S.W.
Ernest Pretto, M.D.
Richard Carmona, M.D.
Jennifer Leanning, M.D.

EMS medical directors differentiate between multiple casualty incidents (MCIs) that can be managed by local EMS systems and those catastrophic events commonly known as disasters, during and after which the local emergency health care system and infrastructure are overwhelmed or destroyed. To be effective the medical response to catastrophic events must be planned and coordinated locally, regionally, statewide, nationally, and even internationally.

The past few years have witnessed a number of catastrophic events such as earthquakes in Mexico, Armenia, California, Iran, the Philippines, Turkey and Egypt; armed conflicts in the Persian Gulf, Somalia, the Balkans and the former Soviet republics; and hurricanes in the United States and Guam. In light of these events, EMS medical directors in the United States should examine six crucial issues to prepare their systems (see box at right).

Many American communities have well-developed EMS systems that are effective, limiting both injury and loss of life in everyday emergencies and MCIs. Most localities, however, are not prepared or equipped to deal with the medical aspects of a truly catastrophic event, because outside assistance would be needed to rescue, resuscitate, and treat the casualties. The most important steps that medical directors can take to prepare their community are to improve the routine operations of the EMS system, plan responses for the most likely events, and realistically test those preparations and plans regularly. For more than a decade the federal government's traditional answer to the sixth crucial question has been, "The National Disaster Medical System."

The National Disaster Medical System

History

In the early 1980s the Department of Defense established the Civilian Military Contingency Hospital System (CMCHS) to use civilian hospitals as a backup for military hospitals during wartime.[1] Some medical professionals and others opposed CMCHS, feeling that it was part of a military buildup for nuclear war. Therefore, the federal government replaced CMCHS with the National Disaster Medical System (NDMS).[16] NDMS like CMCHS was designed to use civilian hospitals to treat the casualties of conventional warfare. Under NDMS, military and veterans hospitals were to backup civilian hos-

Six Crucial Catastrophic Event Issues

1. When and where could catastrophic events occur in the future?
2. What might be the nature of those catastrophic events?
3. What would be the expected morbidity and mortality of various types and scales of catastrophic events?
4. How can the various levels of government organize a timely, coordinated, effective medical response?
5. What sort of outside medical assistance will be required by the local EMS system?
6. What national responses are available?

pitals in the event of a major natural disaster. For the case of both civilian and military casualties a provision to use civilian health professionals was included. Lastly, NDMS provided a more concrete mechanism for participating civilian hospitals to be paid for the care that they provided to military patients.

NDMS planners recognized that combining the civilian and military components would enhance the philosophical acceptability and functional efficiency of NDMS. Conservatives who emphasized defense-related programs could embrace the military aspects of NDMS; liberals, some of whom had opposed the CMCHS, could support the civilian disaster role.

Description

NDMS was intended to be a joint effort of the private and public health care sectors to provide medical care to casualties emanating either from a peacetime disaster such as an earthquake or from a military conflict. The system was jointly developed by the following four federal agencies: the Department of Defense (DOD), the Department of Veterans Affairs (VA), the Department of Health and Human Services (DHHS), and the Federal Emergency Management Agency (FEMA). In addition, voluntary participation was solicited from state and local governments, civilian hospitals, and individual health care professionals.

The medical response component of the overall catastrophic event response included disaster medical assistance teams (DMATs) that would either treat casualties at the disaster site or receive casualties at sites distant from the place of injury. Each DMAT was comprised of physicians, nurses, medical technicians, and other support personnel patterned after the deployable military surgical team. Currently the DMATs are designed to combine and form casualty clearing and staging units. Each such unit includes a 16-person command and support element and approximately three fully staffed DMATs.

Evacuation and transportation of casualties is performed by the military aeromedical evacuation system or the Military Airlift Command (MAC). As of June 1991, the DHHS, which is the lead agency for NDMS development, claimed enrollment of 100,000 beds in hospitals throughout the nation.[9]

Actual Responses

DHHS, DOD, VA, and FEMA have collaborated for nearly a decade to organize NDMS as it is currently structured. During that time, questions were often raised about the feasibility of the concept and the actual degree of personnel readiness; however, federal officials assured local EMS medical directors that NDMS would function in a crisis situation. In June 1991, the FEMA director stated that NDMS would work effectively in a massive California earthquake that caused as many as 20,000 deaths and 100,000 injuries.[9] This assertion was based on the success of the NDMS in deploying a 29-person medical team from Albuquerque to the Virgin Islands after Hurricane Hugo.[26] Obviously, neither Hurricane Hugo nor the Loma Prieta earthquake, both of which occurred in the fall of 1989, resulted in a number of casualties that adequately tested NDMS. However, over the next 3 years the NDMS concept was tested by Operation Desert Storm and Hurricane Andrew. Despite significant progress, NDMS did not live up to its potential or its expectations in either situation. The midwestern floods and California earthquakes of 1993 did not test NDMS, although DMATs were eventually activated and deployed with improved facility.

Operation Desert Storm. Beginning in August 1990, the United States and a number of other allied nations prepared for a war in the Middle East. Although an allied victory was generally expected, it was forecast that a large number of casualties, especially burns, would occur during massive armored battles to free Kuwait.

In truth, this was exactly the type of military situation for which NDMS had been designed and publicized. By the early fall of 1990 the DOD realized that the country was unprepared to process and treat a large influx of wartime casualties. In many cases the civilian hospitals and local EMS agencies expected to supplement the military had not been fully briefed on their roles or accepted them. In other cases the civilian agencies were ready, but the local VA and DOD components were not prepared to access them.[4,19] NDMS was never activated; instead, an older plan (the DOD-VA Contingency Plan) was dusted off, and hurried efforts were made to have it ready for the invasion. The specific local plans were often poorly developed. For example, in Tucson, Arizona, the DOD-VA Contingency Plan called for incoming casualties to be transported to the VA hospital, while the VA patients were sent to the trauma centers.

Ultimately, military action was postponed until there was a full mobilization and yet another totally different and totally DOD controlled medical casualty treatment system was devised. Medical teams organized by the Society for Critical Care Medicine were prepared to be deployed under the direction of the DOD.[13] When the ground attack was finally launched in early 1991, American casualties were much lighter than had been expected. They were handled well by the military system. But the questions remained, "Why was NDMS neither initially ready nor ultimately activated? Why, too, were some hospitals and local EMS agencies dealing with three different plans for the same contingency?"

The General Accounting Office (GOA) reviewed the matter. In February 1992, the GAO reported that during Operation Desert Storm the military system was simply not prepared to treat the projected number of casualties.[18] According to this report,

- Personnel information systems to identify reserve doctors and nurses for assignment to active units contained incomplete and outdated information.
- Many doctors and nurses in active, reserve, and national guard units had not trained during peacetime to perform their wartime mission thus doctors and nurses were not familiar with the mission or equipment of their units.
- Despite a massive logistical effort to supply equipment, hospitals often did not receive equipment and supplies.
- Evacuation of casualties was hampered because of long distances, poor communications, and a lack of navigational equipment.

In March 1992, the GAO submitted further testimony to Congress, this time focusing specifically on the readiness of NDMS and the other hastily revived hospital contingency system.[8,18] According to this testimony,

- DOD did not know enough about the qualifications or readiness of its medical reservists.
- The number of hospital beds in DOD and VA hospitals actually committed and the number of civilian beds physically available had been overstated.
- DOD lacked adequate beds for specialty care such as burn treatment.
- Some communities that were supposed to participate in the NDMS response lacked workable plans to receive, transport, and track casualties.
- By most accounts the Army was able to provide adequate care for those few soldiers in need. However, had the predicted number of casualties occurred or had the ground war started earlier or lasted longer the Army would not have been able to provide adequate care.
- In many cities the EMS resources and local hospital beds were committed to two or more preparedness plans, often without the awareness of the medical providers.

Hurricane Andrew. On the morning of August 24, 1992, Hurricane Andrew made landfall on the east coast of Florida. Winds were estimated at more than 150 miles per hour and extended 45 miles from the storm center. Even though the storm passed rapidly through southern Dade County without a great deal of precipitation, more than 2 million Florida residents were left without power, more than 50,000 homes were damaged, and property destruction was at least $20 billion. The immediate casualties from Andrew were minimal. Though large numbers of people suffered moderate injuries, only 30 persons died as a result of the hurricane.[21] This low number was probably because of an excellent warning system and an adequate evacuation plan. However, according to Dade County emergency management, a hurricane catastrophic event scenario had never been fully tested through the county-state interface and certainly never to the point of the state-federal interface.[7]

In the days immediately following Andrew the plight of the survivors and the inability of government resources to respond effectively on many levels were national concerns. The lack of adequate catastrophic planning and drilling combined with the significant disruption of the local infrastructure, severely hampered relief efforts. Television showed looters, armed residents guarding their homes, relief supplies piling up in puddles, and the emergency manager of Dade County asking, "Where is the cavalry?" These were images that many EMS medical directors had thought possible following a third world disaster but not likely domestically.

The GAO testimony before the Senate on January 27, 1993 concerning response to Andrew made the following statements[21]:

- The federal government's strategy for comprehensively and effectively dealing with catastrophic disasters is deficient.
- The federal government lacks provisions to comprehensively assess damage and provide quick, responsive assistance.
- The federal government does not have explicit authority to adequately prepare for disasters.
- State and local governments do not have adequate training and funding to enable them to respond to catastrophic disasters on their own.
- The military has the capability to respond to the immediate needs of disaster victims in a highly effective manner.

The GAO report focused on the actions of FEMA, the inadequacies of the new Federal Response Plan developed to clarify roles, and the inability of the American Red Cross to determine what assistance was required, and the FEMA Inspector General directly addressed the NDMS response.[5,25] The overall assessment of the use of DMATs was both depressing and hopeful. Although several were actually operating within three days, none came close to seeing patients within 24 hours, which is the longest time one could reasonably wait for critical emergency medical responses. In Dade County the local EMS initially functioned, albeit marginally. Typical of such stressed situations, however, the local EMS systems essentially ran out of personnel in a few days. Lastly, few if any of the DMATs deployed in Florida had self-contained food, medical supplies, and shelter. Most operated from buildings that had survived the storm.[6]

The FEMA Inspector General's report described how 16 DMATs were eventually deployed, two within 36 hours of the storm. However, problems with training, logistics, supplies, and length of commitment were rampant. Simultaneously the DOD deployed considerable medical resources independently of the DMATs. The new Federal Response Plan broke-down in this crucial arena. Finally the inspector general recommended that[5]:

> FEMA needs to work with other federal agencies to realistically evaluate current capabilities as compared to the assumptions for requirements for health and medical services in the Federal Response Plan to determine whether the planned federal response is adequate or if other resources should be used until Disaster Medical Assistance Teams are fully operational.

Current Reality

The current NDMS plan calls for the creation of 150 local DMATs throughout the country. These teams, comprising volunteers from disparate hospitals and health organizations, are to be organized to respond to and operate in disaster areas. In theory, select DMATs should be mobilized within 24 hours and would set up clearing-staging stations within 48 hours; but even that two day time frame is too late to save critically injured victims in the chaos immediately following an incident. In addition, relatively immobile DMATs may be too localized to treat casualties stranded across a wide geographic area such as southern Florida.

In theory, other DMATs would deploy to receive patients transferred to areas far from the disaster site. Although DMATs have been described in planning documents since 1985, barely a dozen are fully functional and most had their first real experience following Andrew. Under NDMS doctrine, casualties resulting from a disaster are to be evacuated to hospital beds in NDMS committed civilian hospitals and VA hospitals. Many of these designated hospitals, however, lack sufficient staff experienced in the treatment of disaster related illnesses and injuries. There still remain a number of unanswered questions about reimbursement and liability for individual volunteers and the hospitals.

Activating and deploying NDMS for a major domestic disaster is complex. Each of the four agencies involved plays a different role, and the interrelationships of these roles are still not clear. The current NDMS plan has minimal framework for incorporating and coordinating the local and regional EMS systems that are critical during the initial response. Although the need for civilian and military collaboration is acknowledged, no established mechanism exists through which military deployment supports regional EMS agencies rapidly enough to significantly impact mortality and morbidity immediately following an event producing many casualties. No national plan exists for training and equipping local survivors to perform the crucial lifesaving tasks in the 24 hours immediately following a disaster, and no one federal agency has overall responsibility and accountability for either NDMS preparations or operations.

Currently, NDMS is unable to initiate and coordinate a comprehensive medical response to a catastrophic event. The fragmented leadership and lack of accountability within NDMS leaves the United States unprepared to address the basic health and medical needs generated by a major disaster. The difficulties that became apparent during a 6-month period of attempting to mobilize appropriate civilian medical resources for the Gulf War were mirrored in those identified in the days following Hurricane Andrew.

Essentials

The primary objective of a practical and workable NDMS must be to maximize the potential for saving lives and reducing morbidity by rapidly mobilizing prepared medical personnel and equipment. As yet, there is no consensus regarding the most effective way to accomplish that objective; as with many MCI or catastrophic event contingency plans, an effective NDMS must have the qualities of flexibility, appropriateness, timeliness, and efficiency.

Flexibility

To be effective, NDMS must be designed as a truly integrated system, not just a collection of federalized response teams. That is, it must include all components needed to support a continuum of medical care for victims of a catastrophic event from the time of the incident until days or even weeks later. Thus ideally a comprehensive NDMS would provide the following:

- Immediate life-supporting first aid and basic rescue by uninjured survivors.
- Advanced trauma life support within the first few hours.
- Heavy rescue and advanced extrication teams within the first 12 hours.
- Resuscitative surgery either at hospitals or in the field within the first 12 hours.
- Ongoing medical care for chronic illnesses and emergent problems within 24 hours and continuing for weeks if necessary.

Beyond these elements, an NDMS system requires comprehensive preparation of the following:

- Catastrophic event planning by community EMS systems, including complete risk assessments and hazard analyses.
- Meaningful training for all NDMS participants, including personnel neither associated with medicine nor EMS.
- Prepared and prepositioned logistical support from the military and other national sources.
- Tested capacity for rapid notification and activation of the system, and continual communication throughout the hierarchy (vertical) and among rescue teams (horizontal). Communication methods must be flexible, incorporating backup mechanisms for use when a primary system fails. For example, how many crucial communication failures will it take before planners stop relying on the telephone?

Appropriateness

Preparation and mobilization of medical manpower and supplies must match the evolving clinical demands during all phases of the operation. For example, there may be a need for medical trauma teams to deal with major life-threatening trauma from serious injuries; another need may be for mobile teams of medical personnel to treat the emergent but noncritical problems of victims spread over a wide geographic area; a third need may be for medical personnel and supplies to treat chronic medical problems that rapidly become critical if untreated. Finally, public health specialists are needed to prevent and treat widespread medical problems related to lack of sanitation, water, food, or other basic necessities.

Meeting these specific challenges mandates an immediate and ongoing area reconnaissance by qualified medical specialists to assess health and medical needs and authorize action. Andrew suggests that these assessment tasks cannot be left entirely to local agencies or the Red Cross. A national catastrophic event medical resource information bank is crucial; it would be accessed to identify, mobilize, and coordinate medical supplies, equipment, and personnel as required from across the country.

Timeliness

The timeliness of medical response after a catastrophic event is critical. Numerous serious injuries can occur both immediately and in the chaotic environment following such an event. An effective NDMS includes plans to provide appropriate life support both immediately and within predetermined time frames. For example, airway obstruction or apnea destroys the traumatized but salvageable brain within 5 minutes, exsanguinating hemorrhage kills within an hour, and resuscitative surgery is most effective within the first few hours after injury. In the case of an earthquake no trapped, severely injured victim will likely be alive if extricated after more than 24 hours.[20,23]

Therefore an ideal NDMS includes a training component to maximize the ability of local survivors to perform critical lifesaving functions during the hours immediately following the event and before the arrival of outside medical assistance. Given adequate training and preparation, first aid can be initiated within minutes by uninjured survivors, if they are taught basic rescue techniques. As proposed by Koenig, medical supplies can be prepositioned in the target area and local health care providers trained to deliver austere emergency care.[11] Slightly later, resuscitative surgery can be performed by expert medical teams either local or airlifted to the scene with the search and rescue teams and their equipment. These teams must be self-supporting and prospectively equipped for their tasks and supplied for their basic living necessities. In addition to emergency specialists, the NDMS response must include general practitioners, epidemiologists, public health specialists, mental health experts, and other health professionals to deal with the numerous ongoing clinical problems during the subsequent days and weeks. Generally, teams will have to be rotated after approximately 2 weeks.

EMS regions should develop DMATs for rapid deployment and backup teams for duties in the region. Having worked together in everyday practice, team members from the same area usually interact more efficiently under chaotic and austere conditions.

Efficiency

Efficiency complements timeliness. The NDMS response must be performed without waste of time, effort, supplies, or personnel. Such efficiency must be facilitated by enlisting the participation of local public safety agencies, the National Guard, the active duty military, and other organizations. Such security personnel must control vehicular traffic, control air traffic in areas surrounding the disaster zone, and take other measures to protect property, survivors, and rescuers. Maximal use of helicopters for transporting teams to the scene and evacuating the injured should increase the lifesaving potential. As much as possible, all planning should encourage nationwide standardization of clinical response techniques, protocols, and equipment.

The Future

The NDMS existing in the first years of the Clinton Administration still fails to incorporate essential organizational and clinical components necessary for an efficient and timely medical response. Based on the scrutiny in the wake of Hurricane Andrew, it is expected that NDMS will be redesigned to allow for more timely and practical national responses. State and county governments should be encouraged to test and improve their responses, including the medical aspects, so local responders can function effectively before the arrival of outside assistance.

Numerous often compatible recommendations have been made concerning catastrophic event medical responses. Pretto and Safar recommend an EMS-based NDMS that stresses rapid resuscitation of salvageable victims, first aid, and rescue training for the general public following by trauma center-based medical resuscitation teams.[22] Leaning and Lewis recommend that FEMA expand its training function for state and local emergency management officials and develop rapid deployment disaster teams comparable to those used by the National Transportation Safety Board after air crashes.[14] Carmona asserts that the everyday medical experience of civilian trauma and burn centers better prepares them than DOD and VA hospitals to deal with a sudden influx of disaster victims or war casualties.[3] Bosner and Jordan state that NDMS must be redesigned with greater input from the emergency preparedness and EMS communities, and a single federal official must be given overall responsibility and authority for developing and implementing NDMS.[2] Kuehl advocates funding a comprehensive academic effort to develop the science and terminology of catastrophic event medicine coupled with the assignment of responsibility and authority for the immediate response to DOD.[12] In February 1993, Senator Mikulski of Maryland suggested that FEMA be given full authority for catastrophic disaster response, including the NDMS component.[15] Obviously the improvement of the national response system requires a consensus solution.

PICE Nomenclature System

Static	Controlled	Local	P	Stage 0
Evolving	Disruptive	Regional	I	Stage 1
Dynamic	Paralytic	National	C	Stage 2
		International	E	Stage 3

The first prefix describes the potential for additional casualties. The second describes the ability of the jurisdiction to respond. The third classifies the geographic extent of the event. The stages indicate the need for outside medical assistance. (that is, Stage 0: None. Stage 1: Put remote medical personnel on alert. Stage 2: Commit remote medical personnel. Stage 3: Commit personnel and prepare remote hospitals for reception of patients.)

Examples of the kind of basic work that will form the foundation of future consensus are the investigations of reanimatology by Pretto and the nomenclature system proposed by Koenig, Dinerman, and Kuehl.[17,23] Using the latter system, any catastrophic event large or small can be accurately described by adding three prefixes and one suffix to the term "potential injury creating event" (PICE). See the Box above.

Using this system the February 1993 World Trade Center bombing would have initially been an "evolving, disruptive, local PICE-Stage 1." Hurricane Andrew initially would have been a "dynamic, paralytic, regional PICE-Stage 1." Obviously, with time the description of these events would change. In the case of Andrew by the third day it would have been described as a "static, disruptive, local PICE-Stage 2", and the bombing on the third day would have been a "static, controlled, local PICE-Stage 0." A Californiawide severe earthquake (Richter 7 or 8) likely would be initially described as a "dynamic, paralytic, regional PICE-Stage 3." The 1993 Los Angeles Basin earthquake was described initially as a "dynamic, disruptive local PICE-Stage 1."

Summary

While as of June 1994 responsibility for NDMS remained at DHHS, it remains to be seen what direction the federal government will take in addressing national disaster response and its medical component. In the meantime the local EMS medical director can improve preparedness for medically catastrophic incidents in his region by taking the following actions:

- Promoting first aid training through local health organizations and in schools.
- Lobbying for improved trauma and EMS services, especially in rural areas and disaster prone regions.

- Encouraging government agencies and professional organizations to support the nationwide compatibility of rescue equipment, medical supplies, training standards, and personnel reciprocity.
- Establishing and training a local DMAT team.
- Demanding a functional and responsive NDMS that will integrate with state and regional EMS activities in a disaster.
- Carefully cataloging and learning to access local, regional, and national resources that would be needed following a local catastrophe.
- Building the best possible local EMS system. After all, if EMS does not work well on a normal day, it will not work well in a disaster. The DMAT capability is evolving very slowly and should not be relied on for the timely availability of health and medical services support needed by a given locality following a catastrophic event.

REFERENCES

1. Bisgard JC and Mullaly CF: The civilian-military contingency hospital system (CMCHS) on the USA, *Prehospital Disaster Medicine* 1:35-38, 1985.
2. Bosner L and Jordan L: Needed: a national program for disaster medical preparedness, *PSQR* 160-164, Sep 1991.
3. Caroma R: The paradox of military trauma and emergency care, *JAMA* 266:217, 1991.
4. Confusion hindered EMS preparations for return of war wounded, *JEMS* 16(5):17, 1991.
5. FEMA's Disaster Management Program: *A performance audit after hurricane andrew,* Washington, DC, Dec 1992, Office of Inspector General, FEMA.
6. Gaffney JK, Schodort L, and Jones G: DMATs respond to andrew and iniki, *JEMS* 17(11):76, 1992.
7. Hale K: Lessons learned panel, Disaster 1993 Conference, Orlando, Fla, Feb 27, 1993.
8. *Health care: readiness of US hospital systems to treat war casualties,* GAO/T-HRD-92-17, Washington, DC, Mar 25, 1992, US General Accounting Office.
9. In the catastrophic disaster: who will help the injured? *Journal of Civil Defense* 16-17, Jun 1991.
10. Jones NP et al: *Preliminary earthquake injury epidemiology report.* In Bolin R,: *The Loma Prieta earthquake: studies of short-term impacts,* A Natural Hazards Center Monograph. Boulder, Colo, 1990, University of Colorado.
11. Koenig KL, Schulz CH, and DiLorenzo R: Crush injury cadaver lab: a new method of training physicians, *Ann Emerg Med* 21:196, 1992 (abstract).
12. Kuehl AE: Developing the science of dealing with disasters, *Rescue-EMS* 11/12:27, 1992.
13. Kvetan V: Operation desert storm: task force critical care, *Crit Care Med* 19:854, 1991.
14. Leaning J and Lewis D: The future of FEMA, *JEMS* 16(3):11, 1991.
15. Mikulski BA: *Keynote address,* Disaster 1993 Conference, Orlando, Fla, Feb 27, 1993.
16. *The national disaster medical system,* Rockville, Md, 1984, Public Health Service.
17. Noji EK et al: The 1988 earthquake in Soviet Armenia: a case study, *Ann Emerg Med* 19:891, 1990.
18. *Operation desert storm: full army medical capability not achieved,* GAO/T-NSIAD-92-8, Washington, DC, Feb 5, 1992, US General Accounting Office.
19. Plan for stateside care of casualties criticized, *Washington Post A26, Feb 7, 1991.*
20. Pollander GS and Rund DA: Analysis of medical needs in disasters caused by earthquakes: the need for a uniform injury reporting scheme, *Disasters* 13:365, 1989.
21. Preliminary report: medical examiner reports of deaths associated with hurricane andrew: Florida, *JAMA* 1644, Oct 7, 1992.
22. Pretto E and Safar P: National medical response to mass disasters in the United States: are we prepared? *JAMA* 266:1259, 1991.
23. Pretto E et al: Disaster reanimatology potentials III: results, conclusions, and recommendations, *Prehospital and Disaster Medicine* Oct-Dec 1992, (in press).
24. Pretto E et al: *The incidence of protracted death after the April 22, 1991, earthquake in Limon Province, Costa Rica,* Second Asian-Pacific Conference of Disaster Medicine, Tokyo, Japan, Oct 1992.
25. *Recent disasters demonstrate the need to improve the nations response strategy,* GAO/T RCED-93-4, Washington, DC, Jan 27, 1993, US General Accounting Office.
26. Roth PB et al: The St. Croix disaster and the national disaster medical system, *Ann Emerg Med 25:391, 1991.*

47

Diversion and COBRA Issues

Stanley Zydlo, J.D., M.D., FACEP

This chapter presents the terms and concepts used in various EMS systems in the United States relative to ambulance diversions and declared limitations of resources. It does not advocate what should or should not be done but merely describes what does exist and offers suggestions to those seeking information on which to craft their own policies.

Background

EMS systems developed as a response to a recognized need for efficient, reliable, and enhanced prehospital care. Until recently, prehospital care generally was rendered via private, municipal or volunteer ambulance services that had neither organized and accountable structures nor training and functional standards. Furthermore, patients were usually transported to either the closest hospital or to the requested hospital with little awareness of the capabilities of the hospital emergency department (ED).

Throughout the 1970s patients were often transported to the hospital that provided direct medical control. The terms *base hospital* and *resource hospital* were and are still used colloquially to denote a direct medical control facility. In this section, the term *base hospital* will be used exclusively to avoid confusion and repetition. The terms *diversion, rerouting,* and *bypass* will be used interchangeably. During the 1980s, the magnitude of these diversions became a nationwide problem requiring decisive action on the part of the prehospital and medical communities.[16,18]

As the EMS concept evolved and expanded, other hospitals within or near the EMS region either were asked to participate or rushed to join the system in an effort to secure patients from the ambulance providers. Two patterns of patient distribution evolved. In one model, all patients requiring prehospital care under direct medical control were transported to the base hospital. In the other model, the additional hospitals were authorized to receive patients.[20,28] These additional hospitals were called associate or monitoring hospitals.

As patient volumes at specific hospitals increased in the 1980s and caused concomitant ED overcrowding, hospitals attempted to limit the influx of patients by requesting that ambulances temporarily bypass their EDs.[3] This practice resulted in prolonged transports to other facilities and allegations of patient dumping.[10] Additionally, some hospitals began to request that specific types of patients be diverted when clinical capabilities to provide services were fully utilized. According to the American College of Emergency Physicians (ACEP), variables to be considered in patient destination decisions should include[1]: patient condition and location, patient request, patient's personal physician request, facility capabilities, and preplanned regional system destinations.

A 1992 study found that paramedics generally identify the closest hospital for trauma transport but bypass some hospitals systematically for reasons not related to trauma score, time of day, day of week, or season of the year. The study found that both the correct identification of the closest hospital and the assumptions made when selecting a receiving facility significantly impacted on the number of times a hospital was bypassed.[21] In an effort to address these inconsistencies, some states enacted legislation that mandated patient transportation only to the nearest hospital, at least under normal circumstances. Others laws empowered EMS systems to develop policies that ensure access to emergency medical care for all consumers in a timely and medically appropriate manner. In some cases such as New York City in 1982 the diversion system was codified operationally by the municipal provider without specific authority, based on the hospital designation system.

The concept of diversion developed to allow a patient who would normally go to a particular receiving facility to be rerouted, either by protocol or by direct medical control instruction to an alternate hospital that was better prepared. For example, if a particular hospital did not possess either the equipment or the staff to handle a specific medical problem, it was logical that patients should not be brought to that facility but rather should be routinely transported to another institution that did have the needed resources.

Additionally, the diversion concept was expanded to incorporate criteria that allowed a hospital to inform the EMS agency if it did not wish to receive patients with a particular problems, or even any patients at all. Thus an ambulance proceeding to a hospital that was on bypass would be diverted by the system to an alternate facility. In an effort to develop uniformity in the content of diversion protocols, ACEP established 18 guidelines for the development of diversion policies. As an outgrowth of system categorization and designation, certain hospitals were placed on permanent bypass status for specific cases such as pediatrics, in diversion of ambulances to other hospitals with the appropriate resources.

Definitions

There are two general categories of rerouting bypass or diversion.

Total

After proper notification by the appropriate party, all ambulances are diverted to other hospital EDs, due to temporary and catastrophic resource limitations such as electrical failures, strikes, or floods.

Partial

After proper notification, all patients requiring selected care (e.g., trauma, burns, critical) are diverted to other hospitals. For example, a hospital may elect partial bypass specifically for trauma patients because of operating and surgical resource limitations but can still accommodate medical patients in its ED. In another case, a hospital may have the all burn-unit beds filled; the facility may request partial bypass so that burn patients will be diverted while it still accepts other categories of patients.

The acceptable reasons for diversion must be determined by the specific EMS system. The mechanics of diversion vary tremendously, depending in part on whether central dispatch decides and directs hospital destinations. The system in cooperation with the medical oversight must decide both how hospital requests for diversion are prioritized and how decisions to grant the requests are made. For example, can the system ever deny the request for diversion?

Controversies

Controversies over bypass arise when a hospital declares a resource limitation for reasons that do not seem valid. For example, a hospital may claim that its intensive care unit beds are fully occupied when it still has ED beds available to receive patients for evaluation and stabilization. A hospital may claim it has inadequate nursing personnel to care for patients needing intensive care beds, yet the ED still has beds and adequate nursing availability. In a third example, a hospital may claim that all its surgical suites are occupied, yet patient assessment and care could be initiated in the ED. The patient may never need surgery or can be stabilized in the ED and then be safely transferred.

Many argue that the critical patients always should be transported to the closest appropriate facility and then stabilized in the ED as long as it does not have a resource limitation of space and/or personnel to care for such patients.[5] During emergency evaluation and stabilization, operations are completed and intensive care unit patients can be moved to other beds. Some emergency patients, once stabilized, can be transferred to other facilities so long as there are clinical benefits to be gained.

Bypass may also be abused by hospitals in attempts to avoid receiving certain categories of undesirable patients, such as nonpaying, uninsured, or intoxicated.[4] This practice has markedly decreased since the enactment of the Consolidated Omnibus Budget Reconciliation Act (COBRA) in 1986 and the Omnibus Budget Reconciliation Act (OBRA) of 1989, which became effective in July 1990.[7,22]

Depending on local politics, resources and protocols, it is advantageous for EMS systems to cooperate with their responsible authoritative health care agencies, such as the local department of health, to monitor and investigate possible misuse of the diversion process. This can be accomplished by evaluating the validity of each bypass request against standards that have been established. Issuing warnings for noncompliance with system standards may be a joint venture or the EMS system may do so itself.

Bypass criteria can be developed by an individual institution or through a cooperative EMS system agreement.[17] Irrespective of the method by which they are established, each hospital should have standardized internal policies stating the thresholds for declaring a resource limitation. In addition, there should exist internal quality improvement processes and strategies to minimize the need for requesting bypass. The system must have an operational plan for the safe, appropriate, and timely care of patients who continue to access the EMS system in spite of numerous hospital diversions.[1]

A software system has been implemented in Portland that allows monitoring of the diversion status of all the hospitals in the EMS system through an integrated computer network. At a glance, providers, dispatchers, and hospitals know if the nearest ambulance destination is on bypass. Known as CHORAL (Computerized Hospital On-line Resource Allocation Link), the software monitors six diversion categories and displays the information system wide. Each hospital enters its own data, and none of the hospitals can change another's entries.[2]

For any type of bypass, specific time limits should be requested and granted. Updates should be given to the operational units and direct medical control continuously.

Generic Operational Policy

Policy Purpose

It is the responsibility of all hospitals in any EMS system to provide emergency assessment and care to all patients presenting to their emergency departments. When exceeded by patient demand or in the event of limitation of resources, a hospital may request bypass status from the system medical or administrative control. Ambulance diversion should only occur after a hospital has exhausted all internal mechanisms to relieve the situation. Hospital decisions must not be based on factors such as protection of beds for elective cases, protection of significant numbers of beds for unforeseen needs, or a desire not to call in overtime staff. No diversion decision should ever be made based on financial resources of patients.

Diversions must occur only after a prospective decision has been made by direct medical control that the transport can be safely accomplished in a timely fashion with available EMS resources, and a physician certifies that it is appropriate to take the patient to a more distant hospital that can provide definitive care for that patient. In busy systems a general policy may be necessary because individual physician decisions cannot be made in a timely manner.

Procedure

When a hospital administrator elects to request bypass status, the following specific steps shall be followed. The hospital administrator or his designee will notify all of the following of the need to request a diversion and the anticipated duration for which the diversion is needed: direct medical control, the dispatch center, the police department, and the Department of Health.

The EMS direct medical control shall be notified of the type of bypass requested (e.g., total or partial, trauma or burns), when it was requested, and the approximate duration for which bypass is needed. Furthermore, the system should be informed that the dispatch center, ambulance providers and the police departments have been notified. If the bypass is requested after normal working hours, the Department of Health should be informed the next business day. The EMS system will immediately accept or reject the request for diversion. Normally, requests will be granted unless the system is in an area-wide overloaded situation.

Written Documents/Diversion Information

1. Name of the administrator who authorized the bypass.
2. The name of the individual making the bypass notification calls and times of notifications.
3. The number of emergency department physicians and nurses on duty.
4. The reason for the bypass, (e.g., CT scanner down, surgery full, no monitors, no stretchers, flooding).
5. The number of patients in the ED at the time the bypass was requested.
6. The number of critical patients in the emergency department at the time bypass was requested.
7. The number of cardiac monitors in the emergency department.
8. The number of monitors in the emergency department in use at the time the bypass was requested.
9. Action taken (e.g., approved or rejected) and the name of EMS official making decisions.

An example of a diversion data document is seen in the box on the following page.

EMS administration or direct medical control should be responsible for notifying other hospitals and ambulance providers of the approved bypass. The EMS system routinely should send a staff member to the hospital to review and document

Emergency Department Bypass Documentation

Date: ______________ Name of Hospital: ______________________________

Individual Authorizing Bypass: ______________________________

Type of Bypass: ______________________________

Reason for Bypass Request (Resource Limitation): ______________________________

____

Time Initiated: ______________ Time of Cancellation: ______________

Supervising Physician on Duty: ______________________________

Charge Nurse on Duty: ______________________________

Bypass Notification Calls:

		Individual
Resource Hospital:	Time: __________	Making Call: __________
Ambulance Dispatch Center (Phone Number):	Time: __________	Individual Making Call: __________
Police Department (Phone Number)	Time: __________	Individual Making Call: __________
Department of Health (Phone Number)	Time: __________	Individual Making Call: __________

Bypass Information:

Emergency Department

Staff on Duty:	#MD: ________	#RN: ________
Patients in Emergency Dept.	#Critical: ________	Total: ________
Functioning Monitors in Emergency Dept.:	#In Use: ________	Total: ________

Individual Authorizing Bypass Cancellation: ______________________________

Time of Cancellation: ______________________________

Bypass Cancellation Calls:

Resource Hospital:	Time: __________	Individual Making Call: __________
Ambulance Dispatch Center (Phone Number)	Time: __________	Individual Making Call: __________
Police Department (Phone Number)	Time: __________	Individual Making Call: __________

the conditions which necessitated the bypass. The hospital may be issued a Department of Health citation, in the event that the bypass request was not warranted. Direct medical control, the dispatch center, and the police department should be notified as soon as the hospital is no longer experiencing a problem.

As EMS systems mature, the need to formalize bypass policies will become more apparent. When hospitals frequently request bypass, the requests must be aggressively verified, and at times actually denied by the EMS system either because specific patients cannot be diverted for clinical reasons or because other hospitals are also in overload situations.

Special Cases

An EMS system, through the medical control board or medical oversight physician, should prospectively determine any types of patients who need transport directly to a specialty referral center. Such facilities include burn centers, trauma centers, pediatric care centers, psychiatric hospitals, replantation centers or hyperbaric facilities. Other prospective diversion agreements should be made concerning specialty units such as neurosurgery, spinal cord, high risk pregnancy, neonatology, or poison control units. In addition to having a detailed plan for sending appropriate patients to these centers, an EMS system must develop a diversion policy to reroute patients elsewhere should a specialty referral center (SRC) have its resources overloaded or otherwise be compromised. However, in the cases of patients in extremis, it is advisable to send them to the closest appropriate emergency facility, even if it has requested a bypass status; although such a policy must be formally developed. Since there remains a problem of identifying appropriate SRC candidates in the field, it is usually operationally most effective to overtriage patients to the SRCs.

Trauma Diversion Policy

Policy Purpose

It is the trauma center's responsibility to provide care for all trauma patients that are directed to the center. If the resources of the trauma center are exceeded by the demands, the trauma center may elect to go on trauma bypass; however, the emergency department of that hospital may continue to be open. Direct medical control should temporarily divert patients from that trauma center to an alternate trauma center, if one exists, or to a facility that can provide care for the patient. In the event of a multiple casualty incident (MCI), the usual trauma diversion policy, and the standard ED diversion policy may be superseded by the requirements of the MCI. All requests for bypass are usually invalidated by a declared MCI, which requires that hospital resources be mobilized to provide care for larger numbers of casualties than under normal circumstances.

Procedure

After proper request and notification, any ambulance transporting a designated trauma patient will proceed to (or be directed to) another facility appropriate to the patient's needs. When a trauma center is on bypass, the system will direct ambulances to the next closest appropriate institution. Trauma diversion may be requested when the hospital administrator determines that his hospital cannot meet the needs of an additional trauma patient. Examples of conditions that would warrant requests for trauma diversions are: no available staffed operating rooms, an inoperable CT scanner, an inoperable piece of equipment required for the routine treatment of a trauma patient, a major physical plant failure, or a lack of blood.

When the trauma center administrator requests trauma bypass, the following procedures must be followed:

1. The hospital administrator or designee notifies the following organizations of the need to institute a trauma diversion and its anticipated duration:
   - Direct medical control is responsible for notifying other hospitals and providers of the initiation of the trauma diversion. Updates must be give to the hospitals regularly.
   - The ambulance dispatch center.
   - The police department.
   - The department of health.
2. Written documentation for the trauma diversion should be prepared and should include the following information:
   - The reason(s) for the request to be on bypass.
   - The name of administrator who requested the bypass.
   - The name of the person making the trauma diversion notification calls to the appropriate authorities.
   - The times of notification.
   - The name of the EMS authority granting or denying the request.
3. As soon as the trauma center is capable of caring for trauma patients, all of the individuals should be made aware of the cancellation of the trauma diversion. The times of these notifications should be documented. Direct medical control is normally responsible for notifying other hospitals of the trauma diversion cancellation. The Department of Health or the EMS system may send a staff member to review and document the conditions that necessitated the trauma diversion request. The hospital may be issued a citation by the Department of Health for failure to comply with the local trauma diversion procedure.

Existing Policies

Although there are many approaches to the design and implementation of systemwide policies, one of the better ones is included in its entirety in the Appendix.

COBRA

In the mid-1980s, hospitals were jolted by a rise in the numbers of uninsured and underinsured patients which developed concurrently with the 1983 adoption of the Medicare prospective payment plan. Together these resulted in decreased hospital revenues and profits. In some states, hospitals were allowed to transfer uninsured emergency patients to public facilities. As a result, EMS systems were placed in the difficult situation of making patient transfers based on economic rather than medical reasons. In 1987, an estimated 250,000 transfers occurred for economic reasons alone.[4]

In an attempt to stop this practice of "patient dumping", Congress enacted the Emergency Medical Treatment and Active Labor Act (EMTALA) of 1986 as a part of COBRA. The primary focus of these laws was to prevent hospitals from refusing to treat either emergency patients or women in active labor because they were unable to pay or exhibited some other undesirable characteristics.

Under COBRA and its amendments, if an individual presents for a purported emergency condition to a hospital with an ED, the hospital must provide an appropriate screening examination to determine whether or not an emergency condition exists. This screening examination must utilize all the appropriate capabilities of the hospital, including laboratory studies, roentgenograms, and whatever else is considered appropriate to reach a conclusion. A simple nursing triage examination is not adequate; the examination content and scope is the ultimate responsibility of the ED physician. If an emergency medical condition does exist, the patient must be stabilized before discharge or transfer to another facility. If the patient is a pregnant woman having contractions, she is considered unstable until delivery of the child and the placenta. If unable to be delivered vaginally, then an appropriate transfer may be made to a facility capable of providing other means of delivery, if such capabilities do not exist at the transferring facility.

Terms Defined by COBRA

Emergency Medical Condition

A medical condition manifesting itself by acute symptoms of sufficient severity (including severe pain) such that the absence of immediate medical attention could reasonably be expected to result in placing the patient's health in serious jeopardy, serious impairment to bodily functions, or serious dysfunction. In the emergency of a pregnant woman having contractions there is inadequate time to effect a safe transfer to another hospital before delivery or the transfer may pose a threat to the health or safety of the woman or the unborn child.

Stabilize

To stabilize an emergency medical condition means to provide such medical treatment as may be necessary to assure, within reasonable medical probability, that no material deterioration is likely to result from the transfer of the individual from the facility.

Transfer

Movement, including discharge, of an individual outside a hospital's facilities at the direction of any person employed by (or affiliated or associated directly or indirectly with) the hospital. It does not include movement of an individual who is dead or who leaves the facility without permission.

COBRA Regulations

The basics of COBRA regulations should be understood and followed since punitive damages for violation entails fines of up to $50,000 for each infraction. None of the fines are covered by malpractice insurance. Originally, COBRA allowed the infractions to expose the involved physician to civil suit, and the transferring institution to a fine of up to $50,000 with exclusion from Medicare participation.

Congress added the OBRA amendments in June 1990, which lowered the maximum fines to $25,000 against hospitals with fewer than 100 beds. Further, OBRA requires peer review organizations (PROs) to review alleged violations for appropriateness; however, the hospital does not have to adhere to the conclusions of the PRO. OBRA allows receiving hospitals that suffer a financial loss from an inappropriate transfer, to file civil suit against the transferring hospital to recover such losses. Finally, it establishes a "whistle blower" protection provision to prevent either the penalizing or the initiation of adverse actions against a "qualified medical person or physician" who "refuses to transfer an individual who has not be stabilized—or against any hospital employee because the employee reports a violation."[26]

The OBRA amendments have made it more difficult to exclude a hospital or physician from the Medicare program unless either they are proven to negligently violate the statute or the violation is "gross and flagrant or is repeated." Violations are investigated by the Health Care Financing Administration and penalties are applied by The Department of Health and Human Services (DHHS). As of 1991, 140 hospitals and three physicians had been cited under COBRA; DHHS had penalized 19 hospitals and barred six from participating in Medicare. Of these, three were reinstated.[15]

If a competent patient gives a written, informed refusal to treatment or transfer after all risks and benefits are explained and the hospital's obligations under the law are provided to them, they are not required to be treated or transferred. A patient or his surrogate can request transfer after being first informed of the risks of the transfer and the hospital's obligations under COBRA. This is generally termed a patient generated transfer.

A physician can order a transfer if he both believes and documents that the medical benefits of the transfer reasonably outweigh the risks to the patient. This must be written in a detailed manner, based on information available at the time of the transfer, and must state the benefits to the patient of the transfer.

Every hospital is required to maintain a list of on call physicians who are available to stabilize a patient after initial examination. If an emergency physician, after the initial exam, determines that the patient requires the expertise and services of one of these on-call specialists and the specialist refuses or fails to appear in a "reasonable" (not defined) amount of time, a transfer may be ordered if the benefits of transfer outweigh the risks of the transfer. Such an on-call physician refusal to respond in a timely manner should be clearly documented.[13,14]

Finally, if the on-call physician is not physically present in the ED but consults with a qualified person who is, together they can make the medical determination to transfer. The documentation can be signed at a later time thus not delaying the transfer.

The "appropriate transfer" aspect of the regulations is of particular interest to EMS personnel. Once a patient is examined and stabilized by the transferring hospital, the transfer can proceed if the receiving hospital agrees to accept the patient, agrees to provide appropriate care, and has available space and qualified personnel to do so. The transferring hospital must send all medical records (or copies), including the emergency condition of the patient, the observed signs or symptoms, the preliminary diagnosis, the treatment rendered, the results of any clinical tests and the informed, written consent of the patient.[13,18] Documentation by the nursing staff is critical in protecting against potential violations. Charting must include both "incoming and discharge vital signs, pertinent physical findings, any change in status, and physician signatures on all charts." Receiving hospitals also want the "name and address of any on-call physician who has refused or failed to appear within a reasonable time to provide necessary stabilizing treatment" to accompany the patient.[9]

The transferring physician has the responsibility for the selection of the appropriate mode of transporting the patient; the equipment, medication, and supplies on the transporting vehicle; and the availability of properly trained and licensed personnel to use all of these to ensure "necessary and medically appropriate life support measure during the transport."[24] Finally, COBRA requires transferring hospitals to "meet other such requirements as the Secretary (DHHS) may find necessary in the interest of the health and safety of individuals transferred." The lack of clearly stated definitions makes these provisions subject to interpretation and continues to generate concern in the medical and prehospital communities.[8] Certainly, additional changes and interpretations can be expected in the near future, which should encourage those charged with EMS medical oversight to be aware, informed, and responsive.

Summary

To avoid failing compliance with COBRA and its regulations, it is critical that the physician responsible for medical oversight adopt and implement a locally tailored diversion policy. In addition, every patient transfer performed by the EMS system must be documented to meet COBRA requirements before leaving the originating hospital.

REFERENCES

1. ACEP: *Guidelines for ambulance diversion/destination policies,* 1991.
2. ACEP: Ambulance diversion/destination policies, *ACEP News* 29-30, January 1992.
3. Andrulis DP et al: Emergency departments and crowding in United States teaching hospitals, *Ann Emer Med 20*(9):980-986, 1991.
4. Ansell DA and Schiff RL: Patient dumping, *JAMA 257*:1500-1502, 1987.
5. Aranosian R: Medical-legal concerns in EMS. In: Roush WR (editor): *Principles of EMS systems,* Dallas, 1989, American College of Emergency Physicians.
6. Bern A: Disaster medical services. In: Roush WR (editor): *Principles of EMS systems,* Dallas, 1989, American College of Emergency Physicians.
7. Consolidated Omnibus Budget Reconciliation Act of 1985: Law of the 99th Congress, 42 USC. Section 1395 dd.
8. Dooley RE: COBRA's hidden venom, *Emergency* Dec, 1989.
9. Frew SA, Roush WA, and LaGreca K: COBRA: Implications for emergency medicine, *Ann Emer Med* 17: 835-837, 1982.
10. Garza MA: Dangerous detours Ambulance diversions staff patient delivery. *JEMS* 14(7):43, 1989.
11. George JE and Quattrone MS (editors): Hospital liability for economic transfers, *Emergency Physician Legal Bulletin* 11(3), 1985.
12. George JE and Quattrone MS (editors): No room at the inn. *Emergency Physician Legal Bulletin* 15(4), 1989.

13. George JE, Quattrone MS and Espinosa JA (editors): Alphabet soup (COBRA, OBRA and PRO), *Emergency Physician Legal Bulletin* 17(3), 1991.
14. George JE, Quattrone MS, and Espinosa JA (editors): I. The COBRA misses: EMTALA protects against "patient dumping", not ordinary negligence. II. COBRA update: beyond the ED, *Emergency Physician Legal Bulletin* 19(1), 1993.
15. Kent C: Patient transfers and the law, *Risk Management Report* 3(2), 1991.
16. Manson T: *EMS system diversions.* Unpublished raw data from a study completed by the American Hospital Association, Chicago, 1990.
17. Megargel RE and Dickinson ET: Prehospital care, *Foresight* 23: 3-4, 1992.
18. Metropolitan Chicago Healthcare Council: *Emergency department overcrowding.* Unpublished raw data from state-wide survey, 1991.
19. Neely KW et al: Computerized hospital on-line resources allocation link (CHORAL): A mechanism to monitor and establish policy for hospital ambulance diversions, *Prehospital and Disaster Medicine* 6:459-462, 1991.
20. Neely KW et al: The effect of base station contact on ambulance destination, *Ann Emer Med* 19(8):906-909, 1990.
21. Norton RL et al: Compliance with closest hospital transport protocol, *Prehospital and Disaster Medicine* 7:243-249, 1992.
22. Omnibus Budget Reconciliation Act of 1990: Amendments to Section 1867 of the Social Security Act, 1990, Law of the 101st Congress.
23. Patient Protection Amendments: 42 USC 1935 dd(C)(2)(D) 1989.
24. Rothenberg MA: Uncoiling COBRA (letter), *JEMS* 14(11): 7-8, 1989.
25. Rubin MS (editor): *Complying with COBRA: a reference handbook of guidelines, forms and compliance recommendations,* Chicago, 1990, Metropolitan Chicago Healthcare Council.
26. Rubin MS: Complying with COBRA: An update on the "patient dumping" Law, Metropolitan Chicago Healthcare Council Correspondence March 1991.
27. Study finds inappropriate transfers, *American Medical News* August 1992.
28. Waddington N et al: The effect of on-line medical control centralization on ambulance destination, *JEMS* 5(4):299-303, 1987.

Appendix

Rerouting Policy

To: D. Directors
Hospital Administrators

From: Andrew G. Wilson, Jr., M.D.
Chairman, Medical Control

Date: May 31, 1988
Subject: Rerouting Policy, effective July 1, 1988

Enclosed you will find the recently approved OAKEMS policy for the rerouting of ambulances. Rerouting has become a necessary evil in the present health care environment. The intent of the policy is to enable rerouting to occur with a minimal impact on patient care. An important secondary objective is to help the EMT/paramedic deal with this problem.

To the end of helping the paramedic, and in this instance indirectly helping out patients, I would draw your attention to "Status C." Status C is defined as that situation where "the emergency department itself is so inundated with patients that it cannot safely accept further patients." A survey I have conducted of some Emergency Departments would suggest that there is considerable variation in criteria used for declaring an Emergency Department as Status C. I would like to draw your attention to the implications of Status C for the paramedics, and enter a plea not to resort to Status C except under unusual circumstances.

Status C carries with it not only the suggestion that it would be inadvisable to bring patients to the Emergency Department in question, but that mere communication with that institution is inadvisable. This, in effect, cuts the EMT/paramedic off from advice and discussion about a case with what may, in fact, be the closest appropriate hospital. Status C, in effect, mandates a call to another hospital. It would seem that a phone/radio consultation with the Emergency Physician could be held and best course of care decided upon.

The Medical Control Committee would strongly suggest that, except under extremely unusual circumstances, an Emergency Department declare itself "Status B to everything" rather than Status C. In this way, the message that the hospital cannot easily handle more patients will be sent, but without the deleterious implication of Status C that the E.D. should not even be called.

General Statement

Patients exhibiting uncontrollable problems in the field will be accepted by the closest appropriate facility regardless of the hospital's rerouting status. Critical patients will be accepted by the closest appropriate hospital when transportation to a more distant hospital could pose a further significant risk to the patient. Serious, but stable, patients may be rerouted by the medical control physician.

Patient Triage

All persons examined will be assigned a priority rating by the EMT/paramedic in charge of the case. As with all triage decisions at all levels of care, the priority assigned may change depending on further assessment, communication with physicians, or overt change in patient's condition.

Priority 1: Critically ill or injured patient who needs immediate attention. Delay in care will threaten life or limb.

Priority 2: An urgent situation where the patient's condition could deteriorate into a Priority 1 prior to arrival at a medical facility.

Priority 3: Illness or injury not meeting the criteria for Priority 1 or 2.

Priority 4: Dead on scene according to SOP's.

Rerouting

1. The decision by a hospital to reroute patients should be made by the emergency department director, or his emergency physician designee. The emergency physician should consult with nursing, administration, and/or with the directors of specialty units as individual circumstances dictate.
2. On-line medical control will remain available at all times from all OAKEMS participating hospitals. If all area hospitals are rerouting, then the rerouting status will not be honored and the patient will be transported to the closest appropriate hospital.
3. It is the responsibility of the emergency department to use the following codes to indicate status:

Status A: Accepting all patients normally appropriate for that hospital.

Status B: Emergency department is open, however, services elsewhere in the hospital are limited. Services or resources that are not available should be specified.

Status C: The emergency department itself is so inundated with patients that it cannot safely accept further patients.

4. Patients will not be rerouted on the basis of ability to pay.
5. The decision to reroute a patient will not be based on a previous relationship with a particular institution, except where it would impact the patient's emergency care.
6. Participating health care facilities shall not reroute a BLS unit transporting a Priority 1 or Priority 2 patient unless it is in a declared disaster mode.
7. If the EMT believes that the ordered reroute will be deleterious to a particular patient, that patient may be brought to the hospital called.

Communications

1. Communications with Hospitals under Status B:
   Units may communicate with the closest appropriate hospital, if:
   - BLS unit with Priority 1 or 2.
   - ALS unit with Priority 1.
   - Patient or family insists on a hospital that would normally be an appropriate destination. The base station physician will communicate with the patient/family.
2. Communication With Hospitals Under Status C:
   The emergency department is overburdened. It would be suggested that a patch to this facility not be made, except under exceptional circumstances. Transportation to and communication with that hospital may not be advisable, other options should be considered.
3. Once Communication Has Been Established Under Status B or C:
   Once communication with a hospital under Status B or C is made and a decision has been made to transport to another facility, the hospital called will communicate with the receiving hospital decided upon.

Notification

1. All OAKEMS participating hospitals shall be notified when another OAKEMS hospital is rerouting. All hospitals are encouraged to post this information by the radio for quick reference.
2. Hospital Rerouting Notification Procedures:
   A. When a unit calls in and requests a patch to a rerouting facility, "O"COM advises the unit, via MED 9, that the hospital is rerouting.

   B. "O"COM phones and advises adjacent communication's centers (i.e., Macomb County MEDCOM, etc.).

   C. In the following instances; UHF communications failure, ALS traffic, BLS traffic, or out-of-county transports; should contact "O"COM, via MEDCOM 340, prior to transport, in order to check the hospital's rerouting status.

   D. Agencies must notify "O"COM in writing requesting that their dispatch center be notified by phone regarding each hospital's rerouting status change.

   E. It is the responsibility of all OAKEMS participating agencies to notify their own personnel when "O"COM advises of a hospital rerouting.

48

Regionalization and Designation of Medical Facilities

Lynne Cooper, J.D., M.A.
Alasdair Conn, M.D.

Regionalization of medical facilities is recognized as critical to the ultimate success of EMS systems. Although great progress has been made in developing truly comprehensive EMS systems during the past 20 years, the degree of effort to regionalize facilities through categorization (review against standards to classify emergency care capabilities) and designation (formal selection for patient referral and transfer) has varied.[16]

Notwithstanding the significant impact of the enactment of EMS system legislation on EMS development in the early 1970s, economic, political, and legal factors contribute to the benign neglect of medical facilities by EMS groups.[11-13] The slow rate of progress in categorizing and designating medical facilities is especially disappointing in the area of regional trauma systems implementation, given the apparent effectiveness of regionalized trauma care.[6,30,36]

The results of a 1987 nationwide survey conducted by the American College of Surgeons (ACS) Committee on trauma, showed that statewide compliance with ACS trauma guidelines is poor. Only two states (Maryland and Virginia) had all of the eight essential components of a regional trauma system. Nineteen states and the District of Columbia either did not have statewide coverage and/or lacked one or more essential components; 29 states had not started the process of designation trauma centers.[35]

Controversy and confusion still surround the concepts of categorization and designation.[1] Proponents of categorization alone argue that it enhances the level of care provided without the need for designation. Supporters of designation, achieved with or without the initial categorization of facilities, point out that designation is even more difficult to achieve than categorization. Although problematic, most concede that emergency department (ED) or specialty referral center (SRC) designation combined with system integration appears to offer a distinct advantage over categorization alone.[32]

Categorization and designation have the same general goals; however, they are markedly different processes. Categorization is a voluntary process not subject to verification and not binding on the system providers. Categorization, while an accepted method of regionalizing certain services such as emergency, obstetrics, psychiatric, and burn care provides for hospital self-assessment of capabilities without limitation on the numbers of hospitals participating in a given system.[8,9,19]

Although it has been shown that categorization reduces the provision of unacceptable care at hospitals,[10] it may not impact on patient outcome, or reduce costs through the elimination of duplication of services.[17] Categorization establishes standards of care and may serve as a preliminary framework for the designation of medical facilities, a component that should be in place before a system can consistently deliver patients to the most appropriate facilities. The categorization process is usually referred to as either vertical (the care for a particular medical problem throughout the institution) or horizontal (the scope of care of an ED).

Designation usually limits hospital participation and is a binding process requiring independent verification of both hospital compliance with standards and adherence to strict patient transport guidelines by prehospital providers. Implementation of designation fosters regionalization through accountability and commitment, which in turn theoretically reduce morbidity by improving the quality of care rendered.[2,4,20]

This chapter describes the regionalization process, its origins, and its evolution. It includes an approach to the designation of medical facilities within an EMS region. While these processes traditionally have begun at a local level, it is anticipated that states will likely enact minimum standards for EDs and SRCs. In a perfect world, the state standards will mirror the locally developed standards that are the basis for the designation guidelines in this chapter, and which are also reflective of the current criteria recommended by national professional organizations.

Historical Background

Regionalization accomplished through designation requires changes on the part of providers and, if an authorized lead agency is not already identified, it also requires enactment of state or municipal laws. For example, in New York State in 1981, facilities in half of the EMS regions were categorized based on guidelines established by the State EMS Council without formal state authority.[18] Since there was no legal authority to designate facilities, the process relied on voluntary participation that was uneven in some regions and nonexistent in others.[16,21]

Without an authorized lead agency to carry out the process, the risk of legal challenges increases since designation often creates de facto monopolies by restricting the number of facilities allowed to participate and by requiring that certain standards of care be met prior to participation.[7,19] In the absence of explicit authority, the designation process may be impeded by physicians, hospitals or other special interest groups.

Initially, the need for explicit authority to designate was not adequately addressed by the EMS system program planners and this shortfall was compounded by the lack of federal funding for upgrading hospital facilities. Individual hospitals were relied upon to make costly improvements on a voluntary basis.[16] Since it was thought that designation of trauma centers would promote the development of regionalized EMS systems, attempts were often made in the 1970s to organize EMS systems around trauma center development.[2]

Under these circumstances, local EMS system program development usually focused on SRCs and rarely on EDs. This approach produced false starts and unbalanced results stemming from the failure to upgrade general emergency care capabilities, as well as from an over concentration on trauma care; when the trauma center process collapsed, so often did EMS system development. Many of the SRC problems were caused by the relaxation of the original strict criteria recommended by the ACS and the premature development of Level II (area) trauma center designations. The competition for designation as Level II centers among smaller community hospitals and the resulting litigation effectively halted development of the designations process in many areas.[24]

Awareness of potential adverse economic effects, mainly the loss of patients by those institutions not designated, occasionally resulted in resistance by hospital administrators and physicians to both categorization and designation. In fact, less than 10% of all trauma patients actually required trauma center care; therefore, the actual loss of patients from non-designated hospitals was minimal.[16] In reality, most trauma center program failures have been attributed to the financial burden caused by the large numbers of uninsured or indigent patients brought to the centers.[34,35] Other factors that act as economic disincentives to continued trauma center participation are the low rate of diagnosis related group reimbursement for trauma care, the increasingly high cost of malpractice insurance premiums, and the perceived increased liability risk to physicians associated with the provision of trauma care.[23,25,35]

EMS systems development is much more difficult when there is fragmentation of authority or no authority for facility designations and regionalization. Legally authorized lead agencies are important since usually they may plan, implement, and operate, without serious legal challenge.[3,26,28] A branch of government with legislative authority to designate is the best suited to serve as the lead agency. Since state government is responsible for setting medical facility reimbursement rate schedules,[21] ideally the designation authority will be with a state agency. Colorado and Pennsylvania utilize an independent foundation for trauma center designation. The effectiveness of such an approach has not yet been fully determined; however, that approach should be followed carefully by system medical directors in other states.

When federal EMS systems funding effectively ended in 1982, program initiatives and necessary legislative changes became the responsibility of individual states. Those responsible for developing or managing EMS systems found that in the absence of both the carrot of federal money and the stick of legal authority, plans for regionalization through facility designation usually failed.

Unauthorized designations expose agencies to antitrust liability. Explicit statutory authority affords the greatest protection against exposure to risk of liability for violation of the Sherman Act when limitations are made on the number of medical facilities used by a system.[32] In Huron Valley Hospital Inc *v.* City of Pontiac the court held that " . . . (State) regulatory actions within the gambit of valid legislation . . . are exempted from the antitrust laws under the 'state action' defense." Proper authorization to designate granted to an agency that enforces state policies through activities closely supervised by state officials would not violate antitrust laws. However, "anything short of properly constituted authority, may run afoul of federal law. To avoid such antitrust problems, the proper authority must perform hospital designation."[19] Although the law is unsettled nationally, it would appear that, in the absence of definitive court decisions or express legislative authority, governmental agencies with 'implied' powers may be considered to be outside of the scope of the antitrust laws.

The system medical director will undoubtedly face the situation where hospitals "self-designate" as trauma, eye trauma, or hernia centers, and then request the delivery of certain types of patients. This problem is best faced with a united physician community. Other than trauma centers, the SRC designations are often not competitive, although in the future more favorable reimbursement programs for specific medical problems may encourage medical centers to competitively develop SRCs dealing with those specific problems.

Public Law 101-590

The enactment in November 1990 of the Trauma Care Systems Planning and Development Act (PL 101-590) the establishment of a federal trauma systems program.[14] However, the 1990 Act, which was supposed to provide grants to states for planning, implementing, and developing comprehensive trauma systems, was not funded when enacted. In November 1991, funding finally was authorized to implement a new federal trauma systems program for 1992 totalled only $5 million. This amount was well below earlier projections, which were as high as $75 million in 1989.[15,27]

PL 101-590 had two primary goals. First, it was designed to remove the barriers and rectify the problems that in many parts of the country prevented timely and efficient EMS from being provided. Second, it provided incentives for states and localities to establish coordinated regionalized trauma care systems that would enable severely injured individuals to receive timely and highly specialized care.

Passage of PL 101-590 ratified the widely held belief that regionalized trauma systems reduced death and disability from trauma. Regionalized trauma care systems were models of health care delivery that could coordinate and integrate prehospital services and hospital resources to assure that optimal care was provided to traumatically injured patients. The 1990 legislation specified that such systems must identify and designate trauma centers with specialized physicians and equipment immediately available on a 24 hour basis. Also required were methods to identify severe trauma victims in the prehospital phase and to ensure that all major trauma victims were transported to trauma centers.

PL 101-590 addressed the issue of authority, effectively diminishing the threat of legal challenges to development and implementation of designation schemes. However, while the threshold issue of legal authority to designate was resolved, the financial burden caused by the large numbers of uninsured or indigent patients brought to designated facilities, along with inadequate reimbursement rates, still presented a great barrier to regionalization.[34,37]

A May 1990 Senate committee report addressing the Emergency Medical Services and Trauma Care Improvement Act revealed that since 1987 many urban trauma systems were threatened by total collapse because of financial losses. The Senate report used the following examples[29]:

- An estimated 20 designated trauma centers had withdrawn from regional trauma systems.
- Inadequate funding of trauma centers resulted in seven level II centers dropping out of the Dade County trauma systems, leaving Jackson Memorial Hospital as the county's only remaining trauma center.
- The Los Angeles trauma system was on the verge of collapse after 11 of the city's 23 trauma centers dropped out because of high uncompensated costs.
- Huntington Memorial Hospital in Pasadena had lost $3.7 million in 1989 and had withdrawn from the system.
- San Diego's trauma system reported a loss of $6.8 million for 1988 for its six designated trauma centers.
- Four out of ten trauma centers in Chicago had dropped out of the system.
- Houston's Hermann Hospital, one of only two level I trauma centers in that city, had withdrawn after losing more than $7 million.
- The MedSTAR Trauma Center at the Washington Hospital in Washington, DC reported losses totalling $8.9 million in 1989 attributed to providing care to trauma and burn victims.

The committee reported the financial strains caused by undocumented persons requiring health and social services in counties that border Mexico. Many trauma centers located in border counties experienced serious financial losses because of the large numbers of undocumented persons needing trauma care. The report stated that "thirteen trauma centers in these areas incurred $8.2 million of bad debts in 1989 as a result of treating seriously injured patients who were undocumented." Additionally, the committee report discussed the findings of a 1989 review conducted by the Office of Technology Assessment (OTA) on rural EMS and trauma care needs that noted that not all states had developed EMS systems extending into rural areas. The report detailed the fact that rural EMS systems lacked adequate numbers of trained personnel, universal coverage by a communications network, and overall systems development. Serious injuries, according to the report, posed special problems to rural communities: "Injury related morbidity and mortality are often higher than in urban areas because of the time delays in reaching trauma victims on isolated roads, homes, or farms. The chance of a severely injured individual dying in a rural area is three to four times higher than in urban areas." The OTA report concluded that "EMS systems that integrate all levels of hospital care within a state promote regionalization and are likely to improve rural trauma patient outcomes."[29]

Another development in the late 1980s was the systems analysis demonstrating improved outcome in trauma systems. Initially, in Orange County, and more comprehensively in San Diego County and in other states, data were collected that demonstrated that a systems approach to trauma dramatically reduced the preventable death rate after implementation.[36] Components of successful system implementation were identified; and in the National Highway Safety Traffic Administration (NHSTA) a technical assistance program was developed that could advise states, compare progress with ten system standards, and make recommendations for change or improvement. Approximately 40 states have gone through this consultation process.

A 1986 document, "States Assume Leadership Role in Providing Emergency Medical Services" produced by the General Accounting Office (GAO) was requested by Senators Cranston and Kennedy. It was to review and analyze the levels of support and proficiency of EMS systems throughout the county following the 1981 repeal of the PL 93-154. The GAO found that[29]

> although many states were assuming a more active leadership role in financing and regulating emergency medical services, there were areas in which gaps in emergency medical services remained and in which federal actions and leadership were desirable.

It made specific recommendations for Congressional action in these areas. Among other things, the GAO found that (1) many states lacked access to the most timely information about EMS developments; (2) many states lacked coordination between agencies with oversight of funds for EMS activities, such as state transportation and EMS agencies; (3) the 9-1-1 emergency telephone number was not uniformly available, particularly in rural communities; (4) the unavailability of funds for the start up and operating costs of a 9-1-1 system was a major barrier to 9-1-1 implementation; (5) overcrowded radio frequencies and outmoded equipment hampered effective and efficient operation of EMS systems; and (6) economic and political factors were preventing the development of trauma services.

In addition, it noted that (1) trauma systems can reduce the trauma death rate by as much as 64%; (2) in the District of Columbia, a 50% reduction in trauma deaths over 5 years has been credited to the development of a trauma care system; and (3) a study of the San Diego trauma system showed that the trauma death rate fell by 55% after the implementation of a trauma care system. The report concluded, in part, that "the failure of many states and local communities to designate trauma centers to care for the most critically injured patients resulted in unnecessary death and permanent disability.[29]

PL 101-590 provided grants to states for development, implementation and monitoring of state-wide trauma systems. The trauma care component included the designation of trauma care regions and centers. The trauma care system concept was premised on the belief that victims of severe trauma require special care and, as a consequence, they were to be transported to designated trauma centers, bypassing the close emergency departments.

In 1992, 26 states were awarded grants adjusted to population and geographical size. The grant program requirements included submission by the state of yearly trauma system plans that took into account guidelines developed by the ACS, the American College of Emergency Physicians, and the American Academy of Pediatrics. While the law specifically provided that grant funds could be used to reimburse designated trauma centers for uncompensated care, the first round of awards did not allow for the funding of uncompensated care. In addition, the law authorized the Secretary of Health and Human Services to (1) establish an information clearinghouse to disseminate information on the experience of state and local agencies with respect to trauma care system development and operation; (2) establish an Advisory Council on Trauma Care Systems to conduct needs assessments on a country wide basis; and (3) establish funding for research and programs that seek to improve rural EMS. In early 1993 there was progress being made in each of those areas.[14]

After more than 25 years of advocacy to enact legislation that would fully address trauma program concerns such as authority, standards, and national coordination, the passage and funding of PL 101-590 was enthusiastically greeted by most of the health care establishment. Unfortunately, enthusiasm has been greatly tempered by an economically constrained environment in which this legislative action is able to attract only token funding. Advocates of trauma care systems are inevitably left with the impression that the 1990 law was meant more to tantalize than to fulfill. The task ahead is to increase federal funding in the long term and to find ways to maximize the benefits of the 1990 Act and the 1991 amendments in the short term.

Increased funding will benefit EMS systems in general since grants may be used to support rural emergency medical services systems, recruit and train EMS personnel, improve communications equipment relating to EMS, improve transportation services for medical emergencies, and conduct public education activities concerning prevention.

A Method for Designation

The mechanism for implementation of designations of medical facilities suggested in this chapter is generic. Although there are other approaches, this general method has been used successfully at local, county, and state levels.

Designations of receiving hospitals and SRCs may occur simultaneously. While designating receiving hospitals is a much more time-consuming process, it is politically easier since the number of designated facilities does not usually need to be limited.

Once an authorized lead agency has been identified, the designation planning process can begin. Planning issues that must be addressed are the development of prehospital triage and transport criteria, hospital care standards, and methodologies for determining geographic locations of SRCs. Additionally, local advisory committees should be drawn from the local medical community to formulate recommendations on all of the above issues.

While all general hospitals may not have services for all categories of patients (for example, psychiatric or obstetric), the EDs of the designated receiving hospitals should be capable of the "initial evaluation, resuscitation and stabilization" of virtually all medical and psychiatric emergencies.[16] Ideally, all of the general hospitals in the jurisdiction are measured against standards of care; those institutions meeting the criteria are offered designation as receiving hospitals for the EMS system. However, the number of SRC designations within each category may need to be limited, since the number of patients may be too diluted to allow the appropriate level of experience and expertise to develop. Decisions to omit "qualified" facilities from a given system are based on the degree of compliance with standards, demographic considerations, and geographic locations.

SRC designations may be made in a number of clinical areas. While all but the most rural EMS systems can usually identify a trauma center, in some areas even trauma center designations may not be available within the geographical area of the local system and may fall to a single statewide center. The following are types of SRCs that may be designated:

1. Trauma
2. Burn
3. Hyperbaric medicine
4. Replantation
5. Venomous bite
6. Spinal cord
7. Neonatal
8. Eye
9. Behavioral
10. Pediatric burn
11. Pediatric trauma
12. Poison

For an institution to pursue SRC designation, the preexistence of a relatively highly developed clinical program is usually necessary to justify the further assembling and organizing of resources needed to meet the required standards. Occasionally, hospitals will attempt to develop a clinical expertise de novo so as to pursue a system designation. This approach is difficult and expensive for the institution. It also tends to create problems for those responsible for the designation process.

An Approach to Implementation

Traditionally, the first two tasks accomplished are (1) the development of categorization guidelines that the facilities use to make self-assessments of their emergency care capabilities, and (2) the formal categorization of facilities. The next step after categorization is to determine the types of SRCs needed for a comprehensive EMS system in the given jurisdiction. In the absence of state minimum standards for EDs and SRCs, local minimum standards are generally developed, based on national professional organization criteria and modified by local medical group consensus.

Once standards of care are established, all medical facilities in the jurisdiction are invited to submit letters of intent to apply for specific designations. The lead agency announces a Request for Proposals (RFP) to meet the standards and the designation policies that detail overall responsibilities of a designated facility. The EMS staff screens the submitted proposals in order to identify applicants that meet the basic parameters required for a site audit. If the RFP minimum requirements are not met, the proposal may either be rejected or the applicant may be asked to submit additional evidence of compliance. Proposals that meet the entry level criteria are then analyzed to determine compliance with all of the standards prior to conducting a site audit. The audit team, usually consisting of local experts, verifies the information submitted in the proposal. An EMS advisory committee reviews the audit results and recommends the institutions that can be considered for designation.

The lead agency medical director should retain the authority to select an adequate number of appropriate institutions from among those in compliance with standards. For example, in the case of trauma centers, designation determinations from among "qualified" institutions may be based on the local incidence of trauma and acceptable transport times for trauma patients. In the case of receiving hospitals, limiting participants is usually neither necessary nor advisable.

Following designation, a contract is executed between the system and each SRC or receiving hospital. The contract should be reviewable after a stated time period and must include the rights and duties of the parties. The lead agency should have the legal right to verify facility compliance with standards without notice. All policies and procedures, including a hearing and appeals mechanism for revocation of designation, should be clear.

The system must monitor both compliance by the designated facility with care standards and by the prehospital providers with the field protocols. Additionally, it is necessary to continually reevaluate the medical care provided by system participants on an outcome basis. Results of ongoing clinical studies should be reviewed for indications that adjustments to the structure or operation of the system are necessary. To confirm compliance with standards, a redesignation process should occur every 2 to 3 years. The evaluation results are considered by the various advisory groups when redesignation recommendations are made.

The Role of Medical Oversight

Regardless of whether statutory authority to designate medical facilities is vested in a governmental, a quasigovernmental, or a nonprofit agency, the role of the EMS system medical director in the implementation of regional designations is critical and complex. Specifically, the medical director must integrate both the administrative and medical aspects of the process at each stage leading to implementation. Following implementation, the medical director must focus on system evaluation to assure the continued provision of timely, high quality patient care and must also serve as the spokesperson for the medical aspects of the system.

When responsibility for medical facility designation is at the state government level, the regional or local medical director must still systematically link the prehospital care components of the system (education, protocols, transportation, and communications) with the statewide hospital and SRC designation process.

The medical director of a local system that has legal authority to designate should rely on consensus medical expertise provided by an EMS advisory committee before and after implementation. The advisory committee, knowledgeable about general and specific emergency conditions, continues to develop recommendations for the system including (1) prehospital triage, treatment and transport; (2) hospital care; and (3) number, location, and level of designated system hospitals.[5] Additionally, the committee reviews the applications that are submitted by designation applicants. Designation recommendations are then made to the medical director based on the degree of compliance with the standards and in the case of SRCs, on the geographic and demographic considerations. If, for political reasons, the system simply designates all the satisfactory SRC proposals, there is a risk, especially for trauma centers, that the resulting network will be unworkable.

The medical director's involvement during the initial review process is generally limited to assuring that it progresses based on strict medical standards with as little political interference as possible.[5] The medical director should only become directly involved when the final selection of acceptable facilities occurs. Facility selections and distribution of patient triage and transportation guidelines are accomplished simultaneously by the medical director in accordance with the overall system plan.

Summary

Generally, all receiving hospitals that meet the standards are designated; however, only enough satisfactory SRCs to meet the projected needs of the system should be initially designated. The continuing commitments of the institutions (compliance with standards) and of the prehospital providers (adherence to patient triage and transport guidelines) must be monitored by the medical director in the same way as direct patient care. PL 101-590 and its amendments will allow EMS systems without trauma programs to initiate them in the near future. It may be possible to "piggyback" designations of other facilities onto the revitalized process.

REFERENCES

1. Bern Al: *Categorization.* In: van de Leuv JH, editor: *Manage-ment of emergency services,* Rockville, Md, 1987, Aspen.
2. Boyd DR and Cowley RA: *Approach to the care of the trauma patient.* In: Boyd DR, Edlich RF, Micik S, editors: *Systems approach to emergency medical care,* Norwalk, Conn, 1983, Appleton-Century-Crofts.
3. Boyd DR: *The history of emergency medical services (EMS) systems in the United States of America.* In: Boyd DR, Edlich RF, and Micik S, editors: *Systems approach to emergency medical care.* Norwalk, Conn, 1983, Appleton-Century-Crofts.
4. Cales RH: *Concepts.* In: Cales RH and Heilig RW, editors: *Trauma care systems: a guide to planning, implementation, operation, and evaluation,* Rockville, Md, 1986, Aspen Publications.
5. Cales RH: *Medical direction.* In: Cales RH and Heilig RW, editors: *Trauma care systems: a guide to planning, implementation, operations, and evaluation,* Rockville, Md, 1986, Aspen Publications.
6. Cales RH, Anderson PG, and Heilig RW: Utilization of medical care in Orange County: the effect of implementation of a regional trauma system, *Ann Emerg Med* 14:853-858, 1985.
7. Chayet NL and Reardon T: *Legal issues.* In: Chayet NL and Reardon TM, editors: *Centers and emergency departments,* New York, 1985, Law and Business.
8. Commission on Emergency Medical Services: *Categorization of hospital emergency capabilities,* Chicago, 1971, American Medical Association.
9. Commission on Emergency Medical Services: *Provisional guidelines for the optimal categorization of hospital emergency capabilities,* Chicago, 1981, American Medical Association.
10. Detmer DE et al: Regional categorization and quality of care in major trauma, *J Trauma* 17:592-599, 1977.
11. Emergency Medical Service System Act of 1973: Law of the 93rd Congress, Public Law 93-154, Washington, DC, 1973.
12. Emergency Medical Service System Act of 1976: Law of the 94th Congress, Public Law 94-573, Washington, DC, 1976.
13. Emergency Medical Service System Act of 1979: Law of the 96th Congress, Public Law 94-573, Washington, DC, 1979.
14. Emergency Medical Services and Trauma Care Improvement Act of 1990: Law of the 101st Congress, Public Law 101-590, Washington, DC, 1990.
15. Esposito TJ, Lazear SE, and Maier RV: *Trauma care systems development: evolution and current trends,* Insert publication.
16. Gann DS (moderator): Panel: Current status of emergency medical services, *J Trauma* 21:196-203, 1981.
17. Gibson G: Categorization of hospital emergency capabilities: some empirical methods to evaluate appropriateness of emergency department utilization, *J Trauma* 18:94-102, 1978.
18. *Guidelines for Emergency Medical Services System Categorization process,* New York, 1981, Emergency Medical Services Council.
19. Heilig RW and Cales RH: *Development.* In: Cales RH and Heilig RW editors: *Trauma care systems: a guide to planning, implementation, operation and evaluation,* Rockville, Md, 1986, Aspen Publications.
20. Heilig RW: *Law.* In: Cales RH and Heilig RW, editors: *Trauma care systems: a guide to planning, implementation, operation, and evaluation.* Rockville, Md, 1986, Aspen Publications.
21. Henry MC and Kresky B: The emergency medical service system in New York State: time for a change, *NY State J Med* 85:2-3, 1985.
22. Huron Valley Hospital Inc *v.* City of Pontiac, 1979 1 Trade Cases/62.520.
23. Jacobs LM: The effect of prospective reimbursement on trauma patients, *Bull Am Coll Surg* 70:17-22, 1985.
24. Kuehl AE: *Coordinating an EMS system: trauma centers and emergency departments.* In: Chayet NL and Reardon TM, editors: *Trauma centers and emergency departments,* New York, 1985, Law and Business.
25. Larsen K et al: Potential impact of the federal prospective payment reimbursement policies on trauma centers (abstract), *Crit Care Med* 12:332, 1984.
26. Micik SH: *Administration and management of EMS system.* In: Boyd DR, Edlich RF, and Micik S, editors: *Systems approach to emergency medical care,* Norwalk, Conn, 1983, Appleton-Century-Crofts.
27. Public Law 102-170, Washington, DC, 1992, Law of the 102nd Congress.
28. Romano TL, Boyd DR, and Micik S: *Medical control and accountability.* In: Boyd, DR, and Edlich RF, and Micik S, editors: Systems approach to emergency medical care, Norwalk, Conn, 1983, Appleton-Century-Crofts.
29. Senate Report No. 101-292, S Rep. No. 292, 101st Congress, 2nd Sess. 1990, 1990 WL 259294 (Leg Hist).
30. Shackford SR et al: The effect of regionalization upon the quality of trauma care as assessed by concurrent audit before and after institution of a trauma system: a preliminary report, *J Trauma* 26:812-820, 1986.
31. Statutes 1 and 2 of Sherman Act, 15 U.S.C. Statutes 1 and 2.
32. Tortella BJ and Trunkey DD: Hospital care. In: Cales RH and Heilig RW, editors: *Trauma care systems—a guide to planning, implementation, operation and evaluation,* Rockville, Md, 1986, Aspen.
33. Uhlar B: Congress addresses trauma network problems, *Hospitals* October 1987.
34. Wallace C: Trauma centers struggling in Los Angeles, Miami, Modern Health Care, July 1987.
35. West JG et al: Trauma systems: Current status—future challenges, *JAMA* 259:3597-3600, 1988.
36. West JG, Cales RH, and Gazzangia AB: Impact of regionalization: the Orange County experience, *Arch Surg* 118:740-744, 1983.
37. Whalar B: Congress addresses trauma network problems, *Hospitals* October 1987.

Epilogue

Alexander E. Kuehl, M.D., M.P.H., FACS

In May of 1989 when the Epilogue of the original text was written, the following four megatrends were discussed as forces that would likely influence EMS in the 1990s:

1. Increased availability of dramatic new technologies.
2. Increased demand for cost efficient *and* medically proven interventions.
3. Increased debate concerning the need for and the role of medical oversight.
4. Continued paradoxical resistance to innovation.

Since those megatrends did not appear to summate in a single vector, we also predicted friction and heat, ultimately to be followed by significant and perhaps cataclysmic changes in prehospital health care delivery. Allow us now to review and to reframe those original four; and to then examine four other trend possibilities for the rest of the millennium:

5. Expanded areas of operational responsibility for medical oversight.
6. Consolidation of EMS activities.
7. More aggressive preparation for catastrophic incidents.
8. Even more friction, heat and cataclysmic change.

Technological Opportunities

Few of us recognized the speed with which the automated external defibrillator (AED) would sweep into and alter our profession; even fewer fully comprehended how rapidly every level of prehospital provider would be given the device and that the entire prehospital approach to the early treatment of sudden cardiac arrest would be changed. We watched in awe as long-standing and restrictive state laws, rules, and regulations simply evaporated in the face of overwhelming provider and consumer demand. As a result of the introduction of the AED, the number of potential EMS system configurations expanded exponentially. New technologies will likely favor specific operational configurations; the evolutionarily favored configurations will be those that are most efficient.

The American Heart Association Statement on Early Defibrillation, written in June 1991, encouraged all EMS responders and vehicles to carry the AED. While early CPR and ACLS are still important, the role of traditional prehospital ACLS as provided by most existing EMS systems must be completely reevaluated with regard to operational objectives, clinical interventions, achievable response times, and logical educational requirements. In reality, if a reliable AED had existed in the late 1960s when the early EMS physicians first took the hospital coronary care unit to the patient, paramedicine, as we currently know it, would never have been invented. Cardiac rhythm recognition and therefore the understanding of cardiac pathophysiology would not have been critical educational objectives.

Another device rapidly spreading throughout the prehospital arena is the pulse oximeter. While its emergency assessment and operational values are impressive enough, it is astounding that the amount of education necessary to put this device reliably, meaningfully, and competently in the hands of all levels of prehospital providers is but a tiny fraction of a standard paramedic curriculum.

Additional technological "future shocks" can be expected throughout the entire decade. How long will it be before an automated venous cannulator (AVC) is marketed? How would an AVC change the practice of prehospital medicine? Already there are airways available that are said to be essentially impossible to use incorrectly. The combitube and AED have been joined to create an entirely new and very efficient universal provider in the province of Quebec. Following such rapid technological developments the only limitations to their clinical proliferation will be the costs of equipment, education, and personnel. While the evaluation and the adoption of new technologies will remain functions of medical oversight, based on our experience with the AED no medical director will be able to stop the routine implementation of cost efficient and medical proven technology.

Increased Requirements for Cost-Efficient and Medically Proven Technology

Although Wall Street did not actually stumble until October 1987, as early as June 1986, looming governmental budget deficits were already a concern for some of the more pessimistic and contemplative EMS medical directors. Since then, most of us have experienced significant budget reductions, painful personnel cutbacks, and severe downward revisions of capital spending plans. With few jurisdictional exceptions, the absolute financial barriers to improved or expanded EMS services have never been greater.

The phenomenally rapid incorporation of AED into our routine prehospital practice was used earlier as an example of the first megatrend; however, it is perhaps an even better example of this second megatrend. The coupled observations that AED is not yet a universal intervention at the First Responder level and that often AED manufacturers must actually assist local systems with the fundraising efforts to sell them crystalize the incredible financial difficulties that currently entangle most systems.

The requirements to prove economical efficiency and clinical efficacy have surged even more dramatically than we predicted in the First Edition; it is likely that they will become even stronger forces. The *current* conventional wisdom in health care is that efficiency, quality care, and customer satisfaction are mandatory by-products of managed care and managed competition; however, in the coming health care environment, the *new* conventional wisdom will be aggressive cost cutting through competition. Unless there is both political and medical consensus, coupled with a real willingness by government to forgo financial support of other deserving and demanding public services, budget directors will simply "just say no" to all unrequired or unproven medical technologies and health service enhancements. EMS is in unrestrained competition with all the other public safety and public health services; it is even in competition with emergency medicine. Make no mistake, most EMS leaders are in the classically awkward political posture of pursuing a larger percentage of a shrinking budget. Of course, this problem is not limited to EMS. Our entire health care system is a runaway train careening down a steep incline; EMS is simply the caboose. The question is not if but rather when the train will plummet off the tracks. Historically, seconds before such an economic derailment, there occurs a political and sometimes cataclysmic solution; however, the solution probably will not appear in the form of a new tax-supported government program. Rather, it will spring from the purchasers of health care, that is, the employers who have been in managed competition for years. They simply will offer Brand X-managed health care, take it or leave it. Whatever the new vehicle and even if there is no new vehicle for the near term, every new clinical addition will have to be proven both medically superior and cost-effective.

Advantages of scale, especially in purchasing, and medically approved clinical pathways will be two of the engines of managed competition; and expanding the role of the prehospital provider will surely be a third.

Increased Debate About Medical Oversight

With 5 years to reflect, some readers of the First Edition may reasonably point to the prediction of increased debate about medical oversight (other than issues of direct medical control) as incorrect. While there is a modest and continuing debate comparing standing orders with direct medical control, of more significance is the fact that several large urban systems have gone for long periods without permanent medical directors. In some cases the delay was caused by difficulties in adequately defining the structural interfaces among medical directors, administrative leaders, and field providers. There has been more turnover of EMS medical directors in the past 5 years than in the preceding 2 decades; these turnovers are not about personalities, they are about the scope of medical oversight.

While the passionate arguments for total prehospital provider independence from medical oversight are currently in remission, there remains a real potential for a gradual philosophical drift by field providers toward independent licensing and away from traditional "Simon Says" medical command. Paradoxically, the increasing presence of physician responders in the field may encourage that drift just as much as the growth of scientific, professional, economic, and political power by the field providers and their organizations. In some jurisdictions this trend has been accelerated by a flagging of interest in medical oversight by the physician community or by the abdication of medical oversight responsibility to nurses, residents, and field supervisors. If this trend continues, EMS could easily evolve into a concept for which medical oversight, at least in a traditionally structured fashion, is irrelevant. For example, the need for extensive direct medical control has ebbed as many EMS medical directors have become content to rely more heavily on the contemporaneous interpretation of cardiac rhythms by providers and the subsequent use of standing orders, rather than on telemetry and contemporaneous physician direction. There has not been a simultaneous balancing expansion of retrospective indirect medical control.

Paradoxical Resistance to Innovation

If only because of the availability of AED, the past 5 years have been marked by significant clinical and structural innovation in EMS, perhaps more than in the entire previous quarter of a century. These innovations have not been limited to clinical interventions but also include organizational, educational, and administrative advances. But increasingly, these changes may be slowing because of the growing difficulty in proving real relevance, efficiency, and need. Innovation is also waning because of organizational inertia, political ossification, and economic paralysis; EMS gridlock may be upon us. This fourth original trend is one that occurs regularly with the maturation of any human endeavor or body of knowledge; status quo sets in and without strong demands for improved efficiency, legitimate threats of litigation or imminent dangers of economic collapse, little happens. While some of these driving elements are present, the inertia and resistance to change is growing as quickly as is the potential for change.

Perhaps the Clinton administration will create the consensus for useful and necessary change. Traditionally, consensus has not come easily to EMS and it is increasingly apparent that consensus is becoming even more elusive. Therefore relatively predictable and constructive evolutionary progress may not occur; instead there may be sudden massive and disruptive mutations that effectively scramble all the traditional rules. Two extreme possibilities are that EMS, perhaps along with the rest of health care, becomes either a government franchised monopoly or, more likely, an operating component of the handful of surviving vertically integrated national managed care providers.

The resistance to evolutionary change in prehospital care is apparent in national organizations, in governmental bureaucracies, and in the providers themselves. Soon, however, we can expect offers of concessions from the various participants, who will try to "vent off steam" so as to avoid a major "explosion." For example, in some jurisdictions the specter of a new type of prehospital provider delivering primary and preventative care from a mobile unit has caused entrenched EMS providers, who have long fought change, now to offer up sacred cows rather than accept a paradigm shift in their profession. Those who blindly resist the winds of change will have the epitaph "save 911 for *real* emergencies" on their gravestone.

Across the country, fire services that avoided EMS involvement for centuries are now embracing this *other* lifesaving role with a passion driven by fewer fires and less money.

New Operational Foci for the Medical Director

A new and fifth megatrend will be increased interest by medical oversight in certain specific operational activities. The first two are the call receiving and dispatching phases of EMS. These aspects of the EMS response have already altered how the public views EMS and how we examine ourselves. The importance of these two inextricably linked phases of the EMS response were recognized and highlighted in the early 1980s; however, they were never packaged together in a fashion that could influence more than a single EMS system at a time. Today, fully integrated call receiving, prearrival instructing, and priority dispatching programs are being implemented rapidly, similarly, and simultaneously in at least three languages.

Another operational activity that the next decade will emphasize is that of the First Responder. This role is rapidly expanding; appropriately, First Responders are being incorporated within the authority of the EMS system administrator and of medical oversight. There is an obvious synergy with the advances in emergency medical dispatching; well-structured and medically approved dispatch and prearrival instructions, coupled with the availability of devices such as the AED, combitube, and pulse oximeter, greatly expands the potential role of the inexpensive first responder. Since the initial education and continued training requirements of First Responders are minute when compared to those required of paramedics, innovative medical oversight, conscientious providers, and responsive government will soon accept the First Responder as an essential fundamental building block of EMS. When that happens, a quarter of a century of preoccupation with federally approved ambulances and nationally certified providers thankfully will come to a close.

Within the first few months of 1993 there were outcries across the EMS spectrum focusing illumination and attention on those two "dirty little secrets" surrounding vehicle operations, use of lights-and-siren, and ambulance accidents. There is an epidemic of inappropriate behavior with regards to ambulance operations; it will take the combination of administrative responsibility, medical oversight and personnel education to establish our credibility in this area. The role of medical oversight will be to define when, if ever, providers can bend or break the automotive laws. Since the consequences of such actions are immense, the exceptions will be few.

The continued use of our current highly trained paramedics may become financially prohibitive, unless their roles can be expanded to increase patient access or to reduce patient care cost. For example, if paramedics could give tetanus toxoid for a puncture wound and then leave the patient at home with access to appropriate follow up, that would be very cost efficient, as long as the additional expenses for education and employment did not surpass the savings. Medical oversight must lead the way.

Lastly, EMS must finally create for its providers an educational and operational continuum that simultaneously provides personal, professional, and clinical advancement, so that our providers can follow an individualized lifelong progressive pathway of continuous enrichment and meaningful contribution. For this to occur, all future national provider levels must be established as practical educational and operational floors and not as either ceilings or as wishful optimals. The graduation to a more advanced clinical level should represent traditional educational success and operational expansion; the advance would simply reflect the attainment of a temporary plateau that is recognized nationally, mainly for reasons of reciprocity.

Greater Consolidation

This sixth megatrend is much more nebulous and more complicated than the editor would like. For years there has been a glacial shift towards the public utility and privatized models of EMS. That shift will continue and those models will thrive in a managed care environment. While it is possible that in some jurisdictions an existing public safety or public health agency provider will become the most economically efficient and therefore the surviving provider, it is more likely that a private-public monopolistic partnership will develop. However, even in a continued pleuralistic EMS system, there will be consolidations of administrative, operational and medical oversight.

There may be a problem caused by these consolidations. Throughout the history of medicine, and more recently in the EMS arena, the marketing, educational, research and clinical components of health have been financially intertwined. The use of thrombolytics for myocardial infarction, the implementation of AED are examples where a new technology led to expansion and profits in many areas of the health care industry. However, consider the example of the simple development of an EMS provider curricula. Sponsoring organizations, authors, textbook publishers, course educators, college administrators, government bureaucrats, and training equipment manufacturers all have financial interests, some not so obvious, in expanding potentially profitable markets by orchestrating the establishment of national standards of provider curricula, equipment and operational levels. As we look back, locally developed and implemented EMS with all its inherent inertia and inefficiencies may be preferable to national EMS standards with all their interlocking corporate, organizational, educational and financial linkages.

A rapid national acceptance and implementation of competitive managed care programs as cost saving devices will initially force efficiencies and price reductions on existing individual EMS providers. Quickly, however, these EMS providers will be fully integrated with every other part of health care into large managed care conglomerates. By the end of the millennium there may be fewer than a dozen ambulance providers nationwide. Even sooner, there will be *no* incentive to perform any intervention or service unless it reduces the overall cost of caring for the patient. There will be no monetary credit for better than average quality, for high patient satisfaction, or for performing lots of high cost services. As an example, the use of a cardiac monitor on a routine call will not generate any increased revenues, only increased expenses; systems that are all paramedic will lose their current reimbursement advantages. In fact, in the future, it may not be cost effective to use paramedics at all, unless they can be shown to lower total annual health care costs through an expansion of their function that somehow keeps patients well.

More Aggressive Preparation for Catastrophic Incidents

The seventh megatrend may be influential in cutting the Gordian Knot that the confluence of the first six megatrends threatens to create. Gradually, the leaders of prehospital, emergency, and disaster medicine are beginning to cooperate in the delivery of a simple message. The message is that EMS systems must organize within themselves and within the entire national health care grid to efficiently prepare for the prevention of, the mitigation of, and the response to medically catastrophic incidents. In large part, that growing awareness is based on the fact that during the initial months of the Desert Shield/Desert Storm operation, local EMS agencies found major tasks and impossible responsibilities inappropriately and unexpectedly thrust upon them. With time, that particular crisis resolved; however, it is irrefutable that both our civilian and military casualty systems *should* have been capable of a full national mobilization in hours not in weeks.

In September 1992, the natural disasters of Hurricanes Andrew and Iniki etched into the national awareness both the fragile nature of our foothold on this planet and the serious shortcomings of many aspects of the existing national disaster medical response system. The Los Angeles Basin earthquake and the midwestern floods did not allay our concerns. Presumably, our concerns and awareness will lead to an expanded national and international focus on disaster medicine. Unlike the federal EMS legislative actions of 1973, which created dinosaurs that all but perished when the climate changed and federal money disappeared, future organizational and legislative efforts in both prehospital and disaster medicine must focus on creating systems that will adequately function in the present and that will evolve successfully into the future.

While we continue to make the same mistakes at each new potential injury creating event (PICE), there is little doubt the public and political reaction to the failures following Andrew have sent a sharply focused demand for competence from those who will be administratively and medically accountable for the responses before, during, and after the next PICE. In order for the catastrophic event emergency medical activities to function well, local EMS systems must be created that can operate efficiently on a good day.

More Friction, Heat, and Change

The continuing cycle of friction, heat, and eventual cataclysmic change in the EMS arena is the eighth megatrend. To those readers with considerable EMS experience, the friction and heat are easily sensed, although the specific causes may not be altogether obvious. However, the near universality of those two natural by-products of every day EMS activity should now be apparent even to those readers with relatively little real-time experience.

Actually predicting into what EMS will gradually evolve or suddenly mutate is a much more difficult task than simply sensing the friction and heat. Few looking ahead from a vantage point in 1973 would have imagined the current state of prehospital and disaster medicine, much less the evolving revolution in health care. That revolution is accelerating and EMS is changing. The chances for personal success, or even for professional survival, are not particularly great; however, as Louis Pasteur reflected over a century ago, "Chance favors the prepared mind."

To Close

Before decisions and plans can be made and before models can be chosen, the physician responsible for EMS medical oversight must identify the business that he and the EMS system really operate. The business is not simply reducing morbidity and saving lives. At the very least, the medical director is in the business of planning and directing the medical aspects of the entire prehospital service or system.

Even if this text is completely on target and even if all the megatrends converge to present accurate indications of the directions of future change, the EMS medical director must still make rapid and difficult decisions without ever really understanding all the rules or all the implications. No matter what occurs, he must be willing to accept full responsibility.

Ultimately, it becomes incumbent on the medical director to convince society that EMS success is less expensive than EMS failure. A solid understanding and appreciation of the public health model of EMS, which invariably places the good of the many over the good of the few (in contradistinction to either the public safety or the emergency medicine models), is probably the single best compass for those who chose in twilight dim to be teachers, designers, and leaders of prehospital medicine.

Glossary

The glossary is a compendium of terminology commonly used in and by EMS systems; it has been expanded, revised, and reframed since the first edition. Where there exist multiple terms describing the same activity or element, we have chosen the most common or most descriptive term. The consistent and universal use of these definitions will lead to increased terminology standardization, better mutual understanding and, ultimately, the stronger professionalization of our field of endeavor. We realize that our vocabulary and our terminology are fluid, evolving almost as rapidly as our form and our function respond to new problems; therefore, we request that you submit new terms, definitions and usages for inclusion in the glossary of the third edition to:

Alexander E. Kuehl, Editor
Prehospital Systems and Medical Oversight
National Association of EMS Physicians
230 McKee Place, Suite #500
Pittsburgh, PA 15213

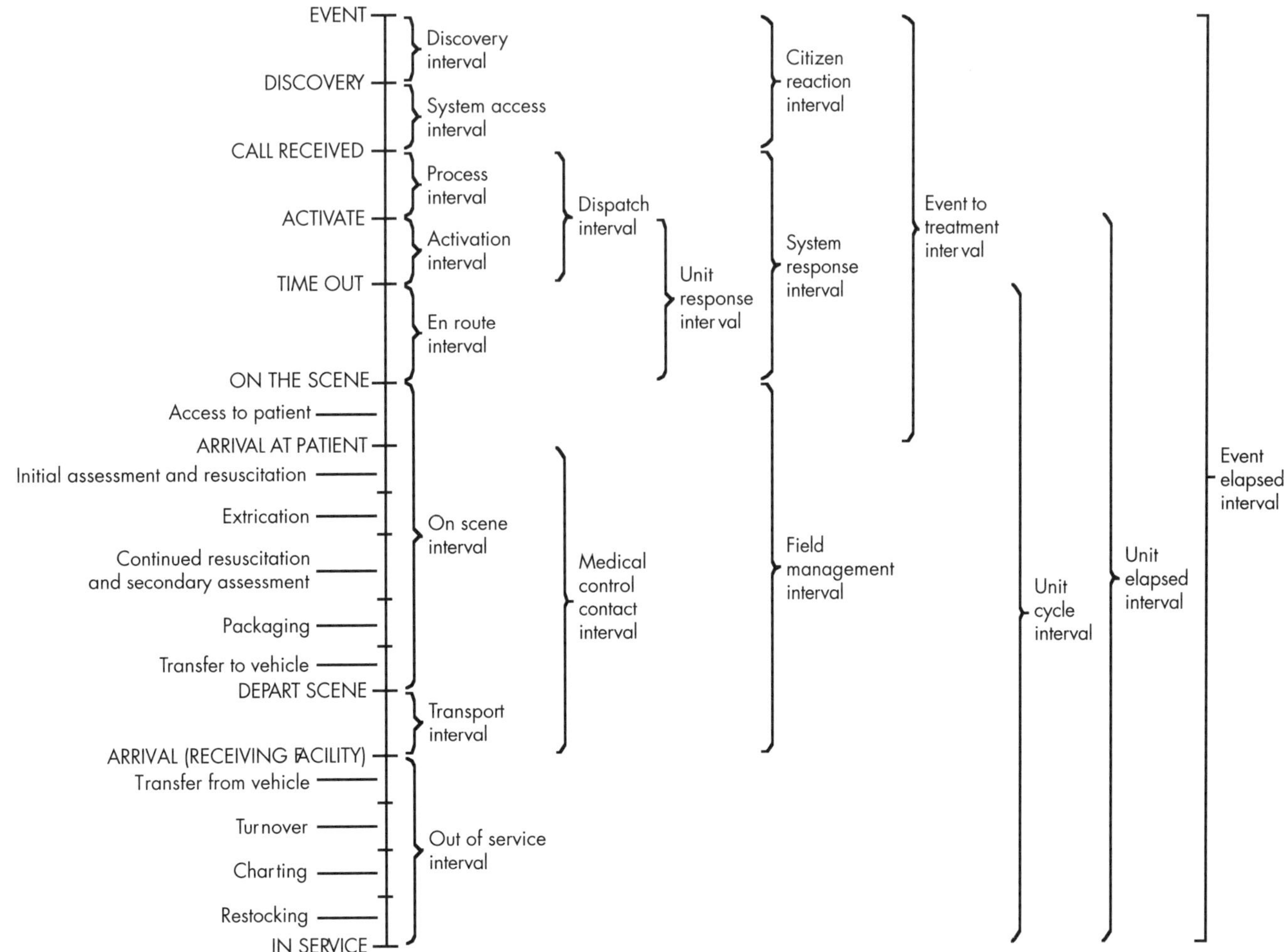

A

Abandonment: The unilateral termination of a patient/care provider relationship by the care provider without an adequate contemporaneous hand-off to another provider.

Access to Patient: The interval from arrival *On the Scene* until *Arrival at Patient* (Fig 1).

Activate: The point when an EMS system begins a standard response to a reported *Event* (Fig 1).

Activation Interval: The time from *Activate* to *Time Out* (Fig 1).

Advance directive: An individual's express advance desire about medical treatment, usually expressed in the form of a living will or durable power of attorney.

Advanced life support (ALS): The unprecise and archaic term to describe the capability of a medical response team to render sophisticated life support procedures beyond basic life support. Traditionally required medical oversight.

Against medical advice (AMA): A phrase used to describe the process and documentation required, when a competent patient refuses offered health care. A standard form which should be signed by a patient when refusing medical assistance.

Air medicine: The study of medicine and physiology in an aviation environment.

Air medical transport: The transport of medical patients by air vehicles.

Air medicine crew (AMC): The members of air medical transport team.

Algorithm: The procedure developed or endorsed by the medical director for prehospital personnel to follow in aid responses.

Allocation: Distribution of finite resources.

AM: Amplitude modulation.

Ambulance: A vehicle certified by federal, state, and local authorities as meeting specifications for transporting and caring for patients. This term generally refers to a wheeled vehicle, but many include boats, planes, helicopters, and other specialized vehicles. A Type I ambulance consists of a truck cab-chassis with a modular body that allows for replacement of the chassis and reuse of the modular body. A Type II ambulance consists of a standard van forward control-integral cab-body unit. A Type III ambulance is a specialty van with forward control and usually with the ability to walk through from front.

Ambulance call report (ACR): A regional name for prehospital care report.

Arrival at Patient: Point when aid team arrives at patient's side, after gaining access, and before initial assessment (Fig 1).

Arrival at Receiving Facility: The point when an EMS unit reaches a receiving facility (most often a hospital) and stops before transferring patient from vehicle (Fig 1).

Associate hospital: A hospital in a designated EMS area, other than the resource hospital, which may on prearrangement with the resource hospital provide medical direction for EMS personnel.

Audio: Pertaining to sounds that can usually be heard by the unaided ear. Usually in the frequency 15 to 20,000 cycles per second.

Autonomy: The person's right to self-determination.

B

Back up: An additional resource, that is, an ambulance or extra personnel available in case the primary resource is unavailable, inappropriate, or inadequate for the situation.

Base communication center: The facility with equipment (radios, antennas, recorders and telephones) and trained personnel to provide community access to the EMS system and ensure communication among the prehospital and hospital components of the EMS system.

Base station: A designated resource responsible for some EMS medical oversight in a defined EMS area. Major functions as delegated by EMS the EMS medical director may include implementing protocols, monitoring compliance (through indirect medical control), offering direct medical control, and providing education to EMS personnel. The base station may be operated from a hospital, which is then referred to as the base station hospital or base hospital.

Baseline bloods: Blood specimens drawn prior to treatment.

Basic life support (BLS): The imprecise and archaic term to describe the EMS procedures (airway positioning, external cardiac compression, and ventilation) to sustain viability of brain and heart in the absence of pulse and/or breathing. The splinting, dressing and other initial care covered in a basic first aid training; traditionally did not require medical oversight.

Beneficence: Acting in the best interest of the patient.

Biotelemetry: The technique of measuring and transmitting physiologic data to a distant terminal, usually the base station or receiving hospital.

Body substance isolation: The procedure of using barriers for self protection when handling blood and body fluids.

Brain death: The cessation of brain stem functions. Also known as biological death.

Break-Break (Breaker): Words used to interrupt ongoing radio communications when another party requests urgent use of that radio net.

Broken up: A term that refers to incomplete understanding of sentences or phrases because of intermittent disruption in communication.

Burn out: A psychological condition caused by various factors with multiple manifestations that results in EMS personnel being unhappy and dissatisfied with their work. A state of fatigue or frustration brought about by devotion to a cause, way of life, or relationship.

Bypass: A regional term for the process by which a hospital requests that an ambulance patient be taken to another hospital; a request that is usually due to a shortage of beds, equipment, or personnel. See Diversion.

Bystander aid: The initial medical assistance provided to a victim by a witness or passerby at the scene of an event.

C

CAD System: A computed aided dispatch system that usually interfaces with enhanced 911 systems and has geo-base verification, and unit recommendation capabilities. More commonly such systems contains a system status management (SSM) program for fluid deployment of resources.

Call: (1) A request for assistance that activates the EMS system. It may come through a variety of mechanisms: voice, regular telephone, 9-1-1, or radio. (2) The overall EMS response best summarized by the events occurring during the Unit Elapsed Interval (Fig 1). May be referred to as run, response, or more properly an incident.

Call Received: The point when an EMS system is first contacted. Ideally, the first ring of the telephone or first call on a radio (Fig 1).

Call receiving operator (CRO): The individual who receives calls for assistance and inputs information for dispatch.

Call screening: The process of determining which requests for assistance require an EMS response, for which a decision is made to provide services, to refuse service, or to refer service to an alternative provider.

Carrier: The microphone of a radio commonly referred to as a hand mike, handset, or mike.

Carrier-open: A term that indicates the microphone is keyed "on."

Case law: A judicial precedent in which an appellate court renders a written decision based on the facts of the specific case as opposed to statutes which establish codifications of law in the abstract.

Categorization: The classification of receiving medical facilities, using standards of medical care, according to emergency medical capabilities. A circular categorization is an agreement between hospitals for providing care and resources. A horizontal categorization indicates the capability of a facility (hospital) to provide general emergency medical care. A vertical categorization indicates the capability of a facility (hospital) to provide special care (for example, burn center, trauma center, and neonatal center).

Central dispatch: (1) An EMS designated mechanism for directing the closest appropriate resources to the scene of a request for assistance. (2) The consolidation of multiple emergency dispatch centers into a single combined dispatch entity.

Centralized medical control: A system wherein all direct medical control, is provided by personnel in the resource center (usually a hospital), often using protocols. The resource center may or may not receive the patients for whom medical control has been provided. Indirect medical control may also emanate from central medical control.

CFR: Certified First Responder

Channel: For EMS this term usually refers to a pair of radio frequencies, one for transmit and one for receive.

Charting: (1) The process of documenting information on ambulance call report (medical incident report). (2) The interval required to complete the prehospital care report, typically occurring after turnover of a patient at the receiving facility (Fig 1).

ChemTrec hot line: A telephone number for chemical industry hazardous material information. (800) 424-9300.

Citizen band (CB): A group of 40 VHF low-band frequencies for use by private citizens.

Citizen Reaction Interval: The time from *Event* to *Call Received.* Includes *Discovery* and *System Access Interval*(Fig 1).

Clinical death: The cessation of respiration with the loss of pulse and blood pressure. (*See also* Brain death.)

Code: (1) Refers to "code status." This term is the process and decision of specifying a patient's legal status and desire for life-sustaining treatment; it is also the process of providing resuscitative measures, that is, cardiac resuscitation (running a code). (2) A commonly used EMS term to describe the nature of a response in relation to use of warning signals and relative urgency of the call. A number accompanying the word refers to the relative priority of the response. Other terms used may include Bell (3 bell, 4 bell). This terminology varies regionally. Some medical directors recommend a "plain language" adaption of a response (for example, transporting a critical patient, transporting a stable patient). Others believe lights and siren should only be used on priority calls, and normal driving without lights and siren should be used at other times. For example, Code 0 includes administrative driving; Code 1 includes routine transport of a stable patient, as in to nursing home (no lights and siren); Code 2 includes using ambulance lights but no siren and driving at normal speed; Code 3 means driving with lights and siren but at normal speed; Code 4 means driving a rapid safe speed with all emergency signaling devices on, in the most expeditious manner (used for such cases as cardiac arrest and shock). Riding HOT means driving with lights and siren, while riding COLD means routine driving.

COLD response: Universal term for emergency vehicle response mode that does not utilize lights and siren.

Common law: Judge-made law; rulings of judicial decisions; also referred as caselaw; a source of law based on custom.

Communication system: A system that links the many interdepartment agencies and facilities involved in emergency response and care.

Computer-aided dispatch (CAD): The process of directing EMS resources to caller locations with the assistance of electronic data concerning system status.

Confidentiality: The assurance that patient information will not be revealed to any source other than those sharing the same duty in the care of the patient.

Continued resuscitation and secondary assess ment: The interval following initial assessment, extrication, and before Packaging (Fig 1).

Coverage: Indicates the geographic area where reliable communications exist. Usually expressed in terms of miles.

Critical incident stress debriefing: The formal decompression and discussion following an emotional EMS event.

D

DAN (Diver's Assistance Network): A telephone number for emergency hyperbaric therapy information. (919) 684-8111.

Dead on arrival (DOA): Patient pronounced deceased shortly after (1) the prehospital providers reach the scene or (2) the ambulance reaches the ED.

Dead spot: An area where radio communications are limited due to geography, terrain, and equipment.

Death: Irreversible cessation of circulatory and respiratory functions or irreversible cessation of all functions of the brain including the brain stem.

Decentralized medical control: A system wherein medical control is provided by more than one resource (hospital) in a designated area. Associate hospitals providing medical control do so by referral or relay, by prearranged agreement and protocol from the Resource Hospital, or upon being called directly by field personnel.

Decibel (dB): A measure of sound intensity.

Dedicated line: A communication system reserved for use specifically from any one resource to another. Generally refers to a reserved telephone line for use between facilities.

Depart Scene: The point when an EMS unit departs from the scene (Fig 1).

Designation: Formally recognizing a resource on its merits including geography, demographics, and capabilities, then permitting it to function within an EMS system.

Direct medical control: (1) The clinical instructions, usually from physicians, or from specially trained medical personnel, to EMS field personnel. This function is delegated by the physician charged with medical oversight. (2) The physician providing immediate and concurrent clinical direction to field personnel.

Disaster: A situation in which the severity of damage or the number of patients exceeds the system's or facility's ability to provide immediate management. Also called a catastrophic event or a PICE.

Disaster plan: Prospective arrangements that are initiated in response to a potentially overwhelming situation.

Discovery: The point when an individual recognizes that EMS assistance is needed (Fig 1).

Discovery interval: The time between *Event* and *Discovery* (Fig 1).

Dispatch: (1) The means by which emergency resources are directed to the scene of an incident or event. (2) The portion of a command center that directs vehicles to a scene.

Dispatch Interval: The time from Call Received until Time Out (Fig 1).

Dispatch priorities: Predetermined, systemized dispatcher interrogation protocols designed to obtain the minimum amount of information necessary to adequately establish the correct level of response and determine the need for prearrival instructions.

Dispatch Time: (1) The interval from when a request for an ambulance is received until the ambulance begins to respond. (2) The time from Call Received to Time Out (Fig 1).

Dispatcher: An individual who alerts an EMS unit to a call for assistance and directs it to the scene.

Diversion: The prefered term for the process of formally directing EMS units to bypass a hospital when the unit has patients for which the hospital is unable to provide optimal care (usually because of an adverse situation, a temporary absence of personnel, needed equipment).

Do not resuscitate (DNR) orders: An order written in a hospital chart by a physician limiting cardiopulmonary resuscitation in the event of arrest. This has recently been expanded in some jurisdictions to encompass portable documents which can be respected by EMS personnel. Also described as do not attempt resuscitation (DNAR) orders.

Down time: The time from a morbid event until resuscitation is begun.

Dual response: A dispatch pattern in which a basic and a more sophisticated EMS team are simultaneously dispatched at the first request for assistance.

Duplex: A radio capable of receiving and transmitting signals simultaneously. This permits information to be sent and received at the same time.

Durable power of attorney: An advance written directive by an individual expressing their desire to have another act as the decision maker in the care they receive if the individual becomes incompetent.

E

Eight hundred (800) MHz: Refers to communication systems using this frequency.

ECG (electrocardiograph or EKG): A visual display of electrical impulses generated by the heart.

EMD: (1) Emergency medical dispatch. (2) Emergency Medical Dispatcher. An individual trained in interrogation techniques, call prioritization and prearrival instructions with a minimum of 24 to 40 hours of training. (3) Electromechanical dissociation.

Emergency rule: Legal and ethical premise which presumes that the patient with a life threatening condition allows the treatment which is necessary to save his or her life.

EMS: Emergency Medical Services. A collective term describing the many agencies, personnel, and institutions involved in planning for, providing, and monitoring emergency care. Frequently refers only to prehospital care.

EMSS: Emergency Medical Services System. Describes the integrated actions of the various EMS components as they relate in a functioning system.

EMT: Emergency Medical Technician. The generic term for any prehospital provider trained to the EMT-A level or above.

EMT-A: Emergency Medical Technician-Ambulance. The original and now obsolete term for EMT-B.

EMT-B: Emergency Medical Technician Basic. A prehospital basic life support care provider with approximately 110 hours of classroom and didactic training based on a national standard training curriculum. Originally referred to as EMT-A.

EMT-D: An EMT who has been taught defibrillation skills, either automated, semiautomated, or manual.

EMT-I: Emergency Medical Technician-Intermediate. An EMT with additional training in one or more advanced methodologies such as intubation and IV access.

EMT-P: Emergency Medical Technician-Paramedic. An EMT with additional training to the full advanced life support level.

En Route: The time when a responder is travelling to or from a scene.

En route Interval: The time from Time Out to On the Scene (Fig 1).

Estimated time of arrival (ETA): The projected moment of reaching a given destination.

Event: A prehospital occurrence, generally considered by an observer or patient to require EMS assistance (Fig 1).

Event Elapsed Interval: The time from Event to In Service (Fig 1).

Event to Treatment Interval: The time from Event until Initial Assessment begins (Fig 1).

Extrication: (1) The process of removing patients from wreckage or other hazardous locations. May require use of special tools and equipment. (2) Extrication; The interval from Initial Assessment and Resuscitation to Continued Resuscitation and Secondary Assessment (Fig 1).

F

False imprisonment: The unjustified detention of a person, so as to substantially interfere with the person's liberty.

Federal Communication Commission (FCC): The United States governmental authority responsible for allocating communication channels and regulating communications systems.

Field: Any locale outside a hospital.

Field Management Interval: The time from On the Scene to Arrival (receiving facility) (Fig 1).

Field release: Non transport situation in which a patient is "released" from the care of EMS provider; the legal authority to detain an adult who is able to make treatment decisions. May also refer to the interaction of the EMS provider with the patient at the scene in which the patient signs a "release" form or waiver form in which the patient releases the EMS provider of liability for the patient's refusal to be transported or treated by EMS provider.

First in: The initially dispatched unit in a tiered response system.

First party caller: A person calling for emergency medical help who is also the patient or victim.

First Responder: (1) The first individual designated to provide medical assistance in an emergency. The degree of training varies by jurisdiction but includes minimum first aid instructions on the airway management, cervical spine control, breathing assistance, circulation assistance, hemorrhage control, and basic patient movement skills. (2) A graduate of a formal approximately 60 hour course in critical emergency medical care. (3) A term that may refer to the first "bystander" or witness to render assistance, no matter what their training. This assistance should more correctly be referred to as bystander aid.

Fixed wing aircraft: Traditional airplanes.

FM: Frequency Modulated. A term referring to radio communications through control of radio wave frequency. Noise and interference are less than in AM (amplitude modulation).

Fourth party caller: A person calling for emergency medical help who is not only remote from the patient but is relaying the information from an associated public safety agency such as a police or fire department dispatchers as well as "medical alert" companies and security dispatcher.

Frequency: The number of cycles per unit of time. Radio frequencies are often measured in megahertz (millions of cycles per second).

Frequency band: A continuous range of frequencies such as VHF low band, VHF high band, and UHF.

G

Garbage: Interference from other radio transmission or electronic interference during a radio communication.

Garbled: A term that describes a radio transmission that is unintelligible or difficult to interpret because of poor transmission or reception.

Geographic assignment: Assignment of a frequency for dedicated use within a geographic area.

GigaHertz (GHz): 1 Billion cycles/second.

Good Samaritan law: A statute that affords immunity to a person who offers assistance to another, without a duty to do so, and without expectation of remuneration. Strictly construed, it does not include the prehospital provider who has a duty to respond or provide care.

Governmental immunity: A statutory provision that prohibits liability for damages where governmental employees, agents, or officers or the governmental entity has been negligent. Generally, such statutes apply only for certain aspects of governmental activities and have exclusions, such as operation of an emergency vehicle and willful misconduct. In addition, claims for violation of constitutional rights also are not effected by immunity provisions.

H

Hand-off: The process of turning the care of a patient over to another appropriately qualified individual. For example, an EMT-B would hand off a patient to another EMT-B, paramedic or physician.

HazMat: Hazardous material.

HEAR: Hospital Emergency Administrative Radio. A VHF communication system for use when telephonic communications are inoperative. Also used for hospital-ambulance communications.

HEMS: Helicopter Emergency Medical Services.

Hertz (Hz): Frequency unit in cycles per second.

Horizontal dispatch: A dispatch configuration where several dispatchers divide individual responsibilities between call interrogation and radio dispatch functions. Also called tandem or team dispatching.

Hospital Time: The interval of time from Arrival at Hospital until Back in Service (Fig 1).

HOT response: Universal term for the emergency vehicle response mode that utilizes red-lights-and-siren; is the current preferred terminology rather than various ten code or code numeric designations. Also referred to as emergency or code response.

Hysteria threshold: The point at which a person changes from hysterical behavior to calm, cooperative action. This threshold varies from individual to individual and may be reached by repetitive persistence.

I

Immunity: An exemption from duties the law generally requires others to perform.

Implementation: The actual use of designated facilities in an organized fashion by an EMS system.

Implied consent: Patient assent to and participation in their care, which notes acceptance of the care.

Indirect medical control: The administrative medical direction of EMS personnel by a physician, usually designated by an medical oversight. This direction includes system design, management, education, critiques and quality assurance. The physician is usually responsible for developing protocols, and medical policies, ensuring compliance, and certifying providers. Some aspects of indirect medical control may be delegated to other physicians or non physicians. Responsibilities may broaden as delegated by medical oversight.

Informed consent: Autonomous decision made by the patient to agree to treatment or intervention after understanding the risks, benefits and alternatives.

Initial Assessment and Resuscitation: Interval from access to patient until either extrication or secondary survey (Fig 1).

Interference: Undesired signals from other radio transmitters or from electromagnetic radiation.

In Service: The point when ambulance and crew are available for appropriate dispatch (Fig 1).

K

Key questions: The predetermined, systemized dispatcher interrogation protocols designed to obtain the minimum amount of information necessary to adequately establish the correct level of response and determine the need for prearrival instructions.

Kilohertz (kHz): 1000 Hertz.

L

Land line: A hand-wired telephone line communication.

Lead agency: The organizational unit established under a federal, state, or regional authority and given the responsibility and authority to plan, implement, evaluate, and generally direct an EMS system.

Lights-and-siren: Using visual and audio warning devices to indicate an emergency vehicle. In some jurisdictions, such use allows traffic laws to be broken.

Living will: An advance written directive by an individual by expressing their desire for medical care if they are no longer competent. The concept is legal in most states.

M

Man down: A generalized dispatch term referring to a request for aid in which the victim has collapsed or fallen for an unknown reason.

Mass casualty incident: An obsolete expression for a disaster. Should not be confused with multiple casualty incident.

MAST: (1) Military Antishock Trousers is the obsolete term for pneumatic anti-shock garment. (2) Military Assistance to Safety and Traffic (military helicopters used by civilian EMS systems).

Maximal response: The credo in public safety agencies that mandates a total HOT initial delivery of resources to the scene.

Mechanism of injury: The exact forces and causes associated with an accident. A serious mechanism of injury, such as a totally wrecked car or a long fall, should be enough indication in and of itself to provide certain care, such as spinal immobilization, even to people who appear initially uninjured.

MEDEVAC: Medical evacuation. Originally used in the military to mean helicopter evacuation, it is now used in civilian settings to refer to any medical evacuation.

Medical command authority (MCA): Direct medical control.

Medical control: The process of performing actions to ensure that care taken on behalf of ill or injured patients is medically appropriate (more appropriately called medical oversight). This includes the prospective, concurrent, and retrospective aspects of EMS and extends to various tasks such as quality assurance, hiring, and education.

Medical Control Contact Interval: The time when direct medical control authority is in contact with prehospital personnel (Fig 1).

Medical Control Terminal Console: A communications device often located in an emergency department for direct medical control of an EMS system.

Medical director: A physician, who by experience or training, handles the clinical and patient care aspects of the EMS system. This position may include one individual with multiple tasks, or several with divided tasks, such as training director, administrative indirect medical control director, clinical direct medical control director, or quality improvement director. There may also be specified state, regional systems, or unit directors.

Medical director (administrative): A physician who has the overall responsibility for quality assurance and control of an EMS service including the physicians providing direct medical control. (See Indirect Medical Control).

Medical director (clinical): The physician who provides effective communication in reference to medical care of patients while the prehospital care is in progress. This physician provides medical orders and scene management orders via radio/telephone to prehospital personnel caring for patients in the field (see Direct Medical Control).

Medical dispatch center: Any agency that routinely accepts calls for emergency medical assistance from the public and/or that dispatches prehospital emergency medical personnel pursuant to such requests.

Medical oversight: (1) The ultimate responsibility and authority for the medical actions taken by a prehospital provider or an EMS system. (2) The physician or medical groups with such authority.

Medical priority dispatch system: A medically approved system used by medical dispatch center to dispatch appropriate aid to medical emergencies, which includes: 1) systematized caller interrogation; 2) systematized Pre-Arrival Instructions; and 3) protocols which match the dispatcher's evaluation of the injury or illness type and severity with vehicle response mode and configuration.

Medical project director: A physician assigned by an EMS authority by the administrative director to direct a specific EMS team. Occasionally used as a term for the physician providing regional medical oversight.

MegaHertz (MHz): One million Hertz.

MICU: (1) Mobile Intensive Care Unit: A specially equipped transport vehicle with sophisticated equipment allowing advanced life support capabilities. (2) A hospital medical intensive care unit.

Mobile intensive care nurse (MICN): A registered nurse with special training in prehospital policies, protocols and procedures. The MICN may have direct and indirect medical care responsibilities. A major role is in answering the radio at the base station, directing field care of patients, and requesting physician consultation as needed. They exist in an official role in only a few states.

Mobile repeater: A fixed transmitter station for relaying and strengthening a transmission from a mobile transmitter.

Mobile transmitter receiver: Vehicle based transmitters/receivers.

Mobile unit: A vehicle. Also a vehicular radio unit.

Multiple casualty incident (MCI): A situation with numerous patients that does not overwhelm the routine capacity of the system.

Multiplex operation: A combination of two or more radio signals for simultaneous transmission on one frequency.

Mutual aid: A term referring to interagency EMS agreements that establish protocols to provide assistance by interacting with other agencies.

MVA: Motor vehicle accident.

N

Negligence: The failure to provide the degree of care (as defined by community or national standard) normally associated with a set of circumstances requiring that care. To establish negligence, the plaintiff must prove four elements: duty to act, breach of that duty, injury, and a clear cause-and-effect relationship between the injury and breach of duty.

Nontransport vehicle: A medical response vehicle that transports medical personnel to the scene of an accident, but is not intended to transport a patient. For example, a rescue vehicle, fire truck, aid car, and a paramedic response unit are all nontransport vehicles.

9-1-1: A telecommunications system devised to centralize and simplify requests for emergency services by channeling all calls to a single 911 number. Calls for true emergencies may then be screened and relayed to appropriate agencies and areas for response.

9-1-1E: 911 "enhanced." A 911 system with computer capability to locate the address and phone number of the originating call, thus allowing more efficient and rapid response to emergency calls.

O

OD: Overdose

Off-line medical control: See Indirect Medical Control.

On-line medical control: See Direct Medical Control.

On-scene Interval: Time from *On the Scene* to *Depart Scene* (Fig 1).

On the scene: The point when an EMS unit arrives (Fig 1).

On your/our own: Driving in routine fashion at normal speed without using warning devices.

Out of Service Interval: The time of Arrival of an ambulance at a receiving facility until the unit is In Service. Includes the turnover of the patient to the hospital staff, charting, and restocking (Fig 1). May also refer to time when a unit is not available because of special situations including mechanical breakdown or personnel breaks.

P

Packaging: (1) Preparing the patient for transfer to a transport vehicle. Includes such tasks as dressing, bandaging, splinting, and immobilization. (2) Interval of time required to package a patient (Fig 1).

Pager: A radio receiving device for alerting personnel, usually by a tone signal.

Paramedic: The generic term for a prehospital care provider with an adequate number of training hours (usually between 300 and 1500 hours) and procedural experience to be certified by local state, and/or national authorities as capable of providing advanced cardiac life support and other medically sophisticated skills.

Paramedic response unit (PRU): A non transporting vehicle used by paramedic providers.

Patch: The process of connecting the communications system of one party into the communications system of another party, usually through a third party such as base station.

Paternalism: Acting according to what the health care provider believes is best for the patient.

Penetration: The ability of a radio signal to go through or around physical obstructions.

Phonetic alphabet: Distinctive words used instead of letters for clarity in radio communication, such as Alpha-A, Bravo-B, and Charlie-C.

Physician option: Possible medical orders from direct medical control, beyond standing orders.

PICE: Potentially injury causing event. A disaster.

Pneumatic antishock garment (PASG): Preferred name for military antishock trousers. A pneumatic counter pressure device applied to lower extremities and abdomen.

Police powers: The power of the state (organized government) to place restraints on the personal freedom and property rights of a person for the protection of public safety, health and welfare or promotion of public good.

Portable transmitter/receiver: A hand carried transmitter/receiver used when away from vehicles. These generally have less power and distance capability than mobile and base transmitter/receiver.

Pre-arrival instructions: Telephone instructions given word for word by trained dispatchers to callers to aid the victim and control the situation prior to arrival of prehospital personnel. They are given from medically approved written protocols.

Prehospital care provider: EMS personnel who are certified and function at any level in actually dispensing prehospital care.

Prehospital care report (PCR): Preferred term for the written documentation of EMS patient contact and assistance. Other names include medical incident report, run report, prehospital care report, patient care report, etc.

Prehospital personnel: Any EMS members, providers of care, or others who are involved in the direct functioning of the EMS system.

Primary Area of Response (PAR): The usual geographic area of responsibility for a specific EMS unit.

Priority dispatch: The process of using a medically approved system to dispatch appropriate aid to medical emergencies, which includes: (1) systematized called interrogation; (2) systematized Pre-Arrival Instructions; and (3) protocols which match the dispatcher's evaluation of the injury or illness type and severity with vehicle response mode and configuration.

Priority system: A spectrum of patient problems that are commonly life-threatening and must be assessed quickly by field personnel. These include abnormal breathing, unconsciousness, chest pain in people of cardiac-disease-susceptible age, dangerous trauma, and dangerous hemorrhage.

Process Interval: The time from Call Received until Activation (Fig 1).

Protocols: Written procedures providing prehospital personnel with a standardized approach to commonly encountered patient problems, thus ensuring consistent care. They may include standing orders to be carried out prior to establishing communication with direct medical control. These procedures usually relate to the assessment, diagnosis, triage, treatment, transfer, and destination of patients.

Push-to-talk: A method of transmission from only one station at a time; the user being required to keep the switch open while talking.

PVC: Premature ventricular contraction.

Q

Quality assurance (QA): The original organized method of auditing, evaluating and improving care provided within EMS systems.

Quality improvement (QI): The concept of a continual cycle of evaluation and improvement.

Quality management (QM): The term embracing and replacing the evolving specific concepts of QA and QI.

R

Radio frequency (RF): A term used in radio communications to designate the cycles per second, or Hertz, for the purpose of identifying specific channels of communications assigned by FCC. Commonly used in EMS are VHF, UHF, and 800 MHz.

Range: The effective transmission distance for radio communication; usually measured in miles.

Rationing: Decisions regarding who will receive aid when there are insufficient resources to care for all in need.

Real time allocations: The sequential assignment of frequencies such as the medical channels as they are needed within a given geographic area.

Receiving center (hospital): A designated medical institution that receives emergency patients under the direction of an EMS system or a base station; usually a hospital.

Refresher course: A standard and often required program to prepare prehospital providers for recertification exams.

Refusal: (1) The ambulance crew member's decision not to provide patient transport. Should involve protocol or a medical decision with the base station supervisor. The decision is based on clinical judgement, community standards, and common sense. (2) The patient's decision not to accept care and/or transport. The patient's mental competence should be evaluated before accepting a patient's refusal.

Recertification: A structured process used to evaluate providers every few years to assure review of skills and maintenance of competency.

RMA: Refuse medical advice or refusal of medical assistance. (See Refusal)

Regionalization: A system that addresses emergency care needs in a defined geographic region through identification and classification of medical resources. It is intended to improve the quality of care in a cost effective way and to facilitate the coordination or handling of responses to emergency medical incidents.

Relay: The rebroadcast of signals by radio station as soon as they are received, enabling transmission of the signal further than could have been accomplished by the originating transmitter.

Relief: New or additional personnel or assistance. The next shift.

Remote center: A facility containing the equipment, personnel, or both to handle EMS communications.

Repeater: A device that relays a radio signal from a transmitter of lower output and transmits it at a higher amplification.

Repeater station: Communications equipment that receives a signal and retransmits it to improve the range and quality of the signal. Generally requires two frequencies, one to receive and one to transmit.

Repetitive persistence: An hysteria controlling technique where the EMD, by repeating in identical phrasing of the same calming message or request, can help most callers regain self control and become able to provide cognate answers on interrogation or deliver prearrival care.

Reroute: A regional term for diversion.

Resource hospital: A hospital in an EMS system that is granted and provides logistical and/or supervising responsibilities for EMS personnel in a geographic area. Often the resource hospital monitors and/or assists direct and indirect medical control functions.

Responder: An individual who assists with scene patient care. May be a citizen trained in first aid and cardiopulmonary resuscitation, or an EMS representative such as a paramedic.

Response configuration: Specific vehicle(s) of varied types, capabilities, and numbers responding to the scene of a medical emergency, also defined as the dispatch priority response assignment.

Response Interval: (1) System - the time from Call Received until EMS vehicle is On the Scene. (2) Unit - the time from Time Out until EMS vehicle is On the Scene (Fig 1).

Response mode: The use of emergency driving techniques, such as lights and siren versus routine driving.

Response zone: Geographical area of service responsibility for a specific EMS unit. Also referred to as primary area of response.

Restocking: (1) The process of refurbishing supplies and preparing equipment after one response and in preparation for another response. (2) The interval required for refurbishing supplies and preparing equipment (Fig 1).

Resuscitation: The combined effect to restore or - maintain ventilation circulation, and/or acceptable physiologic function.

Roger: Radio proword meaning "understood."

Roll: A response by an EMS system to a call.

Rotocraft: Helicopters.

Run: A response by an EMS system to call.

Run review: A quality improvement mechanism that reviews calls for assistance and ambulance requests to determine if proper procedures were followed and proper treatment given. Also referred to as Call Review.

Run tape: A record of audio communication between the field care provider and direct medical control.

S

SAR (Search and Rescue): The initial EMS response where the exact location of the victim is not known.

Saturation: The mobility of an EMS system to respond appropriately to additional requests for assistance.

Say again: Radio proword meaning "Repeat what was just said."

Scene: Geographical area where the event occurred.

Second party caller: A person calling for emergency medical help who is in direct personal contact with the patient.

Simplex: A radio communication system that permits either transmission or reception at any one time.

Skip: The bouncing of signals either off the atmosphere or off buildings causing an abnormal signal projection that may carry great distance and may interfere with radio communications.

Specialty referral center (SRC): A facility dedicated to and recognized as a resource in caring for specific medical problems, such as a trauma center or a burn center.

Squelch: A process or switch used to suppress unwanted noise on a radio frequency.

Stand by: (1) Situation when radio/telephone communication is incomplete and sending party requests receiving party to wait for further information. Similar to wait, wait out, and hold one. (2) Notification from EMS to hospital of the impending arrival of a critical patient.

Standing orders: Instructions approved by medical oversight for prehospital care personnel, directing them to perform certain emergency medical care in the absence of any communication with direct medical control.

Sworn members: Individuals bound by a duly administrated oath to perform actions or powers (e.g., police powers) faithfully and truly.

System Access Interval: The time from Discovery until Call Received (Fig 1).

System Response Interval: The time from Call Received until On the Scene (Fig 1).

T

TA: Traffic accident.

Telemetry: The technique of measuring physiologic data and transmitting it to a distant location for interpretation. Often refers to transmitted tracings.

Telephone aid: Telephone advice provided by dispatchers that is given "ad lib" based on the dispatcher's own training in a procedure or treatment, but not following a written pre arrival instruction protocol. This method exists because either no protocols are used in that center, or protocol adherence is not required by policy and procedure.

Telephone treatment sequence protocols: Specific type of prearrival instruction protocols written as algorithmic scripts that are learned and read by the trained dispatcher to the caller over the telephone during life-threatening emergencies. These instructions include airway control, Heimlich maneuver, cardiopulmonary resuscitation, and childbirth.

Ten codes: A method whereby a number preceded by the number 10 is used to designate a specific message; for example, 10-4 means message acknowledged. Meanings can vary from system to system.

Third party caller: A person calling for emergency medical help who is not in direct personal contact with the patient.

Third service: An EMS responder agency/organization that is independent of police and fire departments.

Tiered response: A multilevel response of emergency assistance, beginning with the closest most basic responder, and progressing to more advanced or more distant responders as needed.

Time out: The point when the EMS unit begins moving to a call for assistance (Fig 1).

Tone: A selective signal used to activate a specific receiver.

Transceiver: A radio capable of both transmitting and receiving radio signals.

Transfer: Moving the patient from one medical facility to another.

Transfer from Vehicle: Interval from Arrival at receiving facility to Turnover of patient (Fig 1).

Transfer to Vehicle: The interval from Packaging to Depart Scene (Fig 1).

Transport Interval: The interval from Depart Scene until Arrival at the receiving facility(Fig 1).

Trauma center: A designated specialty receiving center for specifically defined trauma patients. Such a center should have consistent availability of defined services.

Triage: (1) To assign victims a priority for care and transport based on the degree of injury and the individual's relative salvageability in a given situation. (2) In a non disaster situation, to determine who to transport to the hospital.

Turnover: (1) The process of transferring care of the patient from prehospital personnel to receiving facility personnel. (2) The interval of time from transfer from vehicle until care accepted by receiving facility.

U

UHF: Ultra high frequency. This radio band extends from 300 to 3,000 MHz, with most medical communications occurring in the 450-470 MHz range. UHF has better penetration in dense metropolitan areas and inside buildings. It has a shorter range VHF band and is more readily absorbed by environmental objects.

Unit: An EMS vehicle and crew.

Unit Cycle Interval: The time from Time Out to In Service (Fig 1).

Unit Elapsed Interval: The time from Activate to In Service (Fig 1).

Unit-hour: One EMS ambulance in service for sixty minutes.

Unit-hour utilization: The total number of patient transfers divided by the number of unit hours in a given time period.

Universal precautions: The procedure of using barriers for self protection when handling blood or "certain" body fluids of any patient.

Utilization: The percent of time an EMS unit is on calls.

V

Vehicle response configuration: The specific set of vehicle(s) in terms of types, capabilities, and numbers responding as the direct result of actions taken by the emergency medical dispatch system.

Vehicle response mode: The manner of response used by the personnel and vehicles dispatched which reflects the level of urgency of a particular required treatment or transport (e.g., use of emergency driving techniques such as lights and siren vs. routine driving).

Vehicular repeater: A transmitter incorporated on an ambulance to relay transmissions from portable transmitters.

Vertical dispatch: Dispatcher configuration where a single patcher is responsible for a given geographic area, requiring the dispatcher to handle all functions of interrogation, prearrival instructions, and dispatch for each call. Also called solitary dispatching.

VHF: Very high frequency. The band of electromagnetic energy from 30 to 175 MHz. Arbitrarily divided into low-band (30-50 MHz) and high band (150 to 175 MHz). Characterized by great range capability but may have "patchy" losses of communication because of atmospheric interference.

VHF high band: Frequencies in the 150 to 175 MHz band.

VHF low band: Frequencies in the 30 to 50 MHz band.

Vicarious liability: A legal doctrine in which the negligent conduct of one person is imputed to another person based on the relationship between the two parties, and irrespective of the faultless conduct of the party to whom the negligent conduct is imputed. For example, employer-employee, principal-agent.

Vital signs: The pulse rate and character, breathing rate and character, blood pressure, and relative or exact skin temperature.

Volunteer ambulance corps (VAC): Groups of trained individuals who voluntarily provide EMS services.

W

Wake effect: The disruption of traffic and the accidents that occur as a result of the nearby response of an emergency vehicle traveling in the HOT mode.

Watt: A measurement of transmitter power output.

Willful misconduct: Improperly conducting oneself on purpose, without regard to the consequences of that lack of appropriate behavior or action.

Window phase: The time from exposure to a disease to the time a laboratory test detects the presence of antibody.

Z

Zone: A specific area at an EMS operational site. The cold zone is relatively safe; the warm zone is relatively dangerous; and the hot zone is off limits to EMS personnel.

Index

A

"Accidental Death and Disability: The Neglected Disease of Modern Society," 5-7, 76, 420
Accidents, 5-6, 40, 54-56, 143
Acetaminophen for backpacking first aid, 50
Acquired immunodeficiency syndrome, 36, 317, 353-354
Acute myocardial infarction, 111, 196-197
Adenosine, 112
Advanced cardiac life support, 42,190,207,256
Advanced life support, 29, 36, 67, 87, 105, 178, 196, 425
Advanced trauma life support, 42, 190, 207, 256
Air ambulances, 408
Air Force, EMS training in, 61
Air medical transport, 38, 44-45, 407-416
Airway management, 110-111, 134
Alabama, EMS board of, 69
Alameda County, California, 214-215
Alaska, EMS funding in, 78, 79
Albuterol for airway management, 110
Altered level of consciousness, 113, 114
Ambulance corps, volunteer, 316
Ambulance personnel, 13; *see also* EMT-A
Ambulance service, 4-5, 15, 76, 82, 92-97
  denial of, legal issues involving, 288
  local ordinances affecting, 282
  military and civilian sharing of, 64
  misuse of, 363-364
  regulation of, 15, 322-323
  in risk management, 249
  urban, call volume for, 35
  volunteer, 33, 318-319
Ambulances
  advanced life support, 29-30
  air, 21, 408
  cost of, 77
  emergency deployment of, 29
  equipment for, 190-191, 433
  pediatric equipment in, 426
  wilderness, 54
American Academy of Pediatrics, 423
American Association of Critical Care Nurses, 308
American Association of Orthopaedic Surgeons, 8
American Board of Emergency Medicine, 12-13
American College of Emergency Physicians, 8, 12, 187, 198-199, 382, 423
American College of Nurse Midwives, 308
American College of Surgeons, 8
American Heart Association, 8, 133-134, 472
American Medical Association, 7, 12-14, 423
American Practitioners for Infection Control, 308
American Red Cross, 15, 50
American Society for Testing and Materials, 19
American Society of Anesthesiologists, 8
American Trauma Society, 8
Analgesia, protocol for, 113
Anaphylaxis, protocol for, 114
Andragogy, assumptions of, 260
Antidysrhythmics, controversy over, 111
Arizona, EMS funding in, 78
Aspirin for acute myocardial infarction, 111
Association of Air Medical Services, 408
Association of Operating Room Nurses, 308
Association of Rehabilitation Nurses, 308
ASTM, address and resources of, 56
Asystole, 107, 111, 390-393, 428
Automated external defibrillators, 36, 42, 100, 399-406, 472, 474
  by First Responders, 29, 100, 111-112
  medical oversight of, 209, 401, 403
Automated internal cardiovertor, 399
Automated vehicle locator, 29, 91
Automated venous cannulator, 472

B

Backpacking, first aid for, 50
Barnes, Joseph, 4
Barringer, E.D., 4
Basic cardiac life support, curriculum for, 256
Basic life support, 29, 36, 63, 67, 105, 196, 425
Baxter v. Fulton-DeKalb Hospital Authority, 283
Behavioral disorder, 417-418
Benzodiazepenes, 114
Beta-agonists for airway management, 110
Bishop v. Wood, 322
Block grants, 18, 77
Blunt trauma, 40, 393
Board of Regents of State Colleges v. Roth, 322, 324
Body substance isolation, 357
Boyd, David, 9
Brady, James, 4
Brain damage, 389-390
Breathing management, protocol for, 110-111
Bretylium tosylate, prophylactic, 111
Brooke Army Medical Center, 64
Brooks v. Herndon Ambulance Service, Inc., 285
Bull Run, battle of, 59-60
Burns, 55, 416
Burris v. Willis Ind. School District, 324
Bystander physician(s), 381-387

C

California, 69, 79, 100-101
  legislative rules and regulations of, 70, 71, 73, 182, 300-301
Call screening versus prioritization, 140
Callers, 126-127, 133-135
Calls, 12, 38, 87-88, 208, 287-290
Cardiac arrest, 20, 199-202, 390, 391, 399-406
  discontinuance of resuscitation, 107
  interfacility transport of patient with, 417
  process flow chart for response to, 222, *223*
  as tracer condition, 161-162
Cardiac Arrest Registry Data Entry Form, *232*
Cardiopulmonary resuscitation, 5, 50, 52, 100, 119, 339-400, 428
Case law, 282-283
Catastrophic events, 56, 447-453
Cave rescue, 48, 53, 55
Cellular telephones, 121-122, 442-443
Center for Emergency Medicine of Western Pennsylvania, 47, 56
Center for Rural Emergency Medicine, 41
Center for the Study of Emergency Health Services, 18
Centers for Disease Control, 357, 360, *359*
Certification, 194, 206-207
Charcoal, activated, in-field use of, 114
Chemical Manufacturers Association, HazMat incident video of, 435
ChemTrec, 800 number of, 435
Chicago, 211-212
Child(ren), 21, 417, 420-428
Childbirth, protocol for, 114
Chin lift, telephone instructions for, 133-134
Chronic obstructive pulmonary disease versus congestive heart failure, 106
City(ies), 74, 282
Civil War, 4, 59-60
Civilian Military Contingency Hospital System, 447
Cleary v. American Airlines, 322
Cliff rescue, 48
Climbing accidents, 54-55, *55*
Clinical field supervisor, paramedic as, 303
Clinical Laboratory Improvement Act of 1988, 298
Coded squelch systems, 121
Codeine for backpacking first aid, 50
Colorado, 73, 78
Columbus, Ohio, 212
Commission for the Accreditation of Air Medical Services, 408
Committee on Community Emergency Health Services of the American Hospital Association, 8
Communication(s), 118-124, 191, 200-201, 214
  components of, 24-25
  helicopter, 410
  legislation pertaining to, 72
  in military systems, 63
  in multiple casualty incidents, 442-443
  in rural systems, 43-44
  technologic advances in, 21
  in wilderness EMS, 53-54
Computer-aided dispatch, 29-31
Confidentiality, 278, 283
Congestive heart failure, 106, 112
Consolidated Omnibus Budget Reconciliation Act of 1985, 21, 418, 445, 459
Continuing education, 193-194, 248
Contract(s), 267-269, 291-292, 322
Coronary care, mobilization of, 5, 307
Corpsmen, U. S. Navy, 61
Corpus Christi, Texas, 93
County(ies), EMS ordinances in, 74
Cricothyrotomy, 110
Crisher v. Spak, 377
Critical care units, components of, 25-26
Critical incident stress, 42, 341-345
Cross, Pat, 261
Curriculum(a), 255-259

D

Dalton, Edward, 4
Darnall Army Hospital, 64
Data, 30-31, 153
Data collection, 30-31, 153-157
Dead on arrival, 392
Death, 389-390, 395, 428
Debriefings, 344, 445
DeCicco v. Trinidad Area Health Association, 290
Decontamination, 436, 438
Defibrillation, 8, 20, 399
Defusings, 343
Dehydration in wilderness EMS, 55, 56
Demand pattern analysis, 225, *226*
Deming Cycle, 245, *245*
Demobilizations, 343-344
Dentists, military, 61
Department of Defense, 65, 447
Department of Transportation, 13-16
  curriculum of, exclusion of children by, 421
  EMS funding by, 76
  National Highway Traffic Safety Administration, 186, 307, 421
Deregulation, 18-19
Destination, 286-287, 376-377, 380, 412
Dextrose in children, 114
Diazepam for status epilepticus, 113
Dick, Thom, 338
Disability from injuries, 6
Disaster management, 412-413, 427
Disaster medical assistance teams, 448
Disaster plans, 27, 38, 45, 122-123
Discipline, 321-333

Dislocations, 52-53
Dispatch life support, 134-135, 148
Diversion, 454-464
Diving medicine, 48
Do not resuscitate orders, 108, 274-275, 388-389
Doe v. Borough of Barrington, 283
Droperidol, 114
Drug(s), 50, 174
Drug overdose, protocol for, 114
Due process, 321-333
D_5W for trauma patient, 112
Dwindling heart presentation, 391, *391*
Dysrhythmia(s), 5, 202-204

E

Earthquakes, 447; *see also* Catastrophic events
Economic efficiency, 84-94, 92-94, *85*, *93*
Edema, pulmonary, protocol for, 112
Education, 47, 106, 248, 253-266, 317, 364, 366
  continuing, 193-194
  for emergency personnel, 12-14
  of nurses in prehospital care, 309-310
  for prehospital provider, 190, 193-194
  professional, in rural systems, 41-42
  public, 14, 26-28, 125
Edwin Smith Papyrus, 3
Electrocardiography, 208
Emergency Care First Responder curriculum of Department of Transportation, 52
Emergency Department, 6, 15-16, 294-298
Emergency Department Nurses Association, 8
Emergency medical dispatch, 33, 125-152, 410
  centralized, 14-15
  computer-aided, 29, 128
  medical oversight of, 128-132, 191
Emergency medical dispatcher, 127-133, 145
Emergency Medical Service Systems Act of 1973, 8-9, 12, 72, 76-77, 85-86, 153
  grant activity provided by, 11*t*
Emergency medical services
  access to, 119
  by air, 21
  AMA Commission on, 7
  appropriations authorizations for, 10*t*
  authorizations and appropriations for, history of, 9*t*
  base hospital concept of, 197-199
  beneficiaries of, 81-82
  bystander physician's role in, 381-387
  California legislation pertaining to, 300-301
  communication in, 14-15
  comparing capability of, 89-90
  components of, scope and specificity of, 24-27
  consolidation of, future of, 475
  continuum of care in, 158, *159*
  cost-effectiveness of, 77-78, 103
  court decisions affecting, 282-283
  data handling in, 30-31
  deregulation of, 18-19
  designation of, method for, 469
  economic efficiency of, 84-94
  equal access to, 91, 224
  geographic scope of, 82-83
  goals for, 158-159
  history and development of, legislation in, 67
  history of, 3-23, 420
  lack of personnel for, 12-14
  local planning for, 70-71
  management of, prehospital provider input into, 300-306
  medical director of, 474-475
  medical oversight of, 473-474
  New York public health law on, 178-179
  nonemergent use of, 12, 38, 87-88, 208
  nurses in, 307-315
  on-scene phase of, 29-30
  patient benefits, 81-82
  patient's view of, 86
  pediatric, 21
  physician leadership in, 12-13
  planning process for, 158, *159*
  as point of entry, 35
  policy formation for, 301-302
  political issues in, 347-352
  post traumatic stress disorder, 341
  pre-arrival phase of, 28-29
  professional organizational input into, 8
  public education about, 118-119
  regional councils for, 70
  regionalization of, 465-471
  regions for, 10, 10*t*
  regulations for, coordination of, 16
  resistance to innovation in, 474
  response phases of, 28-31
  rural, 40-46; *see also* Rural systems
  scope of practice in, 66
  state committees or commissions for, 69-70
  supervision and administration of, 302-303
  system models for, 17-18, 32-34
  technology in, 472-473
  third-party reimbursement for, 79
  training for, 20-21
  trends in, 472
Emergency Medical Services and Trauma Care Improvement Act, 467
"Emergency Medical Services at Midpassage," 16
Emergency medical services councils, 70
Emergency Medical Services for children, 420, 421
Emergency medical technician, 51, 52, 67, 102-103, 296, 341, 410
Emergency medical technician-ambulance, 13, 42, 98-101, 253, 255, 415
Emergency medical technician-assistant, 317
Emergency medical technician-basic, 60-61, 105, 186, 208-209, 256, 298
Emergency medical technician-defibrillator, 36
Emergency medical technician-intermediate, 14, 41, 98-101, 186
Emergency medical technician-paramedic, 13, 14, 20, 51-52, 98-102, 186, 255-256, 298
Emergency Medical Training Program, 12
Emergency Medical Treatment and Active Labor Act, 418
Emergency medicine, 12, 13, 13*t*
Emergency Nurses Association, 308
Emergency nursing, establishment of, 13
Emergency Response Handbook: Guidebook for Hazardous Material Incidents, 435
Emergency Response Institute, 57
Emergency vehicles, 143, 361, 415-416
Employee(s), 35-36, 323-325; *see also* Personnel
Endotracheal intubation, 102
Endotracheal tubes, protocols for, 110
End-tidal CO_2 devices, protocols for, 110
Epinephrine, high-dose, studies of, 111
Equipment, 291, 360
Esophageal obturator airways, 101, 110
Ethics, 274-279
Evacuation in wilderness EMS, 56
Evaluation, 158-167
Expectation theory, 335

F

Falls, wilderness, 54-55
Federal AIDS Prevention Act of 1990, 355
Federal Air Regulations, 407
Federal Communications Commission, 15, 122
Federal Emergency Management Agency, 448, 449, 450
Field evaluators, paramedics as, 303
Fifth Discipline, The, 245
Fire departments, 32-33, 316, 437
First aid, 50, 62, 119
First on the Scene: Hazardous Material Safety, 435
First Responder interventions, 20, 21, 29, 33, 36, 42, 51-52, 95-96, 189
First Responders, 98-100, 348, 451, 474
Florida, 78-79, 367
Flow chart, process, 236
Fluid(s), 101, 103, 112, 357
Flumazenil, 113
Fort Wayne, Indiana, 93
Fourteenth Amendment, 283, 322, 324
Fracture(s), open, 52
Funding, 16-17, 33, 42-43, 76-83, 318, 421, 466
Furosemide for congestive heart failure, 112

G

Georgia, 68-73
Glasgow Coma Scale, 163
Goals, setting, 158-159
Good Samaritan statutes, 73, 269, 280
Greatest Management Principle in the World, The, 335
Green v. City of Dallas, 288
Gunshot wounds, 55, 392

H

Hammond, William, 60
HARE traction splint, 44
Hazardous materials, 431-440
Head trauma, fluid administration in, 112-113
Health care, political issues in, 347-352
Health insurance, 17
Health Services and Mental Health Administration, EMS funding by, 7
Health Services Block Grant Program of 1982, 420
Heartmobile program, 8
Heat exhaustion, 50
Heatstroke, 50
Heat-tilt method, 134
Heimlich valve, 110
Helicopter Emergency Medical Services, 407-413
Helicopters, medevac, 21, 38
Hennepin County decision, 284
Hepatitis, non-A/non-B, 355
Hepatitis B, 354-355, *359*
Hialeah v. Weatherford, 288
Highway Safety Act of 1966, 7, 13, 76, 420
Highway Safety Act of 1973, 78
Histogram in quality improvement, 237
Hospital(s), 15-16, 32, 123, 297-298, 376, 454-455
Hospital Authority of Gwinnett County v. Jones, 286
Human immunodeficiency virus infection, 353-354, *359*
Huron Valley Hospital Inc. v. City of Pontiac, 466
Hurricane Andrew, 449-450, 476
Hurricane Iniki, 476
Hydrocodone for backpacking first aid, 50
Hyperglycemia, 114
Hypoglycemia, 114
Hypothermia, 50, 54-55
Hypothesis, formation of, 171
Hypovolemia, fluid administration in, 113

I

Idaho, EMS funding in, 78
Illinois, 207
Immunity laws, 282
Inappropriate use, 363-374
Incident Command System, 431, 433
Indemnification, 73
Indiana, 73, 79
Infection control, 36
Infectious diseases, 353-362
Informed consent, 173-174, 276-278, 375-376
Injury(ies), 6, 54-56

Injury severity score, 162-163
Instruction, 257-258
Insurance, 17, 269
Interfacility transport, 414-418
Intraosseous lines, uses of, 112
Iowa, EMS funding in, 78
Ischemia, diagnosis of, 208
Ishikawa diagrams, 236-237
Isoproterenol for airway management, 110

J

Jablon v. Trustees of the Cal. State Colleges, 324
Journal of Wilderness Medicine, 48
Juan trilogy, 220, *220, 221*

K

Kaizen, the Key to Japan's Competitive Success, 235
Kansas City, Missouri, 224-225
Kentucky, EMS funding in, 78
Keypunching, 156
Knowles, Malcolm, 260
Korean War, 60, 407

L

Labor, interfacility transport of patient in, 417
Labor unions, 36
Lactated Ringer's solution, 112
Larrey, Jean Dominique, 3-4, 59
Law(s), 282-283
Leadership, 334-338
Leadership and the One Minute Manager, 335
Learning, 260-263; *see also* Education
Legal issues, 107, 143-145, 187, 207, 280-293, 418, 427-428
Legislation, 21, 66-75, 281-282, 401, 467-469
Letterman, Jonathan, 4, 60
Liability, 269, 280, 283-285
Licensed practice nursing in military, 61
Licensure, 67, 194
Lidocaine, prophylactic, 111
Life support, 133
Life-threatening dysrhythmia(s), 203-204
Living wills, 275
"Load-and-go situations," 30
Loperamide for backpacking first aid, 50
Lorazepam for status epilepticus, 113
Lubey v. City and County of San Francisco, 324

M

Madigan Army Medical Center, 64
Maine, EMS funding in, 78
Major incident protocols in rural systems, 45
Malcolm v. City of East Detroit, 286
Malpractice, components of, 144
Malpractice litigation, 248-249, 269
Marabian, Albert, 336
Maryland, EMS funding in, 79
Maslow, A.H., human needs theory of, 261, *262*
Massachusetts, EMS funding in, 78
McSwain dart, 110
Medevac helicopters, 21, 38
Media, 123-124
Medical advisory committees, 300-301
Medical arrest, classification of, 107-108
Medical control, 178, 183-216, 418, 425, 456
  legal issues involving, 280-293
  NAEMSP definition of, 148
Medical director, 43, 69, 148, 188, 253, 267-270, 281-285, 321-337, 347-352, 470
  contract for, 291-292
  for children, 424-426
  leadership by, 334-338; *see also* Leadership
  new operational foci for, 474-475
  quality assurance and, 219-220
  roles of, 37-38, 253-254
Medical interventions, 105-117, 385, 387
Medical oversight, 177-187, 401, 403
  dispatch process in, 128-132
  duties of, 89
  effective, 94-95
  increased debate about, 473-474
  legislation pertaining to, 71-72
  physician's role in, 67
  in risk management, 248
Medical records, 123, 248
Medical specialist, military, 60-62
Meningitis, 355, 357
Mentoring, 263-264
Methylprednisolone, 113
Metropolitan Ambulance Services Trust, 224-225
Metropolitan statistical area, defined, 40
Military Airlift Command, 448
Military Assistance to Safety and Traffic program, 60, 64, 407
Military systems, 59-65
Milwaukee, Wisconsin, 210-211, 365
Mine rescue, communications in, 40, 53
Minnesota, EMS funding in, 78
Mississippi, EMS funding in, 78
Missouri, EMS funding in, 78
Mobile intensive care nurse, 67, 206, 207, 211-212
Mocardial ischemia, 208
Monitoring, technological advances in, 30-31
Moore v. Preventive Medicine Medical Group, 377
Moreno v. South Hills Health System, 286
Motivation, 261-263, 319
Mountain rescue, 47-48
Mountain Rescue Association, 53, 57
Mountain sickness, acute, 54-55
Mountaineering First Aid, 50
Mountaintop relays, 121
Multiple casualty incidents, 396-397, 412-413, 441-447
Municipalities; *see also* City(ies), 74
Murden v. County of Sacramento, 324
Mutual aid, 27, 45

N

Naloxone, 113
Natanson v. Kline, 375
National Academy of Sciences-National Research Council, 16, 420
National Association for SAR, 57
National Association of Diver Medical Technicians, 48
National Association of Emergency Medical Technicians, 311
National Association of EMS Physicians creation of, 20, 127-128, 147-150, 207
National Association of Orthopedic Nurses, 308
National Cave Rescue Commission, 57
National Center for Health Services Research, 18
National Demonstration Project on Quality Improvement in Health Care, 219, 220
National Disaster Medical System, 447-452
National Disease Medical System, 65
National Emergency Medical Services for Children Resource Alliance, 421
National Fire Protection Association, Standard 472 of, 431
National Registry of Emergency Medical Technicians, 8, 13, 14, 98, 194
National Rural Health Association, 42
National Safety Council First Aid, 50
National Standard Teaching Curriculum, 190
Needlestick injuries, HIV risk from, 353-354
Needs assessment, 153-154
Negligence, components of, 144
Neonate, interfacility transport of, 417
Neurological emergencies, protocol for, 113
Neuromuscular blocking agents, 208
New Mexico, EMS funding in, 78
New York, 69, 73, 78, 177-179, 209, 380
  on-scene EMS triage procedure of, 368-371
New York City, EMS misuse protocol of, 365
9-1-1, 15, 28, 35, 43-44, 87, 119, 125, 348, 364, 366
Nitrates, 112
Nitroglycerin for congestive heart failure, 112
Nitrous oxide, protocol for, 113
Nixon, Richard, 8, 9
North Carolina, 78, 101
North Dakota, EMS funding in, 78
Nurse(s), 207, 307-315, 410
Nurses Association of the American College of Obstetrics and Gynecology, 308
Nursing, emergency, establishment of, 13
Nursing corps, military, 61, 62

O

Objectives, 159, 257
Occupation(s), high-risk, in rural areas, 40
Occupational Safety and Health Administration, 357, 433
Office of Maternal and Child Health, 421
Office of Technology Assessment, 40
Ohio Department of Natural Resources, 57
Oklahoma, EMS funding in, 78, 79, 94
Omnibus Budget Reconciliation Act, 18, 77, 455-460
One Minute Manager, 334
Operation Desert Storm, 448-449, 475
Organization of Nurse Executives, 308
Outcome analysis, 235-244

P

Paramedic, 8, 73, 196, 280, 303, 307, 410-411
Pareto charts in quality improvement, 237
Patient(s), 26, 38, 86-88, 221-224, 249, 376-379
Patient care incidents, 249-252
Patient rights, transport issues and, 107
Pediatric advanced life support, 42, 190, 424
Pediatric trauma life support, training for, 190
Pediatrics; *see also* Child(ren), 421
Peer review, 305-306
Pennsylvania, EMS councils of, 70
Pennsylvania SAR Council, 57
Percutaneous transtracheal ventilation, 110
Perry v. Sindermann, 322
Personal protective equipment, 357
Personnel, 24, 41-42, 60-61, 72-73, 206-207
Physician(s), 20, 38, 47, 67, 71-72, 187, 280-283
  in Helicopter Emergency Medical Services, 411
  leadership of, 12-13
  military, 61
  in multiple casualty incidents, 443-444
  in quality improvement process, 220
Pinellas County, Florida, 237, 242
Pittsburgh, 210, 365-366
Pneumatic antishock garment, 102-103, 112
Poison control center in HazMat incidents, 435
Poisoning, 114, 417
Political issues, 347-352
Post traumatic stress disorder, 341
Potential injury creating event, 476
Pre-arrival instructions, 132-133, 135, 144, 148
Pre-arrival phase, components of, 28-29
Precepting, 263-264
Pregnancy, 396, 417
Prehospital care; *see also* Emergency medical services, 5-6, 33, 72
  development of, 196-197
  Emergency Department interface with, 296-297
  political issues in, 347-352
  retrospective review of, 304-305
Prehospital care coordinators, 303
Prehospital care report, 153-154, 157, 192, 237-240, 248, 289, 291

Prehospital provider, 98-100, 186, 192-194, 249, 280, 294-306, 341, 415
interaction with bystander physician, 381-387; *see also* Bystander physician(s)
medical director's expectations of, 334
as physician extenders, 181-182
training of, 13-14, 190
in wilderness, 50-53
Prehospital Trauma Life Support, 190
President's Commission on Highway Safety, 7
Preventive Health Block Grant, 18
Procainamide, prophylactic, 111
Process flow chart, 236
Prospectus of the Appalachian Search and Rescue Conference, 47
Protocols, 37-38, 105-114, 135-138, 184, 188-190, 337, 348, 356
Psychiatric disorder, interfacility transport of patient with, 417-418
Psychology of Achievement, The, 335
Public education, 28, 125
Public Health Service, 7
Public information, 26-27
Public Law 101-590, provisions of, 467-469
Public safety, regulation of, 122
Public safety agencies, components of, 26
Public safety answering point, 28
Public safety trunking systems, 121
Public utility model, 79
Pugh v. Sees Candies, 322
Pulmonary edema, acute, protocol for, 112
Pulse oximetry, 10, 472

Q

Quality assurance, 148, 150, 155, 213-244
Quality improvement, 182, 184, 188, 192, 235-244, 248, 303-306, 310-311
Quality management, 129-132, 217-246

R

Radio telephone switching systems, 121
Radioactive spills, 438
Rangers, First Responder training for, 52
Reagan, Ronald, 18
Recertification, 194
Recordkeeping, 26, 153
Refusal of care, 276-277, 287-290, 365, 375-380, 418, 427-428
Registration, 194
Rerouting policy, 462-464
Rescue 3, address and resources of, 57
Rescue squads, volunteer, 316
Research, 168-176
Respondeat superior, concept of, 181
Response phases, 28-31
Response time, 15, 36-37, 40, 90-92, 108, 225, 244
Restraints, guidelines for use of, 417-418
Resuscitation, 107-108, 388-398, 400, 428
Rhode Island, EMS funding in, 78
Right to die, resuscitation decision and, 388
Risk management, 148, 247-252, 287
Robert Wood Johnson Foundation, 8, 12, 76
"Roles and Resources of Federal Agencies in Support of Comprehensive Emergency Medical Services," 8
Rosenthal, Robert, 335
Rural systems, 40-46, 423-424
Ryan White Law, 355

S

Safety, 106, 122
St. George v. City of Deerfield Beach, 288
St. Louis, EMS misuse protocol of, 366-367
Salaries, 35-36
Salt Lake City, EMS misuse protocol of, 366
San Diego, 212
SAR training, 47, 51
Satellite communications, land mobile, 122
Scene time, 109
Screening, 140, 263
Search and rescue, 47-48, 51, 433
Seattle, 209-210
Self-actualization, Maslow's theory of, 261
Shewhart Cycle, 245, *245*
Shimoyama v. Board of Education, 324
Shoulder, dislocations of, in wilderness, 52-53
Simple Triage and Rapid Treatment, 443
Skelly case, 325
Society for Academic Emergency Medicine, 20
Society of Critical Care Medicine, 8
Society of Post Anesthesia Nurses, 308
Society of Trauma Nurses, 308
Sodium bicarbonate, 111
SOLO, address and resources of, 57
South Dakota, EMS funding in, 78
Special Medical Rescue Team, 57
Specialty receiving centers, 106-107
Spinal injury, 113, 416-417
Standing orders, 47, 105-106, 188, 199-202
Statistical tools, 236-237
Status epilepticus, protocol for, 113
Stonehearth Open Learning Opportunities, 57
Stress, 341
Students, 260-263, 294-296
Subsidies, 82, 93-94
Sudden cardiac death, 223, 224
Supraventricular tachycardias, 112
System design, 81-97, 221
System models, 32-39
System status management, 219, 225, 230-231
Systems status management, *236*

T

Tachycardia, supraventricular, 112
Tampa Bay, Florida, EMS system of, 237, 242
Telemetry, ECG, 109, 202-205
Telephone, assistance by, 126-127
Telephone aid, 119, 134
Telephones, cellular, 121-122, 442-443
Ten-minute rule, 376
Tennessee, 69, 73
Terrorist actions, 444
Tests, 258,263
Texas, 70, 72 ,78
Thiamine in altered level of consciousness, 113
Third-party reimbursement, 79
Thrombolytic therapy, 111, 208
Tracy, Brian, 335
Training, 254-255, 295-296, 317, 319
Transport, 30, 277-290, 377-379, 442
hospital selection in, 454-455
hot versus cold, 108
patient and provider refusal of, 107
policies for, 364-365
protocols for, 184
Transportation, 15, 21, 25, 44, 63
Trauma, 112-113, 392-393, 458
classification of, 55-56, 107-108, 161-162
hypovolemic, management of, 189
wilderness, 54-56, *55, 56*
Trauma audit committee, 305
Trauma Care Systems Planning and Development Act, 20, 467-469
Trauma center, 64, 376-377, 416, 428, 467-469
Trauma nurse coordinator, *312, 313*
Trauma nurse practitioner, 314
Trauma score, 162-163, 427*t*
Triage, 396-397, 427, 443-444
on-scene, 368-374
specialty receiving centers and, 106-107
TRISS method, 164
Truman v. Thomas, 377
Tuberculosis, 36, 355
Tulsa Emergency Medical Services Authority, 94

U

UHF radio systems, 121
Uniform Fire Incident Reporting System, 156
U. S. Air Force, EMS training in, 61
U. S. Army, medics in, 62
U. S. Constitution, Fourteenth Amendment of, 283, 322, 324
U. S. Navy, 61, 63
University of Cincinnati, Emergency Medicine residency established at, 12
University of Southern California, Emergency Medicine Department established at, 12
Urban systems, 38, 423
Utah, 78, 145

V

Vaccine(s), hepatitis B, 354-355
Vaughan v. State, 322
Vehicle response configuration, 148
Vehicle response mode, 148
Vehicles, nontransport, 36
Ventricular fibrillation, 8, 20, 103, 111, 399-400
survival of, 202, 222
time course of, 390, *390*
VHF radio systems, 120-121
Vietnam War, 60, 407
Virginia, 51, 53, 78, 101
Virginia SAR Council, 57
Vital signs, assessment of, 165t
Volunteer(s), 41, 280, 285-286, 316-320

W

Walker v. Northern San Diego County Hospital District, 322
War, 5, 60*t*, 447; *see also* Catastrophic events
care of wounded in, 59-60
Washington, local EMS funding in, 79
Washington, D.C., 82
Whitman, Walt, 4
Wideman v. Shallowford Community Hospital, Inc., 283
Wilderness, 44, 47-58
Wilderness emergency medical technician, 51
Wilderness EMS Institute, 51, *55, 56*
Wilderness Medical Associates, 57
Wilderness Medical Society, 48, 50, 57
Wilderness Medicine Institute, 57
Wilford Hall Air Force Hospital as community trauma center, 64
Wilkerson v. City of Placentia, 324
William Beaumont Army Medical Center as community trauma center, 64
Williams v. Department of Water and Power, 324
Wills, living, 275
Workplace, accidents in, deaths from, 5
World War I, 4, 60*t*
World War II, 4, 60*t*
Wounds, gunshot, 55, 392
Wright v. City of Los Angeles, 288
Wyoming, EMS funding in, 78